PSYCHOLOGICAL AND DEVELOPMENTAL ASSESSMENT

PSYCHOLOGICAL AND DEVELOPMENTAL ASSESSMENT

Children with Disabilities and Chronic Conditions

Edited by

Rune J. Simeonsson
Susan L. Rosenthal

THE GUILFORD PRESS
New York   London

Library of Congress Cataloging-in-Publication Data
Psychological and developmental assessment: Children with disabilities and chronic
  conditions / edited by Rune J. Simeonsson, Susan L. Rosenthal.
    p. cm.
  Includes bibliographical references and index.
  ISBN 1-57230-645-9 (hardcover)
    1. Developmental disabilities—Diagnosis. 2. Developmentally disabled
children—Psychological testing. 3. Behavioral assessment of children. I. Simeonsson,
Rune J. II. Rosenthal, Susan L.

RJ506.D47 P795 2001
618.92'075—dc21   00-052781

2003-449

*To Jane, Ted, and all others
who have enriched our
understanding of children's development*

ABOUT THE EDITORS

Rune J. Simeonsson, PhD, MSPH, is Professor of Education and Research Professor of Psychology at the University of North Carolina at Chapel Hill and Adjunct Professor of Medical Psychology at Duke University. He teaches graduate courses in the areas of psychological assessment and child development and disability for students in school psychology and special education. His research interests are in the areas of child development, special education, and public health focusing on the prevention of childhood disability and the promotion of child health and development. He has responsibilities as an investigator with several projects: the North Carolina Office on Disability and Health, a Linkage project (USAID) for graduate education with Cairo University, a subcontract for the National Early Intervention Longitudinal Study (NEILS), and a Centers for Disease Control research grant to measure children's environments. He is actively involved in policy and research on the definition and classification of disability in the United States and is currently serving as chair of the World Health Organization International Task Force on Children and Youth for the revision of the International Classification of Impairments, Disabilities, and Handicaps.

Susan L. Rosenthal, PhD, obtained her doctorate in psychology at the University of North Carolina at Chapel Hill, and completed her pediatric psychology internship at the University of Maryland in Baltimore and her postdoctoral fellowship in psychology at the Yale Child Study Center in New Haven, Connecticut. Dr. Rosenthal is currently Professor of Pediatrics and Director in the Division of Psychology and Behavioral Pediatrics in the Department of Pediatrics at the University of Texas at Galveston. Before assuming her present position, she was Professor of Pediatrics at the University of Cincinnati and Pediatric Psychologist at Children's Hospital Medical Center in Cincinnati, Ohio. Her clinical practice focuses on helping adolescents and their families negotiate the developmental tasks of adolescence in the context of chronic illness, mood disorders, or other life stressors. Her research examining adolescent psychosexual development has been funded by the National Institutes of Health. She has authored numerous articles on adolescent psychological development and the role of the family in protecting adolescent girls from risk.

CONTRIBUTORS

Cassandre Balant, MEd, graduate student, School Psychology Program, University of North Carolina, Chapel Hill, North Carolina

Barbara W. Boat, PhD, Director of The Childhood Trust of Children's Hospital Medical Center, and Associate Professor, Department of Psychiatry, University of Cincinnati, Cincinnati, Ohio

Elizabeth Kelley Boyles, PhD, Assistant Professor of School Psychology, Marshall University Graduate College, South Charleston, West Virginia

J. Lytle Brent, MEd, graduate student, School of Education, University of North Carolina, Chapel Hill, North Carolina

Naeela M. Chaudry, PhD, Instructor, Strong Center for Developmental Disabilities, University of Rochester School of Medicine and Dentistry, Rochester, New York

Cheryl Chase-Carmichael, MA, psychology intern, Department of Psychiatry/Psychology, Children's Hospital of Michigan, Detroit, Michigan

Sheila S. Cohen, PhD, Director of Psychology, Child and Family Division, Central Clinic, and Department of Psychiatry, University of Cincinnati College of Medicine, Cincinnati, Ohio

Carrie Cook, MA, graduate student, School Psychology Program, University of North Carolina, Chapel Hill, North Carolina

Philip W. Davidson, PhD, Professor of Pediatrics and Director, Strong Center for Developmental Disabilities, University of Rochester School of Medicine and Dentistry, Rochester, New York

Deborah Eisert, PhD, Associate Professor, Center on Human Development, University of Oregon, Eugene, Oregon

Sally Flagler, PhD, School Psychologist and Coordinator, Autism Team, Wake County Public School System, Raleigh, North Carolina

Constance J. Fournier, PhD, Senior Lecturer, Department of Educational Psychology, Texas A&M University, College Station, Texas

Gerard A. Gioia, PhD, Director, Division of Pediatric Psychology/Neuropsychology, Mt. Washington Pediatric Hospital, and Assistant Professor, Department of Psychiatry and Behavioral Sciences, Johns Hopkins School of Medicine, Baltimore, Maryland

Steven C. Guy, PhD, private practice, Columbus, Ohio

Deborah L. Halperin-Phillips, PhD, Staff Psychologist, Pediatric Psychiatry, Babies and Children's Hospital, New York Presbyterian Hospital–Columbia Presbyterian Center, New York, New York

Sadarryle Hill, MEd, graduate student, School Psychology Program, University of North Carolina, Chapel Hill, North Carolina

Gail S. Huntington, PhD, Scientist, Frank Porter Graham Child Development Center, and Clinical Associate Professor, School of Education, University of North Carolina, Chapel Hill, North Carolina

Peter K. Isquith, PhD, Pediatric Neuropsychologist, Department of Psychiatry, Dartmouth Hitchcock Medical Center, Lebanon, New Hampshire

Melissa R. Johnson, PhD, Pediatric Psychologist, WakeMed, and Clinical Associate Professor of Pediatrics and Clinical Assistant Professor of Psychiatry, University of North Carolina School of Medicine, Chapel Hill, North Carolina

Kristine Landry, EdS, School Psychologist, Marion County Schools, Marion County, Florida

Lee M. Marcus, PhD, Clinical Director, Chapel Hill TEACCH Center, and Professor, Department of Psychiatry, University of North Carolina School of Medicine, Chapel Hill, North Carolina

Janey Sturtz McMillen, PhD, Investigator, Frank Porter Graham Child Development Center, and Clinical Assistant Professor, School of Education, University of North Carolina, Chapel Hill, North Carolina

Rebecca Pretzel, PhD, Clinical Center for the Study of Development and Learning, University of North Carolina, Chapel Hill, North Carolina

William A. Rae, PhD, Department of Educational Psychology, Texas A&M University, College Station, Texas

Michael C. Roberts, PhD, Professor and Director, Clinical Child Psychology Program, University of Kansas, Lawrence, Kansas

Susan Robinson, MEd, Wake County Public School System, Raleigh, North Carolina

Susan L. Rosenthal, PhD, Division of Psychology and Behavioral Pediatrics, Department of Pediatrics, University of Texas at Galveston, Galveston, Texas

Anita Scarborough, PhD, Investigator, Frank Porter Graham Child Development Center, University of North Carolina, Chapel Hill, North Carolina

Janet R. Schultz, PhD, Professor of Psychology, Xavier University, Cincinnati, Ohio

Rune J. Simeonsson, PhD, MSPH, Professor of Education and Research Professor of Psychology, University of North Carolina, Chapel Hill, North Carolina, and Adjunct Professor of Medical Psychology, Department of Psychiatry, Duke University, Durham, North Carolina

H. Jane Sites, EdD, LSW, Project Director, Therapeutic Preschool Programs, University of Cincinnati Center for Development Disabilities, Cincinnati, Ohio

Tina Smith, PhD, Assistant Professor, School Psychology Program, University of Florida, Gainesville, Florida

Tovah M. Wax, PhD, LCSW, Deaf Service Unit Program Director, Dorothea Dix Hospital, Raleigh, North Carolina

Kathleen White, MEd, Developmental Evaluation Center, Western Carolina University, Cullowhee, North Carolina

Cynthia Wilhelm, PhD, Associate Professor, Rehabilitation Counseling, Allied Health Sciences, University of North Carolina, Chapel Hill, North Carolina

CONTENTS

1 Clinical Assessment of Children: An Overview   1
  Rune J. Simeonsson and Susan L. Rosenthal

I Dimensions and Issues

2 Issues in Clinical Assessment   17
  Rune J. Simeonsson and Anita Scarborough

3 Clinical Assessment in Planning and Evaluating Intervention   32
  Rune J. Simeonsson and Janey Sturtz McMillen

II General Strategies and Measures

4 Quantitative Assessment   53
  Rune J. Simeonsson, Carrie Cook, and Sadarryle Hill

5 A Qualitative Developmental Approach to Assessment   83
  *Rune J. Simeonsson, Gail S. Huntington, J. Lytle Brent,
  and Cassandre Balant*

6 An Ecobehavioral Approach in Clinical Assessment   120
  Rune J. Simeonsson and Elizabeth Kelley Boyles

7 Assessment of Family Context   141
  Susan L. Rosenthal, Sheila S. Cohen, and Rune J. Simeonsson

III Specialized Strategies and Measures

8 Assessment of Trauma and Maltreatment in Children
  with Special Needs   153
  Barbara W. Boat and H. Jane Sites

9   Infant Assessment   176
      Tina Smith, Rebecca Pretzel, and Kristine Landry

10 Assessment of Children with Motor Impairments   205
      Melissa R. Johnson, Cynthia Wilhelm, Deborah Eisert,
      and Deborah L. Halperin-Phillips

11 Assessment of Children with Visual Impairment or Blindness   225
      Naeela M. Chaudry and Philip W. Davidson

12 Assessment of Children Who Are Deaf or Hard of Hearing   248
      Rune J. Simeonsson, Tovah M. Wax, and Kathleen White

13 Assessment of Children with Autism   267
      Lee M. Marcus, Sally Flagler, and Susan Robinson

14 Assessment of Children with Chronic Illness   292
      Janet R. Schultz and Cheryl Chase-Carmichael

15 Assessment of Executive Functions in Children
      with Neurological Impairment   317
      Gerard A. Gioia, Peter K. Isquith, and Steven C. Guy

IV   ETHICAL AND LEGAL ISSUES

16 Ethical and Legal Issues in Assessment of Children
      with Special Needs   357
      William A. Rae, Constance J. Fournier,
      and Michael C. Roberts

Index   377

1

CLINICAL ASSESSMENT OF CHILDREN: AN OVERVIEW

RUNE J. SIMEONSSON
SUSAN L. ROSENTHAL

All children are different, and we need to know the reasons for, and significance of, those differences.
                                                          —ILLINGWORTH (1989, p. 239)

Beth is a 10-year-old girl whose development in the 1st year followed normal milestones. Within the 2nd year of life, she demonstrated significant lags in cognitive and language milestones and repetitive movements of arm and hands. At 3 years of age, Beth presented as a nonverbal child and was diagnosed with Rett syndrome. She has been in a special class since entering school at 5 years of age, and is relatively independent in the personal activities of eating, dressing, and toileting. She does not interact with other children and spends much of her time manipulating selected toys. Management of behavior has become a significant problem at home and at school. Occasionally, she has phases of self-injurious behavior. A developmental evaluation made 2 years ago indicated cognitive, social, and communicative skills in the 10- to 12-month range. In an upcoming follow-up evaluation, an important priority is to document the nature and range of Beth's current level of functioning.

The complex developmental and health problems of children like Beth represent significant challenges for clinical assessment. Fundamental among these challenges is assessment of individual differences in order to provide personalized services and supports. The need for clinical assessment has been a central concern of parents and other advocates on behalf of children with disabilities and chronic health conditions. That need is also evident in the enactment of laws by state and federal governments to insure that the health, developmental, and educational needs of children are met. Representative of these efforts are the Americans with Disabilities Act (ADA; Kalscheur, 1992) and the Individuals with Disabilities Education Act (IDEA) acknowledging rights to accommodation, early intervention, and education. The need for clinical assessment is perhaps best defined by the fact that medical advances have contributed to reduced mortality but changed the picture on morbidity. In the early 1970s, the manifestation of an array of mild but persistent behavioral and developmental problems in children was defined as the new morbidity (Haggerty, Roghmann, & Pless, 1993). With continued advances, survival rates have increased for infants with congenital and neonatal problems and for children having chronic conditions with more severe complications (Darrow & Stephens, 1992). In the developmental years, these children are likely to manifest impairments, experience restrictions in activities, and be at risk for secondary conditions and a diminished quality of life (Simeonsson & McDevitt, 1999).

The development of interventions for children with disabilities and chronic conditions is predicated on comprehensive assessment of the individual characteristics and needs of children. Comprehensive and accurate assessment is important (1) to facilitate diagnostic efforts, (2) to ensure that a match is made between the needs of the child and appropriate intervention, and (3) to evaluate the impact of individualized treatments or interventions. Valid assessment is important, as it takes on increased significance in growing demands for accountability and evidence-based interventions for children with chronic health conditions and disabilities in clinical services, special education, and managed care (Kleinman, 1998; Simeonsson & McDevitt, 1999).

The expansion of early intervention, special education, and related services resulting from the enactment of IDEA, ADA, and other legislation for children with health and developmental problems has highlighted the need for appropriate assessment of children's characteristics and needs. The practical and measurement challenges of assessing such children have been recognized for more than half a century. Addressing the evaluation of the child with cerebral palsy, Bice (1948) cautioned that a numerical and mechanical interpretation of test performances could not be accepted. These challenges still pertain to the assessment of children with disabilities and chronic conditions and are addressed in the chapters of this book. New assessment challenges are also appearing as a function of increased child survival and continuing advances in medicine, pharmacology, and rehabilitation. Cognitive assessment, for example, was used to document a child's recovery of cognitive function following the discontinuation of more than 2 years of treatment with valproate for epilepsy (Guerrini, Belmonte, Canapicchi, Csalini, & Perucca, 1998). Problems of consistent performance and behavior in children who are young or who have severe disabilities continue to raise the need for the development of new tools in the assessment of neuropsychological and neuromotor assessment (Gjaerum, 1997).

Growing recognition of the needs of children with chronic health conditions and disabilities is reflected in a range of implications for assessment that cut across the fields of developmental and behavioral pediatrics, pediatric psychology, and pediatric rehabilitation (Burkett, 1989). Intervention in each of these fields reflects new assessment strategies and tools related to documenting the needs of the child and the family. In developmental and behavioral pediatrics, awareness of the need for inclusive assessment of children's health-related experiences in the form of quality of life is increasing (Drotar, 1998). Representative studies have examined quality of life in children with cancer (Osoba et al., 1996). Technological advances in medicine present opportunities in pediatric psychology for assessment of the impact of cochlear implants on the language development of prelingually deaf children (Bollard, Chute, Popp, & Parisier, 1999). In pediatric rehabilitation, follow-up studies of children with traumatic brain injury have documented changes in child performance and behavior and impact on family (Coster, Haley, & Baryza, 1994). These converging trends are evident in the growing use of combined words that define measurement of neuromotor, psychomotor, and psycholinguistic functioning and performance on neuropsychological and psychoeducational tests. They also highlight the need for assessment procedures that take into consideration characteristics of children with developmental and health problems that are not readily met by traditional measures. A final emerging area with implications for assessment is the need for population-based data on health and disability in children (Halfon & Newacheck, 1999) and the derivation of health utility indices (Lee, Park, Khoshnood, Hsieh, & Mittendorf, 1997).

Although a number of texts are available that cover the psychological and educational assessment of children for whom standardized instruments and traditional approaches are appropriate, coverage of clinical assessment of children with disabilities and chronic conditions has been limited. Further, although psychological assessment of adults in medical rehabilitation is addressed (Cushman & Scherer, 1995), extensions to children and youths, particularly the very young, is lacking. Many assessment instruments and strategies appropriate for children without disabilities are not sufficiently sensitive for children with complex health conditions. This realization has been evident in recent contributions to the periodical literature that target methods and procedures for children who present assessment challenges. The major purpose of this book is to address the limited coverage on this topic by describing objectives, domains, and strategies of clinical assessment appropriate for children with disabilities and chronic health conditions. Through a review of general, as well as specific, approaches, the book focuses on clinical assessment of developmental and psychological characteristics of children and adolescents.

A RATIONALE FOR CLINICAL ASSESSMENT

In introducing this volume, it may be helpful to answer the question, What is clinical assessment, how does it differ from testing, and what does it encompass? Testing defines the common approach of using standardized instruments to define the characteristics and achievements of children relevant to decision making in clinical and school settings. As such, testing typically involves the use of psychometrically precise instruments and procedures to derive values for a child based on normative comparisons with a reference group. The term "clinical assessment" is used in this book with a broader meaning, to encompass the use of varied procedures and tools to document developmental and psychological characteristics of children. The rationale for this approach is based on a recognition that the idiosyncratic and complex nature of problems of children with disabilities and chronic conditions requires appraisal methods that are flexible and comprehensive and that go beyond the reliance on standardized measures. Critical analysis and clinical judgment are central to an assessment approach in which selected measures and procedures are used to document the nature of development, behavior, and emotional characteristics. In the context of this book, clinical assessment encompasses one or more of the activities of screening, testing, observation and interviewing for the purpose of deriving a diagnosis, planning interventions, monitoring progress, or evaluating outcomes. The focus and nature of such assessment is defined by referral concerns about individual children in the context of their unique sensory, health, or developmental status.

A significant premise of clinical assessment is that the physical, cognitive, communicative, emotional, and behavioral characteristics of children with chronic health conditions and disabilities cannot be assessed in isolation. A comprehensive approach to clinical assessment must be built on a framework that integrates conceptions about the nature of child functioning, health, and development. Three contributions seem particularly relevant to such a framework. One is a recognition of the interactive nature of human functioning and development. Valuable contributions in this regard take the form of the "biopsychosocial model" (Engel, 1980) in medicine, "ecobehavioral science" (Barker, 1978) in psychology, and the "bioecological model" (Bronfenbrenner, 1999) in child development. In complementary ways each of these models emphasizes the interactive nature of biological, psychological, and social dimensions of functioning and behavior.

The second contribution to an integrated framework is the fact that functioning is not static but dynamic, varying over time and across situations. The dynamic nature of these characteristics is consistent with a transactional conceptualization of child development (Sameroff, 1975; Sameroff & Emde, 1989). In a transactional model of development, ongoing interactions of the child with the environment across time account for the changing nature of the child's status and the dynamic nature of developmental outcome. In contrast to a main-effects model, in which developmental outcomes are attributed either to biological factors or to environmental factors, a transactional approach defines developmental outcomes as the product of child–environment interactions.

In development, functioning and adaptation are defined by the fact that children continually act upon, and react to, the environment that surrounds them. The environment consists of things, conditions, and circumstances that elicit responses, exert pressure, and provide stimulation or feedback to the child in ongoing interactions. Interactions with an environment that is adequate and accessible promotes development. Interactions with an environment of limited adequacy and accessibility contribute to disablement, defined by a process in which an underlying health condition is exacerbated by experiential restrictions and limitations (Verbrugge, 1994). Interactions thus reflect the child's ongoing adaptation to the environment in processes that contribute to either development or disablement. These interactions are manifested in the performance of daily activities and in participation in personal, social, and communal roles. The nature and extent of activity performance and social participation are thus defined mutually by characteristics of the person and of the environment. To accurately classify and measure human functioning and disability, it is necessary to operationalize each of the dimensions of person, environment, and interaction (Simeonsson, Lollar, Hollowell, & Adams, 2000). As shown in Figure 1.1, the physical and mental characteristics the child brings to interaction may range from intact to limited functions. Interactions are defined by what the person does in terms of performing activities or carrying out social or communal roles. The environment can be defined by its nature (physical, social, psychological) and by its proximity to the person. Bronfenbrenner (1977, 1989) has defined four successive systems with the first being the most immediate and proximal to the person and the fourth being the most distal. Within this conceptual framework of the micro-, meso-, exo-, and macrosystems, the influence of the environment may range from direct to indirect and from adequate to inadequate as a source of stimulation or feedback.

The third contribution to an integrative framework for assessment is differentiating assessment in terms of the components of the person–environment interaction. In earlier perspectives, disability was viewed as a unitary characteristic attributed to the individual. A number of models have emerged in the past 20 years that reflect the changing perspective of disability within a dimensional framework, as shown in Table 1.1. Although the terms used for manifestations of disability differ from one model to another, there is a common recognition that disability is not unidimensional but multidimensional. Two key contributions can be seen as synthesizing these changing views of disability. One is the publication of the *International Classification of Impairments, Disabilities, and Handicaps* (ICIDH) by the World Health Organization (WHO) in 1980. The second is the current draft revision of that taxonomy in the form of the *International Classification of Functioning and Disability* (ICIDH2 B-2; WHO, 1999). The 1980 ICIDH represented a significant break from the earlier medically defined view of disability in two major ways. First,

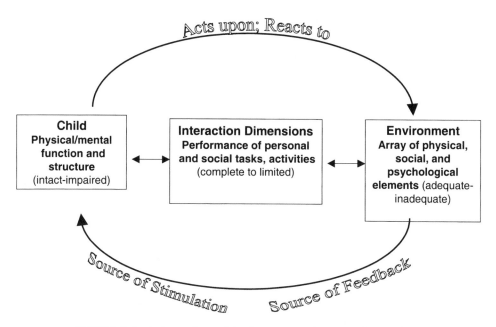

FIGURE 1.1. A dynamic model of person–environment interaction.

it made a distinction between the underlying health condition (illness, injury) and its consequences, which were experienced as disabling by the person. Second, it differentiated those consequences at different planes of human experience. Almost 20 years later, the current revision of the ICIDH2 B-2 represents a similar dramatic shift, with the formalization of the environment as a central factor in defining human functioning and disability (Simeonsson et al., 2000). As shown in Table 1.1, the role of the environment is recognized in three of the most recent models of disability. These conceptual contributions collectively reflect the shift from seeing disability as a medical condition attributed to the person to defining disability as a manifestation of the person's ongoing adaptation to characteristics of the environment.

The models summarized in Table 1.1 provide a basis for operationalizing the purpose and the domain of interest for assessment. The Quebec Classification and the ICIDH2 B-2 can also serve as taxonomies for classification and coding of dimensions of the child's functioning and the environmental context. With this in mind, ICIDH2 B-2 will be described in more detail in Chapter 2. In this regard, it may be particularly useful to document barriers that the child may encounter in the physical environment and the facilitating role of assistive devices and technical aids.

The elements of the framework described herein support clinical assessment of children whose developmental or health conditions are associated with reduced levels of functioning and limited adaptation to environmental demands. This book covers the conceptual, as well as the practical, aspects of psychological and developmental assessment. Although it by no means exhausts all the assessment procedures and instruments, its coverage is representative of comprehensive assessment tools and practices.

TABLE 1.1. Dimensional Models of Disability: Comparison of Terminologies

Models	Health condition	Physical and mental systems	Person-level performance	Social/ communal involvement	Environment
ICIDH	Disease	Impairment	Disability	Handicap	—
Nagi (IOM) Model	Pathology	Impairment	Functional limitation	Disability	—
NCMRR	Pathophysiology	Impairment	Functional limitation	Disability	Disadvantage
ICIDH2 B-2	Health conditions	Function/ structure	Activities	Participation	Environment
Quebec Classification	Risk factors	Organic systems	Capabilities	Environmental factors	Life habits

To this end the book describes measures, tasks, and procedures that can be used in clinical assessment to answer questions such as the following: What procedures and modifications are appropriate in the cognitive assessment of a child with motor impairment? What issues should be considered in the clinical assessment of a child who is nonverbal and who may present with autistic features? What constitutes an appropriate approach to assess the intellectual status of children who are deaf? What are the conceptions of health and coping responses of children with chronic illness? The following section describes the strategies and domains that define clinical assessment.

ELEMENTS OF CLINICAL ASSESSMENT

Assessment Strategies

Clinical assessment of a child's characteristics through informal observation and evaluation has undoubtedly occurred in one form or another since societies first established expectations for children to learn and adapt. The development of more formal and precise assessment procedures, however, appears to be a product primarily of the past century. Cooper (1977) has traced the changing manner in which the development and behavior of children has been documented in the past 100 years, from informal baby diaries and anecdotal records to the later use of standardized tests and ethnograms. As the scope of psychological inquiry continues to evolve, the focus and nature of assessment practices will change as well. An analysis of existing practices suggests that contemporary psychological assessment procedures can be grouped into three major strategies on the basis of the underlying approach to assessment. These are the psychometric, ecobehavioral, and qualitative-developmental strategies. Although each strategy can be found in contemporary settings, they emerged sequentially in the history of psychological assessment in this country. The psychometric strategy became established by the work of Terman on the Binet Scales early in the 20th century. The ecobehavioral strategy operationalized an understanding of the person in context, represented by the work of Barker (1978). The qualitative-developmental approach, although drawing on contributions made by Piaget as early as the 1930s, only began to be advanced as an assessment approach in the late 1960s and early 1970s. Furthermore, domains of child behavior and development such as cognition and communication have also emerged at different points in time, as their relevance to applied concerns was established. To provide a background for the chapters that follow, we give a brief description of the strategies and domains of significance for assessment of special children.

Documentation of Intraindividual Differences

Psychological and developmental assessment is variously concerned with both interindividual differences and intraindividual differences. Assessment concerned with interindividual differences typically focuses on the identification and measurement of factors that differentiate one child from another child or from a group of children. Assessment questions may take the following form: Are the characteristics or performance of this child different from those of a reference group? In what domains and to what degree are those differences found?

Assessment concerned with intraindividual differences, on the other hand, seeks to identify and/or measure the variability of skills and characteristics unique to a particular child. Intraindividual differences reflect the pattern of strengths and weaknesses of a single child relevant to prescribing and implementing intervention activities. In the context of this book, documentation of intraindividual differences is encompassed in clinical assessment.

The distinction between assessment concerned with interindividual differences and that concerned with intraindividual differences may thus be described as a distinction between documenting the manner in which a child is different from other children and documenting the profile of characteristics unique to a single child. In regard to children with disabilities and chronic health conditions, assessment of interindividual differences provides documentation for diagnosis, classification, and labeling—that is, activities intended to confirm the extent to which an identified child differs from other children. Clearly a significant percentage of assessment practice is directed toward this purpose in the form of deriving diagnoses and establishing eligibility for educational and clinical services.

Clinical assessment focusing on intraindividual differences, on the other hand, is essential for documenting the profile of the child's needs and strengths and the development of a valid intervention plan. The major portion of material covered in this book is thus directed toward assessment of intraindividual rather than interindividual differences in children.

A Multivariate Approach

A second assessment strategy is to adopt a multivariate approach in assessing children with complex problems. This can involve analysis of subscores, profiles, and triangulation of data from several measures. A major limitation of traditional assessment with children, particularly intelligence testing, has been an excessive reliance on a single measure or instrument. Given that the characteristics of many children with chronic health conditions and disabilities are expressed in variability and discrepancy of skills across domains, the use of several measures is essential to maximize the validity of assessment. For children with visual, auditory, or motor impairment, for example, it may often be desirable to administer a measure such as the Wechsler Intelligence Scale for Children (WISC), but only one scale may be administered. It is therefore important to administer two or more measures to compensate, at least in part, for the fact that only one-half of what is typically assessed by the measure has been assessed. This recommendation is relevant to any child whose impairment precludes responses involving the affected modality. Assessment thus needs to involve several measures to increase the likelihood that a valid estimate of the child's abilities or skills has been obtained.

Flexibility in Assessment

Clinical assessment of children with chronic health conditions and disabilities requires a comprehensive approach and cannot rely exclusively on a particular strategy or on restricting measurement within a certain domain. The variable manifestation of disabilities or health conditions among children is likely to result in referral questions that emphasize the application of certain strategies and domains with one group and different ones with others. Flexibility of assessment implies a matching of strategies and domains to achieve assessment objectives for a particular child (see Figure 1.2). For children with visual impairment and hearing impairment, for example, assessment concerns may often focus on the documentation of their intellectual status compared with other children both with and without impairments. In such instances, psychometric strategies focusing on the cognitive domain are likely to be applied. For children with motor or hearing impairments, referral questions regarding communicative ability may be appropriately approached through the use of behavioral strategies. Referral questions for hospitalized children or children with chronic illnesses often involve concerns regarding cognitive and emotional adaptations to illness and treatment. These questions may be appropriately addressed through the use of qualitative-developmental tasks to gain an insight into the child's personal understanding of the disease. Psychometric strategies may also be used to permit comparison with healthy peers on measures of coping and adaptation. A frequent goal of assessment with children labeled as autistic or those with pervasive developmental disorders is to determine the nature and level of their social functioning. To this end, behavioral and developmental strategies are often applicable, particularly in cognitive and communicative domains.

Domains

Cognition

Given that a particular strategy has been selected in order to carry out an assessment of a special child, the focus of that assessment may be categorized as reflective of one of four domains: cognitive, communicative, social, and personal functioning. Although these domains are defined somewhat arbitrarily, they do in fact encompass most of the psychological characteristics of interest for diagnostic and prescriptive activities with children with complex problems. Furthermore, as we discuss shortly, the importance of a particular domain may vary as a function of the conditions of the child being assessed.

The cognitive domain of assessment as presented in this book encompasses instruments, tasks, or procedures that focus on the nature and form of a child's cognitive abilities. Broadly speaking, this assessment domain includes measures of intelligence, general cognitive development, and specific cognitive processes such as reasoning. There may be substantial variability in the nature and the format of the instruments, but the defining characteristic of cognitive measures is the fact that they contribute information about a child's cognitive status. Examples of psychometric instruments in this domain may therefore range from the verbal tasks typical of intelligence tests to nonverbal, visual, or tactile stimuli involved

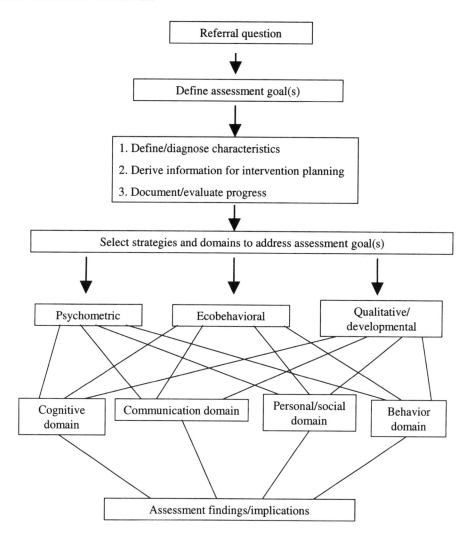

FIGURE 1.2. Matching of assessment strategies and domains with assessment objectives for individual child.

in measures for deaf, motor-impaired, or blind children, respectively. For behavioral and qualitative-developmental strategies, representative items may take the form of discrimination tasks and classification of objects, respectively.

Communication

Measures and procedures in the communicative domain are defined as those that provide documentation of the manner, level, and/or accuracy of a child's expressive and receptive communicative competence. Such communicative competence is not restricted to verbal competence but may include nonverbal forms of communication such as body movements, gestures, or the use of signs. Although measures of communication and cognition obviously overlap substantially and are often used interchangeably, it is particularly important that the clinician distinguish between these two domains in the assessment of specific subgroups of children. When faced with children who have visual, auditory, or motor impairments or who are identified as autistic or who have communicative problems, the distinction between communicative and cognitive competence is often difficult to make. Many children may be characterized by significant deficits in the interpretability and accuracy of their communication skills and yet be cognitively competent. The difficulty of adequately separating these characteristics is, of course, one of the enduring problems of psychological assessment of exceptional children. In order to provide effective assessment, this problem needs to be recognized and carefully documented in assessment and in planning individualized treatment.

A major purpose of this book is to foster clarification of such problems by recommending that the goal of assessment be kept clearly in mind. When a referral pertains to the documentation of a child's ability to communicate, measures should be chosen and results reported that clearly differentiate limitations associated with communication from limitations of cognitive ability. Although the specific measure used will vary with the special child being assessed, formal instruments of expressive and receptive vocabulary, as well as informal documentation of nonverbal signs or gestures, may be appropriate. Because tests of receptive vocabulary are frequently used as indices of intelligence, it is particularly important that, when such instruments are used, the purpose for their use be stated clearly when results are reported.

Personal Functioning

The third domain of assessment instruments, tasks, and procedures focuses on children's personal functioning. Assessment of this domain is reflected by such referral questions as, What is the self-concept of a student with visual impairment? and What defines the behavioral style of a preschooler with hearing impairment? The focus is on measures that reflect different aspects of a child's characteristic traits, emotional status, sense of self, and perceptions of others. Measures in this domain may address areas ranging from self-concept and locus of control to social competence, anxiety, and temperament. Assessment may be based directly on observation or self-report, or it may be secured indirectly through the ratings or observations of a third party such as parents, peers, and teachers. An assumption underlying assessment in this domain is that the personal, emotional, and social characteristics of children are on a continuum rather than a dichotomy of normality and pathology. The premise for the measures and tasks described in this book is that they should document the characteristics, functioning, and behavior of all children, including those with chronic health conditions and disabilities.

Behavior

A fourth domain considered in this book is assessment of behavior. The distinguishing feature of this domain, contrasted with the previous three, is that assessment is made of overt behavior, in simple as well as complex manifestations. In addition to detailed observation, documentation often takes the form of checklists or scales summarizing personal and interpersonal behavior. Chapter 6, on ecobehavioral assessment, emphasizes the importance of assessing not only social behavior but also the context in which social behavior occurs (Scott, 1980).

ASSESSMENT CONSIDERATIONS

In defining the purpose and content of this book, several considerations should be stated at the outset. The first is that the focus of this book is on children whose conditions and characteristics require specialized assessment approaches. The book does not review assessment of the sensory functions of vision and hearing status or visual, auditory, and haptic perception as isolated processes, but they are considered when appropriate in the broader context of clinical assessment. Similarly, assessments of specific motor functions, typically carried out by physical and occupational therapists, also are not considered in detail but are referred to as appropriate in assessment of children with motor limitations. The contributions of related specialty approaches to the multidisciplinary evaluation of children with disabilities and chronic health conditions is recognized and discussed when relevant.

Sensitivity to individual differences is fundamental to comprehensive assessment. The increasing cultural diversity of our society is a factor defining an important individual difference among children seen for assessment in clinics and schools (Solity, 1996). Recognition of that diversity is evident in recommendations for psychological assessment practices that are sensitive to Hispanic American (Cervantes & Acosta, 1992) children, Native American (Dauphinas & King, 1992) children, and children of other minority cultures. The importance of attending to culture and ethnicity is of equal priority in clinical assessment of children with disabilities and health conditions.

A caveat is appropriate here: This book does not provide detailed coverage of psychometric issues such as validity and reliability. Although these issues are important, we assume that the reader has a sufficient knowledge base in this area. However, we need to make two points about psychometric issues relative to the measures and procedures covered in this book.

First, it is important to recognize the significant role of psychometric characteristics of measures in clinical assessment. Thus reliability indices in the form of intratest, test–retest, and interobserver values provide information about the cohesiveness, stability, and rater agreement of measured child characteristics, respectively. Similarly, face, construct, and predictive validity indices reflect the extent to which assessment procedures represent or predict given child characteristics. In either case, the magnitude of such values is a critical factor in determining the confidence that can be placed in the results of assessment. The numerical levels at which such values are judged acceptable may vary as a function of both the nature and the purpose of the assessment, but it is clear that relatively low values will negate the use of some procedures in the assessment of special children.

Second, although reliability and validity are important considerations in assessing children with health conditions and disabilities, their significance has to be viewed in the contexts both of the assessment process itself and of the unique characteristics of the child being evaluated. Given that characteristics of many children with disabilities and chronic conditions may significantly limit their ability to respond to the demands of the assessment situation, a number of instruments may be less than appropriate to administer. However, assessment may need to be carried out in spite of specific concerns regarding reliability or validity. This view should not be taken as an endorsement of using assessment tools that lack reliability or validity. It is, however, a recognition of the problems in assessing children whose unique needs require flexible rather than rigid standards of reliability and validity. It is thus recommended that care be taken to select and apply instruments and procedures with the best psychometric properties relative to the purpose of assessment. In those instances when instruments and procedures with limited reliability or validity have to be used, as they sometimes must, the clinician has an obligation to clearly spell out attendant limitations on obtained assessment results.

In summary, it is our position that the purpose of clinical assessment of children with chronic health conditions and disabilities is first and foremost to solve a problem rather than just to administer tests. The issue, therefore, is not whether to administer certain assessment instruments or tasks but rather to determine what information is needed to address referral questions, assess characteristics, and identify intervention priorities. In the assessment of a child with disabilities, information can be collected by administration of various measures and by systematic observation. It is the inferences that are drawn from such information that define the value of clinical assessment in order to collect information of potential value for identifying the nature of the child's needs and developing appropriate interventions. The strength and validity of inferences are directly dependent on the quality and rigor of assessment methods and procedures. It is therefore essential that assessment results are always accompanied by detailed documentation of conditions under which the results were obtained, including the physical setting, materials, and assessment procedures as well as the child's physical and psychological state. Such documentation provides a basis for recognizing any limitation or qualification that may apply to inferences and interpretation of assessment findings.

ORGANIZATION OF THE BOOK

In order to shed light on these and other concerns in an organized fashion, the content of this book is presented sequentially, beginning with general issues and leading to applications of specific strategies and procedures appropriate for children with particular impairments. In Part I, Chapter 2 addresses developmental and behavioral characteristics of children with disabilities and identifies issues and problems limiting their assessment. The conceptual rationale for a clinical approach to assessment is presented, and a review is made of major strategies and domains for assessment. Chapter 3 is devoted to the integration of assessment data for planning intervention and the relationship of assessment to evaluation of progress in special children. Current concerns about the quality of intervention services, demands by funding agencies for accountability in service programs, and recent advances in evaluative methodology combine to make these topics important considerations in the provision of comprehensive services for special children. Emphasis is on methods that can contribute to the effective planning and evaluation of an individual child's program.

Part II is concerned with general assessment strategies. Chapters 4, 5, and 6 in this section detail the conceptual bases and practical applications of three approaches to comprehensive assessment. Contributions of psychometric, qualitative, and ecobehavioral approaches to clinical assessment are described and selected measures identified. Chapter 7 defines the rationale for and importance of assessing children in the context of the family.

Part III consists of eight chapters devoted to specific subgroups and a consideration of measures, tasks, and procedures unique to their assessment concerns. Chapters cover the topics of children exposed to maltreatment (Chapter 8); infancy (Chapter 9); motor, visual, and auditory impairments (Chapters 10, 11, and 12); autism (Chapter 13); chronic health conditions (Chapter 14); and neuropsychological assessment (Chapter 15). Each chapter in this section follows a similar format, with an overview of the nature of the particular condition and its implications for assessment. Systematic consideration is given to the modification of stimulus materials, content, or response features of measures needed to carry out clinical assessment of children with disabilities and chronic health conditions.

Thus each chapter in Parts II and III provides information on instruments, their applications in assessment of these children, and the manner in which findings can be interpreted and put to use. Part IV concludes with Chapter 16, on ethical issues in assessment of children, a topic of growing concern in the context of test procedures and bias (Koocher, 1993; Koocher & Keith-Spiegel, 1998), as well as informed consent, confidentiality, and access to records.

REFERENCES

Barker, R. G. (1978). *Habitats, environments and human behavior*. San Francisco: Jossey-Bass.

Bice, H. V. (1948). Psychological examination of the cerebral palsied. *Journal of Exceptional Children, 14*, 163–168, 192.

Bollard, P. M., Chute, P. M., Popp, A., & Parisier, S. C. (1999). Specific language growth in children using the CLARION cochlear implant. *Annals of Otology, Rhinology and Laryngology,* (Suppl. 117), 119–123.

Bronfenbrenner, U. (1977). Toward an experimental ecology of human development. *American Psychologist, 32*, 513–531.

Bronfenbrenner, U. (1989). Interacting systems in human development: Research paradigms: Present and future. In N. Bolger, A. Caspi, G. Downy, & M. Moorehouse (Eds.), *Persons in context: Developmental processes* (pp. 25–49). Cambridge, UK: Cambridge University Press.

Bronfenbrenner, U. (1999). Environments in developmental perspective: Theoretical and operational models. In S. L. Friedman & T. D. Wachs (Eds.), *Measuring environment across the life span: Emerging methods and concepts* (pp. 3–28). Washington, DC: American Psychological Association.

Burkett, K. W. (1989). Trends in pediatric rehabilitation. *Nursing Clinics of North America, 24*(1), 239–255.

Cervantes, R. C., & Acosta, F. X. (1992). Psychological testing for Hispanic Americans. *Applied Prevention Psychology, 1*(4), 202–219.

Cooper, M. G. (1977). Observational studies of children from diary to ethnogram: A century of progress. *Child: Care, Health and Development, 3*, 283–292.

Coster, W. J., Haley, S., & Baryza, M. J. (1994). Functional performance of young children after traumatic brain injury: A 6-month follow-up study. *American Journal of Occupational Therapy, 48*(3), 211–218.

Cushman, L. A., & Scherer, M. J. (Eds.). (1995). *Psychological assessment in medical rehabilitation*. Washington, DC: American Psychological Association.

Darrow, D., & Stephens, S. (1992). Interferences in psychosocial development of seriously health-impaired and physically disabled children: Educational implications. *Acta Paedopsychiatrica, 55*(1), 41–44.

Dauphinas, P., & King, J. (1992). Psychological assessment with American Indian children. *Applied Prevention Psychology, 1*(12), 97–110.

Drotar, D. (1998). *Measuring health-related quality of life in children and adolescents*. Mahwah, NJ: Erlbaum.

Engel, G. (1980). The clinical application of the biopsychosocial model. *American Journal of Psychiatry, 137*, 535–544.

Gjaerum, B. (1997). Development of a test battery (NPM-X) for neuropsychological and neuro-motor examination of children with developmental disabilities or mental retardation: A theoretical and clinical study. *Acta Psychiatrica Scandinavica 95*(Suppl. 390), 5–55.

Guerrini, R., Belmonte, A., Canapicchi, R., Csalini, C., & Perucca, E. (1998). Reversible pseudoatrophy of the brain and mental deterioration associated with valproate treatment. *Epilepsia, 39*(1), 27–32.

Haggerty, R. J., Roghmann, K. J., & Pless, I. B. (Eds.). (1993). *Child health and the community* (2nd ed.). New Brunswick, NJ: Transaction Publishers.

Halfon, N., & Newacheck, P. W. (1999). Prevalence and impact of parent-reported disabling mental health conditions among U.S. children. *Journal of American Academy of Child and Adolescent Psychiatry, 38*(5), 600–609.

Illingworth, R. (1989). What matters in developmental assessment? *Pediatric and Perinatal Epidemiology, 3,* 233–241.

Kalscheur, J. A. (1992). Benefits of the Americans with Disabilities Act of 1990 for children and adolescents with disabilities. *American Journal of Occupational Therapy, 46*(5), 419–426.

Kleinman, L. C. (1998). Prevention and primary care research for children: The need for evidence to precede "evidence-based." *American Journal of Preventive Medicine, 14*(4), 345–351.

Koocher, G. P. (1993). Ethical issues in the psychological assessment of children. In T. H. Ollendick & M. Hersen (Eds.), *Handbook of child and adolescent assessment* (pp. 51–61). Boston: Allyn & Bacon.

Koocher, G. P., & Keith-Spiegel, P. (1998). *Ethics in psychology: Professional standards and cases.* New York: Oxford University Press.

Lee, K.-S., Park, S., Khoshnood, B., Hsieh, H., & Mittendorf, R. (1997). Human development index as a predictor of infant and maternal mortality rates. *Journal of Pediatrics, 131*(3), 430–433.

Osoba, D., Aaronson, N. K., Muller, M., Sneeuw, K., Hsu, M. A., Yung, W. K., Brada, M., & Newlands, E. (1996). The development and psychometric validation of brain cancer quality-of-life questionnaire for use in combination with general cancer specific questionnaires. *Quality of Life Research, 5*(1), 139–150.

Sameroff, A. J. (1975). Early influences on development: Fact or fancy? *Merrill Palmer Quarterly, 21,* 267–294.

Sameroff, A. J., & Emde, R. N. (1989). *Relationship disturbances in early childhood: A developmental approach.* New York: Basic Books.

Scott, M. (1980). Ecological theory and methods for research in special education. *Journal of Special Education, 14,* 279–294.

Simeonsson, R. J., Lollar, D., Hollowell, J., & Adams, M. (2000). Revision of the International Classification of Impairments, Disabilities and Handicaps: Developmental issues. *Journal of Clinical Epidemiology, 53,* 113–124.

Simeonsson, R. J., & McDevitt, L. (1999). *Issues in disability and health: Secondary conditions and quality of life.* Chapel Hill, NC: University of North Carolina.

Solity, J. (1996). Reframing psychological assessment. *Educational and Child Psychology, 13,* 94–102.

Verbrugge, L. (1994). The disablement process. *Social Science and Medicine, 38,* 1–14.

World Health Organization (1980). *International Classification of Impairments, Disabilities and Handicaps.* Geneva: Author.

World Health Organization (1999). *International Classification of Functioning and Disability Beta-2 Draft.* Geneva: Author.

PART I

Dimensions and Issues

2

ISSUES IN CLINICAL ASSESSMENT

RUNE J. SIMEONSSON
ANITA SCARBOROUGH

Esperanza is a 14-year-old Hispanic American girl with spina bifida. The lesion is at a high level (T5), resulting in significant impairment of lower extremity function and bowel and bladder incontinence. Motor development was significantly delayed, but with extreme bracing and the use of crutches, she was able to use her legs for very limited movement and transfer by the age of 4. She has adequate upper limb function, but there is some slowness in her movement and response to task demands. She relies on a wheelchair to get around home, school, and the neighborhood, but she is experiencing some difficulty using other forms of transportation. Mental development has been in the normal range, and she has been able to attend regular school with modifications of the environment and attention to her limited mobility. She has a number of self-care skills but needs assistance getting in and out of the bath and dressing the lower part of her body. She is experiencing some difficulties in visual tasks and academic areas of math and science. She has no close friends and is beginning to feel isolated from her peer group, both in class and outside the school setting. She spends much of her time watching television and eating snacks. This pattern is contributing to a number of secondary conditions that are of concern to her family and physician. Hip muscle contractures and some spinal curvature are manifested secondary to muscle imbalance. Furthermore, her sense of being different and isolated is exacerbated by the fact that she has become quite overweight in the last year. Given the current situation, her family and physician are planning to develop a comprehensive plan to assist her in adapting to the changing demands of being an adolescent with spina bifida.

The major goals of clinical assessment of children with disabilities and chronic conditions can be defined in terms of (1) deriving a diagnosis, (2) planning or prescribing intervention, and (3) evaluating progress. A diagnostic goal is evident, for example, when it is necessary to determine whether a child's performance meets established criteria for a specific diagnosis, such as mental retardation. In that case, normative instruments are used that yield information confirming or disconfirming the diagnosis. The goal of planning treatments involves assessment to derive a profile of a child's idiosyncratic strengths and deficits, from which an intervention program can be developed. Evaluation of progress is often a goal of assessment when there is a need to verify change in status following a period of intervention (Maruish, 1994). Whether the goal is to diagnose, plan intervention, or document status, there is an assumption that the instruments used are valid for that purpose and will measure, with some degree of accuracy, the skill, trait, attribute, or behavior of interest. Such an assumption is basic to clinical assessment. However, a variety of factors, considered singly or in combination, may qualify that assumption when children with disabilities or chronic conditions are assessed. These factors may influence the formulation of referral questions, the selection of assessment instruments, and the confidence with which inferences can be drawn about assessment results (Barnett, Macmann, & Carey, 1992). These factors pertain to the assessment of children with a variety of conditions from early childhood through adolescence. The purpose of this chapter is to review these factors and to identify steps that can be taken to reduce their impact. The chapter considers (1) definitional issues, (2) measurement issues, (3) contextual issues, (4) conceptual issues, and (5) classification issues. These issues are generic in nature and are likely to apply to children with various conditions. Issues unique to children with specific chronic conditions and disabilities will be reviewed in subsequent chapters. Finally, a number of steps are proposed to improve the assessment process of children with disabilities

DEFINITIONAL ISSUES

Variability in definitions and classification of children with disabilities and chronic conditions is a central limitation in services. Diagnostic groupings and classification are often specific to disciplines and are not utilized across different service programs. In medical contexts the *International Classification of Diseases*, 10th edition (ICD-10) serves as a primary framework for defining and classifying children. The *Diagnostic and Statistical Manual of Mental Disorders* (DSM-IV; American Psychiatric Association, 1994) and the *DSM-PC—Child and Adolescent Version* (Wolraich, Felice, & Drotar, 1996) serve a similar function in mental health services. In special education, the assignment of children to specific categories is not made on a uniform basis but reflects the primary criteria on which the child's condition is diagnosed. Biomedical, psychometric, or clinical judgment may thus serve as the primary dimension for a given category. Lack of common terminology is also an issue in defining the nature and severity of children's conditions. Although designations of severity represent the degree to which a child's performance or characteristics deviate from normative values, they are usually tied to a fixed age reference group. Thus two children, aged 3 and 7, are alike only in a relative sense (severely impaired); they may differ substantially in terms of actual functioning levels in that one has verbal skills and the other does not. The use of severity labels with children with developmental disabilities may also restrict or distort the expectations of parents and helping professionals.

Labels such as "severely disabled," "moderately impaired," or "multiply handicapped" are frequently used to describe a child who has some form of impairment. Holt (1977) has cautioned that the adjective "multiple" should not be automatically transferred across the terms "defect," "deformity," "disability," and "handicap" because the resulting labels are not similar in meaning. A child with multiple defects, for example, may only be limited in one way (socially), whereas another child with a single deformity may have multiple limitations (e.g., mentally, emotionally, physically). Although labels may often be important in clinical assessment, it is clear that they may also influence the assessment process itself through examiner expectation and test selection. The variability of labels applied to children with developmental disabilities contributes to confusion and to difficulties in generalization of assessment and treatment results.

Clarity in defining and classifying children with disabilities is important in that how children are described and characterized influences every aspect of assessment and treatment (Reynolds, 1994; Simeonsson, Lollar, Hollowell, & Adams, 2000) and is central to documentation and record keeping.

MEASUREMENT ISSUES

Measures designed for typically developing children are often inappropriate instruments to assess children with developmental disabilities and chronic conditions. Many tests present stimuli of a visual or auditory nature that are difficult for the child with a sensory impairment to perceive. Responses requiring speech or manipulation may also not be in the repertoire of children with hearing or motor impairments, such as the motor limitations experienced by Esperanza. A key limiting feature of standardized measures is that they are not well suited for developing prescriptions and planning treatments (Daniel, 1997). A similar case has been made regarding the lack of practical instruments for individuals with severe or profound impairments (Sparrow & Cicchetti, 1978).

Instruments to assess children who are culturally and linguistically different must be customized to adapt to those differences. Hispanic American children with disabilities or chronic conditions, such as Esperanza, may experience cultural bias in the clinical assessment of their developmental status, in addition to their sensory or motor limitations. Traditionally, evaluators have relied heavily on nonverbal tasks for assessment and translated tests (Li, Walton, & Nuttall, 1999; Nuttall, 1987). Culturally sensitive assessment tools have long been recommended for English-speaking minority populations and also for Native American children (Dauphinais & King, 1992) and Asian American children (Goh, 1986). Despite the long-recognized need for culturally appropriate assessment materials, these recommendations are frequently ignored (Desforges, Mayet, & Vickers, 1995; Padilla, 1988).

The lack of comparability of scores from tests with similar content and purpose is an important measurement concern. Beail (1985) showed, for example, that the Bayley Scales of Infant Development (BSID; Bayley, 1969) and the Griffiths Developmental Scales (Griffiths, 1970) yielded substantially different scores for 25 children with more than one impairment. In another study of infants with Down syndrome, Eippert and Azen (1978) concluded that the Bayley Scales and the Gesell Developmental Schedules (Knobloch & Pasamanick, 1974) did not yield similar developmental results and could not be considered interchangeable instruments. This comparison holds true when instruments are revised. The Bayley Scales of Infant Development (1969; revised, 1993), is an example of the lack of comparability between an earlier version and a revision of the instrument (Nellis & Gridley, 1994).

Another measurement concern pertains to methodology employed. Data derived from observation differ from those obtained from testing (Diebold, Curtis, & DuBose, 1978). Accurate identification of problem areas is best achieved by the triangulation of the results of problem-centered interviews, observation (in play, peer, and adult relationships, communicative use of language), and the results of curriculum-based measurements (Barnett, Macmann, & Carey, 1992).

CONTEXTUAL ISSUES

Setting and context variables that may influence child functioning are important factors to consider when interpreting assessment findings with children with developmental disabilities and chronic conditions. The influence of such factors must be considered in several ways. First, characteristics of the physical or psychological setting may enhance or depress assessed behavior. Beyond the standard need for an assessment setting that is quiet, pleasant, and distraction free, unique situational needs must be considered in assessing children with developmental disabilities. For example, an environment that does not include adequate positioning devices (standing boards, wheelchair trays, etc.) may impose serious limitations on the performance of children with motor impairments (Johnson-Martin, Wolters, & Stowers, 1987). Environments that are novel and that have not been tactually explored may constitute an assessment limitation for children with visual impairments, as may settings in which the residual hearing of children who are hard of hearing is not maximized. Lack of familiarity with the assessment setting may be a significant limitation, particularly in assessment of young children with developmental disabilities. Parette, Bryde, Hoge, and Hogan (1995) discuss the advantages of arena assessment, in which a familiar person engages the child in targeted activities in a physical environment adapted to the physical needs of the child in order to elicit optimal behavior from the child.

A second issue to consider in regard to situational factors is reinforcement of performance. As Koegel, Koegel, and Smith (1997) have pointed out, convincing evidence exists that measured ability can be increased substantially if test performance is contingently reinforced. This has implications both for defining the purpose of assessment and for governing the use of assessment results. In the event that reinforcement is used, the nature and purpose of its application should be carefully documented.

A consideration of limitations of a situational nature also must include variables in the larger context beyond those in which direct individual assessment takes place. Indirect assessment of a child's adaptive behavior, behavior characteristics, or personal skills is often obtained through ratings of actual or perceived functioning by proxies such as teachers and parents. Such information is qualified by the settings from which it is drawn and the familiarity of the proxy with the child. For many children with disabilities, problems of mobility or safety severely restrict the number of settings in which they function and can be observed. Generalizations about functioning therefore should be qualified accordingly.

CONCEPTUAL ISSUES

Atypical Development and Disability

The development of children with disabilities is similar to that of all children, and they are, as are all other children, characterized by individual differences. Conceptual contributions, as well as research, continue to add support to these statements and to advocate for alternative approaches based on developmental perspectives of disability. Three concepts in particular contribute to a developmental perspective on disability: the continuum of reproductive casualty, the continuum of caretaking casualty, and the continuum of central nervous system (CNS) dysfunction. These are summarized in Table 2.1 and described in the following sections.

The Continuum of Reproductive Casualty

Beginning in the late 1950s, Pasamanick and Knobloch (1966) and others undertook a systematic analysis of the consequences of pregnancy and delivery complications relative to developmental outcome. The concept of a continuum of reproductive casualty was advanced to express the range of possible outcomes. The range of outcomes was judged to be

TABLE 2.1. A Developmental Approach to Disability: Complementary Contributions of the Continua of Reproductive Casualty, Caretaking Casualty, and Central Nervous System Dysfunction

Continuum	Disability as developmental outcome	Complementary contribution
Continuum of reproductive casualty	Range of developmental outcome as a function of nature and timing of pre/perinatal insult	Disability as variable expression of prenatal interactions
Continuum of caretaking casualty	Range of developmental outcome as a function of transactions between child and postnatal environment	Disability as variable expression of postnatal transactions
Continuum of central nervous system dysfunction	Range of developmental outcome as a function of location, nature, and severity of underlying central nervous system dysfunction	Disability as variable expression of motor/sensory and central/peripheral dysfunction

a function of the nature and degree, as well as the developmental timing, of the insult. Complications at one end of the continuum resulted in death; at the other, the effect on outcome was negligible. For infants who survived the complications, "there must remain a fraction so injured who do not die, but depending on the degree and location of the trauma, go on to develop a series of disorders extending from cerebral palsy, epilepsy and mental deficiency, through all types of behavioral and learning disabilities, resulting from lesser degrees of damage sufficient to disorganized behavior development and lower thresholds to stress" (Pasamanick & Knobloch, 1966, p. 7). Implicit in this concept was the assumption that the range of outcomes expressed in different categories of disability, such as mental retardation, cerebral palsy, or learning disabilities, reflected different manifestations of a common developmental process. This approach is consistent with a developmental perspective in which developmental disabilities are viewed not as unique diagnoses but as outcome variations of a common process, with a focus on similarities rather than differences in children with developmental disabilities and chronic conditions.

The Continuum of Caretaking Casualty

Zeanah, Boris, and Larrieu (1997) emphasized the fact that the reproductive casualty continuum hypothesis needed to be articulated in more specific and precise terms to encompass the complexity of factors contributing to outcome status. In particular, researchers have recognized the fact that the outcome of an infant with prenatal or birth complications can be positively modified postnatally by environmental factors; the development of an infant with an uneventful fetal history, on the other hand, can be seriously delayed or distorted by caregiving experiences. The influence of the caregiving environment has been seen as a factor of major significance in developmental outcome. This emphasis on the caregiver's role in influencing outcome has been central to the articulation of the concept of the continuum of caretaking casualty by Sameroff and Chandler (1975). In this model, developmental outcomes are defined by a sequence of transitions beginning in the prenatal period and continuing into the postnatal period. As in the concept of reproductive casualty, the concept of caretaking casualty proposes that developmental outcomes of children, rather than being discrete entities, are manifested across a continuum. In this manner it extends the continuum of reproductive casualty and conceptualizes differences in children with developmental disabilities and chronic conditions as expressions of similar developmental processes covering both the prenatal and the postnatal periods.

The Continuum of Central Nervous System Dysfunction

A third concept proposed as an alternative approach for viewing exceptionality is the continuum of CNS dysfunction. Capute and Palmer (1980) used the term to emphasize the associated deficits that stem from a common underlying dysfunction of the CNS. Capute and Palmer maintain that for optimal assessment and treatment of the child with a developmental disability, both the spectrum (expressed disability) and the underlying dysfunction must be recognized. Within this model, specific impairments are grouped under three major categories: cerebral palsy, mental retardation, and communicative disorders. Cerebral palsy is considered prototypic of developmental disabilities in that it usually includes cognitive and communicative deficits. Communicative deficits may reflect either central (language disorder, learning disability, autism) or peripheral (hearing or visual impairment) dysfunction.

Distinguishing between the spectrum of disabilities and the underlying dysfunction can facilitate diagnostic efforts with children with developmental disabilities. Detection of atypical development is enhanced through documentation of deviancy, that is, deviations of a child's abilities within a certain domain. Diagnosis of specific disabilities is enhanced through documentation of dissociation, that is, patterns of discrepancy across domains (e.g., motor vs. language, mental vs. motor). Documentation of deviancy can contribute to the detection of a child whose behavior is atypical and whose subsequent development needs careful monitoring. Sensitivity to the dissociation should facilitate the documentation of a child's relative strengths and deficits. Such dissociation is of increasing interest in cognitive neuroscience in differential diagnosis of children with Williams syndrome (Wang & Bellugi, 1993). Dissociation is also applicable for a child such as Esperanza, who is likely to show advanced language abilities relative to her motor abilities.

An underlying premise of the preceding models is that children with disabilities and chronic conditions progress through common developmental stages and are characterized by individual differences. Instead of a diagnostic and categorical conceptualization of disability, a developmental approach focuses on the commonalities and variations of development across major domains. These domains are reflective of the child's interactions with the physical and social environments and can be assessed by measures of cognition, communication, personal and social development, and behavior. In subsequent chapters, these major domains are considered in detail for each of the three assessment strategies and in the assessment of selected groups of children with specific conditions or disabilities.

CLASSIFICATION ISSUES

Children with disabilities have typically been defined by the etiology or impairments associated with their conditions and assigned diagnoses or categories. Some researchers have recommended use of functional and noncategorical approaches with children with developmental disabilities in health (Stein, Bauman, Westbrook, Coupey, & Iveys, 1993) and educational settings (Reynolds, 1994), but diagnostic categorization still appears central to descriptive, diagnostic, and treatment efforts.

Two continuing problems with categorical classification are related to variability of diagnostic criteria and labeling (Reynolds, 1994). Three major types of diagnostic information—biomedical assessment, psychometric assessment, and clinical judgment—have been used singly or in combination to assign diagnostic categories. Biomedical data involve laboratory tests and measures of body structures or functions. Psychometric instruments yield quantitative data, and clinical judgment reflects expert opinions of clinicians. The nature and precision of identification of disabilities or chronic conditions thus varies as a function of the type of diagnostic information used in documentation, with no common dimension cutting across conditions. It is important here to distinguish between diagnostic versus prescriptive purposes in clinical assessment. For most children with disabilities and chronic health conditions, clinical assessment is not primarily designed to provide diagnostic data but rather to generate information from which interventions or treatments can be planned.

Labeling is often a by-product of categorical identification of children with disabilities. Perceptions of dependency and limited functioning are inadvertently reinforced by methods of assessment, with age-equivalent values (mental age, social age) applied to describe a child's functioning. The danger is that an assigned functioning level in one area (e.g., cognition) will be generalized to all areas, producing stereotyped images and promoting invalid generalizations.

TOWARD DIMENSIONAL CLASSIFICATION

An important step in regard to the changing conceptualization of disability would be to reduce the inconsistency of terms that define children with disabilities. The failure to be consistent or precise in the use of such words as "impaired," "disabled," and "handicapped" not only contributes to confusion but also restricts the generalizations that can be drawn in regard to children to whom such labels are applied. In this context it is timely to seek alternative conceptualizations that are suited to assessment, evaluation, and planning of clinical or educational interventions.

As noted in Chapter 1, a number of conceptual and classification systems have emerged that can contribute to more precise terminology for describing children with disabilities and chronic conditions. Of these systems advancing a dimensional view only the Quebec Classification and the *International Classification of Impairments, Disabilities, and Handicaps* (ICIDH) and *International Classification of Functioning and Disability* (ICIDH2) have associated taxonomies, classifying characteristics of functioning and disability, not of persons. This is a crucial difference between these taxonomies and the *International Classification of Diseases* (ICD-10) and DSM-IV that classify individuals on the basis of diagnoses or disease/disorder entities. As the ICIDH and the ICIDH2 are part of the World Health Organization (WHO) family of health classifications, their contribution to clinical assessment can be identified on two levels. First, specific manifestations of the child's condition can be coded along the three major dimensions of the classifications. As summarized in Table 2.2, the dimensions can be operationalized in terms of documenting (1) functions or structures of the body or mind, (2) performance of activities, and (3) participation in life situations or roles. In the 1980 ICIDH, these manifestations were defined at three planes of experience: impairment, disabilities, and handicaps. In the ICIDH2 revision, these manifestations are defined as impairments of body structures/functions, limitations of activi-

TABLE 2.2. World Health Organization International Classification of Impairments, Disabilities, and Handicaps (ICIDH and ICIDH2 B-2): Manifestations of Health Condition Across Dimensions

ICIDH

Disease, injury/ intrinsic condition	Impairment	Disability	Disadvantage/ handicap

ICD-10 codes	Intellectual
	Other
	  psychological
	Language
	Aural
	Ocular
	Visceral
	Skeletal
	Disfiguring
	Generalized/
	  sensory
		Behavior
		Communication
		Personal care
		Locomotor
		Body disposition
		Dexterity
		Situational
			Orientation
			Physical
			Independence
			Mobility
			Occupation
			Social
			  integration
			Economic
			  self-sufficiency
			Other handicap

ICIDH2 B-2

Health condition (disorder or disease)	Body functions, structure (impairments)	Activities (limitations)	Participation (restrictions)	Environmental factors

ICD-10 codes	**Function**
	Mental
	Sensory
	Voice/speech
	Cardiovascular
	Digestive/
	  endocrine
	Genitourinary/
	  reproductive
	Neuromusculo-
	  skeletal
	Skin and related
	  structures
	
	Structure
	Nervous system
	Eye/ear
	For speech
	Cardiovascular
	For digestion/
	  endocrine
	Genitourinary
	Related to
	  movement
	Related to skin
	  and structures
		Learning
		Communication
		Movement
		Activities of
		  moving around
		Self-care activities
		Domestic
		  activities
		Interpersonal
		  activities
		Performing tasks
		  and major life
		  activities
			Personal
			  maintenance
			Mobility
			Exchange of
			  information
			Social
			  relationships
			Home life and
			  assistance to
			  others
			Education
			Work/
			  employment
			Economic life
			Community/
			  social and
			  civic life
				Products
				  and
				  technology
				Natural
				  environment
				  and human-
				  made changes
				  to environment
				Support and
				  relationships
				Attitudes,
				  values, and
				  beliefs
				Services
				Systems and
				  policies

Note. Data from World Health Organization (1980, 1999).

ties, and restrictions of participation. In addition, the ICIDH2 is designed to document factors defining the environmental context of the individual. Such coding of functional characteristics complements classification of the underlying health condition using the ICD or mental disorders using the DSM-IV or the Diagnostic Classification of Mental Health and Developmental Disorders of Infancy and Early Childhood (Lieberman, Wieder, & Fenichel, 1997), a diagnostic framework used to classify maladaptive behavior patterns in infants and young children. It can also yield a profile of the nature and extent of a child's disability. The taxonomies can also be used in a more generic way as a framework for identifying the focus and coverage of assessment tools. The use of the revised ICIDH2 can provide a common language of disability, contributing to precision and clarity of terminology across disciplines and service settings.

Documenting severity of disability is a significant challenge in clinical assessment. The traditional approach has been to designate severity of impairment by levels of mild, moderate, severe, and profound, either on a qualitative basis or tied to a statistical index such as number of standard deviations below the mean. As classifications, the 1980 ICIDH and the ICIDH2 revision both provide qualifiers to indicate severity of impairment, limitations, and restrictions relative to specific dimensions. A measurement approach for practical documentation of the nature and severity of disability in children is the PULTIBEC system, as described by Lindon (1963). The initials stand for eight major functional domains (physical capacity, upper limbs, locomotion, toilet, intelligence, behavior, eyes, and communication); each domain is rated on a 1 (highest) to 6 (lowest) basis to represent the child's status. The resulting matrix can be used to present a profile of the child's functioning levels across domains. Drawing on this approach, the ABILITIES Index was designed to record the nature and severity of major functions (Simeonsson & Bailey, 1991). The initials stand for nine functional domains (audition, behavior, intellectual status, limbs, intentional communication, tonicity, integrity of health, eyes, structural status). As such the index can be used to document intraindividual differences, as illustrated in Figure 2.1 for Esperanza. The index represents an efficient method in which to emphasize a child's profile of abilities and disabilities and provides a way of grouping children on the basis of functional similarity rather than etiology (Simeonsson, Bailey, Smith, & Buysse, 1995). Of particular interest is the fact that it can be used reliably to involve parents in the assessment process (Bailey, Buysse, Simeonsson, Smith, & Keyes, 1995; Bailey, Simeonsson, Buysse, & Smith, 1993).

Another way in which clinical assessment of children with disabilities may be improved is to systematically document their characteristics. Documenting variability of responsivity and disposition, as well as limitations associated with sensory and motor impairments, is important to qualify assessment results and interpretation of findings. A major source of variability in many children with disabilities and chronic health conditions is level of behavioral arousal or state regulation. Drawing on findings from infant research, we have tested the utility of a 9-point rating scale (see Table 2.3) to document state levels in preschool children with disabilities (Simeonsson, Huntington, Short, & Ware, 1982). Landesman-Dwyer and Sackett (1978), for example, have designed a 4-point rating scale appropriate to assess sleep and activity state patterns of children with profound retardation. The concept of state may also be extended to a broader documentation of observable patterns of responsivity and reactivity. The degree to which patterns of responsivity and reactivity are regular and predictable may serve as an index of development and change. In this case, these patterns may be a representation of the child's adaptation to environmental demands in terms of timing of actions (Ashton, 1976).

Other child characteristics, such as variability of disposition and the confounding effects of rhythmic habit patterns, should also be taken into account in a systematic fashion

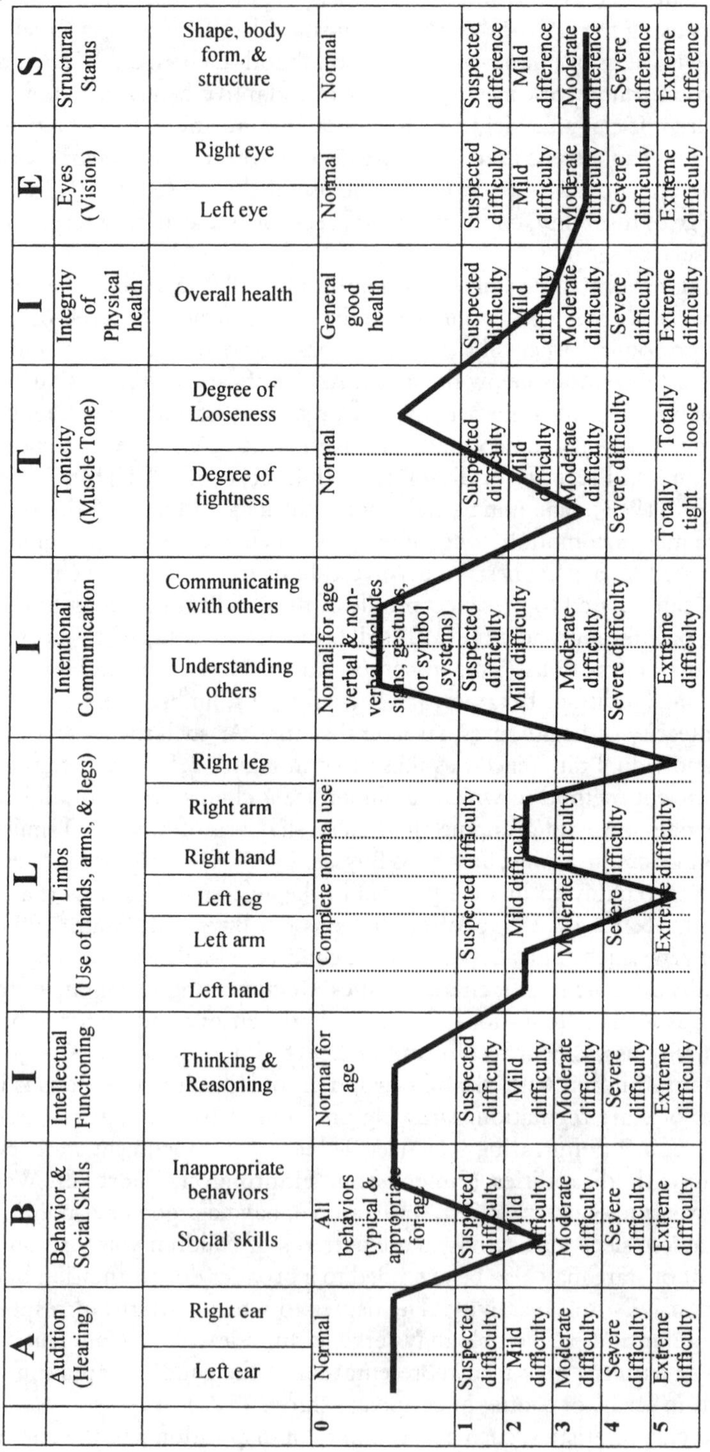

FIGURE 2.1. A.B.I.L.I.T.I.E.S system (Simeonsson & Bailey, 1991).

TABLE 2.3. Documentation of State Levels as Defined in the Carolina Record of Individual Behavior

Level	Child characteristics
State 1	Deep sleep, eyes closed, regular respiration, no movements.
State 2	Intermediate sleep; eyes closed; few minor facial, body, and/or mouth movements; respirations are periodic, alternating periods of shallow and deep breathing.
State 3	Active sleep, eyes closed, irregular respiration, some gross motor activity (stirring, writhing, grimacing, mouthing, or other facial expression).
State 4	Drowsiness, eyes open and closed intermittently, fluttering eyelids, eyes have glassy appearance, frequent relaxation followed by sudden jerks.
State 5	Quiet awake, relatively inactive, eyes open and appear bright and shiny, respiration regular.
State 6	Active awake, eyes open, diffuse motor activity of limbs or whole body, vocalizations of a content nature.
State 7	Fussy awake, eyes open, irregular respirations, diffuse motor activity, vocalizations of fussy, cranky variety.
State 8	Mild agitation, eyes open, diffuse motor activity, moderate crying, tears may or may not be present.
State 9	Marked uncontrollable agitation, screaming, eyes open or closed, tears may or may not be present.

during assessment of children with chronic conditions and disabilities. Dispositional characteristics can be documented through ratings of behavior style, yielding profiles of potential value in interpreting other test findings and planning interventions. In assessment of very young children with disabilities, as well as older children and adults with multiple or severe disabilities, systematic documentation of rhythmic habit patterns such as head rolling and body rocking is important to capture sources of individual variability and record differences among subgroups of children (Short & Simeonsson, 1990).

A final comment pertaining to dealing with child characteristics is the determination of the child's modality preference. The child's modality preference should be ascertained prior to carrying out assessment, both for the sensory modality with which the child receives stimulation and for the motor modality with which the child will respond. For a child with motor impairments, such as Esperanza, cognitive tasks defined by speed of performance would reflect assessment of motor limitations, not her ability to comprehend the task.

IMPLICATIONS FOR CLINICAL ASSESSMENT

There is a lack of assessment tools and procedures that are suitable for children with motor or sensory impairment. Overcoming these limitations in assessment can be accomplished in several ways. The major strategies are to (1) modify the assessment materials (such as test stimuli and format), (2) modify assessment procedures, and (3) expand or vary the content of assessment materials. Specific examples of these strategies are discussed in greater detail in subsequent chapters.

There is general agreement on a whole-child approach in assessment and intervention, with a multidisciplinary team providing a comprehensive perspective. A key element of the team's work is systematic attention to situations and settings in which the child functions, with the need to distinguish between those that are physical and those that are psychological in nature. Physical situations and settings are described in Chapter 6, which focuses on characteristics of environments that may influence child behavior. Psychological situations and settings are those interpersonal contexts, particularly those of the family, that may be associated with child functioning. The importance of the interactive nature of child and family relationships to functioning has been recognized in theoretical and empirical literature and is of particular relevance when considering the families (Simeonsson & Simeonsson, 1993) and siblings (Summers, Hahs, & Summers, 1997) of children with disabilities. Selected measures of family characteristics and functioning that document the psychological context in which children function are described in Chapter 7.

Clinical assessment is variously concerned with interindividual differences and intraindividual differences. Assessment of interindividual differences typically focuses on the measurement of factors that differentiate one child from another child or from a group of children. Clinical assessment of intraindividual differences, on the other hand, is designed to document the variability of skills and characteristics unique to a particular child that are relevant to prescribing and implementing intervention activities. The major focus of this book is on clinical assessment of intraindividual rather than interindividual differences in children with disabilities.

As a final guideline, we advocate a multidimensional approach to the assessment of children with disabilities. This can involve analysis of subscores, profiles, and data from several measures. A major limitation of traditional assessment with children, particularly intelligence testing, has been an excessive reliance on a single measure or instrument. Given the idiosyncratic and variable characteristics of children with disabilities, several measures should be used to maximize valid assessment. For any child with a sensory or motor impairment, at least two separate measures of performance are recommended to compensate, at least in part, for the fact that one measure may be insufficient to capture the child's performance or behavior. This recommendation is relevant to assessment of other subgroups of children with disabilities, whose skills are often assessed in part by only a single measure, emphasizing the importance of assessment that considers the whole child.

This chapter summarized various challenges of clinical assessment of children with disabilities in general. Issues and concerns unique to children with particular impairments or conditions are described in detail in later chapters. As assessment of children with disabilities is challenging but essential for planning interventions, guidelines to improve the process have been proposed. A distillation of some of the guidelines is presented in summary form in Table 2.4, which can be used to complement assessment data. The value of using a form like this is that it provides documentation of factors that may help to qualify assessment findings. For example, similar assessment results obtained for two children with disabilities would be interpreted with different levels of confidence if there was documentation that medication effects were a significant factor for one child and not for the other. The time of day when assessment was carried out may indicate if fatigue or responsivity need to be considered in interpreting findings. Situational variables, modality preferences, and modifications of materials and procedures are additional factors that might qualify assessment findings. In a practical way such documentation provides a way in which the effects of confounding variables can be taken into account.

TABLE 2.4. Inventory of Assessment Variables

Date: _____ Time assessment started: _____ Ended: _____ Examiner: _____

Child's name: _____ Date of birth: _____ Age: ____ Sex: _____

Nature of impairment, if any: _____ Current medication(s): _____

Diagnosis, if any: _____

Etiology, if known: _____ Dosage/frequency: _____

Child's functional status: Circle appropriate entry.

			Limbs		*Body tone*	
Vision	Hearing	Health	Upper	Lower	Hypertonic	Hypotonic
Normal	Normal	Healthy	Functional	Functional	Normal	Normal
Impaired	Impaired	Health	Impaired	Impaired	↑ Tonus	↓ Tonus
Blind	Deaf	impaired	Nonfunctional	Nonfunctional	Rigid	Flaccid
		Incapacitated				

Assessment context: Define physical setting: _____

Describe social setting (no. and function of people present): _____

Describe placement/positioning of child: _____

Preferred receptive modality: _____

Preferred expressive modality: _____

Child's state/responsivity: Circle appropriate entry.

State at time assessment begun: asleep   drowsy   quiet awake   active awake   fussy   agitated

Predominant state during assessment: asleep   drowsy   quiet awake   active awake   fussy   agitated

All states observed: asleep   drowsy   quiet awake   active awake   fussy   agitated

Assessment procedure: Circle appropriate entry.

Modification of standardized test material: None   Minimal   Moderate   High

Modification of standardized procedures: None   Minimal   Moderate   High

Match examiner skills/capabilities
  with child's special needs: Inadequate   Marginal   Good   Excellent

Overall judgment of adequacy of assessment: Inadequate   Marginal   Good   Excellent

Comments: _____

REFERENCES

American Psychiatric Association. (1994). *Diagnostic and statistical manual of mental disorders* (4th ed.). Washington, DC: Author.

Ashton, R. (1976). Aspects of timing in child development. *Child Development, 47,* 622–626.

Bailey, D. B., Buysse, V., Simeonsson, R. J., Smith, T., & Keyes, L. (1995). Individual and team consensus ratings of child functioning. *Developmental Medicine and Child Neurology, 37,* 246–259.

Bailey, D. B., Simeonsson, R. J., Buysse, V., & Smith, T. (1993). Reliability of an index of child characteristics. *Developmental Medicine and Child Neurology, 35,* 806–815.

Barnett, D. W., Macmann, G. M., & Carey, K. T. (1992). Early intervention and the assessment of developmental skills: Challenges and directions. *Topics in Early Childhood Special Education, 12,* 21–43.

Bayley, N. (1969). *Bayley Scales of Infant Development.* New York: Psychological Corporation.

Bayley, N. (1993). *Bayley Scales of Infant Development.* San Antonio, TX: The Psychological Corporation.

Beail, N. (1985). A comparative study of profoundly multiply handicapped children's scores on the Bayley and the Griffiths developmental scales. *Child, Care, Health and Development, 11,* 31–36.

Capute, A. J., & Palmer, F. B. (1980). A pediatric overview of the spectrum of developmental disabilities. *Journal of Developmental and Behavioral Pediatrics, 1,* 66–69.

Daniel, M. H. (1997). Intelligence testing. *American Psychologist, 52,* 1038–1045.

Dauphinais, P. L., & King, J. (1992). Psychological assessment with American Indian children. *Applied and Preventive Psychology, 1,* 97–110.

Desforges, M., Mayet, V., & Vickers, M. (1995). Psychological assessment of bilingual pupils. *Educational Psychology in Practice, 11,* 27–35.

Diebold, M. H., Curtis, W. S., & DuBose, R. F. (1978). Relationships between psychometric and observational measures of performance in low-functioning children. *AAESPH Review, 3,* 123–128.

Eippert, D. S., & Azen, S. P. (1978). A comparison of two developmental instruments in evaluating children with Down's syndrome. *Physical Therapy, 58,* 1066–1069.

Goh, D. S. (1986). Assessing psychological needs of Asian American children: Motivations and precautions. *Asian American Psychological Association Journal,* 7–10.

Griffiths, R. (1970). *The abilities of young children.* Chard, England: Young & Son.

Holt, K. S. (1977). *Developmental pediatrics: Perspectives and practice.* London: Butterworths.

Johnson-Martin, N. M., Wolters, P., & Stowers, S. (1987). Psychological assessment of the nonvocal, physically handicapped child. *Physical and Occupational Therapy in Pediatrics, 7,* 23–38.

Knobloch, H., & Pasamanick, B. (Eds.). (1974). *Gesell and Amatruda's developmental diagnosis.* New York: Harper & Row.

Koegel, L. K., Koegel, R. L., & Smith, A. (1997). Variables related to differences in standardized test outcomes for children with autism. *Journal of Autism and Developmental Disorders, 27,* 233–243.

Landesman-Dwyer, S., & Sackett, G. P. (1978). Behavioral changes in nonambulatory, mentally retarded individuals. In C. E. Meyers (Ed.), *Quality of life in severely and profoundly mentally retarded people: Research foundations for improvement* (pp. 55–144). Washington, DC: American Association on Mental Deficiency.

Li, C., Walton, J. R., & Nuttall, E. V. (1999). Preschool evaluation of culturally and linguistically diverse children. In E. V. Nuttall, I. Romero, & J. Kalesnik (Eds.), *Assessing and screening preschoolers: Psychological and educational dimensions* (2nd ed., pp. 296–317). Boston: Allyn & Bacon.

Lieberman, A. F., Wieder, S., & Fenichel, E. (Eds.). (1997). *Diagnostic classification of mental health and developmental disorders of infancy and early childhood.* Washington, DC: Zero to Three: National Center for Infants, Toddlers, and Families.

Lindon, R. L. (1963). The PULTIBEC system for the medical assessment of handicapped children. *Developmental Medicine and Child Neurology, 5,* 125–145.

Maruish, M. E. (Ed.). (1994). *The use of psychological testing for treatment planning and outcome assessment.* Hillsdale, NJ: Erlbaum.

Nellis, L., & Gridley, B. E. (1994). Review of the Bayley Scales of Infant Development-Second Edition. *Journal of School Psychology, 32,* 201–209.

Nuttall, E. V. (1987). Survey of current practices in the psychological assessment of limited-English-proficiency handicapped children. *Journal of School Psychology, 25,* 53–61.

Padilla, A. M. (1988). Early psychological assessments of Mexican-American children. *Journal of History of the Behavioral Sciences, 24,* 111–117.

Parette, H. P., Bryde, S., Hoge, D. R., & Hogan, A. (1995). Pragmatic issues regarding arena assessment in early intervention. *Infant-Toddler Intervention, 5,* 243–254.

Pasamanick, B., & Knobloch, H. (1966). Retrospective studies on the epidemiology of reproductive casualty: Old and new. *Merrill-Palmer Quarterly, 12,* 7–26.

Reynolds, M. C. (1994). Child disabilities: Who's in, who's out. *Journal of School Health, 64*(6), 238–241.

Sameroff, A. J., & Chandler, M. J. (1975). Reproductive risk and the continuum of caretaking casualty. In F. D. Horowitz, M. Hetherington, S. Scarr-Salapatek & G. Siegel (Eds.), *Review of child development research* (Vol. 4, pp. 187–244). Chicago: University of Chicago Press.

Short, R. J., & Simeonsson, R. J. (1990). Stereotypical behaviors and handicapping conditions in infants and children. *Topics in Early Childhood Special Education, 10*(3), 122–130.

Simeonsson, R. J., & Bailey, D. B. (1991). *The A.B.I.L.I.T.I.E.S Index*. Unpublished manuscript, University of North Carolina, Frank Porter Graham Child Development Center.

Simeonsson, R. J., Bailey, D. B., Smith, T., & Buysse, V. (1995). Young children with disabilities: Functional assessment by teachers. *Journal of Developmental and Physical Disabilities, 7*, 267–284.

Simeonsson, R. J., Huntington, G. S., Short, R. J., & Ware, W. (1982). The Carolina Record of Individual Behavior: Characteristics of handicapped infants and children. *Topics in Early Childhood Special Education, 2*, 43–55.

Simeonsson, R. J., Lollar, D., Hollowell, J., & Adams, M. (2000). Revision of the International Classification of Impairments, Disabilities, and Handicaps: Developmental issues. *Journal of Clinical Epidemiology, 53*, 113–124.

Simeonsson, R. J., & Simeonsson, N. E. (1993). Children, families and disability. Psychological dimensions. In J. L. Paul & R. J. Simeonsson (Eds.), *Children with special needs: Family, culture and society* (2nd ed., pp. 25–50). Fort Worth, TX: Harcourt Brace Jovanovich.

Sparrow, S. S., & Cicchetti, D. V. (1978). Behavior rating scale inventory for moderately, severely and profoundly retarded persons. *American Journal of Mental Deficiency, 82*, 365–374.

Stein, R. E. K., Bauman, L. J., Westbrook, L. E., Coupey, S. M., & Iveys, H. I. (1993). Framework for identifying children who have chronic conditions: The case for a new definition. *Journal of Pediatrics, 122*, 342–347.

Summers, M., Hahs, J., & Summers, C. R. (1997) Conversational patterns of children with disabled and nondisabled siblings. *Applied Psycholinguistics, 18*, 277–291.

Wang, P. P., & Bellugi, V. (1993). Williams syndrome, Down syndrome and cognitive neuroscience. *American Journal of Diseases of Children, 147*, 1246–1251.

Wolraich, M. L., Felice, M. E., & Drotar, D. (Eds.). (1996). *The classification of child and adolescent mental diagnoses in primary care: Diagnostic and statistical manual for primary care (DSM-PC)—Child and adolescent version*. Elk Grove Village, IL: American Academy of Pediatrics.

World Health Organization (1980). *International classification of impairments, disabilities, and handicaps: A manual of classification relating to the consequences of disease*. Geneva: Author.

World Health Organization (WHO). (1989). *International classification of diseases* (10th ed.). Geneva: Author.

World Health Organization (WHO). (1999). *International classification of impairments, activities, and participation: A manual of dimensions of disablement and functioning*. Geneva: Author.

Zeanah, C. H., Boris, N. W., & Larrieu, J. A. (1997). Infant development and developmental risk: A review of the past 10 years. *Journal of the American Academy of Child and Adolescent Psychiatry, 36*, 165–178.

3

CLINICAL ASSESSMENT IN PLANNING AND EVALUATING INTERVENTION

RUNE J. SIMEONSSON
JANEY STURTZ McMILLEN

*The successful experiences of practitioners must be observed, verified, and accumu-
lated through empirical practice and accountability ... without the development of a
cumulative body of knowledge on the effects of interventions ... we are doomed to a
series of never-ending fads and promises.*
                              —Barlow, Hayes, and Nelson (1984, pp. 36–37)

Marcus is a 4-year-old boy with fragile-X syndrome who has been assessed as having
developmental delays in both cognitive and speech areas. He has been receiving preschool
special education services for the past 10 months to address these delays. The interdisciplinary team has recommended that an evaluation be made to determine if the current
intervention activities need to be modified. The school psychologist and the speech language pathologist plan to conduct an evaluation of Marcus's progress using his current
Individualized Education Plan. They will then meet with Marcus's parents to decide on
the next course of action related to Marcus's developmental goals.

Clinical assessment is implemented in response to a variety of concerns about children with
disabilities or chronic conditions. In some situations the same instrument or procedure may
be used to address different concerns. In other instances, similar concerns may require the
use of general measures. Clinical assessment can be carried out for three main purposes:
(1) defining and/or diagnosing child conditions, (2) planning individualized interventions,
and (3) evaluating interventions. This chapter describes the procedures and activities of
gathering and integrating assessment data into intervention plans. A review of strategies
and methods to evaluate child progress and intervention effectiveness follows.

ASSESSMENT DATA AND ASSESSMENT GOALS

Defining/Diagnosing Characteristics

A frequent goal of clinical assessment is to define and/or diagnose a child's specific difficulty or condition. This typically takes the form of specifying child characteristics in order
to determine if they are consistent with a diagnostic entity, such as autism or mental retar-

dation. In this context, clinical assessment is implemented in order to (1) derive diagnostic information, (2) document a child's eligibility for services when a categorical label is required, and (3) provide diagnostic documentation required for reimbursement by third-party payers. An example of a categorical label is the assignment of a child to special education. The use of assessment data to support the diagnosis of a child on one or more axes of the *Diagnostic and Statistical Manual of Mental Disorders* (DSM-IV; American Psychiatric Association, 1994) is an example of documentation for reimbursement. Another common use of DSM-IV diagnoses is in the generation of statistical summaries of children provided diagnostic or intervention services in mental health programs. Assessment results can also be used in other classification applications, such as the *International Classification of Impairments, Disabilities, and Handicaps* (ICIDH; World Health Organization, 1980) and its current revision, the *International Classification of Functioning and Disability* (ICIDH2 B-2; World Health Organization, 1999), described in Chapter 2. An important difference, however, is that the DSM-IV classifies diagnoses, whereas the ICIDH/ICIDH2 B-2 classify functional characteristics.

The use of diagnostic classifications to define placements or determine eligibility for services is likely to increase in health, educational, and social service contexts. Clinical assessment data can be used to confirm that a child meets the diagnostic criteria for mental retardation, autism, or emotional disability in order that special placement or provision of individualized services can be initiated. Applications with children with mental retardation, for example, involve the use of assessment data to determine if the American Association on Mental Retardation criteria for the diagnosis of mental retardation have been met (Luckasson, Schalock, Snell, & Spitalnik, 1996). For children in public schools, state or local criteria define eligibility for special placement and services. With increasing emphasis on interagency collaboration, a priority should be to use classifications that encompass dimensions of disability and chronic conditions in childhood. The diagnostic and functional classifications of DSM-IV and the ICIDH2 B-2, respectively, would provide a comprehensive approach to documentation in this regard (Table 3.1).

In regard to deriving diagnostic labels, we urge the need for caution, particularly with children who are young or who have complex problems. Health settings, schools, and habilitation programs often require some form of diagnostic information to determine eligibility of children with disabilities or chronic conditions for services and for administrative record keeping. Caution should be exercised to minimize the liabilities associated with assignment of a formal diagnosis. One step is to explore criteria that are functional in nature, which may simultaneously serve to reduce the application of a stigmatizing label. A second step is to minimize the possibility of misdiagnosis through verification with multiple sources of information. A third and related step is to identify any limitations that apply to the diagnostic process and to emphasize the need for reassessment of the child to determine if the diagnosis is still appropriate or should be discontinued.

Planning Intervention

The second purpose of clinical assessment is to obtain a base from which to prescribe or plan intervention. Although descriptive informative diagnoses are sometimes derived as independent activities, in practice they are likely to yield integral data on which intervention plans can be developed for a child. The goal of assessment in this regard will thus focus on such referral questions as: What are the learning needs of this child? What intervention will be best suited to facilitate learning? In what sequence should learning activities be presented?

TABLE 3.1. Systems to Classify Diagnoses and Functional Characteristics of Children and Youth with Disabilities and Chronic Health Conditions

DSM-IV multiaxial classification scheme[a]

Axis	Description
Axis I	Clinical disorders
	Other conditions that may be the focus of clinical attention
Axis II	Personality disorders and mental retardation
Axis III	General medical condition
Axis IV*	Psychosocial and environmental problems
Axis V*	Global assessment of functioning

*optional

DSM-IV (PC) Child and Adolescent Version[b]

Environmental situations

Challenges to primary support group
Changes in caregiving
Other functional changes in family
Community or social challenges
Educational challenges
Parent or adolescent occupational challenges
Housing challenges
Economic challenges
Inadequate access to health and/or mental health services
Legal system or crime problem
Other environmental situations
Health-related situations

Child manifestation

Developmental competency
Impulsive/hyperactive/inattentive behaviors
Negative/antisocial behaviors
Substance use/abuse
Emotions and moods
Somatic and sleep behaviors
Feeding, eating, and elimination behaviors
Illness-related behaviors
Sexual behaviors
Atypical behaviors

International Classification of Functioning and Disability (ICIDH2 B-2)[c]

Body functions/structure (impairment)
Activity limitations
Participation (restrictions)
Environmental factors

[a]APA (1994); [b]Wolraich, Felice, & Drotar (1996); [c]WHO (1999)

The essential feature of clinical assessment for intervention planning is a comprehensive and focused picture of the child's strengths and needs. Because the goal is to develop an individualized intervention plan, the clinician should obtain any information that will contribute to a better understanding of the child's characteristics. The nature of the referral question may indicate that a particular domain of assessment (cognition, communication, personal/social, or behavior) and a particular strategy (psychometric, behavioral, or qualitative-developmental) may be best suited to generate information from which to plan intervention. In other instances, several of the domains and several of the strategies may have to be used in combination to derive information specific to a referral question.

Evaluating Progress

A third purpose of clinical assessment is to document the child's progress and evaluate interventions. To this end, a child's characteristics of clinical interest are assessed and summarized to yield descriptive data of current functioning. Progress is commonly documented to provide a current benchmark against which previous and/or future functioning can be compared. In its most typical application, documentation of status is made both pre- and posttreatment to determine the extent of change, if any, that has occurred as a function of a prescribed period of intervention for an individual child.

Another purpose of documenting status is simply to derive data for descriptive statistics. Such data may appear in proposals, surveys, annual reports, or other documents to verify the need for or delivery of services for children with disabilities or chronic conditions. In this regard, diagnostic classifications may of course also be used. The fundamental distinction between assessment for diagnostic purposes and assessment to document status, however, rests on the fact that in the former, assessment data are used to arrive at a diagnosis, whereas in the latter, data are used to describe a child's performance or achievement.

CLINICAL ASSESSMENT AND INTERVENTION

Assumptions

Developing intervention plans for a child requires the clinician to integrate assessment results and translate them into goals and prescriptions for activities. The term "intervention" is used here in a generic sense to define any program or activity prescribed for a child on the basis of assessment results. Intervention thus encompasses treatment and habilitation activities in clinical, as well as educational, settings. Frequently used terms for treatment therapy or intervention, such as "individualized family service plan," "individualized education plan (IEP)," "individualized habilitation plan," and "individualized program plan" are used interchangeably. Each of the terms refers to intervention designed for an individual child and reflects several common assumptions regarding the relationship of assessment to intervention planning: (1) assessment results are assumed to be a valid reflection of the child's current strengths and needs; (2) the intervention will be more effective if assessment data are used in a systematic manner; (3) an interdisciplinary approach is important because the needs of children with disabilities are often complex and multiply determined; (4) assessment data should be translatable into practical terms in order to specify the nature, direction, and sequence of intervention; (5) the intervention plan should include specific procedures for evaluating the intervention; and (6) involvement of the parent and the child, if appropriate, is an essential element in the planning process (Bjorck-Akesson, Granlund, & Simeonsson, 2000; Simpson & Fiedler, 1989; Turnbull & Turnbull, 1990).

These assumptions apply in developing any intervention plan. Such assumptions have recently been formalized to include additional elements and greater specificity in federal and state laws pertaining to special populations, in particular the components of the Individualized Education Plan (IEP) specified by Public Law 105–17. The IEP can be arranged in a variety of formats to document educational programming for a given child.

Integrating Assessment Data

An important step in the integration of assessment data is to review the quality of the obtained assessment results regarding the adequacy of the assessment–child match. As clinical assessment of children with disabilities or chronic conditions may involve nonstandard use of instruments or instruments with limited technical adequacy, it is essential that (1) any limitations are spelled out in detail and (2) the interpretation of findings is qualified accordingly in the report. A related issue of importance in preparing reports and in conducting the treatment planning conference is to distinguish between types of statements or conclusions that can be made about a child's functioning. Swallow (1981) has identified three types of statements that can be made in this context: *factual, inferential*, and *judgmental*. As intervention plans are likely to be based on all three types of statements, recognition of their implications is important. Factual statements summarize the child's performance under specified conditions, derived from informal or formal procedures. The following is an example of a factual statement: "Under standard testing conditions, John obtained a percentile score of 5 on Raven's Progressive Matrices." As Swallow has indicated, "Wording must be clear, exact and precise. Behavior is reported in objective, observable terms— what the child did under these conditions at that moment in time" (1981, p. 65).

Inferential statements, on the other hand, involve inferences and/or interpretations based on assessment results. A statement concluding that John's poor performance on Raven's Progressive Matrices is associated with impulsivity is an example of an inferential statement. A judgmental statement is one in which a judgment is made about interventions that should be initiated for a child. Judgmental statements, according to Swallow, are derived from the facts and interpretations of assessment data and thus flow logically from factual and inferential statements. Drawing on the previous examples, a judgmental statement would take the following form: "A training program to reduce impulsivity is recommended for John in which activities will be structured to promote a more reflective approach to task demands."

The integration of assessment data for planning interventions is derived from the assessment itself and from other sources such as records and reports. Such information about the child is likely to include demographic characteristics, health status, developmental history, current functioning in home and school, and specific performance results. The task of integrating this information requires professional judgment and draws on clinical experience and theory to generate inferential and judgmental statements about the child's difficulties and intervention needs.

Generating Intervention Plans

A set of intervention recommendations is a major product of clinical assessment. Although a clinician may develop and implement interventions individually, in schools and clinical settings these activities are more commonly carried out by an interdisciplinary planning team. By law, these teams in public schools are composed of (1) the child's teacher, (2) an agency representative responsible for providing services, (3) the child's parent(s), (4) the child, if appropriate, and (5) psychologists and other individuals with relevant expertise. Although the composition of interdisciplinary teams in health settings will likely include more specialists, psychologists are likely to play a role on the team. Specifically, psychologists in clinical settings such as hospitals, institutions, or residential programs often have to assume primary responsibility for ensuring that a comprehensive treatment program is carried out. In school settings, this responsibility is typically assumed by teachers. In health settings that serve infants and young children, a pediatrician or nurse may assume the role of coordinator to monitor services and treatments prescribed for the child.

The mission of the interdisciplinary team is to translate assessment results and other information into an intervention program for a child. This involves both identifying and prioritizing goals and writing these goals in a format that lends itself to implementation and evaluation.

Participating in the identification of goals is a key responsibility for psychologists and other evaluation specialists, given their major role in assessment. Securing the participation of teachers, parents, and the child in identifying goals is also an important priority. Although the nature of goals will vary, they should reflect an outcome desired in a specified period of time. The requirement for an IEP is that goals be written on an annual basis, from which intermediate or short-term objectives are derived. Criteria to be considered in selecting annual goals are (1) the child's past achievement, (2) the child's current performance, (3) the practicality of goals and needs of the child, and (4) time required to attain goals.

A practical reality that may hinder the team's identification of a number of intervention goals is that some goals are seen as more important than others. A fixed procedure that takes into account the individual and cumulative perspectives of team members and ensures that treatment plans are developed in an objective and comprehensive manner is of value in the prioritization of goals.

Goal Attainment Scaling in Intervention Planning

Adopting a systematic approach to the development of intervention plans that includes evaluation procedures addresses concerns about accountability of services for children with disabilities or chronic conditions. Issues pertaining to accountability have been raised in the behavioral (Mate-Kole, Danquah, Twum, & Danquah, 1999), educational (Burgee, 1996; Young & Chesson, 1999), and pediatric (Mitchell & Cusick, 1998) fields. Demands for accountability involve a consideration of the effectiveness, as well as the efficiency, of interventions for children. Interventions are required to be documented in a manner compatible with objective evaluation. In spite of the fact that clinicians recognize the importance of documenting intervention effectiveness, attempts to do so have been limited. This may be due not only to the difficulty of documenting change in children with disabilities or chronic conditions but also to the fact that record-keeping systems for intervention plans may not lend themselves to use as evaluation tools. Documentation of intervention plans in a format that includes evaluation elements should contribute to accountability. Goal attainment scaling (GAS) was developed as a planning and evaluation method (Kiresuk & Sherman, 1968) and has been applied in a variety of human services. The flexibility and positive features of the GAS approach have contributed to its widespread use in adult rehabilitation settings (Joyce, Rockwood, & Mate-Kole, 1994; Rockwood, Joyce, & Stolee, 1997; Stolee, Rockwood, Fox, & Streiner, 1992) and, to a lesser extent, with children in mental health and school settings (Palisano, Haley, & Brown, 1992). Studies have investigated its utility with inpatient child psychiatric populations (Holroyd & Goldenberg, 1978; Wallin & Koch, 1978), in a multicategorical preschool project (Shuster, Fitzgerald, Shelton, Barber, & Desch, 1984), and with preschool children in an interdisciplinary treatment program (Case-Smith & Bryan, 1999). Given these features, GAS may be well suited to document interventions for children with disabilities and chronic health conditions.

The GAS method consists of a systematic procedure to evaluate progress toward specified intervention goals. This is accomplished by comparing actual attainment against specified goals across a number of domains using a matrix format (Figure 3.1).

A requirement of the planning process is to identify a child's present status and unique goals in a sequence of projected outcomes (worst to best), as shown in Table 3.2. The fact that it is client-centered promotes the involvement of parent, team members, and the child, if appropriate.

A number of features of GAS recommend its use in the development of individual intervention plans (Simeonsson, Bailey, Huntington, & Brandon, 1991). First, as shown in Table 3.2, its matrix form is uncomplicated and simple to use. Second, it is a flexible method allowing the use of idiosyncratic child information. Third, the requirement that goals or objectives be specified in a sequence of best to worst outcomes lends itself to goal-oriented conceptualizations of treatments for children. This feature avoids the problem of objectives that are defined only in terms of a single specific outcome and that thus fail to provide an index of the extent to which a child exceeds or falls short of achieving a given intervention goal. Fourth, the specification of goals differs from one domain to another as represented by different scales, thus reflecting various intervention goals. Although the GAS method commonly involves specifying goals across five domains, a greater or lesser number of domains can be accommodated. Fifth, the differential importance of one domain over another can be reflected through weighting of domain scales, a feature of special relevance to children with disabilities or chronic conditions. Differential weighting of scales not only permits the highlighting of the unique needs of a child but also serves to reflect the relative importance at-

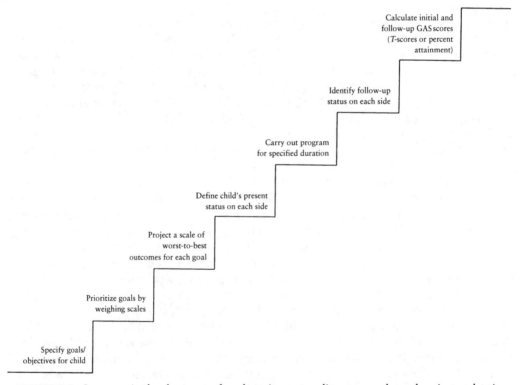

FIGURE 3.1. Sequence in development of goal attainment scaling approach to planning evaluation.

TABLE 3.2. Sample GAS Matrix for a 4-Year-Old Girl with Severe Motor Impairment

Scale attainment levels	Goal 1: Toy play (W1 = 1)	Goal 2: Self-feeding (W2 = 1)	Goal 3: Toileting (W3 = 3)	Goal 4: Manual signing (W4 = 2)	Goal 5: Task persistence (W5 = 2)
2 Best expected outcome	Plays with age-appropriate toys independently.	Eats with spoon independently and with no spilling.	1 accident per day.	Uses 5 manual signs independently. (A)	Attends to task for 1 minute.
1 More than expected outcome	Plays with toys when given verbal directions only.	Eats with spoon independently with some spilling. (A)	2 accidents per day. (A)	Uses 3 manual signs independently.	Attends to task for 30 seconds. (A)
0 Expected outcome	Plays with toys only when given model and verbal instructions. (A)	Eats with spoon independently with considerable spilling.	3 accidents per day.	Uses 1 manual sign independently.	Attends to task for 15 seconds.
−1 Less than expected outcome	Plays with toys only with physical prompts and verbal instructions to play.	Eats with spoon when given physical assistance.	4 accidents per day. (I)	Uses 1 manual sign but only with prompting.	Attends to task for 5–10 seconds.
−2 Worst expected outcome	Does not play with toys at all. Full manipulation required. (I)	Finger feeds only. (I)	5 accidents per day.	Uses no manual signs. (I)	Attends to task for less than 5 seconds. (I)

Note. W, weights; I, initial performance; A, attained level.

tached to prescribed interventions. Sixth, another attractive feature of the GAS method is that the unit of analysis need not be a single child but can be several children, a family, a classroom, or, for that matter, a program. This is important because interventions may sometimes need to be planned and evaluated for groups rather than individuals.

In the actual development of goal attainment scales, the period of intervention is defined, providing a realistic framework for projecting the sequence of best to worst outcomes. This is an important consideration, because the expected goal or outcome for a 6-month intervention period will differ from that proposed for 12 months. School-related goals developed in IEPs are typically defined in annual terms, whereas goals in clinical settings may vary from a period of a few weeks to several months. In either event, defining the time frame is necessary for the projection of realistic goals.

The interdisciplinary team should enter the information into the GAS matrix form based on their identified and prioritized goals for a child with disabilities or chronic conditions. Identified goals should be listed in order of highest priority and entered at the top of each scale. As an example, consider the following goals and priority rankings for a 4-year-old child: self-feeding (4), toileting (1), toy play (5), manual signing (2), task persistence (3).

The priority ranking suggests that toy play and self-feeding constitute less important goals, whereas task persistence, manual communication, and toileting reflect increasingly important priorities. The differential importance of these goals can be reflected by the assignment of weights ranging from 1 to 3, as illustrated in Table 3.2. Although the values chosen for weights are arbitrary, a good rule of thumb is to use values that can convey practical reality. Thus one goal may be assumed to be two or three times more important than another in terms of expenditure of time, money, and/or staff effort. In words, the difference for the weights could be defined as 1 = important, 2 = very important, and 3 = critical. Having identified the domains of each goal and the weight for each domain, the team members should enter expected goals for the proposed period of intervention in operational terms in the horizontal row for each domain. Entries are then also made for the most unfavorable, less than expected, more than expected, and best anticipated outcomes for the period of intervention. The child's current level of functioning relative to the sequence of goals should be recorded to permit comparison against attained level at the conclusion of the intervention. As shown in Table 3.2, the current functioning of a 4-year-old with severe disabilities is at the most unfavorable level for four domains and less than expected for one domain. If regression of functioning is a possibility, the child may be assigned to a less-than-expected level of outcome initially to document the fact that the intervention was effective in maintaining status and preventing decline.

EVALUATING INTERVENTIONS

The emphasis placed on interventions for children with disabilities or chronic conditions in the past decade has been followed by growing demands for demonstration of the effectiveness of such interventions. Providers of educational (Elliott, 1998; Hart & Sciutto, 1996), behavioral (Mate-Kole et al., 1999), and rehabilitative (Mitchell & Cusick, 1998) interventions must answer demands for accountability. Concerns about controversial treatments also serve as the basis for evaluation of interventions (Eberlin, Ibel, & Jacobson, 1994). Parents, clinicians, and funding agencies are all interested in the accountability of intervention programs and services.

Accountability can be defined as giving an account of the services provided for children with disabilities or chronic conditions based on evaluations of the effectiveness and efficiency of such services. The concern for documenting effectiveness is essentially a scientific concern. It raises the question: Can it be demonstrated that the child has changed and/or made progress as a result of intervention? The documentation of progress or change in a child is a necessary but not sufficient condition from which to infer that the intervention, treatment, or program was effective. In this context, professionals who deliver or are responsible for delivery of services are interested in effectiveness. The concern for documenting efficiency is more of a pragmatic or economic concern: Was the progress made by the child effective relative to some cost or expenditure of effort? Cost effectiveness may refer to effectiveness relative to expenditure of time, energy, or funds, as well as utilization of resources and personnel. Efficiency is thus likely to be of interest to those who fund or administer services (such as administrators and legislators). The relationship between these two dimensions of accountability is such that a determination of efficiency is predicated on the fact that effectiveness can be demonstrated. Intervention, on the other hand, may be found to be effective but not necessarily efficient. Although efforts to demonstrate efficiency are desirable and recommended, they may not be required. Psychologists and other clinicians always have continuing responsibility to evaluate interventions for children in order to determine if they should be maintained, discontinued, or modified.

Clinical assessment is related to concerns about accountability of interventions in at least two ways. First, in any determination of child progress, it is assumed that assessment data are reliable and valid at some level. Although assessment limitations often apply to children with disabilities, psychometric information that pertains to the assessment data should be documented and considered in the evaluation of child progress.

Second, assessment data are used as indices to document the effectiveness of intervention. The use of cost–benefit and other utility indices in health-related sectors is growing. To this end changes in IQ scores, age equivalents, or other values from one assessment occasion to the next may be used as indices of progress. A statement such as "Over a 6-month period, a 0.9 mean length utterance (MLU) increase and a change in age from 3 years, 2 months to 3 years, 11 months was found for Marcus, a child with fragile-X syndrome" illustrates the use of assessment data in this manner. In documentation of efficiency, on the other hand, assessment data may serve as numerators in calculations of changes attributable to the intervention relative to some cost measure. The measures of cost may be in terms of dollars expended but may also take the form of personnel, energy, or other resource utilization. Determining how these values should be used to derive appropriate efficiency indices may be a problem.

Although accountability is a high priority, caution must be exercised in deriving efficiency indices from psychological assessment data. Psychologists play an important role in assisting funding agencies and decision makers with appropriate means of applying assessment data to document efficiency of intervention and in minimizing the risk that psychological variables will be used inappropriately in cost–benefit determinations.

IMPLEMENTING INTERVENTIONS

To evaluate clinical interventions, researchers must gather systematic data in order to address issues of accountability to families and to funding sources and the need for program documentation. This systematic approach can be summarized (Simeonsson et al., 1996) in eight questions:

1. What are the intervention expectations of the family and providers?
2. What are the purposes and nature of intervention?
3. How is intervention personalized?
4. Is there fidelity of implementation of planned services?
5. Are anticipated outcomes of intervention specified?
6. Are documented outcomes and other effects attributable to intervention?
7. Are family and provider expectations for intervention met?
8. Are findings generalizable to future efforts?

Accountability to families is addressed by Questions 1, 3, and 7. Questions 2 and 5 address accountability to funding sources. Program documentation is addressed by Questions 4 and 6. Question 8 addresses the overarching issue of providing evidence of the preventive potential of intervention.

Within this approach, interventions may be viewed as a cycle of five sequenced activities that address expectations and facilitate encounters with children and their families: (1) defining intervention expectations, (2) assessing child and family characteristics, needs, and priorities, (3) developing a personalized plan of services, (4) implementing and monitoring services, and (5) evaluating outcomes and satisfaction (Figure 3.2). Each step of the cycle involves data gathering.

At the first step, data should be gathered on the family's and the professional's expectations regarding the content and form of the multidisciplinary evaluation, the assessment of the child, and available intervention and support services. To assess child and family characteristics, needs, and priorities, the clinician should identify the nature and priorities of the child and family and the child's functional abilities. Prior to the development of a personalized plan of services, he or she should gather information regarding the family's preferred level of participation in team development of child and family goals, desired forms

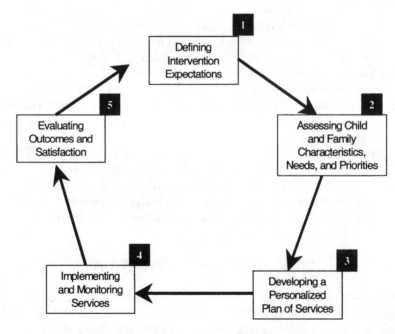

FIGURE 3.2. Elements of the intervention cycle.

of services and support, and outcome expectations. Implementing and monitoring services will also involve gathering data regarding families' collaboration in the implementation of the intervention focus, their preferred level of involvement in implementation, the available resources and supports that can be utilized, and the scaling of goals. Evaluating outcomes and satisfaction requires determining goal attainment levels, validating of the intervention by the consumer, defining the extent to which the intervention has addressed the expectations for the child and family, and informal or structured monitoring of progress toward child and family goals.

IMPLEMENTING EVALUATION

Efforts to document the accountability of intervention with a single child or with a group of children are associated with a number of difficulties that may limit the kinds of conclusions that can be drawn from such efforts. These difficulties can be summarized along the dimensions of the nature, adequacy, and interpretability of assessment information. In regard to the nature of information, it is important to recognize the difference between data and information (Maher, 1979). A key function of evaluation is to transform factual material into information useful for decision making. As we indicated earlier in this chapter, assessment results may take the form of factual, inferential, and judgmental statements (Swallow, 1981), and each of these may have differential utility in the evaluation of child progress. The adequacy of information constitutes a second dimension of difficulties in evaluation of programs for children. One problem area pertains to the fact that data aggregated for evaluation by decision makers may not be collected by those involved directly in the delivery of services. Another area of difficulty involves the interpretability of evaluation information. The most common approach to the evaluation of progress is to document change prior to and following a specified period of intervention. Given that changes in the child's behavior or development can be documented, interpretation is needed to determine (1) if the change can be attributed to the intervention, (2) if the change is relevant to the child's needs, and (3) if the change is significant in some sense.

Attribution of Change

Because psychological assessment and clinical intervention focus on the individual, the evaluation approach will likely involve documenting the child's behavior or characteristics on two or more occasions to determine the direction and magnitude of change. When results of psychological assessment reveal that some change has occurred from one time to another, it is of course desirable to infer that the intervening treatment was responsible for the change. This is basically an issue of causal inference; that is, can the observed change in the child be attributed to the intervention? Unfortunately, difficulties inherent in the pretest–posttest approach have to be considered. The major consideration is to rule out factors other than the intervention that may have accounted for the observed change in the child. Given the fact that time has elapsed during the intervention, it is necessary to realize that progress may be due to maturation, either alone or in combination with the treatment. Another factor that needs to be ruled out in repeated assessment of a child is "test-wiseness," or familiarity with measures or procedures, that contributes to the apparent progress of a child. These and other factors that may provide alternative explanations for change are considered threats to validity in statistical analyses of change.

Relevance of Change

Referral concerns about children with disabilities or chronic conditions often involve problems related to functioning in real-life situations. These functional problems include failure to attend, failure to complete tasks, and difficulties in making friends. However, these referral concerns, when translated into assessment activities, are likely to be redefined as difficulties with distractibility, impulsivity, visual decoding, or self-concept, respectively. Such redefinition of the child's difficulties and associated assessment may be several steps removed from the practical context in which the child's difficulties were originally identified and defined. The point here is not to minimize the value of redefining referral questions in a conceptual way but to emphasize the importance of recognizing the contextual relevance of the child's difficulties. This approach is similar to a methodological position for ecological validity initially advocated by Brooks and Baumeister (1977). Their recommendation in research with children with developmental disabilities is still relevant (Baumeister, 1997). The relevance of change should thus be a central consideration in the scope and context of clinical assessment.

Significance of Change

When evaluation of progress reveals that expected change has occurred, questions may still remain about the significance of that progress. Questions regarding the significance of change are of course dependent on assumptions that the progress is relevant to the child's problems and attributable to the intervention, as discussed previously. Inferences about the significance of change involve judgments about the importance of the child's progress based on statistical or clinical criteria. As these criteria differ, it is possible to find evidence of change that meets statistical, but not clinical or practical, significance. Conversely, it is not uncommon to find research with children with disabilities or chronic conditions in which clinical significance is inferred even in the absence of statistical significance (Kirk, 1996). Resolving the issue of what constitutes important or significant change in some absolute sense is a difficult task. Among the factors that need consideration in this regard are the nature of the intervention, the assessment measures, and the evaluation approach applicable to particular findings.

STRATEGIES IN EVALUATION OF PROGRAMS

In spite of the challenges in evaluating progress of children with disabilities or chronic conditions, steps can be taken to increase objectivity and confidence in the activity. To this end, we review strategies to improve evaluation efforts (Table 3.3.). In reference to the problem of aggregation and synthesis of assessment data, members of the interdisciplinary team must rely on specific guidelines to ensure that the nature of information will be suitable for evaluation. In this regard, the IEP form, skills checklists, graphing, and anecdotal records can be used to document progams. The adequacy of information for evaluation may be of particular significance in the planning and implementation of clinical interventions for children and youth. Along this line, Maher and Barbrack (1980) maintain that it is important to determine the extent to which interventions are implemented, can be evaluated, and can demonstrate consumer satisfaction. The intervention cycle described earlier (see Figure 3.2) may be a useful framework for comprehensive evaluation of services. This cycle involves defining intervention expectations, assessing child and family

TABLE 3.3. Issues and Approaches in Evaluation of Child Progress

Issue	Problem	Approach
Attribution of change	Can progress documented through psychological or developmental assessment be attributed to intervention?	Adopt procedures and carry out analyses designed to rule out alternative explanations for child change or progress.
Relevance of change	Does change assessed with psychological or developmental measures represent real-life change?	Apply principles as ecological validity and social validation to address the issue of relevance.
Significance of change	Should the significance of change be determined on the basis of practical criteria, statistical criteria, or both?	Select procedures yielding appropriate and sensitive evidence of change (such as single-participant methodology, goal attainment scaling).

characteristics, needs, and priorities, developing a personalized plan of services, implementing and monitoring services, and evaluating outcomes and satisfaction.

Attribution of Change

When evaluation results reveal that a child with disabilities or chronic conditions has made progress, that progress can be more strongly attributed to the intervention if we take systematic steps to rule out rival explanations for such progress. A common approach to ruling out the factor of maturation in experimental group designs is to randomly assign children either to an intervention group or to a control group that does not receive the intervention. Because both groups are subject to maturation, any differential effects found in the experimental group can be attributed to the intervention. In the context of clinical interventions with individual children, practical and ethical considerations negate random assignment to experimental and control conditions. However, researchers have explored alternative means to reduce rival explanations for child progress; two of these means are described in the following section.

Relevance of Change

Concerns for the relevance of change may benefit from a consideration of two concepts, ecological validity and social validation. Both concepts relate to the use of instruments and procedures that have demonstrated or probable relevance to the referral concerns for the child with disabilities or chronic conditions. In practice, concern for ecological validity should influence the nature, as well as the context, of assessment and intervention. In some instances this may mean that a criterion-referenced measure should be used instead of or in addition to a norm-referenced measure; in other instances it may mean that a behavioral observation is more appropriate than a formal test. The primary factor guiding the selection of assessment strategies and the interpretation of assessment results should be to maximize the match between the child's presenting difficulty and the development of an individualized intervention plan.

Ecological Validity

Ecological validity of clinical assessment can be enhanced by carrying out assessment in settings in which behaviors of interest are likely to be demonstrated or evident. Although this position may seem obvious for behaviors typically linked to specific settings, such as eating (mealtimes) or gross motor skills (playground), it is equally applicable to less obvious linkages of behavior and settings, such as assertion (group activity) and self-help skills (home setting). Documentation of the characteristics of the setting in which assessment takes place can also provide information to qualify obtained findings. Information that describes the circumstances under which the child was assessed should provide clues as to the confidence that can be placed in the findings. Interpretation of findings for a child with cerebral palsy who was not properly positioned during assessment would differ markedly from assessment findings for another child with cerebral palsy who was properly positioned in an adapted wheelchair with a fixed tray. Minimal confidence would be placed in the findings for the first child, whereas in the latter case prescriptions for intervention can be made with greater assurance.

Social Validation

The goal of the intervention of placing children with disabilities or chronic conditions in least restrictive environments emphasizes the importance of identifying ecologically valid behaviors and outcomes associated with such placements. Kazdin and Matson (1981) have discussed this issue in terms of social validation, that is, examination of the social acceptability of intervention efforts. There are two ways in which they feel social validation is of importance to intervention; one of these pertains to the focus of intervention, and the second deals with the outcome or change due to intervention. Thus, for intervention efforts focusing on social skills and social functioning, the selection of behaviors for intervention and the importance attached to outcome measures should have social and ecological validity. Kazdin and Matson identify two methods, social comparison and subjective evaluation, that may be useful in selecting and evaluating interventions for special populations. The method of social comparison involves the determination of what should constitute acceptable performance by observing the performance of individuals who are functioning adequately in settings of interest. The second method, subjective evaluation, refers to the determination of what should constitute the focus of intervention or outcome measurement, based on the opinions of persons knowledgeable about the clients and the issues of concern. Use of social comparison and subjective evaluation should contribute to the development of intervention programs based on objective data rather than subjective views. With social development constituting an intervention priority, incorporation of social validation is a useful element of evaluation efforts as demonstrated by Oke and Schreibman (1990) in a case study of social training for a child with autism.

Significance of Change

The significance of observed change as a function of interventions for children is a continuing concern in clinical and educational settings. Although helping professionals are often justifiably inclined to infer that intervention has been effective, empirical evidence for effectiveness may be difficult to produce. The problem in such situations is to distinguish between empirical significance and clinical or practical significance. To this end, three approaches are appropriate for evaluation of clinical interventions with children: the case study, the single-participant design, and GAS. These approaches vary in methodology and the manner in which intervention efforts are evaluated. However, each can answer evaluation questions if applied in a systematic method.

Case Study

The case study approach has a long history in medical and allied human services. The definition of a case study can vary, ranging from subjective narratives to objective, analytic reports. It is particularly suitable for documenting clinical interventions, and as such it has been seen as an attractive evaluation tool but has also given rise to concerns regarding its value as an evaluation approach. Wells (1987), in a review of the method's limitations and strenghts, advocated for its use both as a preexperimental and a quasi-experimental design. The adequacy and rigor of this approch as an evaluation tool can be strengthened by applying many of the same standards utilized with group experimental designs. These standards include a theoretically derived framework, detailed documentation, use of multiple assessment sources and different time points, and explicit criteria for evaluating outcomes. Another important step for generalization of case study findings is replication. If attention is paid to these standards, "The quasi-experimental case study research design, that is the intensive study of one case with the application of controls over data collection procedures . . . allows some inferences to be drawn and can properly be used to test some causal hypotheses such as those relating to client change due to treatment" (Wells, 1987, p. 786).

Single-Participant Design

The single-participant-design approach is well established based on the methodology of the functional analysis of behavior. The two essential features of this approach are operationalization of the behavior of interest and recording of the behavior across specified observation and intervention time periods. The ABAB model is the standard design, in which the contingent control of behavior is established across the periods of baseline, intervention, reversal, and reinstatement. When a reversal phase is not desired, multiple baseline designs are used.

Goal Attainment Scaling

The GAS approach, described earlier in this chapter as a method suitable for developing intervention plans, also lends itself to systematic evaluation, yielding a quantitative index reflecting change. The preparation of the GAS form as an intervention document for an individual child, illustrated in Table 3.2, includes the specification of a number of goals, weighting of goals, and sequencing of outcome steps from worst to best. The number of goals specified depends, of course, on a child's needs, but four to five goals may be sufficient for most intervention plans. This number seems typical in that a study of 400 individual education programs has revealed that the average program consisted of four general goals (Anderson, Barner, & Larson, 1978).

At the time the GAS document is developed, the child's status is recorded at the appropriate level for each goal. Following the period of intervention specified in the document, the child's attainment of goals is recorded at the level reflecting follow-up status. A GAS score can then be calculated by entering appropriate values in the equation designed by Kiresuk and Sherman (1968) to yield a standardized T score with a mean value of 50 and a standard deviation of 10 (Figure 3.3). The value of $p = .30$ is used to reflect an estimate of the assumed intercorrelation of goals. This value seems appropriate to use because Maloney, Mirrett, Brooks, and Johannes (1978) have found that substitution of other values (such as $p = .70$) did not alter the derived score substantially.

Drawing on the illustration of the intervention program developed for the child with cerebral palsy described earlier, these steps would be followed in an evaluation of progress based on initial and follow-up status (see Table 3.2). Weighted scores before and after intervention are derived for each goal by multiplying individual goal weights with the level of initial and follow-up status, yielding values of –2, –2, –3, –4, –4, and 0, 1, 3, 4, 2, respectively. Inserting these values into the equation results in GAS scores of 25.5 and 66.3 for initial and follow-up occasions.

These standardized scores can be used for evaluation in two ways. In mental health studies, a common way to apply the procedure has been to focus on the follow-up score, in this case the T score of 66.3, and to interpret its value as a reflection of the extent to which specified goals have been attained. Because a T score of 50 would indicate that the expected level of outcome had been attained, a score of 66.3 would indicate that a higher than expected level was achieved across goals. A second way is to compare the difference between initial and follow-up scores. If the GAS approach is implemented for a number of children served in a program, their GAS scores can be meaningfully compared because they are standardized scores, in spite of differences in the nature and complexity of individual goals, weights, and specified levels of outcome.

The flexibility of the GAS approach in handling idiosyncratic data and its suitability for planning and evaluation make it an attractive methodology to consider in work with children with disabilities or chronic conditions. Further, the GAS approach can be used to complement other data documenting the response of children with disabilities or chronic conditions.

In concluding this chapter, we reiterate the fact that assessment of children and evaluation of their progress is a practical and scientific necessity in clinical contexts. Practical concerns in the form of accountability demands made by consumers and decision makers require that we provide documentation that the needs of children with disabilities or

$$T = 50 + \frac{10 \sum w_j \, x_j}{\sqrt{(1-p)\sum w_j^2 + p\left(\sum w_j\right)^2}}$$

where

w is the weight for subscale and

x is the outcome level value.

$p = .30$

$j = $ item

FIGURE 3.3. Formula to calculate T scores in Global Attainment Scaling.

chronic conditions have been identified and met. From a scientific perspective, there is an ongoing professional responsibility to seek to better understand the complexity of chronic conditions and disabilities and find means whereby their effects can be reduced or ameliorated. To this end we argue for a clinical research model in which every facet of involvement with children with disabilities or chronic conditions is carried out in such a way as to advance knowledge of these children and their needs. In practical terms, this translates into systematic documentation of child, treatment, and setting characteristics that can serve as data for analysis and interpretation. It is our belief that careful and systematic clinical practice can and should advance research, just as research can advance clinical practice. Clinical assessment of children with disabilities or chronic conditions in child and adolescent psychology provides unique opportunities for such advances through innovation and experimentation.

REFERENCES

American Psychiatric Association. (1994). *Diagnostic and statistical manual of mental disorders* (4th ed.). Washington, DC: American Psychiatric Association.

Anderson, L. H., Barner, S. L., & Larson, H. J. (1978). Evaluation of written individualized educational programs. *Exceptional Child, 45,* 207–208.

Barlow, D. H., Hayes, S. C., & Nelson, R. O. (1984). *The scientist practitioner.* New York: Pergamon Press.

Baumeister, A. A. (1997). Behavioral research: Boom or bust. In W. E. MacLean, Jr. (Ed.), *Ellis' handbook of mental deficiency, psychological theory and research* (3rd. ed., pp. 3–45). Mahwah, NJ: Erlbaum.

Bjorck-Akesson, E., Granlund, M., & Simeonsson, R. J. (2000). Assessment philosophies and practices in Sweden. In M. J. Guralnick (Ed.), *Interdisciplinary clinical assessment of young children with developmental disabilities.* Baltimore: Brookes.

Brooks, P. H., & Baumeister, A. A. (1977). A plea for consideration of ecological validity in the experimental psychology of mental retardation [Guest editorial] *American Journal of Mental Deficiency, 81,* 407–516.

Burgee, M. L. (1996). A case study analysis of the intervention effect of goal attainment scaling in consultation. *Dissertation Abstracts International, 56*(8–A), 3053. (University Microfilms No. AAM9539616)

Case-Smith, J., & Bryan, T. (1999). The effects of occupational therapy with sensory integration emphasis on preschool-age children with autism. *American Journal of Occupational Therapy, 53,* 489–497.

Eberlin, M., Ibel, S., & Jacobson, J. W. (1994). The source of messages produced during facilitated communication with a boy with autism and severe mental retardation: A case study. *Journal of Pediatric Psychology, 19*(6), 657–671.

Elliott, S. N. (1998). Performance assessment of students' achievement: Research and practice. *Learning Disabilities Research and Practice, 13*(4), 233–241.

Hart, K. E., & Sciutto, M. J., (1996). Criterion-referenced measurement of instructional impact on cognitive outcomes. *Journal of Instructional Psychology, 23*(1), 26–34.

Holroyd, J., & Goldenberg, I. (1978). The use of goal attainment scaling to evaluate a ward treatment program for disturbed children. *Journal of Clinical Psychology, 34,* 729–732.

Joyce, B. M., Rockwood, K., & Mate-Kole, C. (1994). Use of goal attainment scaling in brain injury in a rehabilitation hospital. *American Journal of Physical Medicine and Rehabilitation, 73,* 10–14.

Kazdin, A. E., & Matson, J. L. (1981). Social validation in mental retardation. *Applied Research in Mental Retardation, 2,* 39–53.

Kiresuk, T. J., & Sherman, R. E. (1968). Goal Attainment Scaling: A general method for evaluating comprehensive community mental health programs. *Community Mental Health Journal, 4,* 443–453.

Kirk, R. E. (1996). Practical significance: A concept whose time has come. *Educational and Psychological Measurement, 56,* 746–759.

Luckasson, R., Schalock, R. L., Snell, M. E., & Spitalnik, D. M. (1996). The 1992 AAMR definition and preschool children: Response from the Committee on Terminology and Classification. *Mental Retardation, 34*(4), 247–253.

Maher, C. A. (1979). School psychologists and special education program evaluation: Contributions and considerations. *Psychology in the Schools, 16,* 240–245.

Maher, C. A., & Barbrack, C. R. (1980). A framework for comprehensive evaluation of the individualized education program (IEP). *Learning Disabilities Quarterly, 3,* 49–55.

Maloney, F. P., Mirrett, P., Brooks, C., & Johannes, K. (1978). Use of the goal attainment scale in treatment and ongoing evaluation of neurologically handicapped children. *American Journal of Occupational Therapy, 32,* 505–510.

Mate-Kole, C. C., Danquah, S. A., Twum, M., & Danquah, A. O. (1999). Outcomes of a nonaversive behavior intervention in intellectually impaired individuals using goal attainment scaling. *Nursing Research, 48*(4), 220–225.

Mitchell, T., & Cusick, A. (1998). Evaluation of a client-centered paediatric rehabilitation programme using goal attainment scaling. *Australian Occupational Therapy Journal, 45*(1), 7–17.

Oke, N. J., & Schreibman, L. (1990). Training social initiations to a high-functioning autistic child: Assessment of collateral behavior change and generalization in a case study. *Journal of Autism and Developmental Disorders, 20*(4), 479–497.

Palisano, R. J., Haley, S. M., & Brown, D. A. (1992). Goal attainment scaling as a measure of change in infants with motor delays. *Physical Therapy, 72*(2), 432–437.

Rockwood, K., Joyce, B., & Stolee, P. (1997). Use of goal attainment scaling in measuring clinically important change in cognitive rehabilitation patients. *Journal of Clinical Epidemiology, 50*(5), 581–588.

Shuster, S. K., Fitzgerald, N., Shelton, G., Barber, P., & Desch, S. (1984). Goal attainment scaling with moderately and severely handicapped preschool children. *Journal of the Division for Early Childhood, 8,* 26–37.

Simeonsson, R. J., Bailey, D. B., Huntington, G. S., & Brandon, L. (1991). Scaling and attainment of goals in family-focused early intervention. *Community Mental Health Journal, 27*(1), 77–83.

Simeonsson, R. J., Huntington, G. S., McMillen, J. S., Dodds, A. H., Halperin, D. L, Zipper, I. N., Leskinen, M., & Langmeyer, D. (1996). Evaluating services for young children and families: Documenting intervention cycles. *Infants and Young Children, 9*(2), 31–42.

Simpson, R. L., & Fiedler, C. R. (1989). Parent participation in Individualized Educational Program (IEP) conferences: A case for individualization. In M. J. Fine (Ed.), *The second handbook on parent education: Contemporary perspectives* (pp. 145–171). San Diego, CA: Academic Press.

Stolee, P., Rockwood, K., Fox, R. A., & Streiner, D. L. (1992). The use of goal attainment scaling in a geriatric care setting. *Journal of the American Geriatric Society, 40,* 574–578.

Swallow, R. (1981). Fifty assessment instruments commonly used with blind and partially seeing individuals. *Journal of Visual Impairment and Blindness, 75,* 65–72.

Turnbull, A. P., & Turnbull, H. R. (1990). *Families, professionals, and exceptionality: A special partnership* (2nd ed.). Columbus, OH: Merrill.

Wallin, R., & Koch, M. (1978). The use of goal attainment scaling as a method of evaluating clinical outcome in an inpatient child psychiatry setting. *Journal of the American Academy of Child Psychiatry, 17,* 439–445.

Wells, K. (1987). Scientific issues in the conduct of case studies. *Journal of Child Psychology and Psychiatry, 28*(6), 783–790.

Wolraich, M. L., Felice, M. E., & Drotar, D. (Eds.). (1996). *The classification of child and adolescent mental diagnoses in primary care: Diagnostic and Statistical Manual for Primary Care (DSM-PC)—Child and adolescent version.* Elk Grove Village, IL: Amercian Academy of Pediatrics.

World Health Organization. (1980). *International Classification of Impairments, Disabilities, and Handicaps.* Geneva: Author.

World Health Organization. (1999). *International Classification of Functioning and Disability Beta-2 Draft.* Geneva: Author.

Young, A., & Chesson, R. (1999). Goal attainment scaling as a method of measuring clinical outcome for children with learning disabilities. *British Journal of Occupational Therapy, 60*(3), 111–114.

PART II

General Strategies and Measures

4

QUANTITATIVE ASSESSMENT

RUNE J. SIMEONSSON
CARRIE COOK
SADARRYLE HILL

Angie and Tim are transfer students and have been referred to the school psychologist for an evaluation. The referral information indicates that both were given a WISC-III at the end of the previous school year. Both of their Full Scale IQ scores are 65. Angie's verbal and performance IQ scores are 76 and 58, and Tim's scores are 58 and 76, respectively. An examination of subtest scores reveals that Angie scored the highest on Information, Similarities, and Vocabulary, and she scored lowest on Picture Completion and Object Assembly. Tim scored lowest on Information, Similarities, and Vocabulary and highest on Picture Completion and Object Assembly. Although both children have the same Full Scale IQ score, they present with different profiles and will require different intervention methods. Angie may need further assessment of visual motor functioning and behavior given an abrupt change in her classroom behavior at the end of the previous year following a head injury sustained from a fall while roller blading.

Quantitative measurement constitutes the major approach to assessment of children's abilities and behaviors in school and clinical contexts in order to determine placements and generate individualized interventions for children such as Angie and Tim. Quantitative measurement also serves as the basis for group testing of student achievement and outcome in schools and for identifying the prevalence of health-related conditions and associated risk factors in population surveys. The defining features of quantitative assessment are measurement of child characteristics with reference to derived numeric values against norms. Although the nature of the numeric value may vary considerably (e.g., standard score, percentile), all are interpreted relative to a norm group. The standard for comparison is the performance of a reference group specified by age, gender, and other demographic characteristics representative of a defined population. The quantitative score for a given child is dependent on age and/or population standards for meaningful interpretation. In this regard it stands in contrast to results obtained with ecobehavioral and qualitative strategies, which are not dependent on age for interpretation.

This chapter provides a review of the quantitative approach, with particular emphasis on the clinical assessment of children with disabilities and chronic health conditions. The review is not exhaustive but representative of measures to assess intelligence, communication, and social and behavioral characteristics. As this book focuses on assessment of children with significant problems of health and development, emphasis is placed on measures particularly suited to documenting their needs. Tests widely used with children are covered thoroughly in other sources and are not detailed in this book. To provide an organized approach for this chapter, we review quantitative strategies and measures using a sequential approach to the domains of cognition, communication, personal and social functioning, and behavioral characteristics. Within each of these domains, we identify measures appropriate for major developmental phases from early childhood through adolescence. In addition to reviewing the quantitative approach in assessment of individual children, we provide brief coverage of its use in the clinical epidemiology of disability.

Quantitative measurement in both clinical and population-based assessment has three main purposes. The first is to derive quantitative indices of a child's functioning, performance, and behavior. The derivation of a quantitative index is important in assessment in that the numeric value (such as age equivalents, scale scores, and percentiles) can be used to identify subgroups of children across relevant dimensions. The results of assessment using quantitative measures thus provide information about a child's abilities and characteristics relative to that of a specific peer group and typically indicate the degree to which such values diverge from the average. Second, a profile of such values can be analyzed to assess variability within an individual child. Assessment results of a quantitative nature are also of value in the derivation of profiles, detailing children's strengths and weaknesses relative to themselves and others. Third, quantitative assessment is useful in that inferences and decisions about intervention may depend on precise values. All other things being equal, for example, the difference between standardized scores of 65 and 73 may be essential in making differential decisions about eligibility for educational placements for two children. In clinical epidemiology, quantitative data in the form of frequencies, proportions, and distributions can serve to estimate the prevalence of disability and chronic health conditions in the population.

CLINICAL ASSESSMENT

Issues

Two issues should be considered in the use of quantitative measures in clinical assessment of children with disabilities. The first is of a conceptual nature, dealing with the concept of age equivalence, a feature central to many instruments. A second is methodological and concerns the comparability of instruments with similar labels.

Age Equivalence

Age equivalents for psychological (cognition, communication) and other developmental characteristics (weight, head circumference) are common in psychometric measurement. These values represent the mean age of a reference group for a particular structure (skeletal age, dental age) or function (mental age, language age, reading age). A 48-month-old child with hypothyroidism, for example, may be described as having a skeletal age of 36 months based on norms of physical development. In another domain, the language abilities of a 5-year-old child with Down syndrome may be described as being at the 18-month level based on norms of cognitive development.

Although the meaning of such descriptions seems clear, several problems are inherent in the use of age equivalents. First, age-equivalent descriptions may lead to generalizations about overall functioning, so that an older (5-year-old) child who functions at a lower level

(18 months) in one domain is assumed to be like an 18-month-old in other domains as well. The 5-year-old is, in fact, different from 18-month-olds physically, physiologically, and experientially, resembling an 18-month-old only in the performance of language tasks. A second problem arises from using an age-equivalent value as a single summary index. The cognitive functioning of a 2-year-old child with autism, for example, may be described as being at a 10-month level. Although it indicates a developmental lag, it fails to reflect the variability of functioning. Such variability may range from failures in some cognitive tasks at 8 months through selected successes up to 19 months.

A third problem has to do with the underlying concept of equivalence of age. The derivation of mental, social, or reading ages is based on a child's performance on tests of intelligence, social maturity, and reading, respectively. When performance is assessed repeatedly over time, differences have been calculated from one time to the next in age equivalents. Such difference scores of age equivalents should not be used as an index of progress relative to a specified period of intervention in that *months of intervention* is a temporal variable, whereas *months of mental-age change* is simply an index derived from a particular measure expressing change in test performance (Simeonsson, 1982). Although the use of age equivalents makes it easy to summarize and communicate test performance, a direct correspondence of test ages to chronological ages should not be assumed. Finally, identical test ages derived from different tests should not be assumed to be identical. The point here is not that such identical test ages lack correlation in some way but rather that the test ages do not reflect absolute similarity simply because they are both expressed in identical age values.

Comparability of Measures

A methodological issue in the use of quantitative measures concerns labeling and comparability of instruments. The labels of instruments sometimes describe the domain they represent, but sometimes they do not. Instruments identified as tests of intelligence may vary widely in their content—for example, from a restricted sampling of one aspect of intelligence (receptive vocabulary), as in the Columbia Mental Maturity Scale (Burgemeister, Blum, & Lorge, 1972) to a differentiated measurement of specific subscales, as in the Wechsler Intelligence Scale for Children—Third Edition (WISC–III; Wechsler, 1991). Tests with similar labels may also differ in the comprehensiveness with which a particular domain is assessed.

We need to identify some practical problems here because they pertain to instruments in common use. Choice of instruments can make a difference in terms of measured performance if there is age overlap of measures. A comparison of Wechsler Adult Intelligence Scale—Revised (WAIS-R; Wechsler, 1981) and WISC-III scores for a group of 16-year-old youths (Thompson & Sota, 1998) revealed that mean scores, variances, and covariances were equal but that subtest scores generally were not equal. Rubin, Goldman, and Rosenfeld (1990) found that WAIS-R scores were consistently higher than WISC-R scores among persons with mental retardation who were between 8 and 26 years of age.

Studies comparing results of different versions of the same test indicate that different versions may tend to provide different scores (Sapp, Abbott, Hinkley, & Rowell, 1997). Slater and Saarnio (1995) found WISC-III Full Scale, Verbal, and Performance IQ scores to be 7.2, 5.8, and 7.5 points lower, respectively, than WISC-R scores in a sample including children with specific learning disorders, children with mental retardation, and children with no disabilities. Additionally, WISC-III scores of children with an EMD (educable mentally disabled) classification may be expected to show a downward trend over a period of three years, as well as a substantial variation in subtest scores (Bolen, 1998).

Comparisons of scores for different intelligence tests have provided varying results (Lavin, 1996; Thorndike, Hagen, & Sattler, 1986). Rust and Lindstrom (1996) did not find mean differences between the WISC-III and the Stanford–Binet—Fourth Edition (SB-IV) to be significant, but differences for some children were substantial. In a group of children between 11 and 17 years of age identified as having mild mental retardation, SB-IV scores were found to be higher than WISC-III scores for 29 of the 31 students (Lukens & Hurrell, 1996). Studies with other children and adults have also demonstrated higher SB-IV scores compared with Wechsler scores (Prewett & Matavich, 1994; Spruill, 1991).

A final practical issue pertains to the fact that similar measures may not be comparable in terms of the entry demands they make on children. In an examination of this issue, Kaufman (1978) found that instruments measuring similar abilities differed dramatically in their demand characteristics. Drawing on the idea of basic concepts essential to understanding test instructions, Kaufman compared the Stanford–Binet, the Wechsler Preschool and Primary Scale of Intelligence (WPPSI), the Illinois Test of Psycholinguistic Abilities (ITPA), and the McCarthy Scales of Children's Abilities (MSCA). The results indicated that the WPPSI required the greatest number (14) of basic concepts in order to understand instructions. The MCSA and the Stanford–Binet required 7 and 5 basic concepts, respectively, and the ITPA required none. An important practical implication of these findings is that the underlying skills required by tests must be examined in order to identify any mediating role those demands may have on child performance.

We have given illustrations of practical problems associated with specific instruments that are reflective of general concerns to be kept in mind when using any quantitative measure. In selecting, administering, and interpreting quantitative measures, a clinician must carefully consider what actually is assessed by a particular instrument, as opposed to the similarity of its label or score with those of other instruments.

Measures

The number of quantitative measures is large, with a particular concentration in the broad area of tests of intellectual abilities. The measures vary widely not only in their sophistication and comprehensiveness but also in their level of acceptance and frequency of use by practitioners.

This chapter identifies and describes a select number of applicable instruments that can be used with children with disabilities. Descriptions of the relevant features of these instruments and their relative assets and liabilities should facilitate the selection of measures appropriate for a particular assessment need.

Cognition

Measures designed to assess cognition and communication frequently overlap, making a distinction between the two domains difficult. A number of measures, particularly those focusing on communication in terms of receptive vocabulary, are often used as substitute measures for intellectual functioning. The distinction between cognition and communication is also blurred in regard to psychological versus developmental assessment in infancy because these two domains are highly intercorrelated, with communication being a strong predictor of intelligence. This chapter therefore includes measures primarily identified as developmental or cognitive but which may also be defined as measures of communication. As a developmental sequence, grouped by broad age categories, measures for assessment in infancy (0–2 years) are covered in Chapter 9. The review here focuses on early childhood (3–5 years), middle childhood (6–10 years), and adolescence (13+ years). Measures that cover more than one developmental phase are assigned to the earliest category for which they are appropriate.

EARLY CHILDHOOD

As is evident in Table 4.1, a variety of measures exist that are suitable for assessing cognition in preschool children. Although several measures have been developed specifically for this age group, many also extend through childhood and adolescence. Furthermore, some measures focus on a very specific function of cognitive ability, whereas others encompass intelligence as more broadly defined.

Boehm's Test of Basic Concepts—Revised (BTBC-R; Boehm, 1986) is a measure that focuses on a specific ability in preschool children, namely, the child's knowledge of basic concepts essential for school readiness. As we have previously mentioned, Kaufman (1978) has shown that some standard psychological instruments for early childhood assume the presence of a number of these basic concepts in children. The value of administering the Test of Basic Concepts to children with disabilities is twofold: (1) An inventory can be made of a child's basic concepts as a measure of cognitive and language ability for its own sake, and (2) the inventory can be used as the basis of determining the appropriateness of administering other measures with known requirements of knowledge of basic concepts. Children whose knowledge of basic concepts is found to be deficient either can be administered measures not requiring those concepts or can be trained in those concepts prior to administration of the test. A downward extension of BTBC for prekindergarten children has been developed and normed on disadvantaged children by Levin, Henderson, Levin, and Hoffer (1975). This modification may be useful to consider as a criterion-referenced measure with low-functioning children. Furthermore, another interesting aspect of measurement in this area is that the Test of Basic Concepts is also available in braille form (Tactile Test of Basic Concepts) for children with visual impairment (Catin, 1975), permitting comparable assessment with this population.

The Miller Assessment for Preschoolers (MAP; Miller, 1982) was developed to measure sensory and motor abilities of children 2½–5½ years of age. A positive feature is the systematic assessment of nine behaviors during testing in the areas of attention, social interaction, and sensory reactivity.

Of the measures designed to assess broadly defined intellectual functioning, five of those listed in Table 4.1 cover only some part of the early childhood period, whereas the other four extend into adolescence or adult levels. The Merrill–Palmer Scales of Mental Development (MPSMD; Stutsman, 1948, 1981) is a dated scale but continues to be used in clinical assessment of children with disabilities (see Chapter 11) when an intermediate instrument is needed between the Bayley Scales of Infant Development (BSID; Bayley, 1993) and such more demanding tests as the Wechsler Preschool and Primary Scale of Intelligence—Revised (WPPSI-R; Wechsler, 1989). A unique feature of the Merrill–Palmer Scales is the inclusion of the Seguin formboard, a task with a long history as a measure of perceptual–motor coordination and spatial reasoning. The WPPSI-R is a well-known measure that shares the conceptual and empirical tradition of the other Wechsler scales and provides the option of full administration of selected subscales. Concerns about prerequisite concepts (Kaufman, 1978) are important to consider in terms of its applicability with young children with disabilities. The McCarthy Scales of Children's Abilities (1972) does cover a substantial age range, incorporates a separate motor scale, and yields a profile of abilities. The McCarthy Scales of

TABLE 4.1. Selected Psychometric Measures of Cognition: Early Childhood

Measure	Age	Format of results	Psychometric properties	Representative applications with children with disabilities
Miller Assessment for Preschoolers (Miller, 1982)	2 yr, 4 mo–5 yr, 8 mo	Standardized scores; overall, neurological foundations, sensory motor coordination, verbal cognitive abilities, nonverbal abilities, complex task abilities	Interrater reliability of core items $r = .98$ (Banus, 1983)	Preschool children with perceptual or language problems (Banus, 1983)
Merrill–Palmer Scales of Mental Development (Stutsman, 1948, 1981)	24–63 mo	IQ scores	Correlation with Stanford–Binet: $r = .89$ and .83 (Magrab et al., 1976)	Young children with Down syndrome (Berry, Gunn, & Andrews, 1984)
McCarthy Scales of Children's Abilities (McCarthy, 1972)	2 yr, 5 mo–8 yr, 5 mo	General cognitive index: 5 T scores; verbal perceptual performance, quantitative, memory, motor	Internal consistency $r = .69$ to .93. Test–retest $r = .69$ to .90 (Nagle, 1979)	Children with neurological impairment (Moore & Burns, 1979)
Coloured Progressive Matrices (Raven, 1991b)	5–11 yr	Percentile scores	Information not found	Children with hearing impairment (Carlson & Dillon, 1978)
Differential Ability Scales (Elliott, 1990)	2½–17 yr	Measure of general intelligence with 17 subtests and a General Conceptual Ability score.	Internal consistency reliability coefficients range from .88 to .92 (cluster scores) to .95 (GCA). Test–retest reliability coefficients range from .83 to .90 (clusters scores) to .93 (GCA).	Children with hearing impairment (Riccio et al., 1997); children who are blind (Hull & Mason, 1995)
Wechsler Preschool and Primary Scale of Intelligence—Revised (WPPSI-R; Wechsler, 1989)	3 yr–7 yr, 3 mo	Intelligence Quotients (IQ) including Full-Scale, Verbal, and Performance IQ are deviation scores with a mean of 100 and SD of 15. Subtest scores are scaled scores with a mean of 10 and SD of 3.	Split-half reliability coefficients for IQ scores range from .86 to .98. IQ score test–retest reliability coefficients range from .88 to .95.	Children with mild mental retardation (Lukens & Hurrell, 1996; Rubin, Goldman, & Rosenfeld, 1990); autism and developmental disorders (Siegel, Minshew, & Goldstein, 1996)

Instrument	Age range	Description	Reliability	Populations studied
Test of Nonverbal Intelligence—Third Edition (TONI-3; Brown, Sherbenou, & Johnsen, 1997)	5–85 years	A nonverbal measure of problem-solving ability with percentile ranks and standard scores (TONI Quotients) with a mean of 100 and SD of 15 provided.	Internal consistency coefficients .90, test–retest reliability .86.	Children with mental retardation (Brown, Sherbenou, & Dollar, 1982); children with autism (Edelson, Schubert, & Edelson, 1998)
Stanford–Binet Intelligence Test—Fourth Edition (SB-IV; Thorndike, Hagen, & Sattler, 1986)	2–23 years	An overall composite score of general intelligence and four area scores (each with mean of 100 and SD of 16) measuring verbal reasoning, quantitative reasoning, abstract/visual reasoning, and short-term memory. Subtest scores are converted to standard age scores.	Composite score internal consistency ratings range from .95 to .99; stability ratings range from .90 to .91.	Children with mental retardation (Lukens & Hurrell, 1996), Williams syndrome (Greer, Brown, Pai, Choudry, & Klein, 1997)
Boehm's Test of Basic Concepts—Revised (BTBC-R; Boehm, 1971, 1986)	Kindergarten—second grade	Measure of knowledge of basic concepts in terms of percentile rank for the total score.	Alternate-form reliability range .65 to .82. Test–retest stability range .55 to .88.	

Children's Abilities may be suitable as an alternate measure to the Stanford–Binet and the WPPSI-R or the WISC-III for children within the 2- to 8-year range. A factor that should be considered in the use of the McCarthy Scales is that the profiles may vary substantially in test–retest situations (Rolfe & Bryant, 1979), thus restricting profile interpretation. Concurrent validity of the General Cognitive Index (GCI) with established IQ tests suggests a lack of comparability (Nagle & Lazarus, 1979).

The Test of Nonverbal Intelligence—Third Edition (TONI-3; Brown, Sherbenou, & Johnsen, 1997) is a language-free measure of intellectual skills suitable for participants ranging from 5 to 86 years of age. It can be administered individually or in a small-group format (fewer than five people) and requires only a pointing response. Instructions are pantomimed, making it appropriate for any child or adult with communication impairment. The TONI-3 is designed to yield a nonverbal IQ with a mean of 100 and a standard deviation of 15. The recent norms make this an especially useful tool. Previous versions have been used in populations with mental retardation, learning disabilities, autism, and dyslexia. The TONI-3 has lowered the ceiling and obtained a new standardization sample. The reliability and validity of the test has remained the same as the TONI-2, and research conducted with TONI-2 is applicable to the TONI-3. The Pictorial Test of Intelligence (PTI; French, 1964) is another nonverbal measure covering the early childhood period. Although dated, the PTI has six subtests, and because it does not require a verbal response, it is particularly appropriate for children with motor and/or speech impairments (Neisworth & Bagnato, 1987).

The Differential Ability Scales (DAS; Elliott, 1990) is a measure of cognitive ability that has been used with children with hearing impairment, specific language impairment, and developmental delays (Riccio, Ross, Boan, Jemison, & Houston, 1997) and with at-risk preschoolers (McIntosh & Gridlay, 1993). Standard scores as low as 25 can be derived, which is of relevance to assessment of children with severe limitations. Additionally, the Speed of Information Processing Scale has been successfully converted into tactile form for use with school children who are blind (Hull & Mason, 1995).

An asset of the Leiter International Performance Scale—Revised (LIPS-R; Leiter, 1953; Roid & Miller, 1997) and the Slosson Intelligence Test—Revised (SIT-R; Nicholson & Hibpshman, 1990) is that cognitive abilities of individuals can be measured across the lifespan, yielding data from repeated assessments. A limitation of the measures, however, is the fact that they tend to be highly verbal in nature, restricting their utility with populations who typically have verbal deficits. The LIPS and the Arthur Adaptation of the LIPS (AALIPS; Arthur, 1949), for children 3–8 years of age, bypass this problem by means of a nonverbal, culture-fair format of assessment. The LIPS and the AALIPS have been of considerable use in the assessment of children with auditory impairments. The concurrent validity of these measures with the Stanford–Binet and the Wechsler scales has been respectable (generally in the .70 range). Scores on the LIPS and AALIPS are likely to be lower than on the Stanford–Binet and Wechsler, and caution should be exercised in the use of such scores for placement decisions (Ratcliffe & Ratcliffe, 1979, 1980). A further caution has been raised by Johnston (1982) in regard to the nature of the LIPS scores for children under 8 years of age. On the basis of research with children with language impairments, she concluded that LIPS scores for children in this age group may represent primarily perceptual rather than conceptual ability.

The Coloured Progressive Matrices (CPM; Raven, 1991b) is one of a series of nonverbal measures of reasoning. Tasks, in the form of matching and analogies, are presented in a series of progressively more difficult plates, with pointing being a sufficient response. The nonverbal nature of the CPM has made its use popular with children and adults with disabilities.

The Kaufman Assessment Battery for Children (K-ABC; Kaufman & Kaufman, 1983) is a measure of intelligence and achievement for children from 2½ to 12½ years of age. The normative data for the K-ABC is based on a stratified sample and includes representative minority and exceptional populations. In addition to subtest scores for mental processing and achievement, four global-scale scores are available summarizing information processing and achievement. The K-ABC has been validated with various subgroups of children with disabilities, and the availability of a nonverbal scale increases its utility for this population.

MIDDLE CHILDHOOD

The most widely used instrument for assessing intelligence of school-age children is the WISC-III (Wechsler, 1991). It is used extensively to diagnose cognitive disabilities (such as mental retardation and learning disabilities) in special education. It also provides a profile for interpreting student strengths and deficits. It should be noted, however, that WISC-III scores and those of the Stanford–Binet are likely to be quite discrepant, as shown in a study by Bloom, Reese, Altshuler, Meckler, and Raskin (1983) with children with mental retardation and learning disabilities. Caution should be exercised when comparing scores from these two instruments. Given the demand in schools and other settings for formal intelligence testing for placement and reevaluation of status of children with disabilities, it is likely that the WISC-III will continue to be used with high frequency among measures for school-age populations (Table 4.2). In reference to the reevaluation issue, Kennedy and Elder (1982) proposed that an abbreviated version of the WISC-R could be used as a cost-effective strategy. Their research with 400 children, ages 6 to 16, indicated that a short form of five subtests (Information, Block Design, Comprehension, Picture Arrangement, Coding) resulted in a multiple $R = .95$ and a standard error of estimate of 4.0. Although Kennedy and Elder's findings are constrained by the characteristics of their sample, abbreviated versions seem appropriate to consider to meet efficiently the reevaluation demands associated with providing services to students with disabilities.

Raven's Progressive Matrices (RPM; Raven, 1991a) is similar to the CPM and is a nonverbal measure of intelligence suitable for older children and adults. The RPM was designed as a nonverbal measure of intelligence and is frequently used with children whose auditory or motor impairments limit verbal comprehension and/or responding and in cross-cultural studies (Aboud, Samuel, Hadera, & Addus, 1991). Its nonverbal nature has contributed to its use with deaf adolescents (Blennerhassett, Strohmeier, & Hibbett, 1994). Carver (1989) used the RPM in a study measuring intellectual growth and decline. Brown and McMullen (1982) reported an innovation in the administration of the RPM to children with motor impairment. Vanderheiden and Grilley (1976) described a special device (ETRAN-N) that requires only simple eye movement responses, rather than pointing.

The Bender–Gestalt Test (BGT; Koppitz, 1964) is an established nonverbal tool that has been variously used as a quantitative measure of cognitive development, of neurological impairment, and of emotional disturbance. The response format of the BGT involves reproduction of designs by the child. The BGT has been used extensively with children with various disabilities. Although the BGT can be scored reliably, clinicians need to exercise caution in specific interpretations. The test may best be used to supplement other assessment data.

ADOLESCENCE

A number of the measures in Table 4.2 are also applicable for assessment of populations of adolescents or adults with disabilities. The Wechsler Adult Intelligence Scale—Third

TABLE 4.2. Selected Psychometric Measures of Cognition: Middle Childhood and Adolescence

Measure	Age	Format of results	Psychometric properties	Representative applications with children with disabilities
Progressive Matrices (Raven, 1991a)	Standard: 6 yr–adult; Advanced: 11 yr–adult	Percentile scores	Information not found	Hearing impaired children (Ritter, 1976)
Wechsler Intelligence Scales for Children—Third Edition (WISC-III; Wechsler, 1991) Wechsler Adult Intelligence—Third Edition (WAIS-III; Wechsler, 1997).	6½ yr–adult	Intelligence Quotients (IQ) including Full-Scale, Verbal, and Performance IQ are deviation scores with a mean of 100 and SD of 15. Subtest scores are scaled scores with a mean of 10 and SD of 3.	Split-half reliability coefficients for IQ scores range from .86 to .98. IQ score test–retest reliability coefficients range from .88 to .95.	Children with mild mental retardation (Lukens & Hurrell, 1996; Rubin, Goldman, & Rosenfeld, 1990), autism and developmental disorders (Siegel, Minshew, & Goldstein, 1996)
Bender–Gestalt Test (Koppitz, 1964)	5–10 yr	Developmental error score; emotionality measures; brain damage indicators	Koppitz score interrater reliability V = .92–.95 (Hustak et al., 1976); Quick-scoring system r = .95–.98 (Pauker, 1976)	Children with epilepsy and mental retardation (Tymchuk, 1974)
Test of Nonverbal Intelligence—Third Edition (TONI-3; Brown, Sherbenou, & Johnsen, 1997)	5–85 yr	A nonverbal measure of problem-solving ability with percentile ranks and standard scores (TONI Quotients) with a mean of 100 and SD of 15 provided.	Internal consistency coefficients .90, test–retest reliability .86.	Individuals with mental retardation (Brown, Sherbenou, & Dollar, 1982)
Stanford–Binet Intelligence Test—Fourth Edition (Thorndike, Hagen, & Sattler, 1986)	2–23 yr	An overall composite score of general intelligence and four area scores (each with mean of 100 and SD of 16) measuring verbal reasoning, quantitative reasoning, abstract/visual reasoning, and short-term memory. Subtest scores are converted to standard age scores.	Composite score internal consistency ratings range from .95 to .99; stability ratings range from .90 to .91.	Children with mental retardation (Lukens & Hurrell, 1996), Williams syndrome (Greer, Brown, Pai, Choudry, & Klein, 1997)

62

Edition (WAIS-III; Wechsler, 1997) is similar in conceptual and statistical properties to the Wechsler scales for younger participants. Although the WAIS-III is certainly a preferred instrument for use in assessing adolescents and adults, its demand characteristics may limit its utility with individuals who have severe mental retardation or with individuals whose sensory or motor impairments restrict their ability to respond. Furthermore, a factor to be considered in the use of any of the Wechsler scales with children with disabilities is the issue of deriving a scale score for a raw score of zero or for scaled scores based on very few responses. The clinician should therefore consult the respective manuals to determine the circumstances under which it is appropriate or inappropriate to compute a subscale score.

Communication

As noted earlier, the distinction among quantitative measures of intelligence, cognition, and communication has been blurred, with the result that the uses of the measures often overlap. This section reviews those measures that appear to focus primarily on expressive or receptive communication. These measures are presented in summary form in Table 4.3. Most of the measures focus on the early childhood period, although some extend into the period of adolescence and adulthood. It should be noted that the measures considered here have a functional focus, addressing the child's use of communication. Measures of the structural elements of speech, such as articulation, are thus not included for review here. We recognize that children with disabilities often have significant speech problems, but these difficulties are assessed by speech and language specialists (Ritterman, Zook-Herman, Carlson, & Kinde, 1982).

A communication measure often used with infants and young children is the Receptive and Expressive Emergent Language Scale—2 (REEL-2; Bzoch & League, 1991). The separate determination of expressive and receptive communication functioning makes the REEL-2 an appropriate measure to document change in language development of young children in early intervention programs.

The Test of Language Development—Primary, Third Edition (TOLD-P3; Newcomer & Hammill, 1997b) is a norm-referenced measure of communicative competence in expressive and receptive language for 4- to 8-year-old children. Its seven subtest scores are converted to language ages, percentiles, and standard scores (M = 10, SD = 3). Six composite scores (M = 100, SD = 15) are derived from subtest groupings. The TOLD-P3 appears adequate for identifying children who may have language disorders. The Test of Language Development—Intermediate, Third Edition (TOLD-I3; Newcomer & Hammill, 1997a) is available for children between 8½ and 11 years of age. It contains six subtests and five composites with the same scoring system as the TOLD-P3. The TOLD's five subtests—picture vocabulary, oral vocabulary, grammatical understanding, sentence imitation, and grammatical completion—provide a basis for determining the component patterns of a child's language skills. Although the TOLD seems applicable to children with disabilities in general, its appropriateness for minority children (both with and without disabilities) whose primary language is not standard American English has been questioned (Wiener, Lewnau, & Erway, 1983).

The Comprehensive Receptive and Expressive Vocabulary Test (CREVT; Wallace & Hammill, 1994) is a norm-referenced measure combining both receptive and expressive language in one test. It yields standard scores with a mean of 100 and SD of 15 for two subtests (Expressive Vocabulary and Receptive Vocabulary) and a composite score (General Vocabulary). The manual includes reliability data for children with learning disabilities, speech–language disabilities, and mental retardation.

TABLE 4.3. Selected Measures of Communication: Early Childhood

Measure	Age	Format of results	Psychometric properties	Representative applications with children with disabilities
Receptive Expressive Emergent Language Scale—2 (Bzoch & League, 1971, 1991)	Birth–3 yr	Three scores: expressive, receptive, combined	Correlation of REEL with Bayley Developmental age .49 and .54; Uzgiris Hunt subscales range .01–.46 (Mahoney, 1984)	Children with PKU (Melnick et al., 1981)
Test of Language Development—Primary, Third Edition (TOLD-P3; Newcomer & Hammill, 1997b)	4 yr, 0 mo–8 yr, 11 mo	Six composites of language development converted from subtest scores (language ages, based on mean performances) percentiles; standard scores ($M = 10$, $SD = 3$). Composite scores are converted to a standard score ($M = 100$, $SD = 15$)	Information not found	Children with specific language impairment (Leonard, 1995); children with brain injury (Jordan et al., 1995)
Peabody Picture Vocabulary Test—Third Edition (Dunn, 1981; Dunn & Dunn, 1997)	2½–40 yr	Standard score and age equivalents; percentile ranks stanines	PPVT-R Split-half reliability, $r = .81$–.84; alternate form reliability .77–.79 (Taylor, 1984)	Educable mentally disabled students (Bracken & Prasse, 1981)
Columbia Mental Maturity Scale (Burgemeister et al., 1972)	3½–10 yr	Percentile ranks; standard score maturity index	Internal consistency $r = .85$–.91; Test–retest range .84–.86	Children with Down syndrome (Henderson et al., 1981)
Expressive One-Word Picture Vocabulary Test (Gardner, 1979, 1990)	2–12 yr	MA, deviation IQ; percentile ranks; stanines	Split-half reliability $r = .87$–.96, validity with PPVT $r = .67$–.78 (Moran, 1983)	Mildly retarded children (Goldstein et al., 1982)
Comprehensive Receptive and Expressive Vocabulary Test (CREVT; Wallace & Hammill, 1994)	4–17 yr	Measure of expressive and receptive vocabulary and general vocabulary standard scores ($M = 100$, $SD = 15$)	Internal reliability .80–.90; test–retest reliability .79–.94	

The assessment of communication beyond the early childhood period has typically taken the form of receptive vocabulary tests covering the span from 2 years of age to adult level. Among the most common measures is the Peabody Picture Vocabulary Test—Third Edition (PPVT-III; Dunn & Dunn, 1997). The Columbia Mental Maturity Scale (CMMS; Burgemeister et al., 1972) is an older measure that may still be used on a selective basis. Both of these measures are nonverbal in nature and yield mental age and IQ indices derived from the participant's comprehension of verbal items. Their concurrent validity with established tests of intelligence has generally been quite good, a fact that has sometimes resulted in their use as substitutes for intelligence tests. These measures provide an estimate of general intelligence, but given their limited scope and format they should not be used as substitutes for comprehensive intelligence measures. The simple, nonverbal format, however, has lent itself to specific adaptations for difficult-to-test children. Levy (1982) administered a standard and a cut-up version of the PPVT to 3- and 4-year-olds without disabilities and to 5- and 7-year-old children with autism, to allow responses other than pointing. This modification resulted in significant improvement of performance among the children with autism but made no difference for children without disabilities. The recency of normative data is important to consider in the use of these measures, given cultural and societal changes. Choong and McMahon (1983), for example, have shown that PPVT scores for a sample of preschool children were significantly higher and more discrepant from chronological age than scores from the revised version (PPVT-R; Dunn & Dunn, 1981).

Although the receptive side of communication has been the major focus of assessment of communication, some measures examine its expressive aspects. The Expressive One-Word Picture Vocabulary Test, 2000 Edition (EOWPVT; Gardner, 1990) is a measure designed to assess expressive vocabulary in children from 2 to 11 years of age. The presentation format is similar to that of the PPVT, the difference being that the child defines the pictorial stimulus verbally. The EOWPVT may be useful as a culturally sensitive measure in that it can also be administered to children whose primary language is Spanish. The use of the EOPWVT in combination with a receptive vocabulary measure may provide an analysis of the total communication skills of children ranging from 2 through 12 years of age, much as the REEL-2 provides similar information for children under 2 years of age.

Personal and Social Functioning

Assessment of personal and/or social characteristics of children with disabilities is an important area. It presents significant challenges in that personality inventories and other forms of assessment may not be appropriate to use with children with disabilities because of verbal response requirements and assumptions about cognitive processes of introspection and projection. If cognitive ability and communication skills are at a level appropriate for the child to serve as a respondent, the use of selected projective techniques may be indicated for some children with disabilities. Some personality measures may be suitable for use with children with disabilities, and personality assessment has been carried out with children with chronic illness and other subgroups. Given the verbal nature of many measures, however, applications with young children and/or children with severe impairments is questionable. Thus any assessment and interpretation of personality functioning in children with disabilities should be undertaken with caution in light of the nature of task assumptions and demands.

If we take a broader approach to personal and social development, however, there are measures that cover a wide developmental range and either have response requirements within the repertoire of many children with disabilities or bypass the child as respondent.

A selected number of these measures are summarized in Table 4.4 according to the major developmental categories defined in this chapter.

EARLY CHILDHOOD

For children with disabilities in the early childhood range, the Behavioral Style Questionnaire (BSQ; McDevitt & Carey, 1978) provides a means of assessing temperament. Four temperament measures have been developed by Carey and his colleagues with each similar in format and content, making it possible to assess the temperament of children repeatedly across different developmental periods. The significance of assessing temperament in young children with disabilities is that it can provide a profile of real or perceived personal characteristics of importance to parents and other caregivers. Values exceeding a standard deviation from the mean in specified directions are interpreted as reflective of significant temperament variability and can be used to derive the diagnostic clusters of *easy, difficult,* and *slow-to-warm-up,* as shown in Figure 4.1.

The Temperament and Atypical Behavior Scale (TABS; Neisworth, Bagnato, Salvia, & Hunt, 1999) is a screening and assessment instrument evaluating dimensions of temperament related to regulatory disorders. It was designed to be compatible with the DC:0–3 (Zero To Three, 1994) classification of infant and early childhood behavior. The four empirical factors of temperament evaluated are related to detached, underreactive, hypersensitive/active, and dysregulated behavioral patterns. Scores have been compared and normed using children without disabilities. Children with raw scores of 5 to 9 are considered to be at risk of aytpical temperament for that factor. Raw scores greater than 10 in any temperamental dimension are considered indicative of atypical temperamental or self-regulation development. The BSQ and TABS provide tools to document individual differences in behavior and their mediating role on the performance and functioning of young children with disabilities and chronic conditions.

The area of social competence has been the focus of assessment for many years. Defining what social competence actually is has been problematic in the fields of child development and developmental disabilities (Simeonsson, 1978). Social competence has often been equated with social maturity and self-help skills, as represented by one of the original measures in this area, the Vineland Social Maturity Scale (VSMS; Doll, 1953). It has been revised as the Vineland Adaptive Behavior Scales (VABS; Sparrow, Balla, & Cicchetti, 1984) and was normed in conjunction with the K-ABC (1983). The Cain–Levine Social Competence Scale is a social competence measure standardized on a population of children with moderate mental retardation (Cain, Levine, & Elzey, 1977). It is a measure with high test–retest reliability and thus may be particularly appropriate in the assessment of children with moderate mental retardation. One of the more interesting measures of social competence is the Children's Adaptive Behavior Scale (CABS; Richmond & Kicklighter, 1980), designed for children between the ages of 5 and 10 years. The CABS was normed on a population of 250 children with mild retardation. The CABS is unique in that it is one of the few measures of social competence that is administered directly to the child rather than deriving the information from the perceptions of a third-party respondent such as parent or teacher. An issue to remember with both the Cain–Levine and the CABS is that, because the standardization samples consist of children with disabilities, generalization of results should be made accordingly. Another self concept measure, described by Stager and Young (1982), was designed for children between 4 and 9 years of age. An attractive feature of this Preschool and Primary Self-Concept Scale (PPCS) is that it includes both verbal and pictorial stimuli in a semantic differential format.

TABLE 4.4. Selected Personal and Social Measures

Measure	Age	Format of results	Psychometric properties	Representative applications with children with disabilities
Behavioral Style Questionnaire (McDevitt & Carey, 1978)	3–7 yr	Rating on 9 temperament dimensions	Test–retest reliability $r = .89$, Alpha reliability $r = .84$ (McDevitt & Carey, 1978)	Children with minimal brain dysfunction, hyperactivity, learning or emotional problems (Carey et al., 1979)
Vineland Adaptive Behavior Scales (Sparrow et al., 1984)	Birth–adult	Various derived scores; 4 domains, 11 subdomains	Median internal consistency across three forms and domains $r = .80–.98$	Standardization samples include populations with disabilities
Cain–Levine Social Competence Scale (Cain et al., 1977)	5–14 years	Five scores; self-help, initiative, social skills, communication, total	Internal consistency, total score $r = .75–.89$; test–retest total score $r = .98$	Children with moderate and severe retardation ages 7–13 (Meador & Richmond, 1980)
Children's Adaptive Behavior Scale (Richmond & Kicklighter, 1980)	5–10 years	Six scores: language, independent functioning, family role performance, economic–vocational activity, socialization, total (Richmond & Horn, 1980)	CABS domain scores correlated with WISC-R FS IQ $r = .42–.51$	Standardization sample includes children with mild mental retardation
Preschool and Primary Self-Concept Scale (Stager & Young, 1982)	4–9 years	Seven scales: happy–sad; strong–weak; good–bad; big–small; liked–not liked; fast–slow; busy–not busy	Test–retest for subsample 55% to 79%	Potential applicability with children with disabilities

	High activity	Arrhythmic	Withdrawal	Slow adaptation	Intense	Negative mood	Low persistence	Low distractibility	Low threshold
6									
5		Diff ↑	SWU Diff ↑	SWU Diff ↑	Diff ↑	SWU Diff ↑			
4									
3		Easy →	Easy →	Easy →	Easy →	Easy →			
2					SWU →				
1	SWU →								
	Low Activity	Rhythmic	Approach	Very Adaptive	Mild	Positive Mood	High Persistence	High Distractibility	High Threshold

FIGURE 4.1. Defining diagnostic clusters of temperament traits (Easy; Diff, difficult; SWU, slow-to-warm-up).

MIDDLE CHILDHOOD AND ADOLESCENCE

The Middle Childhood Temperament Questionnaire is based on the same approach as the BSQ and is designed for children between 8 and 12 years of age. It also involves caregiver responses and demonstrates satisfactory reliability (Hegvik, McDevitt, & Carey, 1982). Gunn and Cuskelly (1991) used this measure to examine the temperament of children between the ages of 8 and 24 with Down syndrome. Schor (1986) utilized this measure to examine the temperament of children with phenylketonuria (PKU).

Locus of control is a widely used measure of personal and social characteristics of children. The Nowicki–Strickland Locus of Control Scale for Children (NSLCS; Nowicki & Strickland, 1973) consists of 40 statements that can be administered orally or in writing and that require only a yes or no response; it is therefore quite easy to administer to children with disabilities. It has been applied with various subgroups of children with special needs (Tolor, Tolor, & Blumin, 1977). A preschool version is also available (Nowicki & Duke, 1974). The Piers–Harris Self-Concept Scale (PHSCS; Piers & Harris, 1969) is another measure that has been widely used with children with and without disabilities. The format of the PHSCS consists of 90 statements, to which the child expresses agreement or disagreement. With children who may lack reading ability, it may be useful to follow the strategy described by Ottenbacher (1981). Scale items were changed from the first person to the second person and read aloud to a group of children and young adults with mental retardation. The constructs measured by the PHSCS have been verified by Wolf, Sklov, Hunter, Webber, and Berenson (1982), who found that factor analysis yielded seven factors amenable to interpretation for research and clinical purposes. The wide age range covered (10–17) and the biracial composition of the sample in this study supports the utility of the PHSCS as a measure of personal functioning.

The locus-of-control construct has been extended to encompass Children's Perceptions of Social Interactions (LOC-CPSI; Dahlquist & Ottinger, 1983). The LOC-CPSI was found to correlate with established measures of locus of control and to predict peer status. The self-appraisal of peer interactions would seem to be an assessment goal of substantial interest as it pertains to children with disabilities, particularly those in mainstreamed settings. The Children's Health Locus of Control Scale (CHLC; Parcel & Meyer, 1978) has been found to have stable reliabilities in a 4-year study of school children across the fourth to sixth grades (O'Brien, Bush, & Parcel, 1989) and particular utility in assessing health beliefs of children with chronic health conditions.

Behavioral Characteristics

The distinction between assessment of social or personal functioning on the one hand and behavior on the other may seem to be arbitrary when an analysis is made of what is observed or rated. This chapter distinguishes between measures that focus on overt behavior and those that focus on traits and characteristics. Most of the measures, as shown in Table 4.5, are based on information derived from observations or ratings of a child's behavior made by others, such as caregivers or teachers.

The systematic assessment of behavior in early childhood has been an area of considerable productivity, as evidenced from the representative measures shown in Table 4.5. A major factor contributing to assessment of behavioral functioning in preschool children is the interest in predicting children who are at risk for behavior problems on entry into school

TABLE 4.5. Selected Psychometric Measures of Behavior

Measure	Age	Format of results	Psychometric properties	Representative applications with children with disabilities
Child Behavior Checklist (Achenbach, 1992)	2–18 years	Emotional and behavioral problems classified in internalizing and externalizing dimensions, as well as 9 syndrome scales	Internalizing and externalizing composites; mean test–retest reliability range .79–.92; mean internal consistency .88–.92.	Children and adolescents with Prader–Willis syndrome (Dykeson et al., 1992; van Lieshout et al., 1998;); children with hearing impairments (Mitchell & Quittner, 1996; Vostanis et al., 1997); children with autism (Boelte, Dickhut, & Poustka, 1999); children with chronic illness (Daltroy et al., 1992; Holmes et al., 1998; Noll et al., 1997).
Behavior Assessment System for Children (Reynolds & Kamphaus, 1992)	4–18 years	14 scales and 5 composites reported in percentile ranks and standard scores (M = 50, SD = 10).	Internal consistency mean .82–.90; test–retest reliability .70–.91.	Children with acute lymphocytic leukemia (Shelby et al., 1998); Children with ADHD (Ostrander et al., 1998; Vaughn et al., 1997)
Devereux Behavior Rating Scales—School Form (DCBS-SF; Naglieri, LeBuffe, & Pfeiffer, 1993) and Devereux Scales of Mental Disorders (DSMD; Naglieri, LeBuffe, & Pfeiffer, 1994)	5–18 years	DCBS-SF gives 4 scales with standard scores (M = 10, SD = 3) and percentile ranks. DSMD gives 6 scales, 3 composites, and a total scale reported in T scores (M = 50, SD = 10) and percentile ranks.	DCBS-SF internal consistencies .83–.94. DSMD total scale internal reliability, .97–.98; composite internal reliability .88–.98.	Children with learning disorders and emotional problems (Naglieri & Gottling, 1995); children with serious emotional disturbance (Gimpel & Nagle, 1996, 1999).
Temperament and Atypical Behavior Scale: Early Childhood Indicators of Developmental Dysfunction (Neisworth, Bagnato, Salvia, & Hunt, 1999)	1–5 years	Four factors of temperament, reported with T scores (M = 50 and SD = 10) and percentile ranks (M = 100 and SD = 15).	Internal consistency using split-half reliability for total of all four factors .88–.95; stability .80–.90.	

(Earls et al., 1982; Harper & Richman, 1979). Some of the measures have focused on a specific age group; others have encompassed a broad age range extending into later childhood and adolescence. The Behavioral Screening Questionnaire (BSCQ; Richman & Graham, 1971), developed for 3-year-old children, has been evaluated in a concurrent validation study by Earls and colleagues (1982). The 12-item BSCQ was found adequate for predicting behavioral adjustment of preschool children. A particularly attractive feature of this study, of potential relevance for work with children with disabilities, is a rating procedure for clinical data in terms of the severity, need for intervention, and prognosis of the behavior problem.

The Behavior Problem Checklist (BPC; Quay & Peterson, 1967) is a teacher-rating scale that has been widely used with school-age children (see Table 4.5). The Revised Behavior Problem Checklist (RBPC; Quay & Peterson, 1987) added 89 new items to strengthen its psychometric properties. Additionally, a Spanish translation is also available that can be used to assess Hispanic children and adolescents (Rio, Quay, Santisteban, & Szapocznik, 1989).

In addition to the RBPC, several other measures of behavior are suitable for use with preschool and school-age children. The multiple forms of the Child Behavior Checklist (CBCL) currently available include the CBCL/2–3 parent report form for ages 2 to 3 (Achenbach, 1992), CBCL/4–18 parent report form for ages 4 to 18 (Achenbach, 1991a), Teacher's Report Form (TRF) for ages 5 to 18 (Achenbach, 1991b), and Youth Self-Report (YSR) for ages 11 to 18 (Achenbach, 1991c). These measures produce a profile of syndrome scales, two broad scales (Internalizing and Externalizing) and a Total Problem score. The normative age groups, reported by gender, permit the derivation of the child's overall behavior profile. The CBCL assesses a child's problem behaviors and competence through items concerning extracurricular activities, social interactions, and school functioning. Applications of the CBCL have been reported for clinical samples referred for mental health services. The CBCL is a well-researched assessment tool and has been widely used with children with multiple disorders and/or impairments (Boelte, Dickhut, & Poustka, 1999; Daltroy et al., 1992; Mitchell & Quittner, 1996; van Lieshout, de Meyer, Curfs, Koot, & Fryns, 1998). The Behavior Assessment System for Children (BASC; Reynolds & Kamphaus, 1992) is a norm-referenced, comprehensive, multimethod, multidimensional assessment system of behavioral problems, emotional disorders, and personality constructs in children from 4 to 18 years of age. Its five forms include a self-report scale, a parent rating scale, a teacher rating scale, a structured developmental history, and a form for recording observed classroom behavior. The manual presents score profiles of clinical groups, including children and adolescents with mental retardation and autism. Advantages of this system are computerized scoring programs and relative speed of completing the forms. A Spanish-language version of the parent rating form is also available. Although this system is psychometrically sound and comprehensive in its use in general, more research using this system in populations with developmental and/or physical disabilities is needed to determine its appropriateness within these populations.

Interest in symptomatic behavior of latency-age children (8–12 years) led to the development and revisions of behavior rating scales at Devereux schools, including the Devereux Behavior Rating Scales—School Form (DCBS-SF; Naglieri, LeBuffe, & Pfeiffer, 1993) and the Devereux Scales of Mental Disorders (DSMD; Naglieri, LeBuffe, & Pfeiffer, 1994). These forms are completed by individuals who know the child on a personal basis. The DCBS-SF was designed for use by teachers to measure behavior problems of children in the context of school. The child and adolescent versions of this form contain four scales, including Interpersonal Problems, Inappropriate Behaviors/Feelings, Depression, and Physical Symptoms/Fears. The DSMD is designed to be completed by a parent or other person who is responsible for caring for the child or adolescent. The DSMD is structured to provide standard scores for a Total scale; three composite scores, including Externalizing, Internalizing, and Critical Pathology composites; and six scales consisting of the Conduct, Attention/Delinquency, Anxiety, Depression, Autism, and Acute Problems scales. The availability of these measures of child behavior that draw on a common conceptual framework can be of value with children with disabilities when longitudinal assessment of problem behavior is desired from early childhood through adolescence.

CLINICAL EPIDEMIOLOGY

Most of this book is devoted to concepts and practices of clinical assessment of individual children with disabilities or chronic conditions. However, we can also approach the assessment of children's characteristics and functional limitations through surveys to estimate the nature and extent of needs for services and supports at a population level. The scientist/practitioner model provides a framework for advancing assessment of children's development and behavior in two ways. One is based on clinical practice with individual children, the other is the use of measures in large-scale efforts to build a science of assessment. There are several elements in the development of a science of assessment. Major goals on behalf of children with disabilities and chronic conditions are not only to address identified intervention needs but also to implement efforts to promote their health and well-being at the population level. Documenting the epidemiology of disability is central to a comprehensive population-based approach. Although health promotion is usually viewed within the public health domain, interventions to prevent or reduce consequences associated with disability should be part of a more inclusive effort that encompasses health, education, and social services sectors. Recognizing the broader role of social and psychological factors that influence children with disabilities and chronic conditions, it would be appropriate to build on elements of psychosocial and psychiatric epidemiology (Kelsey, Whittemore, Evans, & Douglas-Thompson, 1996). The focus of psychosocial epidemiology is on social and psychological factors that contribute to disease and illness. In psychiatric epidemiology, the focus is on defining aspects of mental and psychological conditions. Both of these elements are relevant to building a clinical epidemiology of disability.

The challenges researchers face in psychosocial and psychiatric epidemiology are the same as those they face in developing an epidemiology of disability, namely, what are the phenomena of interest and how should they be measured? To this end at least two key issues should be considered: defining the scope of documentation and specifying variables for measurement.

In regard to the scope of documentation, a major priority is to identify existing surveillance efforts at national and state levels to determine data that are available and data that have to be collected to document parameters of childhood disability and chronic conditions. The National Health Interview Survey (NHIS) and the Disability Supplement (NHIS-D) are administered as household surveys and provide a rich source of primary data on functional status and limitations. Analyses of this data source have been used to generate estimates of functional limitations in the U.S. population of children between 5 and 17 years of age (Hogan, Msall, Rogers, & Avery, 1997). Findings for four functional areas revealed limitations of learning ability to be the most common (10.6%), followed by communication (5.5%), mobility (1.3%), and self-care (0.9%), in descending order. Other applications have provided population estimates for the nature and impact of health-related conditions such as asthma (Newacheck & Halfon, 2000), injury (Danseco, Miller, & Spicer, 2000), and mental health (Halfon & Newacheck, 1999) for children and youth in the United States. In addition to the NHIS/NHIS-D, a number of other national surveys provide data for secondary analyses, including the National Household Education Survey conducted by the Department of Education and the Youth Risk Behavior Survey coordinated by the Centers for Disease Control. Although these two are of particular relevance for studies of children and youth, coverage related to functional limitations and disability in these and other measures is often limited. To this end, a priority is to include indicators related to disability in future administrations of these and other surveys to derive estimates of functional limitations of children in the performance of major life activities in home, school, and community contexts.

A second consideration in clinical epidemiology is specifying variables of interest for measurement. The value of population-based surveys is that results can be generalized to the population; however, items defining the content may not always provide sufficient scope or detail related to a particular domain or application. Hack (1999), for example, has commented on the fact that the global nature of available national surveys and other questionnaires may not be sufficiently sensitive to evaluate the quality of neonatal intensive care and measure outcomes of children. Interesting applications have attempted to enhance the utility of the NHIS-D and other measures by imposing specific definitions as a framework for analyzing available data. To this end, Stein and Silver (1999) analyzed the 1994 Health Interview Survey by applying a conceptually based noncategorical definition of children with chronic conditions and coding for three conceptual domains. These domains were (1) functional limitations, (2) reliance on compensatory devices, and (3) the use or need of services beyond routine care for age. Results revealed that 14.8% of the children had chronic conditions, with 7% meeting criteria in one domain, 5.2% in two domains, and 2.6% across all three domains. In a somewhat similar effort, Newacheck and Halfon (1998) applied a new definition of children with special health care needs to the 1994 NHIS-D. This definition estimated that 18% of the population had a chronic condition of a physical, developmental, behavioral, or emotional nature that required health and related services beyond those typically required by children. These and other applications illustrate that definitional modifications can enhance the utility of national surveys in exploring specific policy and research questions. In more specific applications, surveys can focus on populations identified on the basis of general or specific conditions. The National Longitudinal Transition Study (Blackorby & Wagner, 1996) for example, provides a comprehensive view of the postschool outcomes of students with disabilities. Studies of this nature, utilizing national sampling strategies, are needed to complement experimental and clinical research studies on childhood disability that have restricted generalizability.

To complement national surveys, information is needed on the prevalence of disability, chronic health conditions, and associated problems at local, regional, or state levels. In this regard, surveillance could focus on secondary conditions of impairments and health conditions (Lollar, 1994; Simeonsson & Leskinen, 1999) and factors associated with differential vulnerability in subgroups defined by age, gender, or other indicators. Differential vulnerability can be defined in terms of risk factors and resilience that characterize some individuals and not others and can be documented from prospective cohort studies or retrospective analyses of available data. Knowledge of differential vulnerability provides the basis for targeting prevention efforts for specific subgroups, taking into account the dynamic nature of interactions with the environment. A key consideration in this regard is documentation of the elements of "risk chains" (Simeonsson, 1994) that can identify specific points in development in which prevention efforts are likely to be more effective and efficient than others. The impact of such efforts, encompassing the removal of risk factors or enhancing access and support, should be documented in order to address concerns about generalizability of effects and accountability. Documentation of intervention effectiveness at the level of the individual has been described in Chapter 3. At a population level, surveillance methods may document changes in incidence or prevalence by tracking conditions over time, reflecting the relative impact of prevention or intervention efforts. With the commitment to more comprehensive approaches, impacts should be evident not only in the changes in the targeted condition but also in the promotion of health, sense of well-being, and quality of life for children and youth with disabilities and chronic health conditions.

RECOMMENDATIONS FOR PRACTICE

In concluding this chapter, we reemphasize that the measures reviewed are a selected subset of a much larger pool of measures. The measures selected for consideration are included because of their demonstrated or potential applicability for use with children with disabilities and chronic health conditions. Within this group of measures, the appropriateness or suitability of particular instruments will vary as a function of the assessment focus and examiner preference. In Table 4.6, we have identified a limited set of measures that may be useful across children with varying disabilities.

Two elements should frame the integration and reporting of quantitative assessment data. First, all available quantitative indices should be presented in describing a child's performance. Even though a given performance can be reported by a single index, such as a deviation IQ score, other values should be reported as well to facilitate interpretation of the results. In addition to age and grade equivalents and percentile rank, it is particularly important to describe the range encompassing the first failure and the last success. Although it can be argued that most of the indices only reflect different elements of the same finding, presenting them in several ways emphasizes different aspects of the child's performance and makes the psychological report more complete. A second consideration is to identify and reference any qualifications or limitations that pertain to the assessment process and results obtained. This is particularly important in regard to children with disabilities, because adaptations and modifications may apply to procedures, as well as to derived values. If needed, the rationale for such modifications should be provided in a brief documentation that includes citations of applicable clinical or research studies. Such documentation serves to insure that findings will be interpreted and applied with an appreciation of the particular issues involved in assessing a child with disabilities. Some guidelines for summarizing and interpreting quantitative test results are summarized in Table 4.7.

In the area of interpretation, we must give a word of caution concerning occasions on which measures designed for infants and young children are used with older children or adults with severe disabilities whose level of functioning is within the range of such measures.

1. In general, reference to performance level in terms of age equivalents should be avoided in favor of criterion-referenced descriptions. Describing the performance of an adolescent with a cup and a spoon as reflecting a functional understanding of basic utensils is preferable to describing it as the equivalent of a mental age of 16 months. Such a description emphasizes actual skills rather than an inferred level

TABLE 4.6. Recommended Psychometric Measures by Domain and Functional Level of Child

Cognition	Communication	Personal/social	Behavior
		Early childhood	
Kaufman-ABC WPPSI-III Differential Abilities Scale Leiter Colored Progressive Matrices	PPVT-III TOLD-P3	Behavior Styles Questionnaire Vineland Adaptive Behavior Scales Locus of Control (Preschool)	Child Behavior Checklist Revised Behavior Problem Checklist Behavior Assessment System for Children
		Middle childhood	
WISC-III Standard Progressive Matrices	PPVT-III Expressive One-Word Picture Vocabulary Test	Piers–Harris Self-Concept Scale Nowicki–Strickland Locus of Control Scale Middle Childhood Temperament Questionnaire	Child Behavior Checklist Revised Behavior Problem Checklist Behavior Assessment System for Children
		Adolescence	
WAIS-III Advanced Progressive Matrices	PPVT-III Columbus Mental Maturity Scale		Child Behavior Checklist Revised Behavior Problem Checklist Behavior Assessment System for Children

TABLE 4.7. Recommendations for Summarizing and Interpreting Assessment Results Obtained with Psychometric Measures

Issue	Recommendation	Purpose
1. Quantitative indices to document performance	1. Report all available indices; age/grade equivalents, standardized scores, percentiles, range of first failure to last success.	1. To document nature, range, and variability of performance.
2. Factors qualifying assessment/interpretation.	2. Identify (a) modifications of materials and procedures, (b) relevant child limitations/idiosyncracies, and (c) possible alternate interpretations of assessment findings.	2. To insure that conclusions drawn about child's performance or characteristics are adequately qualified.
3. Concepts of age- or grade-equivalent performance.	3. Describe/interpret results in terms of task demand and functional performance.	3. To insure that conclusions about child performance and functioning are based on considerations of relative (age-equivalent) as well as absolute (task-specific) features.

of ability. Functional descriptions also reduce the likelihood that a person's overall performance will be generalized to a level of 16 months, whereas the range of performance may actually be substantial.

2. Whenever possible, present assessment findings in a profile form, reflecting areas of relative abilities and limitations.
3. In interpreting performance, clinicians should recognize that a particular skill may have a different meaning when observed in an older child or in an adult with a disability than in a young child without a disability. In early development, a skill such as reaching may be a temporary precursor for the more sophisticated skill of pointing, whereas in an adult with profound mental retardation it may be a firmly established, permanent skill.

Quantitative measures have constituted a major approach in the assessment of children with disabilities and chronic health conditions. Limitations inherent in some children (such as sensory or motor impairment), in tests (such as timed tasks), and in standardization data (such as exclusion of persons with disabilities in the norm group) have previously precluded or reduced the use of quantitative measures with children with disabilities. Adapted approaches and measures and improved procedures are likely to increase the appropriateness of quantitative assessment. The norm-referenced basis of the quantitative approach in clinical assessment and in clinical epidemiology is uniquely suited to provide information pertaining to the comparative performance within and across populations that is not inherent in the other approaches reviewed in this book. As such, the selection of the quantitative approach is indicated when its use complements other approaches in documenting the characteristics and needs of children with disabilities.

REFERENCES

Aboud, F., Samuel, M., Hadera, A., & Addus, A. (1991). Intellectual, social and nutritional status of children in an Ethiopian orphanage. *Social Science and Medicine, 33*(11), 1275–1280.

Achenbach, T. M. (1991a). *Manual for the Child Behavior Checklist/4–18 years and 1991 Profile.* Burlington: University of Vermont, Department of Psychiatry.

Achenbach, T. M. (1991b). *Manual for the Teacher's Report Form and 1991 Profile.* Burlington: University of Vermont, Department of Psychiatry.

Achenbach, T. M. (1991c). *Manual for the Youth Self-Report Form and 1991 Profile.* Burlington: University of Vermont, Department of Psychiatry.

Achenbach, T. M. (1992). *Child Behavior Checklist/2–3 Years (CBCL/2–3).* Burlington: University of Vermont, Department of Psychiatry.

Arthur, G. (1949). The Arthur Adaptation of the Leiter International Performance Scales. *Journal of Clinical Psychology, 5,* 345–349.

Banus, B. J. (1983). The Miller Assessment for Preschoolers (MAP): An introduction and review. *American Journal of Occupational Therapy, 37,* 333–340.

Bayley, N. (1993). *Bayley Scales of Infant Development (BSID).* San Antonio, TX: Psychological Corporation.

Berry, P., Gunn, P., & Andrews, R. J. (1984). The behavior of Down's syndrome children using the "Lock Box": A research note. *Journal of Child Psychology and Psychiatry, 25,* 125–131.

Blackorby, J., & Wagner, M. (1996). Longitudinal post school outcomes of youth with disabilities: Findings from the National Longitudinal Transition Study. *Exceptional Children, 62,* 399–413.

Blennerhassett, L., Strohmeier, S. J., & Hibbett, C. (1994). Criterion-related validity of Raven's Progressive Matrices with deaf residential school students. *American Annals of the Deaf, 139,* 104–110.

Bloom, A. S., Reese, A., Altshuler, L., Meckler, C. L., & Raskin, L. M. (1983). IQ discrepancies between the Binet and WISC-R in children with developmental problems. *Journal of Clinical Psychology, 39,* 600–603.

Boehm, A. E. (1971). *Boehm's Test of Basic Concepts*. New York: Psychological Corporation.

Boehm, A. E. (1986). *Boehm's Test of Basic Concepts—Revised*. San Antonio, TX: Psychological Corporation.

Boelte, S., Dickhut, H., & Poustka, F. (1999). Patterns of parent-reported problems indicative in autism. *Psychopathology, 32*(2), 93–97.

Bolen, L. M. (1998). WISC-III score changes for EMH students. *Psychology in the Schools, 35*(4), 327–332.

Bracken, B., & Prasse, D. (1981). Comparison of the PPVT, PPVT-R, and intelligence tests used for placement of black, white and Hispanic EMR students. *Journal of School Psychology, 19*, 304–311.

Brown, L., Sherbenou, R. J., & Dollar, S. J. (1982). *Test of Nonverbal Intelligence*. Austin, TX: Pro-Ed.

Brown, L., Sherbenou, R., & Johnsen, S. (1997). *Test of Nonverbal Intelligence—3*. Austin, TX: Pro-Ed.

Brown, R. J., & McMullen, P. (1982). An unbiased response mode for assessing intellectual ability in normal and physically disabled children. *Clinical Neuropsychology, 4*, 51–56.

Burgemeister, B., Blum, L., & Lorge, I. (1972). *Columbia Mental Maturity Scale*. New York: Harcourt Brace Jovanovich.

Bzoch, K. R., & League, R. (1971). *Receptive and Expressive Emergent Language Scale*. East Aurora, NY: Slosson Educational Publications.

Bzoch, K. R., & League, R. (1991). *Receptive and Expressive Emergent Language Scale—2*. East Aurora, NY: Slosson Educational Publications.

Cain, L. F., Levine, S., & Elzey, F. F. (1977). *Manual for the Cain Levine Social Competency Scale*. Palo Alto, CA: Consulting Psychologists Press.

Carey, W. B., McDevitt, S. C., & Baker, D. (1979). Differentiating minimal brain dysfunction and temperament. *Developmental Medicine and Child Neurology, 21*, 765–772.

Carlson, J. S., & Dillon, R. (1978). Measuring intellectual capabilities of hearing impaired children: Effects of testing the limits procedures. *Volta Review, 80*, 216–224.

Carver, R. P. (1989). Measuring intellectual growth and decline. *Psychological Assessment, 1*(3), 175–180.

Catin, H. R. (1975). *The development and evaluation of a tactile analog to the Boehm Test of Basic Concepts*. Unpublished doctoral dissertation, University of Kentucky, Lexington.

Choong, J., & McMahon, J. (1983). Comparison of scores obtained on the PPVT and the PPVT—R. *Journal of Speech and Hearing Disorders, 48*, 40–43.

Dahlquist, L. M., & Ottinger, D. R. (1983). Locus of control and peer status: A scale for children's perceptions of social interactions. *Journal of Personality Assessment, 47*, 278–287.

Daltroy, L. H., Larson, M. G., Eaton, H. M., Partridge, A. J., Pless, J. B., Rogers, M. P., & Liang, M. H. (1992). Psychosocial adjustment in juvenile arthritis. *Journal of Pediatric Psychology, 17*(3), 277–289.

Danseco, E. R., Miller, T. R., & Spicer, R. S. (2000). Incidence and costs of 1987–1994 childhood injuries: Demographic breakdown. *Pediatrics, 105*(2), E27.

Doll, E. A. (1953). *The measurement of social competence: A manual for the Vineland Social Maturity Scale*. Minneapolis, MN: Educational Test Bureau.

Dunn, L. M., & Dunn, L. M. (1981). *Manual for the Peabody Picture Vocabulary Test—Revised*. Circle Pines, MN: American Guidance Service.

Dunn, L. M., & Dunn, L. M. (1997). *Manual for the Peabody Picture Vocabulary Test—Third Edition*. Circle Pines, MN: American Guidance Service.

Dykeson, E. M., Hodapp, R. M., Walsh, K., & Nash, L. J. (1992). Adaptive and maladaptive behavior in Prader-Willi syndrome. *Journal of the American Academy of Child and Adolescent Psychiatry, 31*(6), 1131–1136.

Earls, F., Jacobs, G., Goldfin, D., Silbert, A., Beardslee, W., & Rivinus, T. (1982). Concurrent validation of a behavior problems scale to use with 3-year-olds. *Journal of the American Academy of Child Psychiatry, 21*, 47–57.

Edelson, M. G., Schubert, D. T., & Edelson, S. M. (1998). Factors predicting intelligence scores on the TONI in individuals with autism. *Focus on Autism and Other Developmental Disabilities, 13*(1), 17–26.

Elliott, C. (1990). *Differential Ability Scales*. San Antonio, TX: Psychological Corporation.

French, J. L. (1964). *Manual: Pictorial Test of Intelligence*. Boston: Houghton Mifflin.

Gardner, M. F. (1979). *Expressive One-Word Picture Vocabulary Test.* Novato, CA: Academic Therapy.

Gardner, M. F. (1990). *Expressive One-Word Picture Vocabulary Test.* Wood Dale, IL: Stoelting.

Gimpel, G. A., & Nagle, R. J. (1996). Factorial validity of the Devereux Behavior Rating Scale–School Form. *Journal of Psychoeducational Assessment, 14*(4), 334–348.

Gimpel, G. A., & Nagle, R. J. (1999). Psychometric properties of the Devereux Scales of Mental Disorders. *Journal of Psychoeducational Assessment, 17*(2), 127–144.

Goldstein, D. J., Allen, C. M., & Fleming, L. P. (1982). Relationship between the Expressive One-Word Picture Vocabulary Test and measures of intelligence, receptive vocabulary, and visual motor coordination in borderline and mildly retarded children. *Psychology in the Schools, 19,* 315–318.

Greer, M. K., Brown, F. R., Pai, G. S., Choudry, S. H., & Klein, A. J. (1997). Cognitive, adaptive, and behavioral characteristics of Williams syndrome. *American Journal of Medical Genetics, 74*(5), 521–525.

Gunn, P., & Cuskelly, M. (1991). Down syndrome temperament: The stereotype at middle childhood and adolescence. *International Journal of Disability, Development and Education, 38,* 59–70.

Hack, M. (1999). Consideration of the use of health status, functional outcome, and quality-of-life to monitor neonatal intensive care practice. *Pediatrics, 103*(1, Suppl. E), 319–328.

Halfon, N., & Newacheck, P. W. (1999). Prevalence and impact of parent-reported disabling mental health conditions among U.S. children. *Journal of American Academy of Child and Adolescent Psychiatry, 38*(5), 600–609.

Harper, D. C., & Richman, L. C. (1979). Preschool screening for behavior problems. *Psychology in the Schools, 16,* 38–42.

Hegvik, R. L., McDevitt, S. C., & Carey, W. B. (1982). The Middle Childhood Temperament Questionnaire. *Journal of Developmental and Behavioral Pediatrics, 3,* 197–200.

Henderson, S. E., Morris, J., & Frith, V. (1981). The motor deficit in Down's syndrome children: A problem of timing. *Journal of Child Psychology and Psychiatry Allied Disciplines, 77,* 426–430.

Hogan, D. P., Msall, M. E., Rogers, M. L., & Avery, R. C. (1997). Improved disability population estimates of functional limitation among American children aged 5–17. *Journal of Maternal and Child Health, 1*(4), 203–216.

Holmes, C. S., Respess, D., Greer, T., & Frentz, J. (1998) Behavior problems in children with diabetes: Disentangling possible scoring confounds on the Child Behavior Checklist. *Journal of Pediatric Psychology, 23*(3), 179–185.

Hull, T., & Mason, H. (1995). The conversion of a psychometric test for use with the blind. *Association of Educational Psychologists Journal, 10*(4), 220–224.

Hustak, T. L., Dinning, W. D., & Andert, T. N. (1976). Reliability of the Koppitz scoring system for the Bender–Gestalt Test. *Journal of Clinical Psychology, 32,* 468–469.

Johnston, J. R. (1982). Interpreting the Leiter IQ: Performance profiles of young normal and language disturbed children. *Journal of Speech and Hearing Research, 25,* 291–296.

Jordan, F. M., Murdoch, B. E., Buttsworth, D. L., & Hudson-Tennent, L. J. (1995). Speech and language performance of brain-injured children. *Aphasiology, 9,* 23–32.

Kaufman, A. S. (1978). The importance of basic concepts in the individual assessment of preschool children. *Journal of School Psychology, 16,* 207–211.

Kaufman, A. S., & Kaufman, N. L. (1983). *Kaufman assessment battery for children.* Circle Pines, MN: American Guidance Services.

Kelsey, J. L., Whittemore, A. S., Evans, A. S., & Douglas-Thompson, W. (1996). *Method in observational epidemiology.* New York: Oxford University Press.

Kennedy, L. P., & Elder, S. T. (1982). WISC-R: An abbreviated version. *Journal of Clinical Psychology, 38,* 174–178.

Koppitz, E. M. (1964). *The Bender–Gestalt Test for Young Children.* New York: Grune & Stratton.

Lavin, C. (1996). The Wechsler Intelligence Scale for Children—Third Edition and the Stanford–Binet—Fourth Edition: A preliminary study of validity. *Psychological Reports, 78*(2), 491–496.

Leiter, R. G. (1953). Part II of the manual for the 1948 revision of the Leiter International Performance Scale. *Psychological Service Center Journal, 4,* 259–343.

Leonard, L. B. (1995). Functional categories in the grammars of children with specific language impairment. *Journal of Speech and Hearing Research, 38,* 1270–1283.

Levin, G. R., Henderson, B., Levin, A. M., & Hoffer, G. L. (1975). Measuring knowledge of basic concepts by disadvantaged preschoolers. *Psychology in the Schools, 12,* 132–139.

Levy, S. (1982). Use of the Peabody Picture Vocabulary Test with low-functioning autistic children. *Psychology in the Schools, 19*(1), 24–27.

Lollar, D. J. (1994). *Preventing secondary conditions associated with spina bifida or cerebral palsy: Proceedings and recommendations of a symposium.* Washington, DC: Spina Bifida Association of America.

Lukens, J., & Hurrell, R. M. (1996). A comparison of the Stanford–Binet IV and the WISC-III with mildly retarded children. *Psychology in the Schools, 33*(1), 24–27.

Magrab, P. R., Burg, C. S., & Scribanu, N. (1976). Stability and comparability of intellectual measures for cerebral palsied children. *Physical Therapy, 56,* 553–558.

Mahoney, G. (1984). The validity of the Receptive-Expressive Emergent Language Scale with mentally retarded children. *Journal of the Division for Early Childhood, 9,* 86–94.

McCarthy, D. (1972). *Manual for the McCarthy Scales of Children's Abilities.* New York: Psychological Corporation.

McDevitt, S. C., & Carey, W. B. (1978). Measurement of temperament in 3- to 7-year-old children. *Journal of Child Psychology and Psychiatry, 19,* 245–253.

McIntosh, D. E., & Gridlay, B. E. (1993). Differential Ability Scales: Profiles of learning disabled subtypes. *Psychology in the Schools, 30,* 11–24.

Meador, D. J., & Richmond, B. O. (1980). Adaptive behavior: Teachers and parents disagree. *Exceptional Children, 46,* 386–389.

Melnick, C. R., Michals, K. K., & Matalon, R. (1981). Linguistic development of children with phenylketonuria and normal intelligence. *Journal of Pediatrics, 98,* 269–272.

Miller, L. J. (1982). *Miller Assessment for Preschoolers Manual.* Littleton, CO: Foundation for Knowledge in Development.

Mitchell, T. V., & Quittner, A. L. (1996). Multimethod study of attention and behavior problems in hearing-impaired children. *Journal of Clinical Child Psychology, 25*(1), 83–96.

Moore, C. L., & Burns, W. J. (1979). The performance of neurologically impaired and normal S's on four screening techniques. *Journal of Clinical Psychology, 35,* 420–424.

Moran, M. P. (1983). Test review: Expressive One-Word Picture Vocabulary Test. *Clinical Neuropsychology, 5,* 7–8.

Nagle, R. J. (1979). The McCarthy Scales of Children's Abilities: Research implications for the assessment of young children. *School Psychology Digest, 8,* 319–326.

Nagle, R. J., & Lazarus, S. C. (1979). The comparability of the WISC-R and WAIS among 16-year-old EMR children. *Journal of School Psychology, 17,* 362–367.

Naglieri, J. A., & Gottling, S. H. (1995). Use of the Teacher Report Form and the Devereux Behavior Rating Scale—School Form with learning disordered/emotionally disordered students. *Journal of Clinical Child Psychology, 24*(1), 71–76.

Naglieri, J. A., LeBuffe, P. A., & Pfeiffer, S. I. (1993). *Devereux Behavior Rating Scales—School Form.* New York: Psychological Corporation.

Naglieri, J. A., LeBuffe, P. A., & Pfeiffer, S. I. (1994). *Devereux Scales of Mental Disorders Manual.* San Antonio, TX: Psychological Corporation.

Neisworth, J. T. & Bagnato, S. J. (1987). Developmental retardation. In V. B. Van Hasselt & M. Hersen (Eds.), *Psychological evaluation of the developmentally and physically disabled* (pp. 179–212). New York: Plenum Press.

Neisworth, J. T., Bagnato, S. J., Salvia, J., & Hunt, F. M. (1999). *TABS Manual for the Temperament and Atypical Behavior Scale: Early childhood indicators of developmental dysfunction.* Baltimore: Brookes.

Newacheck, P. W., & Halfon, N. (1998). Prevalence and impact of disabling chronic conditions in childhood. *American Journal of Public Health, 88*(4), 610–617.

Newacheck, P. W., & Halfon, N. (2000). Prevalence, impact, and trends in childhood disability due to asthma. *Archives of Pediatrics and Adolescent Medicine, 154*(3), 287–293.

Newcomer, P. L., & Hammill, D. D. (1997a). *The Test of Language Development, Intermediate, Third Edition.* Austin, TX: Pro-Ed.

Newcomer, P. L., & Hammill, D. D. (1997b). *Test of Language Development—Primary, Third Edition.* Austin, TX: Pro-Ed.

Nicholson, C. L., & Hibpshman, T. H. (1990). *Slosson Intelligence Test—Revised.* East Aurora, NY: Slosson Educational Publications.

Noll, R. B., MacLean, W. E., Jr., Whitt, J. K., Kaleita, T. A., Stehbens, J. A., Waskerwitz, M. J.,

Ruymann, F. B., & Hammond, G. D. (1997). Behavioral adjustment and social functioning of long-term survivors of childhood leukemia: Parent and teacher reports. *Journal of Pediatric Psychology, 22*(6), 827–841.

Nowicki, S., & Duke, M. P. (1974). A locus of control scale for college as well as noncollege adults. *Journal of Personality Assessment, 38*, 136–137.

Nowicki, S., & Strickland, B. R. (1973). A locus of control scale for children. *Journal of Consulting and Clinical Psychology, 40*(1), 148–154.

O'Brien, R. W., Bush, P. J., & Parcel, G. S. (1989). Stability in a measure of children's health locus of control. *Journal of School Health, 59*(4), 161–164.

Ostrander, R., Weinfurt, K. P., Yarnold, P. R., & August, G. J. (1998). Diagnosing attention deficit disorders with the Behavioral Assessment System for Children and the Child Behavior Checklist: Test and construct validity analyses using optimal discriminant classification trees. *Journal of Consulting and Clinical Psychology, 66*(4), 660–672.

Ottenbacher, K. (1981). An investigation of self conceptual body image in the mentally retarded. *Journal of Clinical Psychology, 37*, 415–418.

Parcel, G. S., & Meyer, M. P. (1978). Development of an instrument to measure children's health locus of control. *Health Education Monograph, 6*(2), 149–159.

Pauker, J. D. (1976). A quick scoring system for the Bender–Gestalt: Inter-rater reliability and scoring validity. *Journal of Clinical Psychology, 32*, 86–89.

Piers, E., & Harris, D. (1969). *Manual for the Piers–Harris Children's Self-Concept Scale.* Nashville, TN: Counselor Recordings and Tests.

Prewett, P. N., & Matavich, M. A. (1994). A comparison of referred students' performance on the WISC-III and the Stanford–Binet Intelligence Scale—Fourth Edition. *Journal of Psychoeducational Assessment, 12*(1), 42–48.

Quay, H. C., & Peterson, D. R. (1967). *Manual for the Behavior Problem Checklist.* Champaign, IL: Children's Research Center.

Quay, H. C., & Peterson, D. R. (1987). *Manual for the Revised Behavior Problem Checklist.* Champaign, IL: Children's Research Center.

Ratcliffe, K. J., & Ratcliffe, M. W. (1979). The Leiter Scales: A review of the validity of findings. *American Annals of the Deaf, 124*, 38–45.

Ratcliffe, M. W., & Ratcliffe, K. J. (1980). A comparison of the Wechsler Intelligence Scale for Children—Revised and Leiter International Performance Scale for a group of educationally handicapped adolescents. *Journal of Clinical Psychology, 36*, 310–312.

Raven, J. C. (1991a). *Progressive Matrices.* New York: Psychological Corporation.

Raven, J. C. (1991b). *Coloured Progressive Matrices.* London: Lewis.

Reynolds, C. R., & Kamphaus, R. W. (1992). *BASC: Behavior Assessment System for Children: Manual.* Circle Pines, MN: American Guidance Service.

Riccio, C. A., Ross, C. M., Boan, C. H., Jemison, S., & Houston, F. (1997). Use of the Differential Ability Scales (DAS) Special Nonverbal Composite among young children with linguistic differences. *Journal of Psychoeducational Assessment, 15*(3), 196–204.

Richman, N., & Graham, P. (1971). A behavioral screening questionnaire for use with three-year-old children: Preliminary findings. *Journal of Child Psychology and Psychiatry, 12*, 5–33.

Richmond, B. O., & Horn, W. R. (1980). Children's Adaptive Behavior Scale: A new measure of adaptive functioning. *Psychology in the Schools, 17*, 159–162.

Richmond, B. O., & Kicklighter, R. H. (1980). *Children's Adaptive Behavior Scale.* Atlanta, GA: Humanics.

Rio, A. T., Quay, H. C., Santisteban, D. A., & Szapocznik, J. (1989). Factor-analytic study of a Spanish translation of the Revised Behavior Problem Checklist. *Journal of Clinical Child Psychology, 18*, 343–350.

Ritter, D. R. (1976). Intellectual estimates of hearing impaired children: A comparison of three measures. *Pyschology in the Schools, 13*, 397–399.

Ritterman, S. I., Zook-Herman, S. L., Carlson, R. L., & Kinde, S. W. (1982). The pass/fail disparity among three commonly employed articulatory screening tests. *Journal of Speech and Hearing Disabilities, 47*, 429–433.

Roid, G., & Miller, L. (1997). *Leiter International Performance Scale—Revised.* Wood Dale, IL: Stoelting.

Rolfe, M. W., & Bryant, C. K. (1979). How reliable are MSCA profile interpretations? *Psychology in the Schools, 16*, 14–18.

Rubin, H., Goldman, J. J., & Rosenfeld, J. G. (1990). A follow-up comparison of WISC-R and WAIS-R IQs in a residential mentally retarded population. *Psychology in the Schools, 27*(4), 309–310.

Rust, J. O., & Lindstrom, A. (1996). Concurrent validity of the WISC-III and Stanford–Binet IV. *Psychological Reports, 79*(2), 618–620.

Sapp, G. L., Abbott, G., Hinkley, R., & Rowell, A. (1997). Examination of the validity of the WISC-III with urban exceptional students. *Psychological Reports, 81*(3, Part 2), 1163–1168.

Schor, D. P. (1986). Phenylketonuria and temperament in middle childhood. *Children's Health Care, 14*(3), 163–167.

Shelby, M. D., Nagle, R. J., Barnett-Queen, L. L., Quattlebaum, P. D., & Wuori, D. F. (1998). Parental reports of psychosocial adjustment and social competence in child survivors of acute lymphocytic leukemia. *Children's Health Care, 27*(2), 113–119.

Siegel, D. J., Minshew, N. J., & Goldstein, G. (1996). Wechsler IQ profiles in diagnosis of high-functioning autism. *Journal of Autism and Developmental Disorders, 26*(4), 389–406.

Simeonsson, R. J. (1978). Social competence. In J. Wortis (Ed.), *Mental retardation and developmental disabilities* (Vol. 10, pp. 130–171). New York: Brunner/Mazel.

Simeonsson, R. J. (1982). Intervention, accountability, and efficiency indices: A rejoinder. *Exceptional Children, 48*, 358–359.

Simeonsson, R. J. (1994). *Risk, resilience and prevention: Promoting the well-being of all children.* Baltimore: Brookes.

Simeonsson, R. J., & Leskinen, M. (1999). Disability, secondary conditions, and quality of life: Conceptual issues. In R. J. Simeonsson & L. N. McDevitt (Eds.), *Issues in disability and health: The role of secondary conditions and quality of life* (pp. 51–72). Chapel Hill: North Carolina Office on Disability and Health.

Slater, J. R., & Saarnio, D. A. (1995). Differences between WISC-III and WISC-R IQs: A preliminary investigation. *Journal of Psychoeducational Assessment, 13*(4), 340–346.

Sparrow, S. S., Balla, D., & Cicchetti, D. V. (1984). *Vineland Adaptive Behavior Scales.* Circle Pines, MN: American Guidance Service.

Spruill, J. (1991). A comparison of the Wechsler Adult Intelligence Scale—Revised with the Stanford–Binet Intelligence Scale—Fourth Edition for mentally retarded adults. *Psychological Assessment, 3*(1), 133–135.

Stager, S., & Young, R. D. (1982). A self-concept measure for preschool and early primary grade children. *Journal of Personality Assessment, 46*(5), 536–543.

Stein, R. E. K., & Silver, E. J. (1999). Operationalizing a conceptually based noncategorical definition: A first look at U.S. children with chronic conditions. *Archives of Pediatric and Adolescent Medicine, 153*(1), 68–74.

Stutsman, R. (1948). *Merrill–Palmer Scale of Mental Tests.* Los Angeles: Western Psychological Services.

Stutsman, R. (1981). *Merrill–Palmer Scale of Mental Tests.* East Aurora, NY: Slosson Educational Publications.

Taylor, R. C. (1984). *Assessment of exceptional students.* Englewood Cliffs, NJ: Prentice-Hall.

Thompson, A. P., & Sota, D. D. (1998). Comparison of the WAIS-R and the WISC-III scores with a sample of 16–year-old youth. *Psychological Reports, 82*(3, Part 2), 1339–1346.

Thorndike, R. L., Hagen, E. P., & Sattler, J. M. (1986). *The Stanford–Binet Intelligence Scale—Fourth Edition.* Chicago: Riverside.

Tolor, A., Tolor, B., & Blumin, S. S. (1977). Self-concept and locus of control in primary grade children identified as requiring special educational programming. *Psychological Reports, 40*, 43–49.

Tymchuk, A. J. (1974). Comparison of Bender error and time scores for groups of epileptic, retarded and behavior problem children. *Perceptual and Motor Skills, 38*, 71–74.

Van Lieshout, C. F., de Meyer, R. E., Curfs, L. M., Koot, H. M., & Fryns, J. (1998). Problem behaviors and personality of children and adolescents with Prader–Willi syndrome. *Journal of Pediatric Psychology, 23*(2), 111–120.

Vanderheiden, G. G., & Grilley, K. (1976). *Non-vocal communication techniques and aids for the severely physically handicapped.* Baltimore: University Park Press.

Vaughn, M. L., Riccio, C. A., Hynd, G. W., & Hall, J. (1997). Diagnosing ADHD (predominantly inattentive and combined type subtypes): Discriminant validity of the Behavior Assessment

System for Children and the Achenbach Parent and Teacher Rating Scales. *Journal of Clinical Child Psychology, 26,* 349–357.

Vostanis, P., Hayes, M., Du Feu, M., & Warren, J. (1997). Detection of behavioural and emotional problems in deaf children and adolescents: Comparison of two rating scales. *Child: Care, Health and Development, 23*(3), 233–246.

Wallace, G., & Hammill, D. (1994). *The Comprehensive Receptive and Expressive Vocabulary Test.* Austin, TX: Pro-Ed.

Wechsler, D. (1981). *WAIS-R Manual: Wechsler Adult Intelligence Scale—Revised.* New York: Psychological Corporation.

Wechsler, D. (1989). *WPPSI-R Manual: Wechsler Preschool and Primary Scale of Intelligence—Revised.* New York: Psychological Corporation.

Wechsler, D. (1991). *Manual for the Wechsler Intelligence Scale for Children—Third Edition.* San Antonio, TX: Psychological Corporation.

Wechsler, D. (1997). *Wechsler Adult Intelligence Scale—Third Edition.* San Antonio, TX: Psychological Corporation.

Wiener, F. D., Lewnau, L. E., & Erway, E. (1983). Measuring language competency in speakers of Black American speech. *Journal of Speech and Hearing Disorders, 46,* 76–84.

Wolf, T. M., Sklov, M. C., Hunter, S. M., Webber, L. S., & Berenson, G. S. (1982). Factor analytic study of the Piers–Harris Children's Self-Concept Scale. *Journal of Personality Assessment, 46,* 511–513.

Zero to Three: National Center for Infants, Toddlers, and Families. (1994). *Diagnostic classification: 0–3.* Washington, DC: Author.

5

A QUALITATIVE DEVELOPMENTAL APPROACH TO ASSESSMENT

RUNE J. SIMEONSSON
GAIL S. HUNTINGTON
J. LYTLE BRENT
CASSANDRE BALANT

As a teenager with Trisomy-21, John has been administered intelligence tests on a fairly regular basis since his infancy. Administration of the WISC at age 12 yielded full scale, verbal, and performance IQ scores in the middle 60s. To explore the nature of cognitive functioning, John was administered conservation tasks of two-dimensional space, number, substance, continuous quantity, weight, and discontinuous quantity. For each conservation task, equivalence was first established, a transformation was made, and John was then asked for a judgment and a justification of the response. On the six tasks, John provided a judgment response for number and space and a justification response for number only. John did not demonstrate the ability to conserve on any of the other tasks. While John's nonconserving responses reflected some intuitive and perceptually based judgments, it was interesting to note that he did vary his problem-solving strategy as a function of the task. On the task of continuous quantity, for example, John agreed to the equivalence of two balls with an equal amount of clay. Following the transformation of breaking up one large ball into five smaller balls, John was asked if there was as much clay in the large ball as in the five smaller balls. John approached the task deliberately, visually comparing the large ball and the five smaller balls. Not satisfied, he tried a second strategy in which he placed his finger in the large ball to see how high it was, followed by the same action with the smaller balls. Still not satisfied, he picked up the large ball with one hand and picked up the five smaller balls in the other hand. At that point, he put all the balls down, and, satisfied that he had solved the problem, pointed to the large ball and said, "More clay here."

Qualitative approaches to the study of behavior and development have had a long and rich history in child psychology. The theories of Piaget, Freud, and Erikson, among others, have contributed substantially both to research on child development and to clinical interventions with children. Applications of a qualitative perspective to psychological assessment have, by comparison, been limited. There is, however, an expanding literature on the application of qualitative approaches to assess children's behavior and development. As the vignette illustrates, qualitative assessment complements the information provided by psychometric testing. Although John's IQ scores provide an estimate of relative intellectual abilities, qualitative assessment indicates that knowledge of qualities of objects and operations on objects is not generalized but specific. This chapter (1) provides a brief overview of a qualitative approach to assessment, with a particular focus on relevant contributions from Piaget's developmental theory; (2) identifies objectives and issues of qualitative assessment; (3) reviews selected measures and tasks; and (4) describes the implications of such assessment for interventions with children.

A QUALITATIVE-DEVELOPMENTAL APPROACH TO ASSESSMENT

The qualitative approach to the study of childhood has been defined by various theorists across a number of developmental domains (Simeonsson & Rosenthal, 2001). The psychoanalytic tradition, exemplified by the work of Sigmund Freud, proposed that the child's affective development could be represented in a sequence of psychosexual stages beginning in infancy and culminating in mature functioning. Anna Freud elaborated this approach in the concept of developmental lines. Emerging from this orientation but focusing more on the role of the ego in development, Erikson identified eight stages reflective of qualitative changes in psychosocial development across the life span.

In the area of cognitive development, qualitative perspectives have been advanced by a number of theorists, including Wemer (1957), Bruner (1965), Kohlberg (1969), and, most notably, Piaget (1970c). There is also increasing interest in Vygotsky's (1978) developmental theory and its implications for assessment and intervention, with particular reference to the importance of the social and cultural context of the child and the concept of the zone of proximal development (Gingis, 1995). Although each theorist has had a somewhat unique focus, all have shared a common assumption that the child's cognitive growth is best understood as a sequence of transitions that reflect qualitative rather than quantitative change. This assumption has been tested in a variety of research studies demonstrating that children progress from primitive to mature stages of cognitive and psychosocial development. Four general features of qualitative approaches, discontinuity, ordinality, symbolic representation, and stage concept, are summarized in Table 5.1 and contrasted with the quantitative and ecobehavioral approaches presented in Chapters 4 and 6, respectively. As Piaget's theory provides the most detailed account of qualitative development, key elements of his theory are reviewed with implications for assessment.

Discontinuity

A feature common to qualitative approaches is the belief that development is not a continuous or cumulative process but is discontinuous in nature. A later stage represents not simply the addition of knowledge or skills from an earlier stage but a structural change in such knowledge and skills. This assumption is in sharp contrast to that of the psychometric approach, in which the conceptual, as well as statistical, assumptions imply that development is continuous and cumulative in nature. The mental-age index common to many psychometric measures implies continuity, with higher ages reflecting quantitative increments. As Furth

TABLE 5.1. A Comparison of the Assessment Implications of Psychometric, Ecobehavioral, and Qualitative-Developmental Strategies

	Psychometric	Ecobehavioral	Qualitative-developmental
Focus of Assessment	Intelligence as fixed characteristic	Behavior in context	Cognition as developing, structural characteristic
Primary Mode of Assessment	Verbal responses and performance on standardized tests	Coding of observed behavior and contexts	Clinical method to elicit performance and explanation
Index of Functioning	Quantitative and/or standardized values	Quantitative, operationally defined values	Qualitative, ordinal values
Intra- versus Interindividual Differences	Normative, focus on differences between individuals	Idiopathic, focus on behavior of individual within specific settings	Idiopathic, focus on performance, and explanation unique to developmental stage
Nature of Assessed Characteristics	Reflects relative average characteristics	Reflects absolute setting-specific behaviors	Reflects absolute stage-specific functioning
Intervention Implications	Decision making relative to normative reference group	Decision making relative to behavior characteristics of the individual	Decision making relative to sequence of developmental stage

(1973) has pointed out, standardized tests of intelligence assume that age defines a constant rate of achievement, determining a child's intelligence. Within a qualitative perspective on development, age may vary relative to transition across cognitive stages (Wadsworth, 1996).

Ordinality of Development

The second feature common to qualitative approaches is ordinality of development. This feature, a logical extension of the assumption of discontinuity, simply conveys the fact that the sequence of development is fixed, with earlier stages followed by later stages in a pre-scribed order. This invariance of developmental sequence implies that progression through developmental stages does not proceed in an erratic fashion but must occur in order. How-ever, although sequence is fixed, rate may vary substantially, reflecting individual differ-ences among children in the acquisition of developmental skills. This premise of qualitative approaches is particularly attractive in the assessment of children with disabilities, whose developmental skills may be very discrepant from those of chronological age peers.

Stage Concept

In this discussion of ordinality it may be useful to call attention to terms often used to define qualitative transitions. Although terms such as "period," "stage," "phase," and "level" are used readily in developmental studies, they are not interchangeable (Von Glaserfeld & Kelly, 1982). Von Glaserfeld and Kelly examined the four terms in reference to several criteria and concluded that the term "level" does not reflect a time dimension, whereas "stage," "period," and "phase," do. Although the terms "period" and "phase" imply a time dimension, they do not imply a progression. "Stage" as a concept, however, implies progression, as well as a time dimension characterized by unique qualitative elements. For the purpose of this book, we use the term "stage" to denote qualitative transition in devel-opment, a practice consistent with its use in the major theories of Freud and Piaget.

CONTRIBUTIONS FROM PIAGET'S THEORY

The contributions of Piaget's theory to the study and understanding of children have been comprehensive in scope and content. His own writings and those of others interpreting or elaborating his theory are extensive and cannot be reviewed comprehensively here. How-ever, we give a brief description of selected contributions of particular relevance to clinical assessment of children with disabilities and chronic health conditions. These contributions encompass assimilation and accommodation in adaptation, the child's construction of reality, symbolic representation, and invariance of stage development.

Assimilation and Accommodation

Central to Piaget's theory is the assumption that development is a reflection of the child's adaptation to the environment. Adaptation involves the complementary processes of as-similation and accommodation. Piaget has defined assimilation as "that aspect of adapta-tion which conserves form or organization. Accommodation is that aspect which modifies form as a function of the external situation. Both notions apply to forms of behavior and thought as well as to organic structures" (1981, p. 4). Although the ratio of these processes may vary from one occasion to the next, adaptation is the relative balance equilibrium of the two. To this point, Piaget has stated, "all behavior is adaptation and all adaptation is the establishment of equilibrium between the organism and the environment. We act only if we are momentarily disequilibrated" (1981, p. 4).

Construction of Reality

Piaget's second concept is that the child's adaptation to environmental demands involves an active, progressive construction of reality. Development is not simply maturational unfolding or the accumulation of learned behaviors; rather, each child constructs meaning in the context of his or her experiences. The availability of objects and stimuli alone is not sufficient for development to occur; there must be action and experience at both physical and mental levels. An important implication of this concept is that variability in the development of children reflects not only the environments children have experienced but also the meaning they have constructed from those experiences. The validity of this concept is readily apparent in the idiosyncratic, prelogical, and sometimes humorous ways in which children explain phenomena. Elkind (1963), for example, in noting children's understanding of religious identity, asked a 5-year-old if a cat could be a Protestant. The child replied "yes," and when asked why, said, "They could fight among themselves. My boyfriend [sic] is a Protestant and he fights" (1963, p. 294).

Symbolic Representation

The child's ongoing adaptation to the environment, the qualitative shift from sensorimotor to preoperational stage, is marked by the emergence of symbolic representation, that is, the ability to mentally represent an object or experience distant in time or space. Such representation is evident in the increasingly complex activities of imitation of an absent model, symbolic play, the use of drawing mental imagery, and ultimately the use of spoken or signed language (Piaget & Inhelder, 1969). In development, representation involves two complementary processes, figurative and operative representation (Piaget, 1970b). In figurative representation, meaning and knowing are based on a correspondence of features or characters, the signifier (e.g., outline of a cat) and the signified object (cat). In operative representation, meaning and knowing are based on actions or transformations involving a signifier (e.g., the word "cat") and the signified object (cat). Figurative representation is thus largely accommodative in nature, whereas operative representation is primarily assimilative in that meaning is achieved at a conceptual rather than perceptual level. Although these two aspects of representation are complementary in typical development, their relative role in symbolic acquisition may differ markedly as a function of specific impairments. Thus, deafness and blindness may be associated with greater roles for figural and operative representation, respectively.

Invariance of Stage Development

The nature and sequence of qualitative stages represents a fourth contribution of Piaget's theory. At certain points in the dynamic balance between assimilation and accommodation, successive adaptations result in qualitative shifts in the way in which the child makes sense of reality. Although the processes of adaptation remain the same throughout development, these qualitative shifts represent different stages of reality construction. Thus earlier stages precede and become incorporated into later stages, each reflecting a more structurally advanced level of understanding.

The first stage, the sensorimotor period, encompasses normal infancy and is defined by the fact that reality for the infant is based on sensory and motor experiences. The infant's understanding is dependent on and governed by actions that begin with reflex activity and progress rapidly to a sixth substage of means and mental combinations to achieve simple objectives (Piaget, 1970c). Achievement of the object concept, the recognition that objects exist in time and space independent of their perceptual immediacy to the child, is a capstone of this stage.

Entry into the preoperational stage, encompassing toddlerhood through the preschool years, is marked by a qualitative transition in which the child's understanding moves to a representative plane. The child's representational competence, however, is very much perceptually based and intuitive in nature. If perceptions are altered or changed, the construction of reality is likely to be altered as well, expressing itself in the egocentric errors children make when faced with tasks in which some transformation takes place. The classic demonstration of the child's failure to conserve amount, number, or weight reflects the centering (unidimensional) quality of preoperational thought. A variety of other tasks, including some with social content (moral judgment), have been used to document this unidimensional, centering characteristic of preoperational thought compared with the decentered nature of concrete operational thought (Figure 5.1), as described subsequently.

The concrete operational stage is marked by yet another qualitative shift in reality construction. Cognitive tasks independent of physical action require the child to decenter and consider multiple dimensions simultaneously without being confused by discrepant cues, perceptual or otherwise. Operations such as grouping, classification, and seriation are all specific expressions of reversibility as a fundamental mental skill. As the term "concrete operations" indicates, however, cognitive development is still on a concrete plane, lacking hypothetical or abstract qualities. Such qualities are demonstrated in the formal operations stage, usually achieved by late childhood. The ability to engage in hypothetical, propositional reasoning reflects the achievement of mature thought, which Piaget (1970c) has labeled "complete equilibrium." Such equilibrium implies that what is objective in nature can be the focus of subjective reasoning and that what is subjective in nature can be understood objectively.

These four conceptual contributions represent a selective consideration of Piaget's comprehensive theory. Good reviews of his theory with practical implications can be found in earlier works by Flavell (1963), Cowan (1978), and Hogg and Raynes (1987) and in more recent contributions by Sexton, Kelley, and Surbeck (1990), Williams (1996), and Wadsworth (1996). Research contributions in the developmental literature in the past four decades also provide a rich source of information on the validity and implications of cognitive-developmental theory. A particularly rewarding and valuable source is Piaget's original writings, which provide intriguing examples of tasks to assess children's concepts of reality (1954), time (1970b), number (1952), and moral judgment (1948). With minimal requirements for materials, these tasks can be modified for administration to children of varying levels of ability and stage of development. Two other sources are lists of tasks and measures described by Formanek and Gurian (1981) and Schmid-Kitsikis (1990). Formanek and Gurian, for example, have assembled an extensive set of tasks covering the concrete operations period with descriptions for administration and scoring. Schmid-Kitsikis

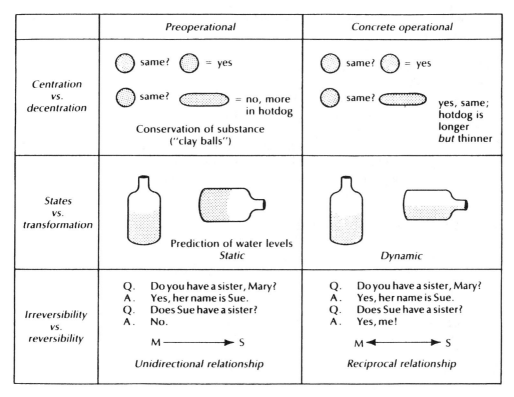

FIGURE 5.1. Contrasts between preoperational and concrete operational thought.

provides a similar list of tasks in four categories: construction of invariants, symbolic constructions, construction of images, and logical reasoning. An array of tasks differentiating figurative from operative aspects of thought of particular relevance for the assessment of children with visual impairment have been described by Hatwell (1985). These tasks cover a 4- to 13-year age range and include spatial representation, displacement, conservation of substance weight and volume, and classification and seriation.

OBJECTIVES IN QUALITATIVE ASSESSMENT

The reasons for carrying out qualitative assessment with children differ in unique ways from those of quantitative and behavioral assessment (see Table 5.1). Qualitative assessment differs from psychometric assessment in that interest resides in analyzing the nature and stage of development, not in a normative comparison of child performance. Although both qualitative and ecobehavioral approaches are nonnormative in nature, they differ in their focus on structural versus functional aspects, respectively. Ecobehavioral assessment thus yields information about functioning of a given child, whereas qualitative assessment yields information about theoretically defined cognitive structures. The value of a qualitative approach is that it is applicable to the assessment of any child, regardless of the nature or severity of impairments or disabilities. Drawing on the contributions reviewed, a qualitative approach can be used to pursue these representative assessment questions.

1. What is the nature of the child's adaptation in terms of assimilation and accommodation?
2. On what basis does the child construct reality?
3. Is there a difference between performance and competence?
4. What is the qualitative level of the child's reasoning?
5. Are there characteristics of thinking unique to diagnostic groups?
6. Is there a discrepancy in figurative and operative representation?

These representative questions can be embedded within three broad objectives for assessment unique to the qualitative approach: (1) analysis of cognitive structures; (2) documentation of competence; and (3) assignment to stage of functioning.

Analysis of Cognitive Structures

An assumption basic to Piaget's theory is that development is a reflection of structural change in the child's understanding of reality. An analysis of what cognitive structures characterize the child thus constitutes a major assessment objective. In qualitative assessment, this translates into an analysis of the cognitive structures the child demonstrates in solving problems, whether through sensorimotor means or through mental operations. Interest is not in the assessment of the child's level of arithmetic achievement, for example, but rather in the operations the child uses to solve problems. In the context of Piagetian theory, assessment might thus encompass analysis of symbolic functioning, decentration, reversibility, or propositional thinking within the sensorimotor, preoperational, concrete operations, or formal operations stages, respectively. Such assessment emphasizes the structural nature of thought independent of a particular content domain.

Documentation of Competence

Documentation of competence has particular relevance for children with disabilities. In the psychometric approach, the focus is on documenting incompetence; the performance of children with disabilities is measured by the extent to which it is less competent relative to normative values. Relative deficits in performance are associated with, or attributed to, impairment or disability. In qualitative assessment, documentation is made of a child's competence at the stage that applies, regardless of the severity of disability. Illustrations of this conceptual distinction can be found in the work of Rogers (1977) and others who have documented the competence of children with profound mental retardation. Within a psychometric perspective, two children sharing similar low IQs would be assumed to function at the same level of profound intellectual deficits. Within a qualitative perspective, however, assessment of the two children might reveal different competencies, as evidenced by performance at different substages of the sensorimotor period. In practical terms, this distinction means that the same psychometric index (e.g., IQ = 30) is relative in nature; it does not necessarily imply a similar level of functioning in children of different ages. Evidence of competence at the substage of secondary circular reactions by two children, however, implies the same level of absolute functioning regardless of age or other characteristics such as IQ.

Documentation of competence is also important in distinguishing between competence and performance. This is of particular interest with regard to children with disabilities whose performance may not be commensurate with competence. The presence of echolalia in children with autism and of social desirability responding in children with mental retardation may yield results that reflect higher levels of performance than of competence. In children who have motor impairments, the reverse may be true, with demonstrated performance being lower than actual competence. The analysis of cognitive structures and processes inherent in qualitative assessment emphasizes the documentation of competence. Inhelder has summarized the issue clearly: "To determine that a subject is capable of solving such and such a problem is one thing, while to understand how he manages to do so is quite another" (1966, p. 300).

Assignment to Stage of Functioning

Qualitative theories are commonly applied in assigning a child's performance to a developmental stage. Although age boundaries can be given for most stages in typical development, the assignment to a stage is independent of age, depending only on evidence of competence reflective of that stage. This feature is attractive in the assessment of children with disabilities and chronic health conditions, whose chronological ages usually exceed those of their peers at similar functioning levels. Identification of children in terms of stages of functioning is useful descriptively in order to plan treatments that are developmentally sequenced. The value of this approach is evident in the fact that a group of children with a homogeneous label, such as severe mental retardation, may in fact be heterogeneous in regard to level of qualitative functioning. Grouping children on the basis of stage of competence, rather than by a shared psychometric label, would facilitate specificity and appropriateness of planned interventions.

ISSUES IN QUALITATIVE ASSESSMENT

Several issues are useful to consider in a qualitative approach to clinical assessment with children. We label these "conceptual" issues and "clinical" issues, reflecting theoretical and applied considerations, respectively.

Conceptual Issues

Piaget's interests were in documenting typical development; others extended his theory to developmental pathology and disability. His colleague, Inhelder (1966), described the implications of cognitive-developmental theory for understanding children with a variety of impairments and disabilities. As early as 1943, Inhelder (1968) wrote on the topic of reasoning in children with mental retardation, presenting concepts and research findings pertaining to this population. One of her central contributions was defining mental retardation within the concept of a false equilibrium; that is, the failure of an individual to achieve formal operations at maturity. Persons who reach only the stage of concrete operations at maturity were defined as being at the level of mild mental retardation. Those who reach only the preoperational stage at maturity were characterized by moderate to severe mental retardation, and those who do not develop beyond the sensorimotor stage at maturity were characterized by profound retardation. This approach to defining the nature and levels of mental retardation differs from the statistical use of deviation IQ scores to define mental retardation. The qualitative approach based on levels of competence offers an alternative way in which to define the phenomenon of mental retardation. Further, in that levels reflect qualitatively different cognitive structures, they provide a basis for differentiating interventions accordingly.

A second concept pertains to the notion of *décalage*, defined as relative lags in the acquisition of similar cognitive skills within a stage. In typical development, for example, the conservation of mass, weight, and volume are acquired in sequence rather than simultaneously. If the *décalage* concept is viewed as a marker of generalization, it would have obvious value in the assessment of children with disabilities. Rogers (1977) has found that children with profound mental retardation were in fact characterized by marked *décalage* of skills within the sensorimotor period. In a comparative study, Volpe (1976) found marked lags in tasks of seriation and conservation of weight, but not in classification or conservation of mass tasks in children with disabilities compared with nonimpaired peers, reflecting the specific impact of motor impairment on cognitive development.

A third concept of relevance for children with disabilities pertains to adaptational imbalances in the reciprocal processes of assimilation and accommodation. If assimilation predominates over accommodation to an excessive degree, reality construction proceeds in an egocentric, autistic-like direction. Inhelder (1966) has described one form of such imbalance, found in children with prepsychotic conditions, as a deforming assimilation of reality. If accommodation predominates over assimilation in an excessive way, the result is likely to be rote imitation rather than comprehension. The situation-specific rote behavior often demonstrated by children with mental retardation when faced with excessive learning demands is likely due to an imbalance of accommodation over assimilation. Interventions to address imbalances of adaptation should take the form of modifying environmental demands faced by the child.

Oscillation is a concept defined by Inhelder as fluctuations from one stage to another in child's reasoning. Although oscillations do not represent distortions of reality, they are seen as symptomatic of a child's anxiety or indecision and may be manifested in children identified with affective problems. The oscillation concept expresses the interaction between cognitive and affective development and may provide a useful frame in which to interpret variations in reasoning among children with disabilities.

Clinical Issues

The central diagnostic tool used by Piaget and his colleagues was the *method clinique*—the clinical interview in which assessment activities and the use of objects can be modified on an ongoing basis to capture the uniqueness of the child's responses. Inhelder (1966) suggested that when it is used with many children it serves as an experimental procedure. The clinical interview is a particularly valuable tool for assessing children with disabilities in that it creates a situation in which the examiner provides minimal structure as the child seeks to solve a problem. In trying to solve the problem, the child demonstrates cognitive processes through manipulation of materials and/or verbalizations, as illustrated in the introductory vignette of John's conservation performance. The clinical nature of such assessment is enhanced in that "the examiner not only participates in an exchange with the child, but is also constantly formulating and testing hypotheses as to the possible significance of the child's replies and behavior" (Inhelder, 1966, p. 300). Such ongoing formulation and hypothesis testing may be a particularly appropriate strategy to adopt in the assessment of a child with disabilities whose performance may be idiosyncratic and not readily comparable to that of other children. Thus, whether there is interest in assessing object permanence in an infant with cerebral palsy (Felters, 1981), moral judgment in a 12-year-old child who is deaf (Sam & Wright, 1988), or health conceptions of a child with spina bifida (Feldman & Varni, 1985), the clinical method as illustrated in many of Piaget's writings offers a flexible and rich approach to clinical assessment.

SELECTED MEASURES AND PROCEDURES

Compared with the wide range of psychometric measures, the number of formal measures based on qualitative theories is quite limited. There are, however, a variety of informal measures and procedures described in the literature that can be applied in assessment contexts. In keeping with the format of previous chapters, we review here selected measures and procedures in the categories of cognition, communication, personal and social functioning, and behavior. Most of the measures come from the literature based on Piaget's theory, but selected measures based on other qualitative perspectives are included as appropriate. Within each category, measures are reviewed developmentally, with those assessing early stages reviewed prior to those assessing later stages. Contributions to the literature indicate that there are several reasons why the administration of qualitative tasks is of value with children with disabilities and chronic conditions. The first and most obvious reason is to examine the nature of thought in the individual child in order to generate information planning or evaluating treatments. Such an approach may yield unique information that complements psychometric data, as illustrated by Halpern's (1966) presentation of conservation performance and IQ scores in the longitudinal case study of a child described as psychotic. The utility of a Piagetian approach to assessment has been recommended for children with visual impairments (Lister & Atha, 1986), emotional and behavioral difficulties (Hill, 1993), and mental retardation (McCormick, Campbell, Pasnack, & Perry, 1990).

A second reason is to document the impact of a specific impairment on the nature and rate of development. This approach has taken the form of research in which the performance of a group of children with the same impairment is compared with that of normally developing peers. Examples of this approach include research with children with visual impairments (Dimcovic & Tobin, 1995; Heller & Kennedy, 1990; Pring, Dewart, & Brockbank, 1998), hearing impairments, motor impairments (Volpe, 1976), mental retardation, and learning disabilities (Fakouri, 1991; Yirmiya & Shulman, 1996). Findings have generally supported the invariant nature of development, although lags or variability in rate have been associated with different disabilities and health conditions.

A third reason for administering qualitative tasks is to interpret performance within a theoretically based approach. Inhelder's (1966) propositions regarding mental retardation as the absence of formal operations at maturity and the distortion of reality construction in severe emotional disturbance represent contributions relevant to children with disabilities. Research on assessment and training of formal operations in adolescents with mental retardation (Kahn, 1974; McCormick, Campbell, Pasnak, & Perry, 1990) and on the relationship of dream conceptions and reality orientation in children who are borderline or psychotic or who have behavior disorders, (Evans, 1973; Hill, 1993; Lister, Leach, & Hill, 1990) illustrates the clinical utility of these diagnostic contributions. Although this theory testing approach has not yet been widely implemented, positive findings by Kahn (1974), Evans (1973), Hill (1993), Lister and colleagues (1990) and others indicate its potential to support differential diagnostic efforts with children with disabilities.

A fourth reason for qualitative assessment is to identify correlates of operational thought. At one level, this could be seen as an extension of assessment to examine the nature of thought in the child with disabilities. The focus is usually much more specific, however, in that elements of the child's cognitive performance are examined relative to achievement or functioning in other domains. Examples of this approach include studies of the correlates of conservation performance in children with mental retardation by Yirmiya and Shulman (1996), Yirmiya, Sigman, and Zacks (1994), and Lister, Leach, and Wheeler (1993). In the section that follows, representative applications provide evidence of the richness and flexibility that the qualitative approach has to offer in terms of assessment of children with disabilities and chronic health conditions.

Cognition

The assessment of cognition represents the area of greatest focus in research based on Piaget's theory. From the emergence of the object concept in the sensorimotor period to the acquisition of propositional logic in the formal operations stage, measures and procedures have built, in one way or another, on the clinical interview. The goals of assessment with various tasks is to identify the nature and level of the child's reasoning. Representative measures and procedures are summarized in Table 5.2 according to developmental stage and domain.

Assessment of sensorimotor functioning has been an area of significant activity with children and adults with disabilities. The most widely used measure of sensorimotor development is the Infant Psychological Development Scale (IPDS) developed by Uzgiris and Hunt (1975). This scale encompasses the areas of object permanence, object means, imitation, causality, objects in space, and schemas. Dunst (1980) has developed a manual describing the utility of this measure for children with disabilities. On the basis of the child's performance, functional levels are defined for each of the areas in terms of one of the six substages of the sensorimotor period. This scale has seen various applications with children with hearing impairments (Best & Roberts, 1976) or mental retardation (Wohlheuter & Sindberg, 1975; Woodyatt & Ozanne, 1993), and with children identified by psychiatric diagnoses (Serafica, 1971). An interesting finding in Serafica's study was that, although severely deviant children showed a normal sequence of object concept development, they differed in that there was a marked time lag (*décalage*) in this development between preferred and neutral objects. In the study of children with Rett syndrome (Woodyatt & Ozanne, 1993), assessed cognitive development remained in the sensorimotor stage over a period of 3 years even though ages range from 2½ through 13½ years.

Although assessment of object permanence usually involves a motor response by the infant, Felters (1981) has described an interesting approach that made it possible to assess infants with motor impairment without requiring manipulation. Using visual searching responses and heart-rate change as outcome measures, Felters was able to show differences in the stage attainment of these infants as a function of traditional and nontraditional assessment of object permanence. Sensorimotor measures permit the profiling of functional levels across cognitive domains (as illustrated in Figure 5.2 on page 96). Furthermore, the ordinal nature of assessment provides a basis for identifying behaviors that have been acquired and those still to be developed.

Assessment of preoperational development focuses on the development of representational competence in the form of deferred imitation, pretense, drawings, symbols, and words. The child's growing use of representation through spoken or signed language makes it possible, for example, to assess the child's emerging concepts of causality, life, and dreams. Preoperational reasoning is characterized by intuitive, perception-based, and egocentric thinking, reflecting the child's difficulty in differentiating between appearance and reality.

TABLE 5.2. Qualitative Developmental Assessment of Cognition and Communication

	Cognition	Communication
Sensorimotor	Infant Psychological Development Scale (Uzgiris & Hunt, 1975)	Sequence of declarative/imperative communication behaviors (Bates et al., 1975, 1977)
		Developmental nature of looking, showing, and hiding (Lempers et al., 1977)
Preoperational (through formal operations)	Concepts of time, reality, movement (Piaget, 1970a, 1970b, 1970c)	Referential communication adequate in two-person task (Krauss & Glucksberg, 1977).
	Causal reasoning: life, dreams, origins of night (Laurendau & Pinard, 1962)	Matrix task of referential communication in first through sixth graders (Greenspan, 1976).
		COMTASK to assess developmental changes in quantity and quality of referential communication (Rosenthal & Simeonsson, 1991)
Concrete operations	Concept Assessment Kit (Goldschmid & Bentler, 1968)	
	Conservation of number, quantity, seriation, classification	
Formal operations	Solubility of liquids	
	Conservation of volume	
	Pendulum problem	

These difficulties are expressed in artificialism, animism, and syncretism. Artificialism is evident in the child's prelogical belief that natural phenomena occur for the benefit of mankind (e.g., it gets dark so children can sleep). Animism reflects the child's attribution of life traits to inanimate objects (e.g., the table is alive because it has legs/stands). In syncretistic thought, events that occurred together by chance are assumed to be causally related (e.g., a visit to the farm should always result in a thunderstorm). In the typical clinical interview procedure, the child is given the opportunity to answer such questions as: "What makes clouds move?" "Is a bicycle alive?" "Where do dreams come from?" Children's responses are scored according to the manner in which they reflect qualitative transitions in reality orientation from preoperational substages into the stage of concrete operations.

The value of assessing these unique concepts is to document the way in which children comprehend the reality of their experiences. The measures in this area are drawn from clinical and empirical literature, with Piaget's original writings on the child's conception of time (1970b), reality (1954), the world (1929), and movement (1970a) providing some excellent illustrations of clinical interviews and procedures (see Table 5.3 on page 97). A good example of the use of Piaget's clinical method is a study by Laurendau and Pinard (1962) on causal reasoning in children ranging in age from 4 to 12. Children were interviewed about four domains (origin of night, dreams, life, and movement of clouds), yielding a summary of qualitative transitions in causal reasoning. If a child has verbal limitations, a picture-sorting approach, for example, can be used to implement the clinical interview in the assessment of animism (Beveridge & Davies, 1983).

SUBSTAGE	PLAY	OBJECT PERMANENCE	MEANING	SPACE	CAUSALITY	TIME	IMITATION	INTENTIONS AND MEANS/ ENDS
VI. Invention of new means								
V. Tertiary circular reactions	Art			Art				
IV. Coordination of 2nd schemata		Art Bob	Art			Art		
III. 2nd circular reactions	Bob		Bob	Bob	Art	Bob		Art
II. Primary circular reactions					Bob		Art Bob	Bob
I. Exercising reflex schemes								

FIGURE 5.2. Sensorimotor profiles of two 7-year-old children (Art and Bob) with severe disabilities.

An illustration of the utility of assessing causal reasoning is a comparative study by Smeets (1974) of children with mental retardation and their chronological and mental age peers. The task assessed the child's attribution of life and life traits to four stimulus categories: animals, plants, objects moving of their own accord (such as a river), and objects not moving of their own accord (such as a clock or a bottle). The questionnaire allowed for scoring of simple "yes" and "no" responses and thus may be appropriate for children with disabilities who would have difficulty with a more subjective interview (such as that of Laurendau and Pinard). Follow-up questions can of course be asked to elicit the child's explanation and understanding of the concept. Smeet administered this questionnaire to children with mental retardation ranging in mental age from 5 years, 10 months to 7 years, 2 months and to their chronological age (CA) and mental age (MA) peers. This assessment approach demonstrated that understanding of life and life traits by children with mental retardation differentiated them from both their CA and MA matched peers, as illustrated in Figure 5.3 on page 98.

Assessment of concrete operations has perhaps been the area of most research interest, with the conservation task being the prototypic task of mental operations to assess the reversibility of thought. In the basic conservation assessment paradigm, equivalence of mass, number, or length is established for two objects by a child. A perceptual transformation is then made of the objects through rearrangement of shape or configuration. The child's task is to determine if the essential quality (mass, number, length) is conserved in spite of the perceptual transformation as illustrated in the initial vignette about John. Conservation is documented if the child makes an appropriate judgment and provides a justification based on reversibility, identity, or compensation. Tasks assessing conservation and other aspects of concrete and formal operational thinking are listed in Figure 5.4 on page 99. Formanek and Gurian (1981) have prepared a book on assessment of a range of concrete operations including conservation, classification, causality, and time, movement, and speed.

TABLE 5.3. A Summary of Qualitative Transitions Observed in Laurendau and Pinard's Study of Causal Thinking in Children 4 to 12 Years of Age

Stage/substage	Concept of dream	Concept of life	Origin of night	Movement of clouds
0	Incomprehension/refusal	Incomprehension/refusal	Incomprehension/refusal	Incomprehension/refusal
1	Complete belief in reality of dream	Life defined in terms of usefulness, movement, or anthropomorphism	Absolute artificialism, explanations based on needs of humans	Human or divine action
a			Explanations in terms of usefulness to humans	
b			Intermingling of finalistic and artificialistic explanations	
2	Alternates between belief in interiorization/exteriorization	Life defined in terms of spontaneous movement	Semiartificialistic, semiphysical, explanations	Autonomous movements; actions of other celestial bodies
a	Attempts to interiorize dream			
b	Balance between realism/ subjectivism			
c	Residual realism in terms of materiality			
3	Realism disappears	Total disappearance of animistic thought	Explanations restricted to physical/natural elements	Action of the wind
a	Selected inclusion of precausal factors		Selected residual animistic/ finalistic factors	Residual precausal reasoning
b	Totally subjective reasoning		Total disappearance of precausal thinking	Total disappearance of precausal thinking

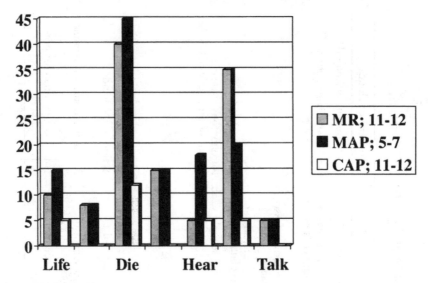

FIGURE 5.3. Percent of life traits to "bottle" by children with mental retardation (MR) and chronological age (CAP) and mental age (MAP) peers.

Various replications have confirmed the utility of the conservation paradigm to assess concrete operational reasoning. Acquisition of conservation skills is sequential in development, with mass conserved earliest, followed by weight and volume. The mental operations of reversibility and decentration (e.g., considering two or more dimensions simultaneously) are also assessed in other tasks associated with the concrete operations stage. These include tasks of classification, grouping, and seriation. In each instance the task is designed to assess the child's ability to set aside intuitive and perceptually based judgments in favor of judgments made from the application of mental operations of reversibility and logical manipulations. Findings pertaining to the diagnostic utility of assessing concrete operations performance have been demonstrated with various clinical groups, including children with visual impairments (Stephens & Grube, 1982), blindness (Dimcovic & Tobin, 1995), mental retardation (Yirmiya & Shulman, 1996), and autism and Williams syndrome (Wang & Bellugi, 1993).

Reasoning at the formal operations stage is characterized by abstract and propositional thought involving the ability to take into account not only the actual, concrete dimensions of the task but also the hypothetical possibilities. Formal operations tasks are designed to assess the child's ability to solve mental problems in which variables have to be manipulated systematically in order to arrive at a solution. Representative tasks of formal operations reasoning are the pendulum task, conservation of volume, and solubility of liquids. In the pendulum task, for example, the child is given the problem of determining the variables (length of string, weight, and release point) that govern the frequency of oscillation. Sommerville's (1974) findings, illustrative of studies on the pendulum problem, revealed that, in a study of 10- to 14-year-olds, full solution of this problem at a formal operations level was not demonstrated by a majority of children until the age of 14. The transition to formal operational reasoning in children can also be assessed through tasks of conservation of volume and solubility of liquids. Table 5.4 on page 100 may serve as a reference source to identify tasks appropriate to pursue specific assessment questions.

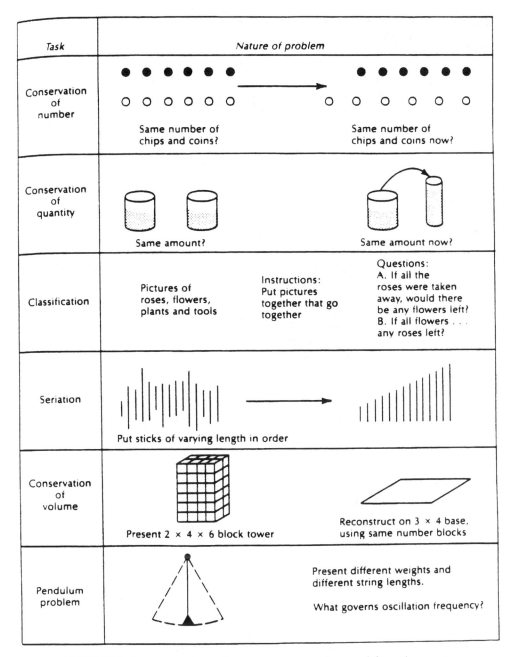

FIGURE 5.4. Representative tasks—concrete operations and formal operations.

Communication

Piaget did not cover communication in detail in his original work. Although he did examine the changing frequency of self-referents with age in children, the focus was on the concept of egocentrism rather than communication per se (1957). More recent contributions, many growing out of a Piagetian framework, illustrate a qualitative-developmental ap-

TABLE 5.4. Qualitative-Developmental Assessment of Self–Other Differentiation and Behavior: Selected Tasks

	Self–Other Differentiation	Behavior
Sensorimotor	Miniature objects used to assess symbolic play in 12-, 15-, 18-, 21-, 24-, 30-, and 36-month-old infants (Lowe, 1975)	Carolina Record of Individual Behavior (Simeonsson et al., 1982)
	Set of 36 toys used in longitudinal study of symbolic play in 14- to 19-month-old infants (McCune-Nicolich, 1976)	Developmental sequence of peer play (Parten, 1932; Whiteside et al., 1976)
Preoperational-formal operations (role-taking, person perception)	Five role-taking tasks used with 3- to 5-year-old children involving four affective roles: happy, sad, angry, and afraid (Urberg & Docherty, 1976)	
	Perceptual, cognitive, and affective role-taking tasks used with K–6th graders (Kurdek & Rodgon, 1975)	
	Person-perception interview (Secord & Peevers, 1973)	
	Perception of recursive/ nonrecursive thinking in others (Barenboim, 1981)	
Defense mechanism		Developmental understanding of psychological causality (Dollinger et al., 1981; Whiteman, 1967)
Self-consciousness		Imaginary Audience Scale (Elkind & Bowen, 1979)
Moral judgment		Intent/consequence paired-story format (Piaget, 1948; Weiner & Peters, 1973)
		Dimensions of moral judgment: reciprocal/expiatory punishment; immanent justice, etc. (Kohlberg, 1964)
		Moral dilemma (Kohlberg, 1969)

proach to assessment of communication (Abrahamsen & Mitchell, 1990). In this section the focus is on the pragmatic nature of communication and the function communication serves rather than on its semantic or syntactic elements. The emphasis is thus on the competence of the child to communicate and not on the linguistic properties of the communication itself. Representative measures and procedures of demonstrated or potential relevance to children with disabilities are summarized in Table 5.4.

The fundamental issue in assessment of communication across stages is to determine the adequacy of the sender's message to the recipient. A developmental sequence of communication skills in the sensorimotor period has been described by Bates and her colleagues (Bates, Benigni, Bretherton, Camaioni, & Volterra, 1977; Bates, Camaioni, & Volterra,

1975). Lobato, Barrera, and Feldman (1981) have drawn on this sequence and on Snyder's (1978) tasks to assess declarative and imperative elements of communication in children and adolescents with severe and profound mental retardation. The measure focuses on the sequence of communication within Stages III through VI of the sensorimotor period. At the earliest stage, declarative and imperative behaviors are defined by the absence of a communicative response. At Stage IV, behavior involves showing or giving objects to adults without adult attention, whereas imperative behavior is defined by "noncommunicative point" (in which the child's pointing is followed by an engagement of the adult's attention). In Stage VI, both behaviors are defined by the use of simple, intelligible words or signs. In their research with a residential population, Lobato and colleagues (1981) found that the presence of simple words was most frequently associated with Stage VI, coordinated gestures with Stage V, and inadequate integration of object-oriented behavior and person-oriented behavior with Stage IV.

Using a somewhat different approach, Lempers, Flavell, and Flavell (1977) identified 27 tasks, categorized as hiding (percept deprivation), looking (percept production), and showing (percept identification), for use with children between 1 and 3 years of age. Their findings with normally developing children revealed that 1-year-olds understood the role of the eyes in seeing, 2-year-olds understood the requirements of showing, and only 3-year-olds demonstrated understanding of the concept of hiding. Blacher (1982) compared the sequence of this communicative skill mastery in children with disabilities and their nondisabled peers matched on the basis of social age equivalents of 2, 3, and 4 years. Her findings revealed a comparable pattern of acquisition in both groups, although individual differences were evident. Communication assessment as described here is of value in that it is appropriate for any child or adult functioning at a basic developmental level; speech is not required to perform the tasks, and nonverbal communication in the form of gestures can serve as an appropriate response. Findings provide information about the nature and level of communicative competence of children with disabilities.

Qualitative assessment beyond the sensorimotor period has focused primarily on the referential nature of communication. A standard paradigm has been to document the communicative adequacy between speaker and listener in a two-person task. Although specific aspects of the task may vary as a function of developmental level, assessment focuses on the extent to which the speaker is able to accurately infer the informational needs of the listener receiving messages. The prototypic task used in this context is that reported by Krauss and Glucksberg (1977), in which a speaker's communicative effectiveness is assessed by placing a visual barrier between the speaker and listener and recording the accuracy with which the listener follows instructions (Figure 5.5 on page 102). In a developmental study of children ranging from kindergarten through the ninth grades, Krauss and Glucksberg (1977) found that the performance of children in kindergarten, first, third, and fifth grades was marked by communication that was to varying extents idiosyncratic and not fully comprehensible to the listener. This was generally true for all the age groups on the first trial, but on subsequent trials, with feedback, there was improvement for all groups except the kindergarten children. Only the performance of ninth-grade children approximated that of adults on this task, and that was found only after a number of trials. Krauss and Glucksberg concluded that inadequate communication of younger children may be an expression of egocentrism, that is, a failure of the speaker to take the listener's perspective into account. For older children a more likely factor was that they are able to assume the perspectives of others but may fail to do so when task requirements are excessive.

Assessment of referential communication in populations with disabilities has been an area of clinical and research interest. The value of this approach is illustrated in a novel study by

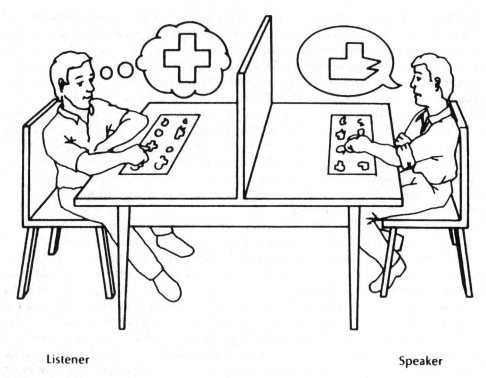

Listener   Speaker

FIGURE 5.5. Referential communication task assessing a speaker's ability to convey information to a listener.

Longhurst (1974), who used the speaker–listener paradigm to examine descriptions given by adolescents with mental retardation. Communicative adequacy was assessed in four speaker–listener combinations: speaker with retardation–listener with retardation; speaker with retardation–normally developing listener; normally developing speaker–listener with retardation; and a listener with retardation listening to her or his own descriptions on tape. The results revealed that the highest communicative adequacy was found for the normally developing speaker–listener with retardation, followed by the person with retardation listening to his or her own descriptions on tape. This finding indicated that poor performance on the task was accounted for by speakers with retardation who gave idiosyncratic and noncommunicative descriptions. The nature of communicative problems and the identity of the speaker have also been studied by Abbeduto, Short-Meyerson, Benson, and Dolish (1997) to document the performance of children and adolescents with mental retardation. Such information has diagnostic value in distinguishing between speaker-versus-listener contributions to communicative effectiveness (Abbeduto, Short-Meyerson, Benson, Dolish, & Weissman, 1998), with implications for defining the level and focus of communication intervention.

Schwartz (1983) compared the referential communication skills of children with visual impairment and sighted children between 7 and 9 years of age on a task in which the participant was to provide a description of novel forms to a nonpresent peer. Schwartz found that children with visual impairment verbalized more but that the nature of their encodings did not differ from sighted peers.

A limitation of the two-person task is the requirement for participation by two subjects. To bypass this problem, Greenspan (1976) developed a task that could be administered to one child. We have developed a similar task that can be used to assess referential communication skills of children and adolescents with disabilities, including those with sensory impairments. The COMTASK consists of two shelves, on each of which are inverted eight different containers varying along these dimensions: size (large/small), shape (round/square), color (yellow/blue), and texture (rough/smooth). The child's task is to place ten small objects under different containers and then fully describe the locations of those objects to the examiner, who is in another room and who has not seen the placement of the objects. The child's descriptions are scored in terms of figurative (form, size, color) or operative (location, direction, number) referents. A comparative study revealed poorer communication performance with lower use of figurative responses by emotionally disturbed adolescents compared with nondisturbed peers (Rosenthal & Simeonsson, 1991). Tasks of this nature can yield diagnostic information about specific elements of difficulties in referential communication, providing the basis for targeted intervention. The utility of such application has been demonstrated in a study comparing the referential communication skills of children with and without mental retardation at the mental ages of 5, 8, and 11 years (Brownell & Whitley, 1992). Results revealed that messages of children with mental retardation were less informative than those of their peers without mental retardation. However, directed training involving perceptual feedback improved their communication skills, supporting the utility of such assessment for planned interventions.

Personal and Social

Assessment of personal and social characteristics from a qualitative developmental perspective can be defined as focusing primarily on the manner in which the developing child constructs social reality. In practical terms, this has taken the form of assessing the emergence of self–other differentiation from infancy through adolescence (Table 5.4).

At the sensorimotor level, emerging self–other differentiation can be assessed through observation of the child's use of toys, as described by Lowe (1975). Using a variety of standard toys (toy trucks, toy furniture, dolls, etc.), it was found that the nature of children's play began to change around 20 months, in that doll-related play increased and self-related play decreased. The symbolic play of infants without disabilities follows a developmental sequence beginning with banging in 7-month-olds, simple relational acts in 9-month-olds, accommodative relational acts for 13-month-olds, and the demonstration of symbolic play in all 20-month-olds (Fenson, Kagan, Kearsley, & Zelazo, 1976). Generally, between 2 and 6 years of age, play progression has been found to become increasingly decentered, decontextualized, and integrated (Lyytinen, 1991). To document this changing complexity of symbolic play, Lewis, Boucher, and Astell (1992) have developed the Warwick Symbolic Play Test to extend assessment through age 6. The task is designed to be administered using minimal language and assesses spontaneous, modeled, or instructed play. Studies of children with mental retardation, autism, and deafness have demonstrated the value of assessing symbolic play given its association with mental and language development (Casby & Ruder, 1983; Gould, 1986; Spencer, 1996). These findings indicate that assessment of symbolic play in children with disabilities has value both as an index of the child's representational competence and as a marker of language development (Casby, 1997).

The emergence of symbolic skills in the preoperational period provides a basis for assessing self–other differentiation through representation of human figure drawings. As with other skills, this form of representation follows a developmental sequence reflecting progress toward more realistic drawings of the human figure. Referring to earlier work by Piaget, and Inhelder (1969) emphasized that the drawings progress from what the child knows to what he or she sees. The first stage in this progress, around two years of age, is defined as "fortuitous realism," in that the child develops what is drawn in the act of drawing it. A year or two later, the child draws recognizable elements resulting in the "tadpole" person. This is a stage of "failed realism" in that only selected elements (head and legs) are included. Around age 5 years or so, drawings reflect "intellectual realism" in that the drawing is conceptually complete, but fails to take into account visual perspective or proportionality. It is only around age 8 or 9 that the child's drawing reflects "visual realism," accurately conveying a visual perspective and proportional dimensions.

This developmental progression in the child's ability to represent self and others through drawings is a common approach useful for children with disabilities. Cox and Howarth (1989) provided a good example of this approach in a study that compared the human figure drawings of 8- to 9-year-old children with mental retardation with their mental age (MA) and chronological age (CA) peers. The human figure drawings of children with mental retardation were generally of the tadpole form, resembling the performance of their MA rather than their CA peers.

Self–other differentiation through the use of human figure drawings has been demonstrated in the differential performances of adolescents with psychic-spectrum or conduct-disordered diagnosis (Miller, Atlas, & Arsenio, 1993). In a somewhat different application, the utility of assessing object drawings has been extended to studies of children with specific visual-motor integration problems, such as Williams syndrome (Berthand, Mervis, & Eisenberg, 1997). A novel human figure drawing application, described by Tryphon and Montangero (1992), may be useful in the assessment of children with disabilities and chronic conditions. Building on the child's concept of historical and personal time, the task uses their drawings to measure children's diachronic thinking. Following their drawing of a human figure, the child is asked if he or she always drew that way. Then the child is asked to draw one or more drawings to indicate how he or she drew when they were younger. The analysis of the children's drawings involved quantitative elements (size, number of elements), and qualitative elements (realism and perspective). The child was also encouraged to assign dates to the drawings. Not only do these analyses document developmental progress in the child's representation of time, but also they provide a window on the child's understanding of chronology as a factor defining his or her own development. As such, assessment of diachronic thinking yields a marker of self–other differentiation in the child as defined by levels of awareness of self as a developing individual with a history.

Assessment of self–other differentiation at the preoperational and later stages has involved a variety of perspective-taking tasks (Table 5.4). The development of role taking has been of some controversy as to age/stage of accomplishment and whether egocentrism is a unitary construct (Liotti, 1992; Serra, Minderaa, Van Geert, & Jackson, 1995). Perspective-taking tasks, however, have been found useful to assess the development of self–other differentiation, with a substantial literature documenting the emergence and nature of role taking from preoperational through formal operational stages.

A classic study by Selman and Byrne (1974) of role-taking performance of children 4, 6, 8, and 10 years of age demonstrated four levels of role-taking ability coinciding with stage transitions in cognitive development. Level 0, labeled egocentric role taking, was associated with the preoperational stage. Levels I and II, labeled as subjective and self-reflective role taking, respectively, were associated with children in the concrete operational stage. From Level I to Level II, children progressed from understanding the subjectivity of others' perspectives to the ability to assume the perspectives of others sequentially. Only at Level III, labeled mutual role taking, were children able to assume their own and others' perspectives simultaneously. Level III was associated with formal operations.

Research has provided evidence that perspective-taking skills can be assessed in children with various disabilities documenting performance in sequential qualitative levels. As the nature of tasks vary, it is important that inferences about perspective-taking abilities are qualified in terms of the specific tasks used in assessment. The value of assessing perspective-taking skills in children with disabilities is twofold; one, it documents the child's awareness of self and others; second, it provides markers of social-cognitive development.

At the earliest level, this awareness takes two forms: recognition of self as the object of knowledge and recognition of self as the subject of experience (Bullock & Luetkenhaus, 1990). The tasks used to document typical development of self-recognition on this approach are applicable to young children with disabilites. Self-recognition in a mirror task has been found to be consistent with developmental age in children with mental retardation (Loveland, 1987) but associated with a significant deficit in children with autism (Mitchell, 1997).

An alternative way in which to assess the development of self–other awareness in children is through the use of person-perception measures. Person perception refers to the manner in which an individual describes attributes, qualities, traits, and characteristics in another person. A common method for assessing person perception is to analyze the words a child uses to describe someone else. This approach has been examined developmentally by Secord and Peevers (1973), who asked participants at five age levels (kindergarten, 3rd, 7th, and 11th grades, and college) to describe three liked and one disliked acquaintances. Findings revealed a developmental sequence, with descriptions of others becoming more differentiated, less egocentric, more mutual and other-oriented, more dispositional, abstract, and qualified with age. Using a similar approach, Barenboim (1981) has documented a developmental sequence encompassing behavioral comparisons, psychological constructs, and psychological comparisons from childhood to adolescence.

The assessment of person perception in children with disabilities can document the developmental dimensions within which they differentiate liked and disliked peers or adults. Applications with special populations include studies on children with hearing impairments (Weisel & Bar-Lev, 1992), children and adolescents with mental retardation (Cates & Shontz, 1990), and children with conduct disorder (Matthys, Walterbos, Nijo, & Van Engeland, 1989). These studies have demonstrated that children with developmental disabilities have delays in person perception and limited insight into the attributes and characteristics of others. Assessing person perception may be particularly useful with children whose physical or sensory impairments may limit interpersonal experiences or whose emotional problems may be defined by relationships that are inappropriate or problematic.

Because limited awareness of self and others is often a common characteristic of children with disabilities, perspective-taking and referential tasks provide a practical way to document their personal and social development. With the current emphasis on social integration in regular classrooms and the community settings, assessment of social awareness is an important priority in planning interventions.

Assessment of moral understanding has been a topic of interest in child development research for many decades. The development of moral judgment was the focus of one of Piaget's major books (1948). From a qualitative-developmental perspective, assessment of moral understanding has been considered in two ways, each of which has been employed with children with disabilities. One of these derives from Piaget's original work focusing on the child's understanding of intent and consequence. The second approach, developed by Kohlberg (1969) utilizes a moral dilemma to evaluate the level of moral reasoning displayed by a child.

The classic paired-story format described by Piaget (1948) asks the child to determine which of two story characters is naughtier and should be punished the most for a particular act. The child's task is to choose between a child with good intent (wanting to help with dishes) but a poor consequence (breaking five dishes accidentally) and a child with a bad intent (not wanting to help) but a less serious consequence (breaking one dish intentionally). The pattern of children's responses in Piaget's research led him to conclude that children at the preoperational stage based their judgments on consequences, whereas children at the concrete operations stage took intent into account when making moral judgments. The first kind of moral judgment was labeled "heteronomous," whereas the second kind was labeled "autonomous." Subsequent research has taken issue with the assumption that preoperational children are necessarily restricted to a focus on consequences. Other factors to consider include the form of presentation, the sequence in which reference to intent and consequence is presented, and the systematic presentation of all four combinations of intent and consequence. This latter point addresses the limitation inherent in Piaget's original story format, in which a positive intent is coupled with a major negative consequence, whereas a negative intent is coupled with a minor negative consequence. A developmental interpretation of the difference between heteronomous and autonomous judgments may well be that the child centers on one dimension in the former and is able to decenter and consider two or more dimensions in the latter.

In this context, developmental studies of children without and with disabilities have applied a broader approach to the study of moral judgment. A basic format involving all possible combinations of intent and consequence is typically used to present verbal and/or pictorial vignettes to which the child responds in the form of a moral judgment. Responses of children can be scored quantitatively, as well as qualitatively. On a quantitative dimension, the child can be asked to make a judgment as to how good or bad a portrayed character is in a vignette, using a dimensional scale involving numbers or faces. The child's verbal explanation for the judgment can then be scored qualitatively as to references to intent or consequences. Weiner and Peters (1973) have used this approach in a study of typical children ranging in age from 5 to 18 years. Their findings indicated developmental transitions in the manner in which consequence-based judgments changed to explanations relying more on intent.

In a study of 6-year-old children with adults with mental retardation of comparable mental age, Blakey (1973) used an array of stories to assess moral judgment. These stories focused on the themes of intention versus consequence, reciprocal versus expiatory punishment, and physical consequence versus adult reaction and immanent justice and could be used to address assessment questions. Foye and Simeonsson (1979) carried out a study of moral reasoning of first-graders in public school and adolescents and adults with mental retardation, all with a comparable mean mental age of about 7 years. The results indicated that the three groups performed in a similar pattern along both quantitative and qualitative dimensions. Analyses of the two discordant intent–consequence combinations revealed that the performance of all three groups was influenced by the consequence dimension, with positive intent–negative consequence and negative intent–positive consequence yielding essentially the same numerical score. This was in contrast to the moral judgment of typical fourth-graders, who assigned a rating twice as large to the former than to the latter, suggesting greater attention to the dimension of intent.

The value of administering moral judgment tasks lies in the information they can provide about the moral reasoning of the child or adolescent with disabilities. This can be illustrated by comparing the individual profiles of four adolescents with mental retardation who participated in the Foye and Simeonsson (1979) study. Although they had essentially the same mental age, chronological age, and IQ, their moral judgments varied dramatically, from patterns indicative of total consequence-based judgments to a clear recognition of the mediating role of intent (Figure 5.6). Assessment of moral judgment and other aspects of social understanding may thus provide unique diagnostic information about children with disabilities. Nucci and Herman (1982), for example, demonstrated the difficulty experienced by children with behavior disorders differentiating among moral, conventional, and personal issues.

The second major strategy to assess moral judgment has involved the use of Kohlberg's moral dilemmas (1969), based on three major stages of preconventional, conventional, and postconventional reasoning. Kohlberg's approach has not been without some controversy with particular reference to gender differences as the basis for moral reasoning (Gilligan, 1982). A large body of research, however, has yielded evidence supporting the qualitative progression of moral reasoning in developmental and cross-cultural studies. The verbal nature of Kohlberg's tasks may restrict their use with children who are young or have severe mental limitations. Their application may be indicated with older children and adolescents and those with adequate verbal skills when moral reasoning is of interest in defining individualized interventions. An interesting study compared children with moderate (organic) and mild (sociocultural factors) mental retardation with nonretarded peers of the same mental age (Kahn, 1976). The performance of children with mild mental retardation was comparable to that of their nondisabled mental-age peers, whereas qualitative differences were found for children with moderate mental retardation. The findings suggested the interpretation that mental retardation due to sociocultural factors reflected only quan-

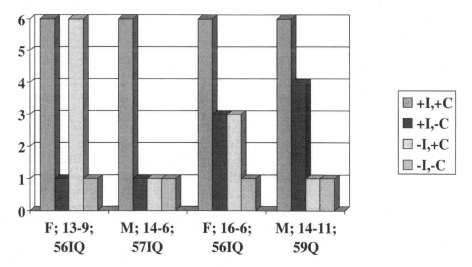

FIGURE 5.6. Individual differences in moral judgment of four adolescents with mental retardation: ratings of stories (very good –6 to very bad –1) counterbalancing positive or negative values for intent (I) and consequence (C).

titative differences (that is, IQ), whereas observed qualitative differences reflected moderate mental retardation associated with organic etiologies. The use of Kohlberg's test with students with hearing impairment supported a relationship between structure of moral reasoning and language development (Sam & Wright, 1988). Findings of this nature support the diagnostic and prescriptive utility of identifying the basis of moral reasoning using either the traditional paired-story format or Kohlberg's dilemma approach.

Behavior

The assessment contributions of Piaget's theory have primarily focused on the quality of children's cognitions about the physical and social world around them. To the extent that cognitions influence social relationships, extensions of Piaget's theory have also included such domains as referential communication, person perception, and role taking. The assessment of behavior is not based directly on Piaget's work, but there are a number of assessment measures and strategies of behavior that are qualitative in nature and that are included for review here because of their demonstrated or potential applicability with children with disabilities and chronic conditions. Measures of behavior are defined as those that assess what children actually do or say they will do. This serves to differentiate them from measures focusing on thoughts or perceptions of their physical and social world. Furthermore, these measures will be considered in terms of Piaget's developmental stages, even though some were not developed specifically within that frame of reference. Within the context of this chapter, measures of behavior are defined as those that assess what children in various settings do. This may seem to be a narrow and arbitrary definition, but it is important to differentiate measures of behavior from other measures focusing on children's thoughts or perceptions of their physical and social world. A list of selected tasks is presented in Table 5.4.

Behavioral assessment of children's functioning within the sensorimotor stage presents a challenge when they have mental, motor, and/or sensory impairments. As we indicated in Chapter 3, valid assessment of such populations is problematic due to diagnostic ambiguity, instrument limitations, examiner limitations, and limited response capability of the child (Simeonsson, Huntington, & Parse, 1980). To address some of these problems, we developed an instrument with a qualitative focus and ordinal scales. The Carolina Record of Individual Behavior (CRIB; Simeonsson, Huntington, Short, & Ware, 1982) is an observational measure. It consists of three sections (A, B, C); A addresses developmental characteristics, and B and C document behavioral characteristics. The CRIB was designed to capture the sensorimotor level of functioning and is thus suitable for young children with disabilities or for older children whose functioning is at a very basic developmental level. The CRIB was derived in part from items on the Infant Behavior Record (Bayley, 1969) and can be used with individuals of any age. A unique feature of the CRIB is that it addresses a major assessment concern with children with disabilities mentioned in Chapter 3, namely, child responsivity defined by states of arousal. Systematic assessment of state has been found important to document in newborn behavior (Brazelton, 1973) and seems equally important with infants and children who have disabilities, given the likelihood of CNS dysfunction associated with the impairment or with medication or both (Simeonsson et al., 1982). To this end, the CRIB requires the documentation of initial and predominant state of arousal, as well as a record of all the shifts in responsivity (states) observed for the period of assessment. Such documentation can serve to qualify overall assessment findings in terms of the responsivity of the child. Thus assessment of a child whose predominant performance state was one of drowsiness would be less valid than that of a child whose predominant state was one of quiet alertness. It may also serve as a marker of development in its own right, in that response variability should decrease and state consistency and organization should increase with development (Simeonsson et al., 1980). As an observational measure the CRIB can be completed either on the basis of observing the administration of developmental scales or on the basis of a period of systematic interaction with the child. The CRIB has been used in a number of studies involving young children with varying disabilities and severity levels (Bagnato & Mayes, 1986; Beckman, Thiele, Pokorni, & Balzer, 1986; Short & Simeonsson, 1990). This documentation takes the form of profiles of individual characteristics, as shown in Figure 5.7. Factor analysis has provided support for the designation of Section A items as developmental and Section B items as behavioral (Simeonsson, Huntington, Short, & Ware, 1982). Repeated assessment with the same children has also yielded evidence that Section A items, such as object orientation and receptive and expressive communication, are ordinal in nature and do reflect change with development. The importance of assessing state as a mediating variable on functioning of students with profound disabilities has also been advocated by Guess and his colleagues (1993).

A qualitative measure of behavior that includes the sensorimotor, as well as the preoperational, stages is peer-play development. Assessment involves the observation of the manner in which the infant and young child interacts with peers. This interaction is scored along physical dimensions such as proximity and use of objects and along social dimensions such as reciprocity and communication. The classic assessment framework for this

• Initial state	1 2 3 4 5 6 7 8 9	_____
• Predominant state	1 2 3 4 5 6 7 8 9	_____
• All states observed	1 2 3 4 5 6 7 8 9	_____
• **Section A**		
• Social orientation	1 2 3 4 5 6 7 8 9 NA	_____
• Participation	1 2 3 4 5 6 7 8 9 NA	_____
• Motivation	1 2 3 4 5 6 7 8 9 NA	_____
Endurance	1 2 3 4 5 6 7 8 9 NA	_____
• Expressive Communication	1 2 3 4 5 6 7 8 9 NA	_____
• Receptive Communication	1 2 3 4 5 6 7 8 9 NA	_____
• Object Orientation	1 2 3 4 5 6 7 8 9 NA	_____
• Consolability	1 2 3 4 5 6 7 8 9 NA	_____
• **Section B**		
• Activity	1 2 3 4 5 6 7 8 9 NA	_____
• Reactivity	1 2 3 4 5 6 7 8 9 NA	_____
• Goal Directedness	1 2 3 4 5 6 7 8 9 NA	_____
• Frustration	1 2 3 4 5 6 7 8 9 NA	_____
• Attention span	1 2 3 4 5 6 7 8 9 NA	_____
• Responsiveness/caregiver	1 2 3 4 5 6 7 8 9 NA	_____
• Body tone	1 2 3 4 5 6 7 8 9 NA	_____
• Responsiveness/examiner	1 2 3 4 5 6 7 8 9 NA	_____
• **Section C**		
• Rhythmic habit patterns	1 2 3 4 5 6 7 8 9 NA	_____

FIGURE 5.7. Carolina Record of Individual Behavior (CRIB): Summary dimensions.

OBJECT PLAY (*)	PEER PLAY (#)	PRETEND PLAY (+)
Banging, stereotypical play (7 months)		Nonpretend play
Simple relational play (9 months)		
Accommodative relational play (13 months)		Self-directed acts
Symbolic play (20 months)	Looking (1½–2 yrs)	Decentration; Passive other-directed acts; object-directed acts
	Parallel play (2 yrs)	Short sequences; 2–3 play themes
	Fleeting contact (2–2½ yrs)	
	Rigid contact (2½–3yrs)	Active other-directed acts
	Associative play (4 yrs)	Decontextualization; Substitutive acts, inventive acts
	Cooperative play (5 yrs)	Integration; Single-scheme combinations; multischeme combinations
		Events/episodes; 4, 5, 6 play acts

FIGURE 5.8. Developmental transitions in object, peer, and pretend play in the first 6 years of life. Data from (*) Fenson, Kagan, Kearsley, & Zelazo (1976); (#) Whiteside, Busch, & Horner (1976); (+) Lyytinen (1991).

domain was developed by Parten (1932). The developmental sequence of peer play she described is similar to the sequence observed by Whiteside, Busch, and Horner (1976). The emergence of social play in the child, along with symbolic play, is clearly an important marker of cognitive and communicative development. The developmental sequence of symbolic play is paired with that of peer play (Figure 5.8), indicating that on the basis of physical and cognitive skills the young child first develops mastery of play with objects and then acquires mastery of play with peers. Because inappropriate or delayed symbolic and social play is frequently observed in infants and young children with disabilities, systematic assessment of these domains is of value diagnostically and in the development of intervention activities. Cornelius and Hornett (1990) and Erwin (1993) have illustrated the value of assessing peer play in children with learning impairment and visual impairment, respectively.

Problem solving is an assessment domain applicable for children with disabilities functioning at or above the preoperational stage. The focus here is on assessing how children say they would solve a specific situational problem. An area of substantial interest in this regard has been that of theory of mind (TOM) tasks with both children and adults. This approach consists of structured interpersonal situations described or illustrated to a child, who is then asked to solve the problem. The prototypic task is the "Sally and Anne Task" (Baron-Cohen, Leslie, & Frith, 1985) in which one of two story characters has information that the other does not. The child's task is to recognize this distinction in solving an interpersonal problem. Because these problems are often representative of the interpersonal conflicts that occur in everyday situations, assessment of this domain may provide a good index of the problem-solving skills possessed and implemented by the child with disabilities. Application of TOM measures have included children with deafness (Peterson & Siegal, 1995), autism (Buitelaar, Van der Wees, Swabb-Barneveld, & Van der Gaag, 1999), and mental retardation (Tager-Flusberg & Sullivan, 2000). In general these studies have supported TOM deficits associated with persons with autism and mental retardation. To the extent that problem-solving skills require cognitive strategies and social insight, performance on TOM measures can provide useful insights on social understanding and skills of individual children. Further utility may derive from the distinction between social-cognitive and social-perceptual components of TOM, as noted by Tager-Flusberg and Sullivan (2000) in a study of children with Williams syndrome.

A measure of problem-solving behavior assessing the stage transition from concrete to formal operations is a scale developed by Elkind and Bowen (1979) on the expression of self-consciousness in children. This scale was based on the concept of social egocentrism in early adolescence, expressed in children's preoccupations with the thoughts of others about themselves. Drawing on cognitive-developmental theory, Elkind (1967) has labeled two of these expressions of self-consciousness as the "imaginary audience" and the "personal fable" of early adolescence. The Imaginary Audience Scale (IAS; Elkind & Bowen, 1979) presents vignettes about social situations focusing on the transient self (e.g., appearance) and the abiding self (e.g., traits). Elkind hypothesized that this form of self-consciousness would be most evident in early adolescence, reflecting entry into the stage of formal operations. It would not be evident prior to this phase because of the cognitive limitations of the younger child in regard to insight and would cease to be an issue in older adolescents given increasing cognitive sophistication. Elkind and Bowen (1979) found support for their hypothesis in a cross-sectional study, which found that 8th-grade students were more self-conscious than either 4th-graders or 12th-graders. In a later study, using the IAS, Adams and Jones (1981) found that self-consciousness was not unique to younger adolescents but characterized 10th- and 12th-graders, a result that may have been due to differences in the nature of the samples in the two studies. Taken collectively, however, the findings suggested that the self-consciousness and independent behavior seen in adolescence have a significant cognitive component. Elkind maintains that the give and take of social experience and feedback subsequently contribute to a more realistic appraisal of self and others.

Measures such as the IAS and others by Enright, Shukla, and Lapsley (1980) and Lapsley (1993) tap areas of personal awareness pertaining to self-appraisal and self-identity that are usually not included among traditional instruments of personal behavior. As such, they represent an approach that may be useful to consider in the assessment of adolescents and young adults whose impairments and limited social experiences may contribute to unrealistic perceptions of themselves and their peers. The value of the IAS approach lies in the assessment strategy, in which the presentation of common social situations requires the respondent to indicate feelings about the resolution of a personal dilemma (e.g., unaffected, accepting, self-conscious). An added feature of potential significance with special populations is that half of the IAS items measure abiding self (permanent traits) and half measure transient self (situational factors). Analyses along these dimensions may be useful in identifying the extent to which self-appraisal of adolescents with disabilities is a function of factors seen as permanent and unchangeable (e.g., impairment) and those seen as situational and changeable (e.g., social experiences). This premise was tested in a study using the IAS with emotionally disturbed adolescents and their nondisturbed peers (Simeonsson & Rosenthal, 1989). Differences in self-consciousness, mediated by gender, were found between the two groups. These and other findings demonstrate that measures of this type are suitable to administer, yielding both quantitative (resolution choice) and qualitative (explanation) data. For children and adolescents with disabilities who are verbal, measures of self-appraisal may be useful to administer in that they contribute information about their social understanding and self–other differentiation.

RECOMMENDATIONS FOR PRACTICE

Assessing children with disabilities from a qualitative-developmental perspective differs from that of standardized psychometric testing in several ways. The fundamental purpose of assessment differs in that the former seeks to document the child's quality of reasoning regardless of age, whereas in the latter strategy comparability to age norms is central. Although the number of formal instruments for qualitative-developmental assessment is limited, many tasks are described in writings by Piaget and in works based on his theory. Both quantitative and qualitative assessment have assets and limitations. The purpose of assessment should dictate the selection of the strategy most appropriate to answer an assessment question. In many instances data obtained with one approach complements the other.

In summarizing the material reviewed in this chapter, two points need consideration regarding the integration of qualitative-developmental assessment data and its implementation in intervention plans. First, it is clear that the formal instruments and nonstandardized procedures place limitations on generalization of qualitative assessment results. Although some of the tasks and measures described in this chapter have been used with some frequency in research or clinical contexts, others have seen only limited application. There are, however, studies examining the psychometric properties of qualitative-developmental measures as illustrated by the reliability determination of social intelligence tasks (Mathias & Nettlebeck, 1992). The inclusion of measures in this chapter was based on their demonstrated or perceived appropriateness for the assessment of children with disabilities. It is likely that many clinicians use a variety of measures that may be based on qualitative approaches. In the assessment of a child, it may be that a measure of play not described in this book may be as appropriate as those described here, as long as both measures were derived from a similar conceptual base and differ only in administrative details. The qualitative findings and the implications for intervention may ultimately be the same. Because there is continued interest in the clinical and research applications of cognitive-developmental theory, further development and refinement of assessment measures can be anticipated.

A second consideration pertains to the conceptual framework of the assessment process. The conceptualization of the child's assessment needs, the purpose of the assessment, and the interpretation of the assessment results must all be tied together logically. Although this statement applies to any assessment approach, it is particularly applicable when assessment is couched in theory-specific terms, such as conservation, egocentrism, or symbolic play, as distinct from the generic terms of intelligence, language, or personality, respectively. Inhelder (1966) has spoken clearly to this issue: "From our point of view we should not dissociate these diagnostic tools from the theory on which they are based. For this reason, the practitioner who desires to employ them must back up his procedures with an interpretation that is within the theoretical system. It is only in this way that he can realize the full significance of the many details he observes in the behavior of the child" (pp. 301–302). Increasing efforts are being made to develop conceptual models based on an integration of theoretical and empirical contributions that can be drawn upon in the selection and interpretation of assessment measures. Greenspan and Granfield (1992), for example, have developed a multidimensional model of personal competence. The value of such models lie not only in their theoretical derivation but also in their implications for systematic assessment of distinct elements of social intelligence.

In closing, the following guidelines are recommended when summarizing findings from qualitative-developmental assessment (Table 5.5). In writing the assessment report, the first

TABLE 5.5. Guidelines for Summarizing and Interpreting Qualitative-Developmental Assessment Results

Step	Example
1. Define domain/focus of assessment	1. Assessment of one specific facet of cognition, namely that of causality to determine the quality of nature of reasoning.
2. Define specific task or procedure employed	2. Causal reasoning assessed by administering a set of questions pertaining to the attribution of life and life traits to animate and inanimate objects.
3. Describe assessment results in nontechnical, nontheoretical terms	3. Responses reflect whether child has attributed life and life traits only to plants and animals or included inanimate objects.
4. Limitations of the assessed domain should be made clear	4. The child's understanding of causality in regard to life and life traits represent a selected and limited aspect of cognitive reasoning abilities.
5. Present implications of assessment results within theoretical framework from which it is derived	5. Responses may indicate precausal animistic reasoning in which life or life traits are inferred on the basis of movement of any kind (preoperational thought) or is restricted to spontaneous movement (operational thought).

step should be to define the domain or focus of assessment within its theoretical framework. Conservation or moral judgment, for example, would be defined developmentally as expressions of a cognitive or social-cognitive characteristic particular to a qualitative stage. Second, the specific elements of the assessment procedure or task should be described in detail because even the same concept (role taking, for example) may be operationalized and measured differently from one task to the next. Relevant supporting literature can be cited to reference the procedure or task involved. The third step is to describe assessment results in such a way that the findings are interpretable by someone not knowledgeable about the theory. It is particularly important to avoid the use of terms that are idiosyncratic to a particular theory and therefore of limited value to consumers of the report. The interpretation of results should, as in all psychological reports, include a clear statement of any limitations, that may apply to the findings. Finally, the diagnostic and/or prescriptive implications of the findings should be presented within the context of the theoretical framework in which the purpose of the assessment was developed. The strength of theory-based assessment is the derivation of a logically consistent intervention plan for promoting physical or social cognitive development related to everyday functioning. To this end, the richness of qualitative assessment can complement and extend other forms of assessment and seems particularly well suited to document the developmental characteristics of children with disabilities and chronic health conditions. Its focus on the individual and its emphasis on development contribute to the essential principle of developmental interpretation "that all behavior is to be seen as the result of an active elaboration on the part of the subject. This elaboration more over, has a different aspect at each level of attainment" (Inhelder, 1966, p. 302).

REFERENCES

Abbeduto, L., Short-Meyerson, K., Benson, G., & Dolish, J. (1997). Signaling of noncomprehension by children and adolescents with mental retardation: Effects of problem type and speaker identity. *Journal of Speech, Language, and Hearing Research, 40,* 20–32.

Abbeduto, L., Short-Meyerson, K., Benson, G., Dolish, J., & Weissman, M. (1998). Understanding referential expressions in context: Use of common ground by children and adolescents with mental retardation. *Journal of Speech, Language, and Hearing Research, 41,* 1348–1362.

Abrahamsen, E. P., & Mitchell, J. R. (1990). Communication and sensorimotor functioning in children with autism. *Journal of Autism and Developmental Disorders, 20*(1), 75–85.

Adams, G. R., & Jones, R. M. (1981). Imaginary audience behavior: A validation study. *Journal of Early Adolescence, 1,* 1–10.

Bagnato, S. J., & Mayes, S. D. (1986). Patterns of developmental and behavioral progress for young brain-injured children during interdisciplinary intervention. *Developmental Neuropsychology, 2*(3), 213–240.

Barenboim, C. (1981). The development of person perception from childhood to adolescence: From behavioral comparisons to psychological constructs to psychological comparisons. *Child Development, 52,* 129–144.

Baron-Cohen, S., Leslie, A. M., & Frith, U. (1985). Does the autistic child have a "theory of mind"? *Cognition, 21*(1), 37–46.

Bates, E., Benigni, L., Bretherton, I., Camaioni, L., & Volterra, V. (1977). From gesture to the first word: On cognitive and social prerequisites. In M. Lewis & L. A. Rosenblum (Eds.), *Interaction, conversation and the development of language.* New York: Wiley.

Bates, E., Camaioni, L., & Volterra, V. (1975). The acquisition of performatives prior to speech. *Merrill–Palmer Quarterly, 21,* 205–226.

Bayley, N. (1969). *Bayley scales of infant development.* New York: Psychological Corporation.

Beckman, P. J., Thiele, J. E., Pokorni, J. L., & Balzer, M. L. (1986). Stability of behavioral characteristics in preterm infants. *Topics in Early Childhood Special Education, 6*(2), 57–67.

Berhand, J., Merris, C. B., & Eisenberg, J. D. (1997). Drawing in children with Williams syndrome: A developmental perspective. *Developmental Neuropsychology, 13*(1), 41–67.

Best, B., & Roberts, G. (1976). Early cognitive development in hearing impaired children. *American Annals of the Deaf, 121,* 560–564.

Beveridge, M., & Davies, M. (1983). A picture sorting approach to the study of child animism. *Genetic Psychology Monographs, 107,* 211–231.

Blacher, J. (1982). Assessing social cognition in young retarded and non-retarded children. *American Journal of Mental Deficiency, 86,* 473–484.

Blakey, R. S. (1973). Moral judgements in subnormal adults and normal children. *British Journal of Mental Subnormality, 19,* 85–89.

Brazelton, T. B. (1973). *Neonatal Behavioral Assessment Scale.* London: Heinemann Medical Books.

Brown, A. L. (1973). Conservation of quantity in normal, bright and retarded children. *Child Development, 44,* 376–379.

Brownell, M. D., & Whiteley, J. H. (1992). Development and training of referential communication in children with mental retardation. *American Journal on Mental Retardation, 97*(2), 161–171.

Bruner, J. S. (1965). The growth of mind. *American Psychologist, 20,* 1007–1017.

Buitelaar, J., Van der Wees, M., Swaab-Barneveld, H., & Van der Gaag, R. J. (1999). Theory of mind and emotion-recognition functioning in autistic spectrum disorders and in psychiatric control and normal children. *Development and Psychopathology, 11,* 39–58.

Bullock, M., & Luetkenhaus, P. (1990). Who am I? Self-understanding in toddlers. *Merrill–Palmer Quarterly, 36*(2), 217–238.

Casby, M. W. (1997). Symbolic play of children with language impairment: A critical review. *Journal of Speech and Hearing Research, 40*(3), 468–479.

Casby, M. W., & Ruder, K. F. (1983). Symbolic play and early language development in normal and mentally retarded children. *Journal of Speech and Hearing Research, 26*(3), 404–411.

Cates, D., & Shontz, F. (1990). Role-taking ability and social behavior in deaf school children. *American Annals of the Deaf, 135*(3), 217–221.

Cornelius, G., & Hornett, D. (1990). The play behavior of hearing-impaired kindergarten children. *American Annals of the Deaf, 135*(4), 316–321.

Cowan, P. A. (1978). *Piaget with feeling: Cognitive, social and emotional development.* New York: Holt, Rinehart & Winston.

Cox, M. V., & Howarth, C. (1989). The human figure drawing of normal children and those with severe learning difficulties. *British Journal of Developmental Psychology, 7,* 333–339.

Dimcovic, N. (1992). Why is the change in the task difficult for blind children? *European Journal of Psychology of Education, 7*(3), 231–244.

Dimcovic, N., & Tobin, M. J. (1995). The use of language in simple classification tasks by children who are blind. *Journal of Visual Impairment and Blindness, 89*(5), 448–459.

Dunst, C. J. (1980). *A clinical and educational manual for use with the Uzgiris and Hunt scales of infant psychological development.* Baltimore: University Park Press.

Elkind, D. (1963). The child's conception of his religious denomination: 3. The Protestant child. *Journal of Genetic Psychology, 103,* 291–304.

Elkind, D. (1967). Egocentrism in adolescence. *Child Development, 38,* 1025–1034.

Elkind, D., & Bowen, R. (1979). Imaginary audience behavior in children and adolescents. *Developmental Psychology, 15,* 36–44.

Enright, R. D., Shukla, D. G., & Lapsley, D. C. (1980). Adolescent egocentrism, sociocentrism and self-consciousness. *Journal of Youth and Adolescence, 9,* 101–116.

Erwin, E. J. (1993). Social participation of young children with visual impairments in specialized and integrated environments. *Journal of Visual Impairment and Blindness, 87,* 138–142.

Esposito, B. G., & Koorland, M. A. (1989). Play behavior of hearing impaired children: Integrated and segregated settings. *Exceptional Children, 55*(5), 412–419.

Evans, R. C. (1973). Dream conceptions and reality testing in children. *Journal of the American Academy of Child Psychiatry, 12,* 73–92.

Fakouri, M. E. (1991). Learning disabilities: A Piagetian perspective. *Psychology in the Schools, 28*(1), 70–76.

Feldman, W., & Varni, J. (1985). Conceptualizations of health and illness by children with spina bifida. *Children's Health Care, 13*(3), 102–107.

Felters, L. (1981). Object permanence development in infants with motor handicaps. *Physical Therapy, 61,* 327–333.

Fenson, L., Kagan, J., Kearsley, R., & Zelazo, P. (1976). The developmental progression of manipulative play in the first two years. *Child Development, 47,* 232–236.

Flavell, J. H. (1963). *The developmental psychology of Jean Piaget.* Princeton, NJ: Van Nostrand.

Formanek, R., & Gurian, A. (1981). *Charting intellectual development* (2nd ed.). Springfield, IL: Charles C. Thomas.

Foye, H., & Simeonsson, R. J. (1979). Quantitative and qualitative analyses of moral reasoning in children, adolescents and adults of similar mental age. *Journal of Pediatric Psychology, 4,* 197–209.

Furth, H. G. (1973). Piaget, IQ and the nature-nurture controversy. *Human Development, 16,* 61–73.

Gilligan, C. (1982). New maps of development: New visions of maturity. *American Journal of Orthopsychiatry, 52*(2), 199–212.

Gingis, B. (1995). The social/cultural implication of disability: Vygotsky's paradigm for special education. *Educational Psychologist, 30*(2), 77–81.

Goldschmid, M. L., & Bentler, P. M. (1968). *Concept assessment kit—conservation.* San Diego, CA: Educational and Industrial Testing Service.

Gould, J. (1986). The Lowe and Costello Symbolic Play Test in socially impaired children. *Journal of Autism and Developmental Disorder, 16,* 199–213.

Greenspan, S. (1976). Matrix test of referential communication. In O. G. Johnson (Ed.), *Tests and measurements in clinical development: A handbook* (Vol. 2, pp. 74–75). San Francisco: Jossey-Bass.

Greenspan, S., & Granfield, J. M. (1992). Reconsidering the construct of mental retardation: Implications of a model of social competence. *American Journal on Mental Retardation, 96,* 442–443.

Guess, D., Roberts, S., Siegel-Causey, E., Ault, M., Guy, B., Thompson, B., & Rues, J. (1993). Analysis of behavior state conditions and associated environmental variables among students with profound handicaps. *American Journal of Mental Retardation, 97*(6), 634–653.

Halpern, E. (1966). Concept development in schizophrenia: The use of traditional intelligence scales and Piagetian tasks. *Journal of the American Academy of Child Psychiatry, 5,* 66–74.

Hatwell, Y. (1985). *Piagetian reasoning and the blind*. New York: American Foundation for the Blind.

Heller, M., & Kennedy, J. (1990). Perspective taking, pictures and the blind. *Perception and Psychophysics, 48*(5), 459–466.

Hill, J. (1993). The use of the Piagetian method of critical exploration in understanding the cognitive development of children with emotional and behavioural difficulties. *Early Development and Care, 95,* 105–124.

Hogg, J., & Raynes, N. V. (1987). *Assessment in mental handicap: A guide to assessment practices, tests, and checklists*. Cambridge, MA: Brookline Books.

Inhelder, B. (1966). Cognitive development and its contribution to the diagnosis of some phenomena of mental deficiency. *Merrill–Palmer Quarterly, 12,* 299–319.

Inhelder, B. (1968). *The diagnosis of reasoning in the mentally retarded*. New York: John Day.

Kahn, J. V. (1974). Training EMR and intellectually average adolescents of low and middle SES for formal thought. *American Journal of Mental Deficiency, 79,* 397–403.

Kahn, J. V. (1976). Moral and cognitive development of moderately retarded, mildly retarded, and non-retarded individuals. *American Journal of Mental Deficiency, 81,* 209–214.

Kohlberg, L. (1964). Development of moral character and moral ideology. In M. L. Hoffman & L. W. Hoffman (Eds.), *Review of child development research* (Vol. 1, pp. 383–432). New York: Russell Sage Foundation.

Kohlberg, L. (1969). Stage and sequence: The cognitive-developmental approach to socialization. In D. A. Goslin (Ed.), *Handbook of socialization, theory and research* (pp. 347–408). Chicago: Rand McNally.

Krauss, R. M., & Glucksberg, S. (1977). Social and nonsocial speech. *Scientific American, 236,* 100–105, 138.

Kurdek, L. A., & Rodgon, M. M. (1975). Perceptual, cognitive and affective perspective taking in kindergarten through sixth grade children. *Developmental Psychology, 11,* 643–650.

Lapsley, D. (1993). Toward an integrated theory of adolescent ego development: The "new" look at adolescent egocentrism. *American Journal of Orthopsychiatry, 63*(4), 562–571.

Laurendau, M., & Pinard, A. (1962). *Causal thinking in the child, a genetic and experimental approach*. New York: International Universities Press.

Lempers, J. D., Flavell, E. R., & Flavell, J. H. (1977). The development in very young children of tacit knowledge concerning visual perception. *Genetic Psychology Monographs, 95,* 3–54.

Lewis, V., Boucher, J., & Astell, A. (1992). The assessment of symbolic play in young children: A prototype test. *European Journal of Disorders of Communication, 27,* 231–245.

Liotti, G. (1992). Egocentrism and the cognitive psychotherapy of personality disorders. *Journal of Cognitive Psychotherapy: An International Quarterly, 6*(1), 43–58.

Lister, C., & Leach, C., & Hill, J. (1990). Sequence and structure in the concept development of children with emotional and behavioral difficulties. *Journal of Genetic Psychology, 151*(3), 287–300.

Lister, C., Leach, C., & Wheeler. (1993). Developing quantity concepts in children with special needs. *Early Child Development and Care, 95,* 125–141.

Lister, C. M., & Atha, G. (1986). The use of a Piagetian approach in work with the visually handicapped child. *Early Child Development and Care, 23*(1), 63–74.

Lobato, D., Barrera, R. D., & Feldman, R. S. (1981). Sensori-motor functioning and prelinguistic communication of severely and profoundly retarded individuals. *American Journal of Mental Deficiency, 85,* 489–496.

Longhurst, T. M. (1974). Communication in retarded adolescents: Sex and intelligence level. *American Journal of Mental Deficiencies, 78,* 607–618.

Loveland, K. (1987). Behavior of young children with Down Syndrome before the mirror: Finding things reflected. *Child Development, 58,* 928–936.

Lowe, M. (1975). Trends in the development of representative play. *Journal of Child Psychology and Psychiatry, 16,* 35–47.

Lyytinen, P. (1991). Developmental trends in children's pretend play. *Child: Care, Health and Development, 17*(1), 9–20.

Martlew, M. (1989). Observations on a child with cerebral palsy and her twin sister made in an integrated nursery and at home. *Child: Care, Health and Development, 15*(3), 175–194.

Mathias, J. L., & Nettelbeck, T. (1992). Reliability of seven measures of social intelligence in a sample of adolescents with mental retardation. *Research in Developmental Disabilities, 13*(2), 131–143.

Matthys, W., Walterbos, W., Njio, L., & Van Engeland, H. (1989). Person perception in children with conduct disorders. *Journal of Child Psychology and Psychiatry and Allied Disciplines, 30*(3), 439–448.

McCune-Nicholich, L. (1976). A longitudinal study of representational play in relation to spontaneous imitation and development of multi-word utterances. *Dissertation Abstracts International, 36*(7-B), 3580–3581.

Miller, A. L., Atlas, J. A., & Arsenio, W. F. (1993). Self-other differentiation among psychotic and conduct disordered adolescents as measured by human figure drawing. *Perceptual and Motor skills, 76*(2), 397–398.

Mitchell, R. W. (1997). A comparison of the self-awareness and kinesthetic-visual matching theories of self-recognition: Autistic children and others. *Annals of the New York Academy of Sciences, 818*, 38–62.

McCormick, P., Campbell, J. W., Pasnack, R., & Perry, P. (1990). Instruction of Piagetian concepts for children with mental retardation. *Mental Retardation, 28*(6), 359–366.

Nucci, L. P., & Herman, S. (1982). Behavioral disordered children's conceptions of moral, conventional and personal issues. *Journal of Abnormal Child Psychology, 10*, 411–426.

Parten, M. B. (1932). Social participation among preschool children. *Journal of Abnormal and Social Psychology, 27*, 243–269.

Peterson, C., & Siegal, M. (1995). Deafness, conversation and theory of mind. *Journal of Child Psychology and Psychiatry, 36*(3), 459–474.

Piaget, J. (1929). *The child's conception of the world.* New York: Harcourt, Brace.

Piaget, J. (1948). *The moral judgment of the child* (M. Gabain, Trans.). Glencoe, IL: Free Press.

Piaget, J. (1952). *The child's conception of number* (C. Gattegno & F. M. Hodgson, Trans.). London: Routledge & Paul.

Piaget, J. (1954). *The construction of reality in the child.* (M. Cook, Trans.). New York: Basic Books.

Piaget, J. (1957). *The language and thought of the child.* New York: Meridian Books.

Piaget, J. (1970a). *The child's conception of movement and speed* (G. E. T. Holloway & M. J. Mackenzie, Trans.). New York: Basic Books.

Piaget, J. (1970b). *The child's conception of time* (A. J. Pomerans, Trans.). New York: Basic Books.

Piaget, J. (1970c). Piaget's theory. In P. H. Mussen (Ed.), *Carmichael's manual of child psychology* (Vol. 1). New York: Wiley.

Piaget, J. (1971). *Science of education and the psychology of the child.* New York: Viking Press.

Piaget, J. (1981). *Intelligence and affectivity: Their relationship during child development* (T. A. Brown & C. E. Kaegi, Ed. & Trans.). Palo Alto, CA: Annual Reviews.

Piaget, J., & Inhelder, B. (1969). *The psychology of the child.* New York: Basic Books.

Pring, L., Dewart, H., & Brockbank, M. (1998). Social cognition in children with visual impairments. *Journal of Visual Impairment and Blindness, 754–768.*

Rogers, S. (1977). Characteristics of the cognitive development of profoundly retarded children. *Child Development, 48*, 837–843.

Rosenthal, S. L., & Simesonsson, R. J. (1991). Communication skills in emotionally disturbed and nondisturbed adolescents. *Behavioral Disorders, 16*(3), 192–199.

Sam, A., & Wright, I. (1988). The structure of moral reasoning in hearing-impaired students. *American Annals of the Deaf, 264–269.*

Schmidt-Kitsikis, E. (1990). An interpersonal approach to mental functioning: Assessment and treatment. In D. Kuhn (Ed.), *Contributions to human development* (Vol. 20, pp. 1–104). Basel, Switzerland: Karger.

Schwartz, T. J. (1983). Social cognition in visually impaired and sighted children. *Journal of Visual Impairment and Blindness, 77*, 377–381.

Secord, B. H., & Peevers, P. F. (1973). Developmental changes in attributions of descriptive concepts to persons. *Journal of Personality and Social Psychology, 27*, 120–128.

Selman, R. L., & Byrne, D. E. (1974). A structural-developmental analysis of levels of role-taking in middle childhood. *Child Development, 45*, 803–806.

Serafica, F. C. (1971). Object concept in deviant children. *American Journal of Orthopsychiatry, 41*, 473–482.

Serra, M., Minderaa, R., Van Geert, P., & Jackson, A. (1995). Emotional role-taking abilities of children with a pervasive developmental disorder not otherwise specified. *Journal of Child Psychology and Psychiatry and Allied Disciplines, 36*(3), 475–490.

Sexton, D., Kelley, M. F., & Surbeck, E. (1990). Piagetian-based assessment. In A. F. Rotatori, R. A. Fox, D. Sexton, & J. Miller (Eds.), *Comprehensive assessment in special education: Approaches, procedures and concerns* (pp. 54–88). Springfield, IL: Charles C. Thomas.

Short, R., & Simeonsson, R. J. (1990). Stereotypical behaviors and handicapping conditions in infants and children. *Topics in Early Childhood Special Education, 10*(3), 122–130.

Simeonsson, R. J., Huntington, G. S., & Parse, S. A. (1980). Assessment of children with severe handicaps: Multiple problems, multivariate goals. *Journal of the Association for the Severely Handicapped, 5,* 55–72.

Simeonsson, R. J., Huntington, G. S., Short, R. J., & Ware, W. (1982). The Carolina Record of Individual Behavior: Characteristics of handicapped infants and children. *Topics in Early Childhood Special Education, 2,* 43–55.

Simeonsson, R. J., & Rosenthal, S. L. (1989). Emotional disturbance and the development of self-consciousness in adolescence. *Adolescence, 24*(95), 689–698.

Simeonsson, R. J., & Rosenthal, S. L. (2001). Developmental models and clinical practice. In C. E. Walker & M. C. Roberts (Eds.), *Handbook of clinical child psychology* (3rd ed.). New York: Wiley.

Smeets, P. M. (1974). The influence of MA and CA on the attribution of life and life traits to animate and inanimate objects. *Journal of Genetic Psychology, 124,* 17–27.

Snyder, L. (1978). Communication and cognitive abilities and disabilities in the sensorimotor period. *Merrill–Palmer Quarterly, 24,* 161–180.

Somerville, S. C. (1974). The pendulum problem: Patterns of performance defining developmental styles. *British Journal of Educational Psychology, 44,* 266–281.

Spencer, P. (1996). The association between language and symbolic play at two years: Evidence from deaf toddlers. *Child Development, 67,* 867–876.

Stephens, B., & Grube, C. (1982). Development of Piagetian reasoning in congenitally blind children. *Journal of Visual Impairment and Blindness, 76,* 132–143.

Tager-Flusberg, H., & Sullivan, K. (2000). A componential view of theory of mind: Evidence from Williams syndrome. *Cognition, 76,* 59–89.

Tryphon, A., & Montangero, J. (1992). The development of diachronic thinking in children: Children's ideas about changes in drawing skills. *International Journal of Behavioral Development, 15*(3), 411–424.

Urberg, K. A., & Docherty, E. M. (1976). Development of role-taking skills in young children. *Developmental Psychology, 12,* 198–204.

Uzgiris, L. C., & Hunt, J. M. (1975). *Ordinal Scales of Intellectual Development.* Urbana: University of Illinois Press.

Volpe, R. (1976). Orthopedic disability, restriction and role-taking activity. *Journal of Special Education, 10,* 371–381.

von Glaserfeld, E., & Kelly, M. F. (1982). On the concepts of period, phase, stage and level. *Human Development, 25,* 152–160.

Vygotsky, L. (1978). *Mind in society.* Cambridge, MA: Harvard University Press.

Wadsworth, B. J. (1996). *Piaget's theory of cognitive and affective development* (5th Ed.). White Plains, NY: Longman.

Wang, P. P., & Bellugi, U. (1993). Williams syndrome, Down syndrome, and cognitive neuroscience. *American Journal of Disease and Children, 147,* 1246–1251.

Webb, R. A. (1974). Concrete and formal operations in very bright 6–11-year-olds. *Human Development, 17,* 292–300.

Weiner, B., & Peters, N. (1973). A cognitive developmental analysis of achievement and moral judgments. *Developmental Psychology, 9,* 290–309.

Weisel, A., & Bar-Lev, H. (1992). Role-taking ability, nonverbal sensitivity, language and social adjustment of deaf adolescents. *Educational Psychology, 12*(1), 3–13.

Werner, H. (1957). The concept of development from a comparative and organismic point of view. In D. Harris (Ed.), *The concept of development: An issue in the study of human behavior.* Minneapolis: University of Minnesota Press.

Whiteside, M. F., Busch, F., & Horner, T. (1976). From egocentric to cooperative play in young children. *Journal of the American Academy of Child Psychiatry, 15,* 294–313.

Williams, K. C. (1996). Piagetian principles: Simple and effective applications. *Journal of Intellectual Disability Research, 40,* 110–119.

Wohlheuter, M. J., & Sindberg, R. M. (1975). Longitudinal development of object permanence in mentally retarded children: An exploratory study. *American Journal of Mental Deficiency*, *79*, 513–518.

Woodyatt, G. C., & Ozanne, E. (1993). A longitudinal study of cognitive skills and communication behaviours in children with Rett syndrome. *Journal of Intellectual Disability Research*, *37*, 419–435.

Yirmiya, N., & Shulman, C. (1996). Seriation, conservation, and theory of mind abilities in individuals with autism, individuals with mental retardation, and normally developing children. *Child Development*, *67*(5), 2045–2059.

Yirmiya, N., Sigman, M., & Zacks, D. (1994). Perceptual perspective-taking and seriation abilities in high-functioning children with autism. *Development and Psychopathology*, *6*(2), 263–272.

6

AN ECOBEHAVIORAL APPROACH
IN CLINICAL ASSESSMENT

RUNE J. SIMEONSSON
ELIZABETH KELLEY BOYLES

I'm in the tenth grade at school. I got straight A's the last five years. To get into the high school I'm going to, I really had to fight because they said they did not allow anyone in wheelchairs. One counselor said, "It's against our policy." Some of the classrooms are upstairs, all my Social Studies and English. I really had to fight them. Then I found out that another girl had gone there ten years ago. How she got upstairs was really neat. The football team—they made arrangements ahead of time—whenever she had classes upstairs they met and carried her up and down the stairs.

In the fourth grade I had the same fight. Then, I was on crutches. They said, "You can't go because somebody might knock you over and hurt you." They said, "Use a wheelchair." So I bought a wheelchair just to make them happy and never used it. This year it was just the opposite. They said they didn't allow wheelchairs. Finally I just showed up at the beginning of the year and they had to let me go. (Goodman & Krauss, 1977, p. 46)

In the study of children, three approaches share a common recognition of the significant influence of the environment on behavior and development. These three approaches are functional analysis of behavior, ethology, and ecobehavioral science. A major difference between the behavioral approach and the other two approaches resides in the manner in which the influence of the environment is defined and assessed. The influence of the environment in the functional analysis of behavior model is defined by specific environmental stimuli (S) that elicit and/or reinforce behavior (B). The behavioral position as expressed by Bijou and Baer (1961) can thus be formulated as $B = f(S)$, in which behavior is seen as a function of eliciting or reinforcing stimuli. Within the functional analysis of behavior model, assessment and intervention procedures are inseparably linked. The flexibility and versatility of behavioral technology is evident in the fact that it has been applied widely with populations ranging in age from infancy to senescence and for problems ranging from academic achievement to self-injurious behavior.

A survey of the periodical literature focusing on children with disabilities indicates that unique and complex problems of these children have been successfully dealt with through behavior modification procedures and contingency management. There is also a very substantial literature drawing on this perspective to assist teachers, parents, and clinicians serving special populations. This extensive literature on behavioral assessment and intervention has been described elsewhere and will not be reviewed here. Sundel and Sundel (1999) and Beck (2000) have provided substantial coverage of assessment issues from a behavioral perspective.

In contrast to the perspective of the functional analysis of behavior, ecobehavioral science, building on the ecological psychology tradition (Barker, 1965), views child behavior as an interdependent part of the total setting. In this context, Scott (1980, p. 284) has defined a behavior setting as "a specific set of time, place and object props, and an attached standing problem of behavior. Both clusters are necessary and they are interdependent." A similar focus on the pervasive role of the environment on behavior in natural contexts is found in the ethological approach (Richer, 1979). Thus both the ecological and the ethological approaches advocate for assessment of behavior in natural environments (Berkson, 1978). Defined in terms of Lewin's (1951) original formulation, behavior (B) is seen as a function of the person (P) in the environment (E)—that is, $B = f(PE)$.

The purpose of this chapter is to draw on the literature related to ethology and ecobehavioral science as a framework for assessment of the environmental correlates of child behavior. To this end, we focus on the identification of instruments and strategies uniquely suited to assess the behavior of children and on the relationship of behavior with environmental contexts. Within this chapter, the contributions of these two frameworks will be defined as an ecobehavioral approach.

DEFINING AN ECOBEHAVIORAL APPROACH

Ecobehavioral assessment has evolved as a form of behavioral observation and assessment of environmental factors that draws on the theoretical contributions and research findings.

The following are features of an ecobehavioral approach relevant for assessment:

1. Ecobehavioral assessment relies on systematic observation of the child as a means of assessment. The focus, precision, and methods of observation do differ, as is shown later in this chapter.
2. Both ecological and ethological approaches are age irrelevant as assessment strategies in that they can be used to assess any individual without regard for age or maturity. The content of observation may be age specific, but the process of observation is age independent.
3. In both approaches, assessment is criterion referenced rather than norm referenced. The commonality of this feature is based on the fact that both approaches strive to define the role of the environment relative to a specific child rather than in terms of a normatively defined population.
4. Neither approach makes inferences about the meaning of behavior or situations. Environmental variables and behaviors are recorded directly and "purely" as samples of the factors in question. There is no a priori search for underlying or hidden causes or explanations.

The use of ecobehavioral assessment is important because the information obtained differs from that gained from other assessment strategies. Hartmann, Roper, and Bradford (1979), for example, have identified a variety of differences between traditional and behavioral assessment. The information derived from the use of quantitative measures (see

Chapter 4, this volume) focuses on assessed or inferred characteristics based on standardized procedures. The contextual or functional role of the environment on such assessment is either controlled through standardized assessment procedures or regarded as random variability. The qualitative assessment (see Chapter 5, this volume), with a central focus on documentation of cognitive competence, similarly does not attend to environmental correlates in a systematic manner.

The value of an ecobehavioral approach is that it provides means whereby the contextual and functional influences of the environment can be assessed. To this end, the major objective of ecobehavioral assessment, as considered in this chapter, is to define the environmental correlates of behavior. Pursuit of this objective is predicated on the fact that behavior is not assessed in a vacuum, nor can assessment results be assumed to be generalizable across a variety of settings. Ecobehavioral assessment is a method of observation in which the behavior of a child can be described and its relationship with environmental variables analyzed. This method, for example, provides a means to provide meaningful comparisons across settings and to analyze behavioral outcomes of students, as they are associated with various instructional or setting variables. At times, ecobehavioral assessment may add a situation-specific normative slant to the data by looking at multiple individuals within a larger shared system, such as analyzing and comparing mainstreamed and regular education students' experiences with a given classroom. The success with which assessment results can be used to prescribe intervention is in no small part dependent on the degree to which environmental factors are taken into account in the implementation of that intervention. Research has clearly shown that children's behavior varies across settings. Achenbach, McConaughy, and Howell (1987) conducted a meta-analysis in which they found marked differences in reports of children's behaviors in different situations and with different informants. Reports were most consistent when assessed by similar informants in similar settings.

CONTRIBUTIONS FROM ECOLOGICAL SCIENCE

A contribution of importance in regard to assessment is the emphasis on the concept of naturalness. Scott (1980), for example, has included four elements of dimensions of naturalness (natural behavior, setting, treatment, and a match between theoretical and empirical aspects and behavior in environmental contexts). Translating this concept of naturalness into assessment practice requires that documentation of behavior settings be done with the least degree of predetermined criteria by which observations are recorded. In this context Schoggen (1978) has emphasized the role of the observer as a transducer, recording events in as unbiased and noninferential a manner as possible. Along an applied line, Field (1981) has discussed the issues of examiner bias and ecological factors in the assessment of preschool children with disabilities. Only after all recording has been completed is an attempt made to analyze the records to determine what patterns and sequences may emerge. Illustrative of this approach is the use of the chronolog, a systematic time-referenced recording of behavior within its context (Scott, 1980). Inspection and evaluation of chronologs ultimately yields units of analysis, such as Activity Units (AU), through which the interdependence of behavior and the environment can be understood.

A second and related contribution from ecological science pertains to the methodology of assessment. Given the emphasis on naturalness, observations are to be made in as unintrusive a manner as possible and should be comprehensive rather than selective in scope. The result is data that are extremely complex and rich in information providing archival material. Thus, in regard to the ecological strategy, assessment is designed to reflect naturalness and to minimize the use of inference in obtaining data. As data are divided into units and categorized, however, they can provide information about a number of salient issues and relationships—for example, the structure of behavior in children, the effectiveness of teachers, and the pattern of activities of child advocates (Scott, 1980). The particular relevance of ecological science for assessment of children with disabilities is that it provides a systematic means of examining the direct influence of the environment on behavior.

The major characteristic of ecological methods is the focus on naturalistic observation. Naturalistic in this sense refers to the fact that observation is as natural and unobtrusive as possible, "an ongoing part of the subjects' lives which would occur with or without the experimenter" (Scott, 1980, p. 280). Applications to assessment can be made in terms of an ecological analysis of either groups or individuals. In regard to groups, focus is placed on defining the behavior setting. As Scott has indicated, a behavior setting is defined not only by time, place, and object characteristics but also by a specified pattern of behavior. Both elements of the definition are essential to describe a behavior setting.

Two general methods involved in an ecological approach to assessment are the specimen record and the chronolog. The specimen record and the chronolog are in fact similar in nature, the chronolog having evolved from the specimen record. Both methods require the narrative recording of observable behaviors. The specimen record involves recording descriptions of behaviors and speech at a detailed molecular level. The chronolog, on the other hand, although restricted to observable behaviors, yields narrative statements that have a more molar focus, summarizing the situation. Scott (1980) has defined the chronolog as a "running narrative record of all of a given individual's behavior at the molar level. The observer simply records everything that the individual says and does and everything that is said and done to him/her. Context for the behavior and the behavior of others in the environment is also recorded" (p. 285). Implementation of the chronolog method of observation requires that the person or person to be observed be informed of the procedure and that several sessions be carried out prior to actual data gathering to permit coordination. Scott reports that acclimation can usually be achieved in three to five sessions and that interrater reliability of observations has been consistently high.

Once the narrative record has been obtained in the form of the chronolog, it can be analyzed to provide information about behavior within environmental contexts. Scott (1980) describes two separate steps in the analysis of chronology: unitization and categorization. Unitization is a procedure whereby the narrative record is divided into structural units reflecting naturally occurring segments of behavior. These units are called Activity Units (AUs) and are characterized by a beginning and end point. The AUs are marked on the chronolog by inclusive bracket lines and are given descriptive titles. Within a given situation it is, of course, possible that several AUs are proceeding simultaneously. Such situations are reflected by overlapping bracket lines, as shown in the excerpt of a hypothetical chronolog for a 9-year-old girl with mild mental retardation in an inclusive classroom in Table 6.1. Examples of the AUs in the chronolog are "talks to classmate" and "teacher gives assistance."

The second step in the analysis of the chronolog is categorization of the AUs. The categories chosen depend on the purpose of the observational assessment. As Scott (1980) has pointed out, categorization should facilitate description, identification, and definition of the behavior as it occurred and was recorded. She has identified ways in which AUs can be categorized: the goal of the AU, such as the initiation or termination of the AU; the nature of involvement of others in the AU; and the temporal duration of the AU. These

TABLE 6.1. A hypothetical chronolog for a 9-year-old girl with mental retardation

Waiting in school cafeteria lunch line	Talks to classmate	12:00 Lunch bell rings and Mary gets in line at cafeteria with her lunch box.
		12:01 Her friend Sue comes up and says, "Guess what I have for lunch?"
		12:02 Mary turns around and says, "Let me see."
		12:03 Sue shows her the contents of her lunch bag.
		12:04 After looking at the contents Mary says, "That's neat. Guess what I got."
	Drops lunch box	12:05 Mary moves her lunch box from her left hand to her right hand.
		12:06 As she tries to open the lunch box, Mary drops it on the floor and all the contents fall out.
		12:07 Mary says, "Oh no!" and gets on the floor to pick up the contents.
Teacher gives assistance		12:08 The teacher gets up from the table and comes over to help Mary.
		12:09 The teacher helps Mary pick up the contents.
		12:10 Mary looks at the teacher and says, "Thank you."
		12:11 The teacher helps her get all the food back in the lunch box.
		12:12 The teacher returns to her table.

categorical data can then be summarized in various ways, such as numerical percentages, to convey the findings. Although the number of studies using an ecological approach has been limited, the unique focus and comprehensiveness of findings emphasize the value of this approach compared with methods that have not systematically sought to examine behavior as an integral part of the environmental context. In this context, for example, Scott reviews findings showing that (1) the focus of both ecological and ethological methods is on nonintrusive, or minimally intrusive, observations; (2) the nonintrusive nature of observations lends itself to the need for data gathering procedures with children with disabilities that are not complicated or difficult to implement; (3) the nonintrusive observations allow the derivation of naturalistic information regarding common behaviors and common environments; and (4) such naturalistic information has direct therapeutic implications for changing environments and behavior (Richer, 1979).

ECOBEHAVIORAL ASSESSMENT

Ecobehavioral assessment draws from the preceding contributions and can be used to view the child's experiences within the environment. This method seeks to identify and analyze those variables that shape the child's performance. Molar variables are those that are broad, are less amenable to manipulation, and have an indirect effect on the child's behavior. Molar variables can include socioeconomic status, gender, and disability (McEvoy & McConnell, 1995). Molecular variables, interactional or instrumental variables, are narrower in scope, are generally more amenable to manipulation, and have more direct effects on the child's behavior (McEvoy & McConnell, 1995).

This model can be used to formally analyze the ecology of children's learning experiences, of which the major ones are home, neighborhood, and school. Ecobehavioral systems may analyze the physical and social environment of the school (grouping of students, instructional materials utilized, instructional methods utilized, schedule of the school day, physical location, etc.) and the teacher's behavior (physical location, verbalizations, response to the student's behavior, etc.; Greenwood, 1996).

An analysis of any environment needs to take into account both molecular and molar dimensions. Darvill (1982) has identified molecular dimensions as easily recognized features of a child's environment such as people, toys, and other nonsocial objects. Molecular dimensions may also include less readily recognizable aspects of the environment, such as the social or spatial density of the space in which the child is found. The molar dimensions of the environment are more broad-based variables, such as socioeconomic status and other cultural indices. The focus of much of the recent literature on the ecological approach, and hence this chapter, will be on the molecular dimensions of the environment. This focus is reflected in Ulvund's (1984) emphasis on the need to consider the psychological basis of physical environmental parameters in cognitive development. As Ulvund has pointed out, parameters of the physical environment, such as variety, complexity, and responsiveness, have been found to be associated with competence in children. To this end there is a need to assess the physical environment to extend knowledge on the association of experience and cognitive development.

ASSESSMENT DOMAINS

In this section we identify assessment procedures and measures that have been used in specific domains. In addition to the four domains of cognition, communication, personal/social functioning, and behavior, we also focus on the environment as a domain of assessment. The procedures and measures reviewed are often not commercially available but rather are drawn from clinical or research literature.

Environments

In recent years, the impact of ecological psychology and the recognition of the important role of the environment in mediating outcomes for children (Sameroff & Chandler, 1975) have contributed to a strong interest in systematically assessing the nature of the environment. Such assessment focuses on characteristics of the environment itself rather than on the behavior of individuals within environments. Assessment of the latter is discussed under a subsequent heading.

Assessment of environments has primarily focused on home and school settings. Although the number of measures is limited and their content varies, each shares a common objective of documenting the extent to which a setting stimulates and/or supports the development of the child. As shown in Table 6.2, the assessment procedures differ as a function of the setting to be observed. The PHSI (Wachs, 1979; Wachs, Francis, & McQuiston, 1978), the HOME Inventory (Caldwell, 1972), and the CIE (Yarrow, Rubenstein, & Pedersen, 1975) reflected the growing interest in the 1970s to document the nature of the home environment in early intervention. This interest in examining the relationship of the home environment and the development of children with disabilities is illustrated in a study by Best and Roberts (1976) with hearing-impaired infants. The utility of the HOME Inventory has been extended beyond infancy to encompass versions for early and middle childhood. Applications with families of children with different disabilities revealed low to moderate relationships of the HOME with other measures of family status and child competence (Bradley, 1994; Bradley, Rock, Caldwell, & Brisby, 1989). The Early Child-

TABLE 6.2. Selected measures to assess environments

Measure	Age/stage	Format of results	Psychometric properties	Applications with children with special needs
Purdue Home Stimulation Inventory (Wachs, 1979; Wachs et al., 1978)	Infancy	30 item scores, 12 factors	Mean interobserver agreement: 85%	Potential applicability with families with infants with disabilities
HOME Inventory (Bradley, 1994)	Infancy and preschool	Infancy: 6 subscales Preschool: 8 subscales	Infant scale: correlations of 6- and 24-month scores with 54-month Binet: $r = .44$ and $.57$ Preschool scale: correlations with achievement in primary grades: $r = .26-.47$	Infants with hearing impairments (Best & Roberts, 1976); children with various disabilities (Bradley et al., 1989)
Characteristics of the Inanimate Environment (Yarrow et al., 1975)	Infancy	Responsiveness Complexity Variety	Interobserver reliability: $r = .88-.99$	Potential applicability with families with infants with special needs
Early Childhood Environment Rating Scale (Harms & Clifford, 1980)	Preschool	Ratings from inadequate (1) to excellent (7) for each of 37 items, as well as a total score	Interrater reliability: $r = .79-.90$ Test–retest reliability: $r = .96$ (Bailey et al., 1982)	Preschool children with disabilities (Bailey et al., 1982)
Classroom Environment Scale (Moos & Trickett, 1974)	School age	Nine classroom dimensions	Internal consistency: $.67-.86$ Test–retest reliability: $r = .72-.92$	Students with emotional and behavioral problems (Trickett et al., 1993)

hood Environment Rating Scale (ECERS), a 37-item scale, was used by Bailey, Clifford, and Harms (1982) to compare preschool programs for children with and without disabilities. Their results revealed that, on 12 of the 37 items, classrooms for nondisabled preschoolers were rated significantly higher than those for children with disabilities. As the authors noted, the findings point to concerns about the quality of settings for children with disabilities and the importance of identifying environmental features relevant to planning and implementing intervention programs.

A somewhat different approach has been applied in the analysis of environments for school-age children. The Classroom Environment Scale (CES) developed by Moos and Trickett (1974) allows the derivation of information along nine dimensions, which Forness, Guthrie, and MacMillan (1982) found could be presented in a four-cluster profile (see Table 6.2). Their findings indicated that the dimension of classroom structure was associated with on-task behavior of students. The CES has been revised for use in special education classrooms for students with behavioral or emotional problems (Trickett, Leone, Fink, & Braaten, 1993). Findings revealed support for seven of the nine original domains. In addition to established measures, environments can also be assessed with informal, observer-designed procedures.

Although the assessment of environments is currently a low-frequency activity in comparison with assessment of individual child behavior and development, it is a domain that is likely to increase in importance in services involving children with disabilities or chronic conditions. The value of assessing environments may lie along several lines. First, one value of assessing environments is that it provides a formal method by which to define and evaluate settings in which children with disabilities are served. In an evaluation of a special education program, DeSouza and Sivewright (1993) described the importance of measuring both the static and dynamic dimensions of classroom environments. Second, from a practical standpoint, assessment of environments allows a determination of the general adequacy of the environment as a human service setting. Efforts in this area reflect the expanding interest in issues of access to the built environment for persons with disabilities (Imrie & Kuman, 1998). An example of such environmental assessment is the Instructional Environment Scale (TIES) developed by Ysseldyke and Christenson (1987) for describing the environmental context of student behaviors and to suggest potential starting points for behavior interventions to modify those behaviors. Third, and perhaps most relevant to the concerns of this book, assessment of environments can serve programmatic goals for children with disabilities. In this regard, the goal of assessing environments is to insure that environments are arranged to optimize the learning and development of an individual or group of children. At the current time there is not a well-established literature on the exact manner in which environments can be arranged or manipulated to effect specific behavior change. As the research in social psychology, child development, and other fields of study sheds further light on this topic, it is likely that more precise forms of environmental engineering can be followed in matching characteristics of the child with those of an environment to achieve desired outcomes for the child. Rettig (1998), for example, has described how environments can be designed to promote play development of young children with disabilities. Another is the use of a self-assessment measure by adults with physical disabilities to describe accessibility of their housing environment (Faenge & Iwarsson, 1999). In a different context, Cotton and Geraty (1984) have discussed the translation of clinical goals into the design of therapeutic space for children who are emotionally disturbed. For those interested in assessing environments of children with disabilities, a review of the information in Table 6.2 and of the primary literature from which that information is derived may assist in the selection of a procedure most suited to a particular assessment need.

Cognitive Domain

The assessment of cognition through observation of behavior has been operationalized in ethological, as well as behavioral, approaches. Within the ethological approach, Charlesworth (1979) described the importance of assessing intelligent behavior, not in test settings but rather as it is observed in everyday situations. Such behavior is assumed to be cognitively mediated and serves individual adaptation through problem solving. Adaptation in turn is assumed to involve progressive acquisition of skills from early to later development. Charlesworth has developed a method called PROBA (Problem Behavior

Analysis) by which problem-solving behavior can be observed in the ongoing activities of children. Problems, blocks, or interruptions are categorized and recorded in six cells of three dimensions of content (social, physical, informational) and two sources (external versus internal impositions on the individual). Additional features that are recorded include (1) the ongoing behavior that was disrupted, (2) the response to the problem, (3) the effectiveness of the response in dealing with the problem, and (4) the final status of the behavior. Activities in which the child was engaged and the presence of others during the problem sequence are also recorded. Agreement among observers has ranged from 75% to 95% depending on the nature of the problem observed.

Charlesworth has observed both children without disabilities and a child with Down syndrome in the 20- to 48-month range using this approach and obtained a number of interesting findings. Children were found to experience between 29 and 40 problems per hour, and the majority of these (80–90%) were social in nature. Many of the problems were essentially interruptions of the children's ongoing behavior, and very few were of a complex nature, as might be found in psychological testing. Children often solved the problems (30–40% of the time), and they returned to their ongoing behavior about one-third of the time. Of particular interest was the fact that although the child with Down syndrome experienced fewer problems, minimal differences were found in the nature of the problems and responses to them.

Charlesworth has also applied the method to infants and adults. Although he recognizes that PROBA is not without limitations in terms of procedural elements, he concludes that it can be of value for clinicians and others interested in the relationship of behavior and stimuli in everyday contexts. More specifically, he feels that the procedure reveals: "(a) features of everyday living that are problematic; (b) who or what was responsible for these features; and (c) how the individual responded to them" (1979, p. 215). To this end, an ethological approach may be a uniquely appropriate means for investigating the interactions of children with disabilities or chronic conditions with their environments.

Communication Domain

Communication, like cognition, has been examined broadly using behavioral approaches in a variety of studies that involve some aspect of communicative behavior. More narrowly, the assessment of communication as a domain of behavior has been quite limited. Applications of behavioral strategies, however, do hold promise as a useful and practical tool in assessment of children with disabilities. In an interesting study of children with cleft lip and cleft palate, Long and Dalston (1982) recorded the gestural and vocalization communicative skills of ten children without disabilities and ten 12-month-old infants with disabilities. Significant differences were obtained between the two groups, indicating communicative deficits in children with cleft lip and palate problems. An analysis of categories of communicative gestures revealed that the giving gesture, accompanied by vocalization, was the strongest variable discriminating between the two groups. The value of this observational approach, as the authors noted, is that it permits documentation of a phase of communicative development reflecting a transition from nonverbal to verbal communication. Early communicative behavior was the focus of a similar observation study of young children with cochlear implants (Lutman & Tait, 1995). An analysis of interactions of children with adults revealed one factor on turn-taking and gazing behavior by the child. These procedures may have potential utility for other infants and young children whose development is associated with communicative deficits.

Personal/Social Domain

Although the extent of deficits in children with disabilities may vary widely from one child to another in such domains as cognition, motor functioning, or communication, almost all children with disabilities are characterized by deficits in the personal/social domain. In some populations, such as children with emotional or behavioral disorders, these deficits may be the primary features of the condition. In other children, such as those with mental or physical impairments, they may be secondary to children's restricted abilities and/or experiences. In any case, immature or atypical personal/social behavior constitutes a pervasive characteristic of children with disabilities, making it increasingly a focus for more intense and precise assessment. In a review of behavioral assessment of personal/social functioning in children with disabilities, we examine two representative areas. One area in which there has been substantial research is social behavior patterns. Representative research in this area has focused on identifying the nature and timing of social play behaviors of children with hearing impairment exposed to either oral or sign communication (Cornelius & Hornett, 1991). Results indicated that higher social play behavior and lower levels of aggression were found in children in the sign-based group. A study of children with Down syndrome, ranging in age from 5 to 6½ years, and of children without disabilities in approximately the same age group, involved time sampling (30-second intervals) of behavior over a period of 8 weeks using the Preschool Observation System for Social Interaction—Research Edition (Rogers-Warren, Ruggles, Peterson, & Cooper, 1981). Analyses were made of the play areas the children occupied, the type of play behavior exhibited, and the type of playmate with whom interaction occurred. In general the results revealed minimal differences between the two groups in terms of preferred play areas. Although distribution of play behavior was found to be similar for both groups, differences were found in the frequency of solitary play as a function of setting, a finding also obtained for playmate preference. With the growing focus on inclusion there is interest in children's behavior in context. In a comparison of preschool children with and without disabilities, Kontos, Moore, and Giorgetti (1998) found that those children with disabilities spent most of their free time in manipulative activities, whereas children without disabilities spent most of their time in dramatic play. These results illustrate the importance of examining the pattern of social interaction of children with disabilities in various settings to accurately assess both developmental and situational characteristics.

A second area in which behavioral assessment strategies have been applied is in personal relationships, such as friendship patterns. Earlier research in this area has involved adult populations, but the relevance of assessing these patterns in children with disabilities is clear and should lead to applications in the future. The work of Landesman-Dwyer, Berkson, and Rosner (1979), for example, was carried out in the context of behavioral and ecological studies of group homes for persons with mental retardation and has included analyses of affiliation and friendship patterns. The researchers classified observed behavior as social if it met the criteria of reflecting interactive activities or if it involved some form of communication. The results were examined in terms of informal grouping behavior, affiliation patterns, and friendships of the participants.

The value of a social ecology perspective (Ramey, Dossett, & Echols, 1996) for psychological assessment of children with disabilities is threefold. First, the findings provide evidence for the fact that affiliation and friendship patterns are an appropriate and important domain to assess even in individuals with severe disabilities. Second, these patterns can be observed and recorded readily in the everyday lives and environments of children with disabilities. Third, the obtained relationship between social behaviors and environmental variables provides support for manipulating environments as a form of intervention. In this context, the importance of peer relations and friendships have been identified as key components for the development of social competence by Bebko and colleagues (1998).

Behavior Domain

The strategies and procedures considered in this section are restricted to those dealing with the relationship of behavior to specific environmental contexts. In this regard a growing literature on the observation and analysis of behavior in a number of settings addresses a variety of questions. For the purpose of this chapter, studies are grouped according to the following topics: (1) mobility, (2) territoriality, and (3) spacing and density.

Observation of mobility and exploratory behavior in a specific context has been advocated for children who are difficult to test using traditional test measures. Hutt, Hutt, and Ounsted (1963), in an early and intriguing study, utilized an ethological approach to investigate attention span and mobility in children who were hyperactive and had suffered brain damage. The method involved the observation of children in an unfurnished room (12 ft. × 12 ft.) marked into 16 equal-sized squares, which were numbered for easy recording as the child moved from one square to another. This approach is analogous to the open-field test used in animal research in which a box is marked off in checkerboard fashion, to record movement or exploratory behavior of an experimental group and a control group. With children, this approach may be used to document movement patterns, as illustrated in Figure 6.1. In the research reported by Hutt and colleagues, one variable of interest was the effects of treatment with drugs. The mobility patterns observed in a 4-year-old child were found to be associated with different conditions of drug treatment. The measurement strategy is quite simple and consists of recording the child's changing position relative to the numbered squares and the type of activity in which the child is engaged (Figure 6.2). As Hutt and colleagues have noted, the test environment can also be altered in terms of complexity by adding nonsocial, as well as social, stimuli, yielding additional levels of complexity across which behavior can be compared. This approach has also been used in subsequent research to investigate the effectiveness of psychotropic medication with children who are hyperactive (Routh, Schroeder, & O'Tuama, 1974).

A second means of observing situation-specific behavior also relies on ethological theory. The concept of territoriality—that is, "behavior by which an organism characteristically lays claim to an area and defends it against members of its own species" (Hall, 1966, p. 79)—has been applied in a number of observational studies of persons with mental retardation. A hypothesis for its relevance with children with mental retardation is that it represents a primitive form of social behavior; hence, it would be likely to be inversely related to intelligence (Paluck & Esser, 1971). In a study of boys with severe mental retardation ranging from 7 to 10 years of age (IQ range 31–37), Paluck and Esser (1971) compared territorial behavior on two occasions over a period of 20 months. Their procedure was similar to that reported by Hutt and colleagues (1963) in that an experimental dayroom in an institutional setting was marked off into 137 squares to permit the recording of movement and territorial ownership. Paluck and Esser concluded that change in territorial behavior appeared to be associated with clinical improvement. Rago (1977, 1978) has extended this focus on territoriality by demonstrating its utility in differentiating subtypes of adults with profound mental retardation and as a means to document environmental interventions in the form of increased space (Rago, Parker, & Cleland, 1978).

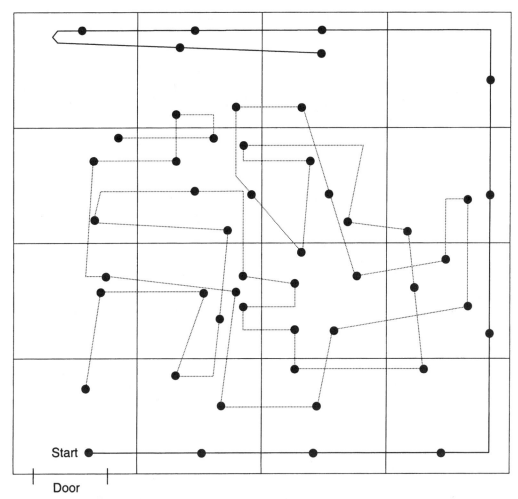

FIGURE 6.1. An illustration of activity assessment using an open-field methodology. ——— Child A: 12 squares entered in 3 minutes; movement along periphery. -------- Child B: 38 squares entered in 3 minutes; movement appears random; central rather than peripheral areas traversed. Observation room is marked off in 4' × 4' squares.

A third means of examing behavioral contexts with special populations is through analyses of spacing and density patterns. Drawing on comparative studies, Burgess and Murphy (1982) investigated the developmental nature of social spacing patterns in the free-play behavior of children from 6 to 60 months of age. Interval data obtained through remote-controlled photography yielded measures of spacing distance, spacing pattern, and spatial variability. The results indicated that social distance to adults increased and that to playmates decreased with age. Variability of spacing also showed a general decrease with age both to adults and to peers. The findings provide a framework in which to examine the pattern and development of social behavior in children with disabilities. Burgess (1981) has in fact applied this approach to studying social spacing patterns of school-age children with and without mental retardation. A time-sampling procedure (15-second interval) was used to observe spacing distance and physical contact during free-play behavior on an outdoor playground. Analyses revealed that younger children (Grades 1–3) played closer

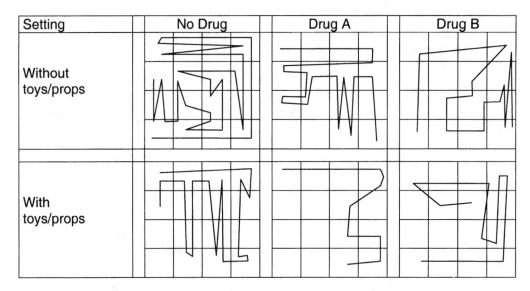

FIGURE 6.2. Movement patterns of a hypothetical 6-year-old epileptic child in a standardized "open field" setting under two experimental conditions and across different drug treatments.

to their peers than older children (Grades 4–6) and that children with mental retardation played significantly closer than nonretarded peers. Touching was observed significantly more in younger than in older nonretarded children, whereas touching was significantly absent among children with mental retardation as a group. Taken collectively, the findings from Burgess's research demonstrate that unobtrusive measures of the development of social orientation in children can be obtained in naturalistic settings. Other ways in which to assess personal space have been described and compared by Cronje and Mollen (1976).

Population density is a concept that has been of interest with particular regard to settings in which individuals are provided institutional or other group-care services. In a review of prior research on institutionalized individuals, Repp, Barton, and Gottlieb (1983) concluded that increasing density was likely to be associated with decreasing appropriate behavior. The inappropriate behavior emitted, however, may vary as a function of the characteristics of the participants. Hutt and Vaizey (1966), for example, found that increased density resulted in more aggression among children with brain damage, whereas in children with autism withdrawal behavior increased. Repp and his colleagues (1983) sought to determine group size and group behavior in a naturalistic study of adolescents who were severely or profoundly retarded and of adults living in an institution. Density was defined as the number of persons present within a 1.5-meter radius of the individual being observed. Thus the units of analysis were the size of the groups observed and the behavior of individuals as a function of group size. The results indicated that the participants spent about 22% of their time in the presence of one or more staff, 24% alone, 22% with another resident, and 33% in groups of two or more. Analyses of density and behavior relationships revealed some limited patterns in that staff presence was associated with reduced self-stimulation and increased physical and verbal interactions, whereas in the presence of peers these effects were not observed. Although nonpurposeful activity did decrease, more activity was observed, leading Repp and his colleagues to conclude that peer proximity was not correlated with greater social interactions (Repp et al., 1983).

Documentation of situation-specific behavior has also been made of children with and without disabilities ranging from 1 to 19 years of age. Phemister, Richardson, and Thomas (1978) compared typical 1- and 2-year-olds in home and nursery settings with children with severe disabilities (functioning in the 1- to 2-year range) in home, day care, and residential settings on dimensions of object availability, adult availability, and social and nonsocial activities. A time-sampling procedure was used to observe behavior across the child's activities for a day in the specific setting. Among findings of interest was the fact that time spent interacting with adults did not exceed 20% for any group in any setting. The lowest percentages, 5.5% and 12.4%, were observed for children with disabilities in residential settings. Furthermore, using a classification in which time was defined as full (such as productive, interactive activities) or empty (such as self-stimulation, inactivity), it was found that children with disabilities in all settings had significantly fewer full times than typical peers in both home and nursery settings. These findings for children with disabilities and those of Repp and colleagues (1983) for adults with disabilities demonstrate the feasibility of assessing situation-specific behavior and indicate the utility of such assessments for planning ecologically valid interventions.

Documenting situation-specific behavior is important in developing effective interventions. For children presenting with challenging behaviors of aggression and self-injury, assessment of environmental influences can serve as the basis for developing individualized interventions. In a review of studies of functional communication training, Miranda (1997) described the use of Motivation Assessment Scale—MAS (Durand & Crimmins, 1992) to document environmental influences on behavior. The MAS is a 16-item instrument for rating the extent to which four dimensions (tangibles, attention, escape, and sensory) influence a specific behavior and are applicable for a variety of behaviors across age groups (Miranda, 1997).

RECOMMENDATIONS FOR PRACTICE

Much of this chapter is devoted to a review of methods and procedures that focus on the assessment of ecological contexts of behavior. A distinctive feature of ecobehavioral strategies is that they are used primarily to derive descriptive and prescriptive information, whereas the use of psychometric strategies may often have diagnostic classification as a primary goal. It should be noted, however, that some classification efforts have emerged based on behavioral approaches.

Although these classification systems may be applied and refined in the future, at the present time the value of ecobehavioral assessment is the prescriptive information it yields. Drawing on this distinction, we consider means whereby the results of ecobehavioral assessment can be translated into intervention plans for children. Issues germane to this consideration include reporting assessment results and modifying environments.

Reporting and Interpreting Results

As the narrative and graphic material in this chapter indicates, the manner in which ecobehavioral assessment data are recorded may vary widely. Ecobehavioral assessment often relies on the use of specific units of analysis derived from observation and data, including specimen records. Thus the presentation of results to a large degree depends on the specific assessment method used and the unit of analysis in which the behavior is recorded. In any event, however, in order to achieve some consistency in reporting ecobehavioral data, the format proposed in Table 6.3 may be useful to follow. Preparation of assessment results in this format should insure that the unit of analysis, the nature of the findings, and the manner and context in which the findings were obtained will be available to the consumer of the report.

Means of interpreting the results of behavioral assessment range from simple visual inspection of the data to complex analyses of theoretical constructs, such as EFUs (environmental force units). The more sophisticated the unit of analysis, the more important it is that the evaluation report be accompanied by a sufficiently detailed explanation of what it is and how it should be interpreted. Increasingly more sophisticated analytic procedures are available to evaluate and interpret data.

Modifying Environments

Although a substantial literature exists on the direct modification of behavior through behavior modification procedures, more indirect and general modification of behavior through manipulation or engineering of the environment appears to be a less developed area. This is surprising in that alteration of the larger environment in this general sense may be both as effective as more precise modification of stimulus–response elements and, at the same time, less intrusive and more efficient in terms of effort and control. A typical approach to modifying aggressive behavior, for example, usually takes the form of a specific program in which a child's inappropriate behavior is ignored and appropriate behavior is reinforced by adult praise according to a determined schedule. Modification of behavior, however, could alternately be approached through environmental engineering in which density and spacing characteristics are changed through rearrangement of people and/or physical props. Although research on this topic is limited, available evidence suggests that environmental alteration is an approach of significant promise in planning interventions for children with developmental problems. Three selected applications are used

TABLE 6.3. Proposed format for reporting ecobehavioral assessment results

Report element	Illustration
1. Define purpose of assessment in ecobehavioral terms	1. To assess the extent to which an ecological factor (place of testing) influences performance of child on referential communication task.
2. Specify unit of analysis	2. Number and accuracy of references provided by a child in 10 trials.
3. Identify manner and context of assessment	3. Referential communication task administered in three settings (home, day care center, and laboratory), differentiated on the basis of familiarity of props.
4. Summarize assessment results	4. Performance was higher and more accurate in home and day care center than in laboratory setting.
5. Identify implications within an ecobehavioral conceptual framework	5. Referential communication appears to be influenced by the degree to which situation is familiar or unfamiliar to child.

to support this premise by illustrating the manner in which deliberate alteration of the physical environment can contribute to behavioral changes in special populations. Specifically, environments can influence behavior through alteration involving (1) space reduction or restriction, (2) space expansion, and (3) material availability.

In regard to space reduction, Jones, Barrett, Olonoff, and Anderson (1969) reported an intriguing approach with preschoolers ranging in age from 28 to 39 months who had physical or behavioral problems. Over a period of 6 weeks, five to eight children were placed briefly as a group in a confined space arranged by adjustable, movable walls to provide 2½ square feet per occupant. An adult also occupied the confined space as recorder and "peace keeper." Each session lasted from 10 to 24 minutes, and during this time observations were made of the children's overall state, communication, and social interaction. Although individual differences were evident in the responses of children, the authors concluded that gains were made in nonverbal communication, as well as in social interaction. In an earlier study with 10 preschoolers with cerebral palsy, Barrett, Hunt, and Jones (1967) also concluded that the confined space experience was beneficial. These studies, although dated, call for systematic experimentation to determine how space reduction can be used as a strategy for promoting the experience of physical and social proximity of children with limited motor abilities. A related technique, namely that of space restriction, has been explored with children with autism. In a small experimental study, eight children with autism were randomly assigned either to a standard ward (control) setting or to a setting of Restricted Environmental Stimulation Therapy (REST; Suedfeld & Schwartz, 1983). The theoretical assumption underlying the REST treatment is that sensory overload may be a factor in the behavior of children with autism. Thus the experimental REST treatment involved placement for 48 hours in a dimly lighted, sparsely equipped room with very limited social contact. Assessment made during and following the REST treatment revealed some expected changes in learning and social measures. Positioning of children with severe neuromotor impairments can also be seen as a form of space restriction. In a study of 10 children with profound multiple disabilities, McEwen (1992) compared communicative interactions under three environmental placements (wheelchair, sidelyer, and floor mat). Different effects were found for adult and child behaviors as a function of environmental placement and session structure. These findings, although exploratory in nature, suggest that selected alterations of the environment may constitute a parsimonious way in which to effect behavior change in children with disabilities.

Alteration of the environment to modify behavior has also been demonstrated through space expansion. In a rather unusual study combining an ethological orientation (territoriality) and a behavioral design (baseline, intervention, reinstatement phases), Hereford, Cleland, and Fellner (1973) recorded bedwetting and soiling in institutionalized nonverbal persons with profound mental retardation as a function of changes in personal space characteristic of institutional life. It was hypothesized that bedwetting and soiling constituted forms of territorial defense associated with limitations of personal space. Systematic expansion of personal space by reducing crowding 64% during the intervention phase resulted in a marked decrease of enuresis and encopresis. A reinstatement phase in which original space limitations were again imposed yielded evidence that wetting and soiling behavior were influenced by environmental changes. Although the investigators' premise that these behaviors represent primitive forms of territoriality and communication is open to debate, the procedures and findings of the study support the value of alternate conceptualizations and approaches to common behavior problems. In particular, the findings document the relevance and utility of an ethological approach to assessment and intervention with a special population with whom traditional assessment is inappropriate or of limited value. Research is needed to determine how space alteration can serve as an efficient means of bringing about behavior change in individual and group interventions.

Another example of environmental alteration involves the dimension of material availability. Under the rubric of socioecological programming, Jones, Favell, and Risley (1983) have defined material and activity availability as the proportion of materials and activities to the number of clients in a setting. Providing toys and other materials is an element that Jones and colleagues identify as important in altering environments for clients with profound multiple handicaps. Focusing on play as a behavior of interest, the researchers reported that settings with more rather than less toys and preferred rather than nonpreferred toys resulted in increased play. Toy preference tended to be idiosyncratic among clients.

Proponents of the ecobehavioral approach have used this model to explore the classroom ecology for students with at-risk status, cultural and linguistic differences, and various disabilities (Arreaga-Mayer, 1999; Bulgren & Carta, 1992; DeSouza & Sivewright, 1993; Greenwood, 1996; Logan, Bakeman, & Keefe, 1997; Logan & Malone, 1998; McDonnell, Thorson, McQuivey, & Keifer-O'Donnell, 1997). By studying the relationships between variables across time, conditional probabilities can be developed that examine how instructional environment variables (such as student grouping or type of instructional materials used) influence teacher and student variables (such as teacher feedback or student verbal responding). These variables can be further compared with outcome measures (such as achievement test scores) to determine which environmental, instructor, or learner behaviors are related to higher degrees of learning success. According to Greenwood, Delquadri, Stanley, Terry, and Hall (1985),

> an ecobehavioral interaction approach in classroom settings offers the potential of studying students' academic achievement or failure in terms of their performance in relation to opportunities to learn, the attempts made to teach them, and the classroom learning interactions in which students engage. This approach to assessment offers enhanced precision by revealing the structure of teaching events in relation to students' behavior. Thus, questions of how instruction affects student behavior from moment to moment, or how teachers may efficiently alter instruction at specific points in time to obtain desired changes in students' performance, are more likely to be answered with this approach to assessment. (p. 332)

Using the ecobehavioral method, Greenwood (1996) found that mainstreamed students with learning disabilities showed less academic growth when they "spent more time in music instruction, in small rather than large instructional groups, in instruction provided by a special rather than a regular education teacher, and in instruction when the teacher focused more often on the target student with LD (p. 54)." This study provided evidence that was used to make and evaluate changes in both instructional methods (implementing a classwide peer-tutoring program) and teacher training (having a teacher with effective procedures instruct a peer in her method of instruction; Greenwood, 1996).

Several ecobehavioral evaluation systems have been developed and have begun to gain research support. The Code for Instructional Structure and Student Academic Response (CISSAR) was developed by Stanley and Greenwood (1981) and is a "momentary time-sampling observations system that allows the recording of students' opportunities to engage in active academic responses as a function of different features in their instructional environments" (Bulgren & Carta, 1992, p. 183). The Code for Instructional Structure and Academic Response—Mainstream Version (MS-CISSAR) is an adaptation of the CISSAR that measures 99 ecobehavioral variables in three areas: (1) teacher variables such as teacher identification, behavior, and focus; (2) student variables such as engaged behavior, competing behavior, and task management; and (3) classroom ecological variables such as grouping, materials used, and activity (Logan et al., 1997; McDonnell et al., 1997). The Ecobehavioral System for Complex Analyses of Preschool Environments (ESCAPE) was developed to examine ecobehavioral variables within the preschool setting (Carta & Atwater, 1990; Greenwood, Carta, Kamps, Terry, & Delquadri, 1994). The Ecobehavioral System for the Contextual Recording of Interactional Bilingual Environments (ESCRIBE) brings these concepts to the bilingual instructional context and adds teacher, materials, and student language to the variables examined for their effects on student behavior and learning (Arreaga-Mayer, 1999).

These examples are described to illustrate the manner in which environmental engineering can be applied to effect behavior change. To the extent that altering an environment in terms of physical dimensions of space reduction or expansion is relatively easy and inexpensive, it offers an efficient approach with significant potential in interventions for children with disabilities. Although research applications in this area are still limited, there is every indication that increasing attention will be given to the practical implications of ecobehavioral science. To this end, it is important that assessment and intervention efforts build on the theoretical and empirical contributions of this approach. The concept of the behavior setting defined as an environment with both physical (milieu) and behavioral (program) characteristics (Gump, 1975) may be valuable to specify in detail for children with disabilities. As Gump has pointed out, an important feature of behavior settings is that "the ratio of number of persons to some measure of behavioral opportunity clearly influences the actions and experiences of a setting's inhabitants" (1975, p. 117). Drawing on ecological research findings pertaining to "manning theory" Schoggen (1978) has presented the concepts of undermanned and overmanned environments as having particular relevance for special populations. In overmanned environments the ratio of behavioral opportunities to individuals is low, resulting in limited participation and involvement. In undermanned environments the ratio of behavioral opportunities to individuals is higher, resulting in greater expectations and demands for involvement. The psychological benefits of an undermanned environment include the development of competence and a sense of responsibility, satisfaction, and self-worth. The concept of the undermanned environment can thus serve as a guiding principle in the development of intervention plans for children with disabilities. Designing environments that meet criteria of being undermanned may be a practical and efficient way in which to promote developmental and personal growth of children with chronic conditions and disabilities.

REFERENCES

Achenbach, T. M., McConaughy, S. H., & Howell, C. T. (1987). Child/adolescent behavioral and emotional problems: Implications of cross-informant correlations for situational specificity. *Psychological Bulletin, 101*, 213–232.

Arreaga-Mayer, C. (1999). *Ecobehavioral assessment of exceptional culturally and linguistically diverse students: Evaluating effective bilingual special education programs*. Paper presented at the Third National Research Symposium on Limited English Proficient Student Issues [Online]. Available: http://www.ncbe.gwu.edu/ncbepubs/symposia/third/mayer.htm

Bailey, D. B., Clifford, R. M., & Harms, T. (1982). Comparison of preschool environments for handicapped and non-handicapped children. *Topics in Early Childhood Special Education, 2,* 9–20.

Barker, R. G. (1965). Explorations in ecological psychology. *American Psychologist, 20,* 1–14.

Barrett, M. L., Hunt, V. V., & Jones, M. H. (1967). Behavioral growth of cerebral palsied children from group experience in a confined space. *Developmental Medicine and Child Neurology, 9,* 50–58.

Bebko, J. M., Wainwright, J. A., Brian, J., Coolbear, J., Landry, R., & Vallance, D. D. (1998). Social competence and peer relations. *Journal of Developmental Disabilities, 6*(1), 1–31.

Beck, S. J. (2000). Behavioral assessment. In M. Hersen & R. T. Ammerman (Eds.), *Advanced abnormal child psychology* (2nd ed., pp. 177–195). Mahwah, NJ: Erlbaum.

Berkson, G. (1978). Social ecology and ethology of mental retardation. In G. P. Sackett (Ed.), *Observing behavior: Vol. 1. Theory and applications in mental retardation* (pp. 403–409). Baltimore: University Park Press.

Best, B., & Roberts, G. (1976). Early cognitive development in hearing impaired children. *American Annals of the Deaf, 121,* 560–564.

Bijou, S. W., & Baer, D. M. (1961). *Child development: Vol. 1. A systematic and empirical theory.* New York: Appleton-Century-Crofts.

Bradley, R. H. (1994). The HOME Inventory: Review and reflections. In H. W. Reese (Ed.), *Advances in child development and behavior* (Vol. 25, pp. 241–288). San Diego, CA: Academic Press.

Bradley, R. H., Rock, S. L., Caldwell, B. M., & Brisby, J. A. (1989). Uses of the HOME Inventory for families with handicapped children. *American Journal of Mental Retardation, 94*(3), 313–330.

Bulgren, J. A., & Carta, J. J. (1992). Examining the instructional contexts of students with learning disabilities. *Exceptional Children, 59,* 182–192.

Burgess, J. W. (1981). Development of spacing in normal and mentally retarded children. *Journal of Nonverbal Behavior, 6,* 89–95.

Burgess, J. W., & Murphy, D. (1982). The development of proxemic spacing behavior: Children's distances to surrounding playmates and adults change between six months and five years of age. *Developmental Psychobiology, 15,* 557–567.

Caldwell, B. (1972). *HOME Inventory.* Little Rock: University of Arkansas.

Carta, J. J., & Atwater, J. B. (1990). Applications of ecobehavioral analysis to the study of transitions across early educational settings. *Education and Treatment of Children, 13,* 298–315.

Charlesworth, W. R. (1979). An ethological approach to studying intelligence. *Human Development, 22,* 212–216.

Cornelius, G., & Hornett, D. (1991). The play behavior of hearing impaired children. *American Annals of the Deaf, 135*(4), 316–321.

Cotton, N. S., & Geraty, R. S. (1984). Therapeutic space design: Planning an inpatient children's unit. *American Journal of Orthopsychiatry, 54,* 624–636.

Cronje, F., & Mollen, A. (1976). Comparison of different procedures to assess personal space. *Perceptual Motor Skills, 43,* 959–962.

Darvill, D. (1982). Ecological influences on children's play: Issues and approaches. In D. J. Pepler & K. H. Rubin (Eds.), *Contributions to human development: Vol. 6. The play of children: Current theory and research.* Basel, Switzerland: Karger.

DeSouza, E. R., & Sivewright, D. (1993). An ecological approach to evaluating a special education program, *Adolescence, 28,* 517–525.

Durand, V. M., & Crimmins, D. (1992). *The Motivation Assessment Scale (MAS) administration guide.* Topeka, KS: Monaco & Associates.

Faenge, A., & Iwarsson, S. (1999). Physical housing environment: Development of a self-assessment instrument. *Canadian Journal of Occupational Therapy, 66*(5), 250–260.

Field, T. (1981). Ecological variables and examiner biases in assessing handicapped preschool children. *Journal of Pediatric Psychology, 16,* 155–163.

Forness, S. R., Guthrie, D. S., & MacMillan, D. L. (1982). Classroom environments as they relate to mentally retarded children's observable behavior. *American Journal of Mental Deficiency, 87,* 259–265.

Goodman, R. B., & Krauss, B. (Eds.). (1977). *An exceptional view of life: The Easter Seal story.* Los Angeles: A Child's Point of View.

Greenwood, C. R. (1996). Research on the practices and behavior of effective teachers at the Juniper Gardens children's project: Implications for the education of diverse learners. In D. L. Speece & B. K. Keogh (Eds.), *Research on classroom ecologies: Implications for inclusion of children with learning disabilities* (pp. 39–67). Mahwah, NJ: Erlbaum.

Greenwood, C. R., Carta, J. J., Kamps, D., Terry, B., & Delquadri, J. C. (1994). Development and validation of standard classroom observation systems for school practitioners: Ecobehavioral Assessment Systems Software (EBASS). *Exceptional Children, 61,* 197–211.

Greenwood, C. R., Delquadri, J. C., Stanley, S. O., Terry, T., & Hall, R. V. (1985). Assessment of eco-behavioral interaction in school settings. *Behavioral Assessment, 7,* 331–347.

Gump, P. V. (1975). Ecological psychology and children. In M. Hetherington (Ed.), *Review of developmental research* (Vol. 5). Chicago: University of Chicago Press.

Hall, E. (1966). *The hidden dimension.* Garden City, NJ: Doubleday.

Harms, T., & Clifford, R. (1980). *The early childhood environmental rating scale.* New York: Teachers College Press.

Hartmann, D. P., Roper, B. C., & Bradford, P. C. (1979). Some relationships between behavioral and traditional assessment. *Journal of Behavioral Assessment, 1,* 3–21.

Hereford, S. M., Cleland, C. C., & Fellner, M. (1973). Territoriality and scentmarking: A study of profoundly retarded enuretics and encopretics. *American Journal of Mental Deficiency, 77,* 426–430.

Hutt, C., Hutt, S. J., & Ounsted, C. (1963). A method for the study of children's behavior. *Developmental Medicine and Child Neurology, 5,* 233–242.

Hutt, S. J., & Vaizey, M. (1966). Differential effects of group density on social behavior. *Nature, 209,* 1371–1372.

Imrie, R., & Kumar, M. (1998). Focusing on disability and access in the build environment. *Disability and Society, 13*(3), 357–374.

Jones, M. H., Barrett, M. L., Olonoff, C., & Anderson, E. (1969). Two experiments in training handicapped children at nursery school. *Clinics in Developmental Medicine and Child Neurology, 13.*

Jones, M. L., Favell, J. E., & Risley, T. R. (1983). Socioecological programming of the mentally retarded. In J. L. Matson & F. Andrasik (Eds.), *Treatment issues and intervention in mental retardation.* New York: Plenum Press.

Kontos, S., Moore, D., & Giorgetti, K. (1998). The ecology of inclusion. *Topics in Early Childhood Special Education, 18*(1), 38–48.

Landesman-Dwyer, S., Berkson, G., & Rosner, D. (1979). Affiliation and friendship of mentally retarded residents in group homes. *American Journal of Mental Deficiency, 83,* 571–580.

Lewin, K. (1951). *Field theory in social therapy.* New York: Harper Row.

Logan, K. R., Bakeman, R., & Keefe, E. B. (1997). Effects of instructional variables on engaged behavior of students with disabilities in general education classrooms. *Exceptional Children, 63,* 481–497.

Logan, K. R., & Malone, D. M. (1998). Comparing instructional contexts of students with and without severe disabilities in general education classrooms. *Exceptional Children, 64,* 343–358.

Long, N. V., & Dalston, R. M. (1982). Paired gestural and vocal behavior in one-year-old cleft lip and palate children. *Journal of Speech and Hearing Disorders, 47,* 403–406.

Lutman, M. E., & Tait, D. M. (1995). Early communicative behavior in young children receiving cochlear implants: Factor analysis of turntaking and gaze orientation. *Annals of Otology, Rhinology, and Laryngology* (Suppl. 166), 397–399.

McDonnell, J., Thorson, N., McQuivey, C., & Kiefer-O'Donnell, R. (1997). The academic engaged time of students with "low incidence" disabilities in general education classes: A pilot study. *Utah Special Educator, 17* [Online]. Available: http://www.usoe.k12.ut.us/SARS/INCLUSION/library/spedarticles/engagedtime.html

McEvoy, M. A., & McConnell, S. R. (1995). Understanding the emotional and behavioral development of young children: 3–6 years. In T. J. Zirpoli (Ed.), *Understanding and affecting the behavior of young children* (pp. 60–81). Englewood Cliffs, NJ: Prentice-Hall.

McEwen, I. R. (1992). Assisstive positioning as a control parameter of social-communicative interactions between students with profound multiple disabilities and classroom staff. *Physical Therapy, 72*(9), 634–646.

Miranda, P. (1997). Supporting individuals with challenging behavior through functional communication training and AAC: Research review. *Augmentative and Alternative Communication, 13,* 207–225.

Moos, R. H., & Trickett, E. J. (1974). *Classroom environmental scale manual.* Palo Alto, CA: Consulting Psychologists Press.

Paluck, R. J., & Esser, A. H. (1971). Territorial behavior as an indicator of change in clinical behavioral condition of severely retarded boys. *American Journal of Mental Deficiency, 76,* 284–290.

Phemister, M. R., Richardson, A. M., & Thomas, G. V. (1978). Observations of young normal and handicapped children. *Child: Care, Health and Development, 4,* 247–259.

Rago, W. V. (1977). Identifying profoundly mentally retarded subtypes as a means of institutional grouping. *American Journal of Mental Deficiency, 81,* 470–473.

Rago, W. V. (1978). Stability and aggressive behavior in profoundly mentally retarded institutionalized male adults. *American Journal of Mental Deficiency, 82,* 494–498.

Rago, W. V., Parker, R. M., & Cleland, C. C. (1978). Effects of increased space on the social behavior of institutionalized profoundly retarded male adults. *American Journal of Mental Deficiency, 82,* 554–558.

Ramey, S. L., Dossett, E., & Echols, K. (1996). The social ecology of mental retardation. In J. W. Jacobson & J. A. Mulick (Eds.), *Manual of diagnosis and professional practice in mental retardation* (pp. 55–73). Washington, DC: American Psychological Association Press.

Repp, A. C., Barton, L. E., & Gottlieb, T. (1983). Naturalistic studies of institutionalized profoundly or severely mentally retarded persons: The relationship of density and behavior. *American Journal of Mental Deficiency, 87,* 441–447.

Rettig, M. (1998). Environmental influences on the play of young children with disabilities. *Education and Training in Mental Retardation, 33*(2), 189–194.

Richer, J. (1979). Human ethology and mental handicap. In F. E. James & R. P. Smith (Eds.), *Psychiatric illness and mental handicap* (pp. 103–113). London: Gaskell Press.

Rogers-Warren, A. K., Ruggles, T. R., Peterson, N. L., & Cooper, A. Y. (1981) Playing and learning together: Patterns of social interaction in handicapped and nonhandicapped children. *Journal of the Division for Early Childhood, 3,* 56–63.

Routh, D., Schroeder, C., & O'Tuama, L. A. (1974). Development of activity levels in children. *Developmental Psychology, 10,* 163–168.

Sameroff, A. J., & Chandler, M. J. (1975). Reproductive risk and the continuum of caretaking casualty. In F. D. Horowitz, M. Hetherington, & S. Scarr-Salapatek (Eds.), *Review of child development research* (pp. 187–245). Chicago: University of Chicago Press.

Schoggen, P. (1978). Ecological psychology and mental retardation. In G. P. Sackett (Ed.), *Observing behavior: Theory and application in mental retardation* (Vol. 1, pp. 33–62). Baltimore: University Park Press.

Scott, M. (1980). Ecological theory and methods for research in special education. *Journal of Special Education, 14,* 279–294.

Stanley, S. O., & Greenwood, C. R. (1981). *CISSAR: Code for instructional structure and student academic response: Observer's manual.* Kansas City: University of Kansas, Bureau of Child Research, Juniper Gardens Childrens' Project.

Suedfeld, P., & Schwartz, G. (1983). Restricted environmental stimulation therapy (REST) as a treatment for autistic children. *Journal of Developmental and Behavioral Pediatrics, 4,* 196–201.

Sundel, M., & Sundel, S. S. (1999). *Behavior change in the human services: An introduction to principles and applications* (4th ed.). Thousand Oaks, CA: Sage.

Trickett, E. J., Leone, P. E., Fink, C. M., & Braaten, S. L. (1993). The perceived environment of special education classrooms for adolescents: A revision of the Classroom Environment Scale. *Exceptional Children, 59*(5), 411–420.

Ulvund, S. E. (1984). The psychological basis for the identification of physical environmental parameters in the development of early cognitive competence. *Scandinavian Journal of Educational Research, 25,* 125–140.

Wachs, T. D. (1979). Proximal experiences and early cognitive intellectual development: The physical environment. *Merrill-Palmer Quarterly, 25*(1), 3–41.

Wachs, T. D., Francis, J., & McQuiston, S. (1978). *Psychological dimensions of the infant's physical environment.* Paper presented at the meeting of the Midwestern Psychological Association, Chicago.

Yarrow, L. J., Rubenstein, J. L., & Pedersen, F. A. (1975). *Infant and environment: Early cognitive and motivational development.* Washington, DC: Hemisphere.

Ysseldyke, J. E., & Christenson, S. L. (1987). Evaluating students' instructional environments. *Remedial and Special Education, 8*(3), 17–24.

7

ASSESSMENT OF FAMILY CONTEXT

SUSAN L. ROSENTHAL
SHEILA S. COHEN
RUNE J. SIMEONSSON

This urgent need for support arises from many sources . . . parents have suddenly been thrust into a vacuum with previous expectations unmet and no knowledge to fill the void. . . . We try to balance our needs as fully functioning adults with her needs as a developing child. The evaluations are less frequent, but the questions raised in the early months continue to be raised, as we try to assess the directions our lives are taking as a family.

—Reisz (1984, pp. 37, 51)

A 9-year-old boy named Andrew was in the hospital with a foot amputated due to complications of a chronic condition. He would be wheelchair bound until his feet healed and prostheses were fitted. Andrew and his parents live in a townhouse in which the only bathroom is on the second floor. Only his father is strong enough to carry him to the second floor. His father is a truck driver, so the mother is often alone with Andrew. As a receptionist, Andrew's mother has limited flexibility in her work hours. Andrew needs to be reintegrated into both his home and school environments.

This chapter defines the objectives associated with assessment of the family and how they complement the comprehensive assessment of children with complex needs. Anyone engaged in the provision of psychological care for children with complex problems holds implicit or explicit assumptions about the nature of families and the way they function. Because these assumptions influence both assessment and intervention activities, it is important to recognize that the "framework that we bring to understanding how families behave can facilitate or retard our work. If we have too narrow a view of family functioning, the types of questions, goals, and strategies we can use become more of a disservice than a help to families" (Freeman, 1976, p. 746). How we observe families is affected by our cultural framework. The qualities that we believe are important for healthier family functioning are those that are associated with the kinds of qualities we believe healthier adults require in our culture (Cole-Kelly & Kaye, 1993). Evaluation of families cannot take place without the consideration of the culture; for example, even the word "family" may mean something different for different ethnic groups (Goldenberg & Goldenberg, 1985). We need to be aware of these frameworks and be willing to incorporate them in order to insure appropriate assessment of families and their roles in the development and adaptation of their children.

As we have indicated elsewhere, the family has been conceptualized in a number of ways (Simeonsson & Simeonsson, 1993). Many approaches have a psychopathological orientation, with the family perceived in terms of dysfunctional relationships. Although psychopathology may be present in the family of a child with special needs, it should not be assumed that the presence of a child with disabilities will, in and of itself, be a marker for psychopathology. The presence of a special child may or may not impose demands or adaptations that will differentiate one family from another in terms of pathology. It is, therefore, important that the assessment of families be approached through frameworks that encompass normality, as well as deviation, of structural and functional characteristics. Families with children with special needs may function in unique ways without being pathological. Family patterns associated with psychiatric difficulties within families of children who do not have special needs are likely also to be associated with such difficulties within families with children with special needs. If parental depression is related to poorer child functioning in families that do not have a child with special needs, then it should be related to decreased functioning within families that have children with special needs as well. An example is a study of children with mental retardation or developmental disabilities that found that those children who experienced depression had mothers who indicated depression on the Parenting Stress Index (Kobe & Hammer, 1994).

One additional consideration of particular relevance for families with children with complex needs is the fact that both child and family are characterized by development and change. For example, the stress on the family of a child with developmental delays may vary according to the age of the child (Orr, Cameron, Dobson, & Day, 1993; Warfield, Krauss, Hauser-Cram, Upshur, & Shonkoff, 1999). A developmental perspective builds on the assumption that changes within and outside the family are transactional in nature, such that one change contributes to another that in turn leads to yet other changes over time. This perspective is consistent with a family life cycle model that focuses on the developmental path of families (Carter & McGoldrick, 1989; McGoldrick, Heiman, & Carter, 1993). The model proposes that families go through a progression of stages. The model incorporates the power of both horizontal stressors (i.e., predictable events or life cycle transitions, such as the child beginning school or getting a driver's license, and unpredictable events, such as untimely deaths or the diagnosis of a chronic illness or condition) and vertical stressors (i.e., family patterns, myths, secrets, and legacies). All of these events occur within the context of the nuclear and extended family, as well as the social, economic, and political climate.

Families with children with complex problems go through a progression of stages in adjusting to the child's disability or chronic illness. The timing of this adjustment occurs in the context of horizontal and vertical stressors. The adaptation to the initial diagnosis or other changes in the child's functioning will be affected by the interaction between the developmental stage of the family and horizontal and vertical stressors. Some families may utilize a coping style that worked previously for predictable horizontal stressors but that may have lost utility when confronted with unpredictable horizontal stressors (Rolland, 1989). For example, a family may be preparing to send their adolescent son to a residential school to study music. They are preparing themselves for the horizontal stressor (a child leaving home) and preparing to address grandfather's lifelong desire to have a concert-level violinist in the family (vertical flow). The son's diagnosis of arthritis results in his being too ill to leave home to attend the residential school and may prevent him from becoming a professional violinist. The family also may have been counting on a music scholarship for college for this adolescent. The timing of this diagnosis may result in poorer adaptation for this family than if the son had been diagnosed as a younger child. The grandfather may have been able to shift his need for a musician to another family member, and the family would not have had expectations that the child was ready to leave home. Considering these issues allows the psychologist to aid the family in reestablishing the developmental momentum (Simeonsson & Rosenthal, 2000).

OBJECTIVES FOR ASSESSING THE FAMILY CONTEXT

Every family presents the opportunity to explore a wealth of information beyond what is realistic for any assessment. Therefore, psychologists must focus their assessments on answering specific questions. However, efforts to address specific questions often need to be broad based. Family assessment can be used to understand better why, despite good intentions, the family has not been able to follow through on treatment recommendations or presents barriers to treatment success. Family assessment may be important at the beginning of program planning because it can help the psychologist and the family choose among intervention options. Comprehensive and integrated care is valued by many families of children with chronic illness (Walders & Drotar, 1999). For example, if the parents of a child with motor impairments are overwhelmed by the financial demands and missed work days resulting from caring for their child, adding a daily trip to the physical therapist may not be effective. It may be more effective to begin by determining additional sources of financial support and teaching the parents activities that they can do in the home to facilitate motor development.

Another aspect of choosing what areas to assess among the wealth of possibilities that families provide is to be cognizant and sensitive to the expectations and needs of the families (Simeonsson, 1996). Families enter the assessment process with expectations; failures to meet these expectations may result in dissatisfaction, distress, or uneasiness. As with all interpersonal experiences, there is an interactive effect, with the professionals affecting the parents and the parents affecting the professionals. However, with time given to establish everyone's expectations and to clarify the potential for meeting those expectations, the experience can be mutually satisfying and can lead to the development of a working alliance. Also, families' expectations and behavior may vary as a function of the age of their child. The family may have very different needs when coping with the initial diagnosis of a chronic illness than when preparing their adolescent with a chronic condition for group care.

In addressing specific questions, at least two distinct domains can be identified as of interest: family culture and family interactions. The overriding objective is to use the understanding of these domains of functioning to develop relevant and supportive interventions for children and families. The information can be useful in maximizing intervention success by developing plans that are compatible with the family's goals and realistic for them to implement.

Documentation of Family Culture

One important assessment objective with the family is to document its psychological characteristics. The objective here is to identify attitudes, values, beliefs, personal traits, and adaptation styles of family members, as well as of the family as a unit. Two types of assessment data are needed. One focuses on differentiating families along such dimensions as coping with stress, accepting a child with special needs, and perceiving control in their lives; and the other type of data describes the family's values and environment.

Documentation of Family Interactions

A second objective of assessing families is to ascertain the nature of relationships among family members. Such assessment can reveal the frequency and quality of verbal and social interactions within the family unit, including the management of boundaries. Historically, the mother–child relationship typically has been investigated with the highest frequency; however, father–child and sibling relationships are also of critical importance to examine.

SPECIAL ISSUES IN THE ASSESSMENT OF FAMILIES

The need to assess families of children with special needs is obvious. However, several issues need to be considered prior to carrying out the actual assessment. Two of these issues are the choice of methodology and the role of significant others.

The Choice of Methodology

The choice of methodology is an important issue in the assessment of the family context. To some extent, this choice may depend on the conceptual framework adopted, in the sense that certain methodologies have grown out of specific frameworks. For example, examination of family culture often relies on structured rating scales of stress or family environment, whereas documentation of family interactions often uses observation of family interactions, either in a structured fashion or during an interview. It is, therefore, important to recognize that the methodology employed may impose limitations on the assessment process and the nature of the data that are derived. Clinical interviews, although they are widely used and provide an extremely rich source of information, yield information that is idiosyncratic and subjective in nature. Self-ratings are potentially confounded by the literacy demands of the instrument and may reflect socially desirable responses. The use of self-ratings may also be confounded by the lack of independence between raters, as in the case of husband and wife ratings of family stress. Third-party ratings may be subject to clinical bias, and observational procedures are often restricted to specific controlled settings that limit the generalizability of the findings. There are, of course, methodological steps, such as test–retest and alternate forms procedures, that can be taken to reduce these limitations. As a further step, we recommend that, whenever possible, a particular domain be assessed in several ways to increase the scope and reliability of findings. Assessment of family functioning could thus be evaluated by interviewing family members, by making systematic observations of family behavior, and by asking family members to complete rating scales. The combination of two or more methodologies can serve to corroborate results, as well as to identify discrepancies of potential importance in interpreting findings.

Another important aspect of choosing the methodology is the purpose of the data collection. The focus of this chapter is on using information to develop intervention plans, but it is also important to be able to document the need for services, or change and progress.

Payers of services require psychologists to justify the need for services and to be accountable for the services that they deliver. In order to document the effectiveness of services, one needs to utilize measures that are as objective and quantifiable as possible. Measures that provide standard scores based on comparing families with a normative sample may be most useful for this purpose. For example, documentation of the amount of parental stress related to medical interventions that may have become routine within the medical community (e.g., apnea monitors; Phipps & Drotar, 1990) could be used to alter treatment plans. Similarly, measures of coping and stress could be used to document whether interventions such as respite care have an impact on a family's life (Rimmerman, 1989; Sherman, 1995).

The Role of Significant Others

A second issue to consider in the assessment of families is the influence of significant others. Families themselves consist of siblings, grandparents, aunts, and uncles. For example, how siblings adjust to a child with disabilities may influence overall family functioning or that of individual members within the family. In addition, the family is a system nested within larger ecological systems (Bronfenbrenner, 1977). The variability in the ways families function may reflect, to different degrees, the influence of significant others in formal and informal systems. Although the potential number of sources of influence is large, those of significance are likely to be immediate rather than distant to the family. In regard to informal systems, friends, relatives, and neighbors may play important roles in the adaptation and functioning of families. The church, other organizations, and private and public agencies constitute more formal systems that may have significant impact on the family.

ASSESSMENT INSTRUMENTS AND PROCEDURES

Family Interviews

Family interviews differ in degree of structure and organization. General clinical interviewing skills apply to working with families as well. In addition, interviewing the family provides opportunities to involve other members of the family, for example, siblings, grandparents, aunts, or uncles. By asking them to participate in the process and by collecting information about their lives, one can assess their adaptation in general and the special demands placed on them and the family, by the needs of the child with complex problems.

One format for collecting information about the family culture is a genogram, which is a method for displaying family information graphically. It allows one to examine family patterns and develop hypotheses about how a problem may be connected to the family context (McGoldrick, Gerson, & Shellenberger, 1999). A system to make the construction of a genogram more uniform is well described by McGoldrick and colleagues (1999). Genograms usually cover a minimum of three generations, allowing a clinician to assess the role of grandparents, aunts, uncles, and cousins in the family's life. Significant others who are not family members are included in the genogram as triangles on the side. This could include organizations, such as churches, support groups, or persons such as nannies or close family friends.

Genograms are a useful tool for helping both the psychologist and family begin to see both the current and historical context of problems and how the horizontal and vertical pressures affect the family. The vertical flow includes patterns of relating and functioning that are transmitted historically down the generations. The genogram of the family of a child with a chronic condition allows one to assess how the family has handled chronic conditions in the past. For example, the family may describe an uncle with a seizure disorder who has never functioned independently. It may then be clear why the family appears concerned that their child will not attain independent functioning or, conversely, why they do not appear to expect independent functioning from their child. The genogram can be used to aid the family in understanding such patterns. Horizontal flows result from current stressors in the family. Again, when creating the genogram with the family, one may find that the grandmother has recently become ill, the father has had to work overtime, and that the mother's friends are all returning to work because their children are at ages at which they can function independently. Yet the mother of the identified child has decided not to return to work because her child with complex problems frequently needs to go to doctor appointments or physical and occupational therapy and because no one else in the family can share these responsibilities. The mother is then in a situation in which the expected developmental processes of families has been disrupted.

Genograms are most useful for understanding family culture, and just the process of collecting the information can provide valuable information. For example, the mother may be silent when the psychologist is collecting information about the father's family, but the father may be vocal and interrupt the mother when the psychologist is collecting information about the mother's family. Observation of this behavior might generate several hypotheses, including that the family may be closer or more involved with the mother's than with the father's family or that the family expects that the father will "speak" for the family. Evaluating these hypotheses may lead to the development of successful interventions.

Another assessment technique is the eco-map (Hartman, 1978). The eco-map has been proposed as a tool to assess and plan intervention for families. Families are asked to identify social networks outside of the immediate family (both formal and informal networks). Those often identified for families with children with special needs include health care systems, educational systems, places of employment, social welfare systems, extended families, neighbors and friends, and church affiliations (Valentine, 1993). It involves line drawings that represent a family and the systems in their environment. The lines are drawn to represent the different kinds of relationships, for example, supportive, stressful, and tenuous relationships. An illustration of the ways in which the relationships between the family and these systems can be differentiated to reflect both strength and quality is illustrated in a report of a hearing-impaired student (Skyer, 1982). The eco-map also has been used to assess and identify intervention strategies for families with children with developmental disabilities (Valentine, 1993). Using the eco-map with 25 families, four family profiles were developed: the well-supported family, the stressed family, the isolated family, and the overextended family. Interventions were then recommended for families that matched the various profiles.

Objective Measures

The range of instruments that can be considered here is large, because there may be interest in any number of characteristics common to most families, or unique to families with children with complex problems. Some of these measures focus on traits, others on adaptation, and others on family environment. Obviously, all three of these aspects of families may influence family interactions.

Traits in this context are defined as characteristics of a personal nature, such as attitudes, values, beliefs, and temperament. Logically, as well as theoretically, the assumption that there are relationships between these traits and child and family outcomes seems reasonable. For example, documentation of parent locus of control (Nowicki & Duke, 1974) may be useful in gaining a more comprehensive picture of the family but may also contribute to a more precise calibration of family intervention based on a recognition of a family's perception of control over events. For example, when a father complained about his frustration with the variability of his child's juvenile rheumatoid arthritis, the father pointed out that he was a mechanic and would lose his job if he did not "fix" the problems presented to him at work.

Assessment of adaptation includes a variety of attempts to assess the family's response to general demands, as well as those specific to raising a child with disabilities. These concepts have been investigated extensively in medical and mental health contexts. Two well-known instruments of stress and/or coping that are applicable to families of children with special needs are the Parenting Stress Index (PSI; Abidin, 1995) and the Questionnaire on Resources and Stress (QRS; Holroyd, 1974). Unlike some of the methods described previously, the PSI focuses on a parent (often the mother) rather than on the family. It can be used, however, to understand the difference between mother's and father's stress responses to a child with special needs (Beckman, 1991; Darke & Goldberg, 1994) and has been used to document the relationship of maternal stress to other measures of the child's functioning, such as adaptive level (Hanson & Hanline, 1990; Robbins, Dunlap, & Plienis, 1991). The fact that a lower level of adaptive functioning was related to parental stress and the child's cognitive level was not (Hanson & Hanline, 1990) points to the importance of considering the relationship between a child's behavior and the functioning of the family but does not suggest a causal direction. The PSI also allows one to differentiate stress associated with child-related issues and those related to aspects of the parent domain (e.g., health, spousal relationship; Orr et al., 1993). The QRS has been useful in a variety of contexts and across populations with different disabilities or chronic conditions. The QRS considers the bidirectional impact between family systems variables and child behavior, as well as development (Dunst, Trivette, Hamby, & Pollock, 1990; Dyson, 1991; Dyson, Edgar, & Crnic, 1989).

Assessment of the family environment includes an evaluation of what the family values and its daily activities. One of the best examples of this approach is the Family Environment Scale (FES; Moos & Moos, 1986). This measure describes family functioning in terms of variables such as cohesion, expressiveness, conflict, organization, and control. A profile of standard scores can be derived indicating the family's relative strengths and deficits in the particular domains. Factor analyses have yielded three higher order factor scales: support, conflict, and control (Kronenberger & Thompson, 1990). Scores on this measure are related to many aspects of adaptive functioning in children and adolescents. An example of its use with families with children with special needs is an examination of the dietary practices of families with and without children with hypercholesterolemia (Rosenthal, Knauer-Black, Stahl, Catalanatto, & Sprecher, 1993). The finding that dietary practices were related to family functioning and not to whether or not the family had a child with hypercholesterolemia may help practitioners identify key focuses of intervention to improve the health of children with hypercholesterolemia. Others have found the scale useful in discovering similarities between families of children with chronic conditions and matched comparison families (Noll et al., 1994).

There is substantial variability in psychometric properties and format of measures of family culture and interaction. The measures described previously are summarized in Table 7.1. A consideration when choosing a measure should include whether one desires a measure used only with certain populations, such as families with children with chronic

TABLE 7.1. Selected Tools to Assess Family Context

Measure/procedure	Form and focus	Format of results
Genogram (McGoldrick, Gerson, & Shellenberger, 1999)	Semistructured—family culture/interaction	Visual representation of family structure/relationships
Eco-map (Hartman, 1978)	Semistructured—family culture/interaction	Visual representation of family structure/relationships
Parent locus of control (Nowicki & Duke, 1974)	Objective—single trait	40 items answered in external direction
Parenting Stress Index (PSI; Abidin, 1995)	Objective—stress	Total stress index and stress scores related to child–parent characteristics and life stress events
Questionnaire on Resources and Stress (QRS; Holroyd, 1974)	Objective—stress and coping	15 scales, 3 clusters of parent, child, and family problems
Family Environment Scale (FES; Moos & Moos, 1986)	Objective—family culture	Profile of 10 subscales

illnesses (Stein & Reissman, 1980), or one used with families either with or without children with special needs (Moos & Moos, 1986). The selection of an assessment instrument also requires consideration of the response format (true/false vs. multiple choice), content orientation (pathology–normality), reading level, and time required for completion. The importance of considering time required for completion is evident in the multiple efforts to shorten the original QRS. The original measure is quite long (285 items), and various efforts have been made to develop a reliable and valid shorter version in order to make its use more feasible (Glidden, 1993; Konstantareas, Homatidis, & Plowright, 1992).

IMPLICATIONS FOR PRACTICE

The importance of understanding the family culture and interaction of families of children with complex problems should be clear. As indicated in this chapter, assessment of families should be carried out in complement to the assessment of the child with special needs in order to improve intervention planning and to evaluate progress. To this end, we must specify some essential points in the assessment of families:

1. Approach the family objectively; avoid a prior assumption of pathology. Be sensitive to cultural, religious, and personal values of families.
2. Specify the purpose of the assessment to the family and involve them in the process of determining overall goals.
3. Select assessment instruments or procedures suited to assessment goals and client characteristics. Develop competence in unstandardized procedures and evaluate the psychometric characteristics of standardized instruments.
4. When feasible, verify the assessment data by obtaining information from several sources and through several means.

In planning interventions for families, it is particularly important that professionals recognize that the values and position they themselves advocate may not be unilaterally endorsed by families. For example, although parent involvement, deinstitutionalization, and mainstreaming are issues strongly advocated by professionals for families in general, they may be neither desired nor appropriate for certain families. Professionals must be particularly aware of the subjectivity of their own philosophies and value systems in order to avoid imposing demands on families that are incompatible with the adaptation of a particular family. Semistructured methods such as the genogram or eco-map may be most useful when the interviewer is well aware of his or her own personal biases. Genograms and eco-maps allow the family to "tell their own story." As the psychologist begins to listen to the family's unique story, hypotheses can be presented to the family for verification and clarification. Regardless of the method, all assessment results should be interpreted in terms of both the theoretical and empirical frameworks from which they are drawn and placed in the practical reality of everyday life. The roles and values of families as consumers may differ from those of professionals as providers (Simeonsson & Simeonsson, 1993). Because most professionals are not likely to have the personal experience of raising a child with complex problems, careful perspective taking on the part of professionals may be an important step to make the assessment process more congruent and thereby more productive for families.

REFERENCES

Abidin, R. R. (1995). *Parenting stress index* (3rd ed.). Odessa, FL: Psychological Assessment Resources.

Beckman, P. J. (1991). Comparison of mothers' and fathers' perceptions of the effect of young children with and without disabilities. *American Journal on Mental Retardation, 95,* 585–595.

Bronfenbrenner, V. (1977). Toward an experimental ecology of human development. *American Psychologist, 32,* 513–531.

Carter, B., & McGoldrick, M. (1989). *The changing family life cycle* (2nd ed.). Needham Heights, MA: Allyn & Bacon.

Cole-Kelly, K., & Kaye, D. (1993). Assessing the family. In M. I. Singer, L. T. Singer, & T. M. Anglin (Eds.), *Handbook for screening adolescents at psychosocial risk* (pp. 1–40). New York: Lexington Books.

Darke, P. R., & Goldberg, S. (1994). Father–infant interaction and parent stress with healthy and medically compromised infants. *Infant Behavior and Development, 17,* 3–14.

Dunst, C. J., Trivette, C. M., Hamby, D., & Pollock, B. (1990). Family systems correlates of the behavior of young children with handicaps. *Journal of Early Intervention, 14,* 204–218.

Dyson, L., Edgar, E., & Crnic, K. (1989). Psychological predictors of adjustment by siblings of developmentally disabled children. *American Journal on Mental Retardation, 94,* 292–302.

Dyson, L. L. (1991). Families of young children with handicaps: Parental stress and family functioning. *American Journal on Mental Retardation, 95,* 623–629.

Freeman, D. S. (1976). The family as a system: Fact or fancy. *Comprehensive Psychiatry, 17,* 735–749.

Glidden, L. M. (1993). What we do not know about families with children who have developmental disabilities: Questionnaire on resources and stress as a case study. *American Journal on Mental Retardation, 95,* 585–595.

Goldenberg, I., & Goldenberg, H. (1985). Patterns of family interaction. In I. Goldenberg & H. Goldenberg (Eds.), *Family therapy: An overview* (2nd ed., pp. 3–27). Monterey, CA: Brooks/Cole.

Hanson, M. J., & Hanline, M. F. (1990). Parenting a child with a disability: A longitudinal study of parental stress and adaptation. *Journal of Early Intervention, 14,* 234–248.

Hartman, A. (1978). Diagrammatic assessment of family relationship. *Social Casework, 59,* 465–476.

Holroyd, J. (1974). The questionnaires on resources and stress: An instrument to measure family responses to a handicapped family member. *Journal of Community Psychology, 2,* 92–94.

Kobe, F. H., & Hammer, D. (1994). Parenting stress and depression in children with mental retardation and developmental disabilities. *Research in Developmental Disabilities, 15,* 209–221.

Konstantareas, M. M., Homatidis, S., & Plowright, C. M. S. (1992). Assessing resources and stress in parents of severely dysfunctional children through the Clarke modification of Holroyd's questionnaire on resources and stress. *Journal of Autism and Developmental Disorders, 22,* 217–234.

Kronenberger, W. G., & Thompson, R. J. (1990). Dimensions of family functioning in families with chronically ill children: A higher order factor analysis of the Family Environment Scale. *Journal of Clinical Child Psychology, 4,* 380–388.

McGoldrick, M., Gerson, R., & Shellenberger, S. (1999). *Genograms: Assessment and intervention* (2nd ed.). New York: Norton.

McGoldrick, M., Heiman, M., & Carter, B. (1993). The changing family life cycle: A perspective on normalcy. In F. Walsh (Ed.), *Normal family processes* (2nd ed., pp. 405–443). New York: Guilford.

Moos, R. H., & Moos, B. M. (1986). *Family Environment Scale Manual* (2nd ed.). Palo Alto, CA: Consulting Psychologists Press.

Noll, R., Swiecki, E., Garstein, M., Vannatta, K., Kalinyak, K., Davies, W. H., & Bukowski, W. (1994). Parental distress, family conflict, and role of social support for caregivers with or without a child with sickle cell disease. *Family Systems Medicine, 12,* 281–294.

Nowicki, S., & Duke, M. P. (1974). A locus of control scale for college as well as non-college adults. *Journal of Personality Assessment, 38,* 136–137.

Orr, R. R., Cameron, S. J., Dobson, L. A., & Day, D. M. (1993). Age-related changes in stress experienced by families with a child who has developmental delays. *Mental Retardation, 31,* 171–176.

Phipps, S., & Drotar, D. (1990). Determinants of parenting stress in home apnea monitoring. *Journal of Pediatric Psychology, 15,* 385–400.

Reisz, E. D. (1984). *First years of a Down's syndrome child.* Iowa City: University of Iowa.

Rimmerman, A. (1989). Provision of respite care for children with developmental disabilities: Changes in maternal coping and stress over time. *Mental Retardation, 27,* 99–103.

Robbins, F. R., Dunlap, G., & Plienis, A. J. (1991). Family characteristics, family training, and the progress of young children with autism. *Journal of Early Intervention, 15,* 173–184.

Rolland, J. S. (1989). Chronic illness and the family life cycle. In B. Carter & M. McGoldrick (Eds.), *The changing family life cycle: A framework for family therapy* (2nd ed., pp. 443–456). Boston: Allyn & Bacon.

Rosenthal, S. L., Knauer-Black, S., Stahl, M. P., Catalanotto, T. J., & Sprecher, D. L. (1993). Psychological functioning of children with hypercholesterolemia and their families: A preliminary investigation. *Clinical Pediatrics, 32,* 135–141.

Sherman, B. R. (1995). Impact of home-based respite care on families of children with chronic illnesses. *Children's Health Care, 24*(1), 33–45.

Simeonsson, R. J. (1996). Family expectations, encounters, and needs. In M. Brambring, H. Rauh, & A. Beelmann (Eds.), *Early childhood intervention: Theory, evaluation, and practice* (pp. 196–207). Berlin: Walter de Gruyter.

Simeonsson, R. J., & Rosenthal, S. L. (2000). Developmental models and clinical practice. In C. E. Walker & M. C. Roberts (Eds.), *Handbook of clinical child psychology* (3rd ed.). New York: Wiley.

Simeonsson, R. J., & Simeonsson, N. E. (1993). Children, families, and disabilities: Psychological dimensions. In J. L. Paul & R. J. Simeonsson (Eds.), *Children with special needs: Family, culture and society* (2nd ed., pp. 97–110). Fort Worth, TX: Harcourt Brace Jovanovich.

Skyer, S. C. (1982). Psycho-social aspects of deafness course as a counseling tool for the hearing impaired. *American Annals of the Deaf, 123,* 115–121.

Stein, R., & Reissman, C. (1980). The development of the Impact on Family Scale: Preliminary findings. *Medical Care, 18,* 465–472.

Valentine, D. P. (1993). Children with special needs: Sources of support and stress for families. *Journal of Social Work and Human Sexuality, 8,* 107–121.

Walders, N., & Drotar, D. (1999). Integrating health and mental health services in the care of children and adolescents with chronic health conditions: Assumptions, challenges, and opportunities. *Children's Services: Social Policy, Research, and Practice, 2,* 117–138.

Warfield, M., Krauss, M., Hauser-Cram, P., Upshur, C., & Shonkoff, J. (1999). Adaptation during early childhood among mothers of children with disabilities. *Developmental and Behavioral Pediatrics, 20,* 9–16.

PART III

Specialized Strategies and Measures

8

ASSESSMENT OF TRAUMA
AND MALTREATMENT IN CHILDREN
WITH SPECIAL NEEDS

BARBARA W. BOAT
H. JANE SITES

Brianna, age 4 years, 3 months, was referred for evaluation through the local develop-mental assessment center by her preschool teacher and her mother. The assessment of this child focused on the following behaviors: aggressive interactions with peers and adults, frequent screaming outbursts, severe articulation problems with language delays, and ter-rified responses to motor vehicles and equipment such as trucks, lawn mowers, and vacuum cleaners. The teacher noted that Brianna preferred to play alone and refused to go on local walking field trips in her inner-city community. The teacher mentioned that she also was concerned about Brianna's reaction to her mother when her mother arrived late each after-noon to take her home. Brianna appeared fearful and whiney and sometimes cried and flinched when her mother attempted to put on her coat. When the clinician asked the teacher if she suspected emotional or physical abuse at home, the teacher admitted that she was worried. The clinician suggested that the teacher take advantage of the frequent changing of clothes and toileting activities that occur in the preschool environment to observe Brianna's body for signs of bruises or cuts. Significant bruising of the buttocks was noted several days later and a referral was made to protective services.

Brianna is one of an increasing number of children of all ages who are experiencing maltreatment in their lives (Westat, Inc., 1993). We know that maltreatment affects chil-dren throughout the developmental range, and we know that the stakes are high. We also know that abuse and neglect of all children, including children with disabilities, is under-reported (Finkelhor, Hotaling, Lewis, & Smith, 1990). For example, it has been estimated by researchers who compared reporting data and population sample interview data that only 3%–5% of all abuse cases are ever reported to authorities. Most abuse occurs in se-cret and is often kept skillfully hidden from teachers, therapists, physicians, and even caregivers. Therefore, we must learn to ask questions and make observations that are not generally covered in standard assessment texts or clinical coursework. Through a system-atic approach to maltreatment assessment, we provide the child and caregivers an opportunity to share, or discover, possible abusive or traumatic histories that are affecting the child's life in ways that may be more disabling than the child's diagnosed disability. In order for effective prevention and intervention efforts to be provided, it is important to identify assessment strategies and measures on which to base these diagnostic efforts.

This chapter focuses on assessment of children with special needs who are at risk for, or who have experienced, abuse or neglect. We present a brief discussion on the prevalence of child abuse and neglect in the general population and among children with special needs; review the effects of trauma and maltreatment on child development; highlight selected issues in reporting suspected abuse or neglect; and describe specific approaches to assessing possible maltreatment in children.

SCOPE OF THE PROBLEM

Prevalence of Maltreatment among Children

When we look at the National Child Abuse and Neglect Statistical Fact Sheet (U.S. Department of Health and Human Services, 1995, 1996), the regrettable statistics alert and alarm us concerning the high incidence of child maltreatment in the general population.

- Investigations by child protective services agencies in 48 states determined that 1,012,000 children were victims of child abuse and neglect in 1994. This figure represents a 27% increase since 1990, when approximately 800,000 children were found to be victims of maltreatment.
- In 1994, state child protective services agencies received and referred for investigation an estimated 2 million reports alleging the maltreatment of 2.9 million children.
- Among the children for whom maltreatment was substantiated or indicated in 1994, about 53% suffered neglect, 26% physical abuse, 14% sexual abuse, 5% emotional abuse, 3% medical neglect, and 19% other forms of maltreatment. Some children were victims of more than one type of maltreatment.
- During the 5-year period from 1990 to 1994, state child protective service agencies reported that a total of 5,400 children died as a result of abuse or neglect.
- In 1994, almost half of all reported victims of child maltreatment (47%) were under age 6 and almost equally divided between boys and girls.
- Several studies suggest that more than twice as many children suffer from abuse or neglect than are noted in official statistics from state child protective services agencies.

Abuse among Children with Special Needs

Children with disabilities are overrepresented in statistics on abuse (Ammerman, Hersen, & Van Hasselt, 1989). One large school district in the Midwest noted that nearly 45% of its reported child abuse cases involved children who were receiving special services (PACER Center, 1988). Information on 1,834 children nationwide, taken from 35 child protective services agencies that were statistically selected to be nationally representative, revealed that the incidence of maltreatment among children with disabilities was 1.7 times higher than maltreatment of children without disabilities (Westat, Inc., 1993). Unidentified prior abuse may have caused the disabilities, created new disabilities, or worsened already existing difficulties.

Recently, Sullivan and Knutson (1998) looked at the association between child maltreatment and disabilities in a rigorous pediatric hospital-based epidomiological study. Disabilities were twice as prevalent among the maltreated hospital sample as among the nonmaltreated hospital controls, consistent with the hypothesis that maltreatment contributes to disabilities (Jaudes & Diamond, 1985; Sandgrund, Gaines, & Green, 1974) as well as with the hypothesis that disabilities increase the risk for maltreatment. Prevalence of a behavior disorder in the abused hospital sample was 20 times greater than in the nonabused control sample. Among abused children, behavior disorders, speech and language disorders, mental retardation, learning disabilities, and hearing impairments were the most common types of disabilities. Children with communicative disorders were at greater risk for physical and sexual abuse. Mentally retarded participants experienced the most severe combinations of physical and sexual abuse. Children with multiple disabilities were at the greatest risk and more likely to have experienced the most severe forms of sexual and/or physical abuse and longer durations of abuse and neglect than children with a single type of disability. Children with disabilities, like children in general, were at greatest risk for maltreatment by perpetrators within the family. A large proportion of children had been maltreated most of their lives. With the majority of abused children with disabilities being maltreated under the age of 5, the need for early assessment and intervention services with young children is obvious.

Boys with disabilities have been found to be more likely victims of sexual abuse than boys without disabilities in the general population, and more male victims are identified in studies of maltreatment among children with disabilities (Sullivan, Brookhouser, Knutson, Scanlan, & Schulte, 1991; Sullivan & Knutson, 1998; Westat, Inc., 1993).

The fundamental question of why children with disabilities should be more vulnerable to abuse remains unanswered (Wescott, 1991) and involves a complex interaction of biological, familial, and sociological variables (Garbarino, Brookhauser, & Authier, 1987; Sobsey & Varnhagen, 1989). Studies have described the "social construction" of disability through disabling attitudes, behaviors, and environments (Sobsey, 1994; Sobsey, Wells, Lucardie, & Mansell, 1995). For example, once a disability is identified, females are at increased risk of maltreatment and abuse (Groce, 1997; Nosek, Howland, & Young, 1997). Some characteristics that are believed to make children with disabilities more vulnerable to abuse appear to be related to their dependency on others for their basic needs (Tharinger, Horton, & Millea, 1990). These children often lack control and choice over their own lives. Compliance and obedience are instilled as good behavior and the unequal power relationships encourage children to heed the instructions of any adult (Sobsey & Varnhagen, 1989). Many of these children lack knowledge about sexualized behaviors and may not understand sexual advances by caregivers. Furthermore, their isolation and rejection by others can increase their responsiveness to attention and affection, as well as a desire to please, making them an easy target for sexual exploitation. The inability to distinguish among different types of touching, as well as problems in reasoning, impulse control, and predicting the consequences of their actions, heightens the vulnerability of many of these children.

In general, children find it difficult to directly disclose abuse. Sorenson and Snow (1991) found that the majority of children disclose sexual abuse accidentally or tentatively and advise that many children will not tell about abuse unless questioned directly. Children with expressive language and other communication disorders often are at even greater disadvantage in describing the acts of abuse and establishing their credibility as accurate reporters (Ammerman, Van Hasselt, & Hersen, 1988; Monat-Haller, 1992). Some children lack sufficient receptive and attentional skills to even process the questions.

There is a body of research that suggests that the child's characteristics may play more than a passive role in abuse and neglect (Cohen & Warren, 1990). The "degree of disability" can affect abuse potential. For example, parental expectations are frequently higher for the more able-bodied or capable-appearing child whose disability is not easily diagnosed. Because of their expectations for normality, a parent may experience more frustration and stress and become abusive or neglectful of a child who is not easily identified as impaired or disabled. In addition, the disability may be a source of embarrassment, failed aspirations, or perceived punishment. Family resources may be strained, increasing levels of family stress with a potential for long-term family crises that place the child at risk for longer periods of time (Morgan, 1987; Zirpoli, 1986).

The care and treatment of a child with disabilities may require educational and caregiving situations that put a child in harm's way, such as unaccompanied bus rides to and from school and the lack of close supervision in residential treatment centers. There is evidence that children with hearing impairments who are educated in residential schools are more likely to be sexually abused than children in inclusionary settings and have more difficulty finding a trusted adult in residential settings to tell about the abuse (Sullivan et al., 1991; Westat, Inc., 1993).

The demands of rearing a handicapped child can be unrelenting. Special attention must be directed toward identifying neglect and being alert to such behaviors as a parent's failure to keep appointments for their child's medical or audiological care, weight loss or failure to thrive in younger children, and poorly informed or uninterested caregivers. When these problems occur with parents who are mentally ill and/or low functioning, appropriate responses to possible neglect of a child are essential.

Although the indicators of child abuse and neglect in children with disabilities are much the same as for the general population, there is an additional problem. Child behaviors that could signal abuse may be inappropriately attributed to the child's disability, and the possible abuse etiologies of such behaviors may never be explored (Horton & Kochurka, 1995). These behaviors include elective mutism, withdrawal, changes in eating or sleeping habits, increased physical aggression, onset of sexual aggression or sexual behaviors, self-destructive behaviors, urinary or bowel problems, and sexually transmitted disease and pregnancy. For example, a young girl with developmental disabilities who wears multiple layers of clothing may be thought of as dressing inappropriately due to a lack of understanding of social norms or weather conditions, rather than the desire to protect her body from sexual assaults. Clinicians need to be aware of these "soft signs" as indicators of possible abuse, as in the teacher's observations in the case of Brianna, and not prematurely attribute such behaviors to the child's disability.

Based on the rationale that we will have more information about the child if we ask relevant questions, the premise of this chapter is that all child assessments should screen for past and current stressors, as well as for traumas and abusive incidents in the lives of children and their caregivers. In addition, child behaviors that may alert us to possible maltreatment must be recognized, evaluated, and referred for investigation whenever maltreatment is suspected.

DEVELOPMENTAL EFFECTS OF TRAUMA
AND MALTREATMENT

Abuse and neglect can have significant effects on children with disabilities and their families. Among the major sequelae of maltreatment and trauma are neurological dysfunction, developmental deficits, and related academic problems.

Neurological Dysfunction in Maltreated Children

A high incidence of central nervous system dysfunction in children with histories of abuse and neglect has been reported over the past 30 years (Elmer & Gregg, 1967, 1979; Gil, 1970; Greene, Voeller, Gaines, & Kubic, 1981; Morse, Sahler, & Friedman, 1970). However, the etiology of the neurological impairment of these children remains controversial. Some studies point to the specific relationship between severe head trauma and brain damage (Brandwein, 1973; Kempe, Silverman, Steele, Droegemueller, & Silver, 1962). Recently concerns have been expressed that children whose mothers are victims of battering during pregnancy may suffer central nervous system damage in utero. Hitting or kicking the abdomen of a pregnant woman is an unfortunately common scenario in domestic violence. Referral for complete neuropsychological evaluations should occur when battering has included assault to the abdomen of a pregnant woman or has included violent shaking or head trauma to a child (Olafson, 1999).

Other studies suggest that brain damage alone is not sufficient to explain the neurological dysfunction frequently found in children with histories of abuse and neglect (Freidrich & Boriskin, 1976; Martin, 1976). Chronically maltreated children with a diagnosis of posttraumatic stress disorder (PTSD) manifest alterations of major biological stress systems. Smaller intracranial and cerebral volumes have been documented by magnetic resonance imaging (MRI) relative to matched controls (DeBellis, 1999). A significant number of abused children without head injury have exhibited neurological defects. Neglect has been implicated in adverse neurological functioning, with neglected children suffering even greater intellectual deficits and language delays than abused children due to a lack of stimulation. The incidence of emotional neglect among maltreated children with disabilities is 2.8 times greater than among maltreated children without disabilities (Westat, Inc., 1993).

Malnutrition and failure to thrive have been cited as causing irreparable damage to the nervous system (Berge, 1972; Chase & Martin, 1970; Martin, 1972; Martin, Beezley, Conway, & Kempe, 1974). A high incidence of malnutrition has been noted in children with histories of abuse and neglect.

Developmental Deficits in Maltreated Children

Findings suggest that the causal factors for developmental deficits are rooted both in the abusive environment and in the child's resulting adaptive survival behaviors. We saw an example in the case of Brianna when her Head Start teacher noticed Brianna's exaggerated fear of motorized objects and vehicles. The teacher discovered that Brianna's mother used Brianna's intense fear of vacuum cleaner noise and the sucking action to frighten Brianna into compliance when the mother became frustrated with Brianna's behaviors. The mother would turn on the vacuum cleaner and run it directly toward Brianna.

Research available on the intellectual functioning of maltreated children usually focuses only on their performance on standardized intelligence tests. Unfortunately, a single test score does not measure the ability of the child to cope and adapt to abusive or neglectful environments. A standard score does not inform effective intervention and treatment nor provide significant evidence regarding how abuse and neglect has altered that child's total development. However, we must not minimize the impact of maltreatment on intellectual functioning. More than 30 years ago we had evidence that 57% of physically abused children who had sustained multiple bone injuries had IQs below 80 (Elmer & Gregg, 1967).

In a normal population we would expect approximately 11% to have IQs below 80 (Sattler, 1998). In a sample of children with less severe injuries (soft tissue damage only), 35% scored below 80 on IQ tests (Martin et al., 1974), and almost half the sample of preschool children with histories of abuse and neglect had IQs below 80 in yet another study (Sites, 1983). Studies have found consistently that when the effects of known brain damage were controlled, abuse and neglect continued to be significantly related to the children's lower IQ scores.

A number of studies support findings of impaired speech, language, and learning skills in children with histories of maltreatment. Abused children appear significantly delayed relative to nonabused peers in personal social skills, hearing and speech, eye–hand coordination performance, practical reasoning, reading skills, and verbal performance (Bladger & Martin, 1976; Oates, Peacock, & Forrest, 1984; Sullivan & Knutson, 1998). Sites (1983) compared 22 school-age children with previous histories of abuse and neglect but without medical or neurological problems to a matched group of children who were not abused or neglected. The abused/neglected children were significantly impaired in the areas of language and reading comprehension skills. Reading and math skills also have been found to be significantly impaired for maltreated children in regular school settings (K–12) regardless of socioeconomic status (SES) (Eckenrode, Laird, & Doris, 1993).

Child neglect is considered by some to be the critical type of maltreatment associated with language delays (Allen & Oliver, 1982). Child maltreatment has been documented as placing low-SES children at even greater jeopardy for compromised communication skills (Beeghly & Cicchetti, 1994; Coster & Cicchetti, 1993). Martin (1976) commented on the prevalence of low intelligence and language scores for children with histories of abuse and neglect in the absence of sufficient neurological problems. Gray and Kempe (1976) noted the children's passivity and striking lack of exploratory activities and postulated that these behaviors resulted from maladaptive survival skills developed in abusive or neglectful home environments.

Psychosocial Problems in Maltreated Children

Psychosocial impediments to learning have been demonstrated in maltreated children. Martin and Beezley (1977) described nine behavioral characteristics that were prevalent in more than half of physically abused children aged 2–13 years. Characteristics included chronic mild depression and impaired capacity to enjoy life; behavioral symptoms such as enuresis, tantrums, and hyperactivity; and low self-esteem. The behaviors were rated independently by clinicians, parents, social workers, and teachers of the children. Five environmental factors were related to the severity and frequency of the rated behaviors: (1) the number of home changes experienced; (2) the child's sense of impermanence in his or her present home; (3) the instability of the home (such as poor household management); (4) the use of punitive practices and excessive physical punishment in the home; and (5) the presence of parental emotional disturbance. The abused child's development appeared to be related to the nature of the environment and the adaptive behavior the child used to survive in the environment.

The adaptive behaviors exhibited by children from abusive and neglectful environments have an impact on both their current and future social interactions. Doren, Bullis, and Benz (1996) found that children with serious emotional disturbances who demonstrated low personal and social adaptive skills were more likely to experience victimization at some time in their school careers than were those with other disabilities. Cicchetti (1984) noted that 70% of the abused children he studied exhibited anxious–avoidant attachment to their mothers. Cicchetti attributed this problem to maternal rejection that resulted in the children being conflicted—both wanting their mothers' attention and fearing their mothers' rejecting responses. He hypothesized that the children would generalize this expectation to other adult relationships. Abused toddlers (ages 1–3) have been found to be significantly more likely to use approach–avoidant behaviors in their interactions with their peers and adult caregivers in a day care environment, approaching adult caregivers only half as often as nonabused toddlers when the caregivers made friendly overtures toward them (George & Main, 1979). Approach–avoidant behaviors included side-, rear-, or back-stepping approaches, with the child frequently moving his or her head in opposition to the body.

As this review indicates, there are no distinct disabilities associated with children with histories of maltreatment and no disability profiles that are definitively correlated with the potential for maltreatment. However, research points to relationships between maltreatment and disabilities and supports screening of children with disabilities for possible trauma and maltreatment.

REPORTING SUSPECTED CHILD ABUSE OR NEGLECT

The act of reporting suspicions of child abuse and neglect by all professionals working with children and families is a fundamental first step in the prevention of the ongoing and long-lasting developmental consequences of child maltreatment. The involvement of a children's services worker as a respected and integral team member in the community interdisciplinary treatment of the child and family is essential. Without the legal backup of children's services departments, the important steps of detection, prevention, and treatment of child abuse and neglect cannot occur. The initial call to a children's services worker when one suspects abuse or neglect is a critical step that may result in saving a child's life or protecting the child from further victimization and its lasting developmental consequences.

Personal Barriers to Eliciting and Reporting Information about Possible Child Maltreatment

Professionals, generally, are not trained to confront and deal with issues, such as child abuse, that arouse anger, pity, loathing, shame, and helplessness. Denial of maltreatment can preserve our sense of the world as a safe place. Child abuse may remind us that we once were young and vulnerable, and we may avoid revisiting that time of extreme dependency or possible maltreatment in our own lives. For children with disabilities, abuse issues can add another layer of isolation. Nurses describe experiencing greater discomfort in dealing with children with disabilities who are abused than with children without disabilities who are abused (Stanton, Seidl, Pillitteri, & Smith, 1994). We must understand when working with special needs children that our tendency may be *not* to question, assess, or report child abuse and neglect. In sidestepping this issue, we may voice the following rationales:

- "Screening for maltreatment is not my job; it is not what I was trained to do."
- "I have reported suspicions in the past and ended up with the child harmed further."
- "The caregivers and child will wonder why I am asking these questions and be affronted and angry."

- "This is a powerful prominent family. I can't risk exposing my suspicions. Besides, I'm not sure something is going on."
- "I will be ostracized in my work setting if I report."

Hopefully, these concerns will be alleviated by understanding more clearly the process of reporting suspected abuse or neglect.

Definitions of Child Abuse and Neglect

Definitions of physical abuse, sexual abuse, neglect, and emotional abuse are presented in Table 8.1. All professionals, paraprofessionals, or other employees who are in a paid capacity when interacting with children are mandated to report suspected child abuse or neglect. All professionals need to be familiar with the child abuse reporting law in their state.

Reports may be made by telephone or in person. Some states require a follow-up written report. Reports should contain the following information (if available):

1. The name of the child and parents or guardian, if known.
2. The nature or extent of the neglect or the child's injuries.
3. Any evidence or knowledge of previous injuries or neglect or family disturbances that further support the suspicion of abuse or neglect.
4. The present location of the child.
5. Any additional information or possible informants who can help establish the case for abuse or neglect because of personal or professional interactions with the family or child.

Most states require immediate medical evaluation of reports of physical or suspected sexual abuse. Photos will be taken during a medical evaluation, but this does not preclude other professionals, as mandated reporters, from also taking photographs (e.g., of a bruised cheek or blackened eye). Taking photographs of genitalia in suspected cases of sexual abuse is not advised unless directed by the mandated reporting agencies or physician.

It is important to remember that all laws have an immunity clause. One need not be trained in the investigation and substantiation of child abuse and neglect to have reasonable cause to suspect child abuse and neglect. It is often helpful if pediatric clinics, schools,

---

TABLE 8.1. Definitions of Child Maltreatment

Emotional abuse: Pattern of behavior that attacks a child's emotional development and sense of self-worth.

Neglect: Withholding of or failure to provide a child with the basic necessities of life: food, clothing, shelter, medical care, attention to hygiene, or supervision needed for optimal physical growth and development.

Physical abuse: Nonaccidental injury including beatings, burns, bites, strangulation, immersion in scalding water, which results in bruises, welts, broken bones, scars, or serious internal injuries.

Sexual abuse: Sexual contact or use of a child by an adult or older child for the sexual gratification of the offender.

---

child care centers, and private practitioners state in their policy handbooks that they are mandated to report suspicions of child abuse and neglect. Such statements support the fact that it is appropriate for the professionals to be aware of, and assess for, the possibility of child abuse and neglect. A policy statement might be followed by a list of resources available within the community or within the agency to address these concerns for families. Sometimes the professional statement alone enables a parent to disclose concerns about possible neglectful or abusive situations. If a report is made, parents need to be reassured that children's services agencies try to keep the family intact and work for the welfare and well-being of all family members, but especially the children. Many parents panic and view children's services agencies as existing to "take my child away."

Although most states offer the option of making an anonymous report, this practice is not recommended. When appropriate, professionals need to be available to the caseworker, parent, and child for interagency and interdisciplinary assessment and possible interventions. In addition, parents frequently figure out who has made the report of child abuse or neglect and feel angry, rejected, and betrayed. They are also left without a forum for further discussing their concerns when reports are made anonymously.

Some professionals have problems consulting with a parent about a call to children's services. These professionals wait to report their suspicions of abuse or neglect until the child has left their care, or they make the call at the end of the day, possibly after guilt has overwhelmed them. This practice makes it more difficult for children's services staff to begin a timely evaluation (most are mandated to investigate within 48 hours). Teachers frequently are ambivalent about making a call on a stressed or overwhelmed family. Furthermore, the appearance of a children's services worker at the school or clinic carries its own stigma and may contribute to after-hours reporting. Anonymous and late reports hamper effective investigation and may preclude the interviews being conducted in a "safe" environment, such as the school.

What responsibility do professionals have in reporting their suspicions to the parent, as well as to the children's services agency? Although none is mandated, discussing suspicions can elicit more information regarding the frustrations, stress, hardships, mental illness, substance abuse problems, and so forth that might be contributing to abuse or neglect. Such a discussion conveys to the parent that a problem has been observed and that the issues must be addressed. This can be done with empathy for the stigma attached to the possible charges. The professional can model the ability to speak and act openly about sensitive issues and may be seen as a future resource by that parent. Parents remember and trust professionals who are honest with them, especially when dealing with difficult subjects during difficult times. In Brianna's case, the teacher was advised to call Brianna's mother at work and ask to speak with her at the end of the day. In a private conversation between mother and teacher, the teacher told the mother of her observations of bruises on Brianna and the mandate that required her to report this incident to children's services. The teacher also commented sympathetically on her observations of the mother's high stress and frustration levels at dismissal time, when she was trying to prepare Brianna for the bus ride home. The teacher was careful to point out how difficult it is for a mother to work all day and then have to struggle with a noncompliant child. She told her that the school program had a "mothers' helper" senior volunteer program and that the mother might like their assistance at the end of the day. Initially, the mother was angry and defensive about the child abuse report, but later she called the teacher for the phone number of the volunteer program. Brianna stayed enrolled in the preschool.

There is an important caveat to the practice of notifying the parent before calling children's services. When dealing with possible sexual abuse, do *not* contact parents unless you can obtain an *immediate* victim interview by a children's services worker. The disclosing child must be protected from harm or coercion, intentional or unintentional, by either the alleged perpetrator or nonoffending parent. A more prudent practice is to call the children's services agency and, if possible, meet with the worker, and later with the parent, and explain your concern for the child and family.

As a professional, to protect and support your relationship with a child, we advise that you tell the child that you have concerns about his or her safety or well-being and that you need to call in other adults whose job it is to keep children safe. Sometimes this statement will elicit responses and reactions from the child that further corroborate your suspicions or shed light on the risk factors the child may face as a result of reporting. Be sure to document the child's concerns and tell him or her that you will advise the caseworker to be careful about these issues.

It is important that institutions and agencies that routinely work with families and children discuss the reporting system among their employees. Although state laws mandate reporting by professionals, the laws are not clear on the reporting system recommended for larger agencies and institutions. Some schools or hospitals require that a particular department, frequently the counseling or social work department, be the mandated entity to make such reports. Other systems require that each person individually report to the appropriate police department or children's services department within their community after appropriate child abuse and neglect training. There are advantages and disadvantages to each system. Mandating a particular department to report frequently results in fewer reports being made and in the minimizing of the facts and issues surrounding the report.

CLINICAL ASSESSMENT FOR TRAUMA AND MALTREATMENT

There are two major ways for professionals to identify cases of physical, sexual, and emotional abuse and neglect. One way is to recognize possible indicators of abuse and neglect; the second is to use screening and assessment tools in a systematic approach.

Knowing Possible Indicators of Abuse and Neglect

The first method of identifying cases of abuse and neglect is to be aware of the physical and behavioral signs and symptoms that may be indicators of sexual abuse. A cluster or pattern of indicators, although never providing conclusive evidence of abuse or neglect, can support a concern and a call to a mandated reporting agency. A key factor in determining whether the child may have been victimized is to know the child. Be alert to any sudden or gradual behavior and health changes. Be willing to explore your concerns by talking to the child or referring the child to another professional. It may also be useful to document the troubling behaviors noted in a child, a parent, or adult caregiver. Possible indicators of child abuse or neglect are listed in Table 8.2.

Using General Screening and Assessment Tools

A second approach to identifying abuse, neglect, and trauma histories is to screen for incidents and behaviors that raise concern as part of the assessment of the child. None of the following suggested assessment tools should be used as a sole basis for a determination

TABLE 8.2. Indicators of Child Maltreatment

Child neglect

Does the child . . . ?
- frequently miss school
- beg or steal food or money from friends or classmates
- lack needed medical or dental care, immunizations, or glasses
- appear consistently dirty or have severe body odor
- lack sufficient clothing for the weather
- abuse alcohol or other drugs
- state that there is no one at home to provide care

Does the parent or adult caregiver . . . ?
- appear to be indifferent to the child
- seem apathetic or depressed
- behave irrationally or in a bizarre manner
- abuse alcohol or other drugs

Physical child abuse

Does the child . . . ?
- have unexplained burns, bites, bruises, broken bones, or black eyes
- have fading bruises or other marks noticeable after an absence from school
- seem frightened of the parents and protest or cry when it is time to go home from school
- shrink at the approach of adults
- report injury by a parent or another adult caregiver

Does the parent or adult caregiver . . . ?
- offer conflicting, unconvincing, or no explanation for the child's injury
- describe the child as "evil" or in some other very negative way
- use harsh physical discipline with the child
- have a history of abuse as a child

Sexual child abuse

Does the child . . . ?
- have difficulty walking or sitting
- suddenly refuse to change for gym or to participate in physical activities
- demonstrate bizarre, sophisticated, or unusual sexual knowledge or behavior
- have a venereal disease, or has the child become pregnant (particularly if under age 14)
- run away from home
- report sexual abuse

Does the parent or adult caregiver . . . ?
- appear unduly protective of the child, severely limiting the child's contact with other children, especially of the opposite sex
- seem secretive or isolated
- describe marital difficulties involving family power struggles or sexual relations

Emotional child maltreatment

Does the child . . . ?
- show extremes in behavior, such as overly compliant or demanding behavior, extreme passivity, or aggression
- display behaviors that are inappropriately adult (e.g., parenting other children) or inappropriately infantile (e.g., frequently rocking or headbanging)
- seem delayed in physical or emotional development
- speak of suicide, or has the child attempted it?
- report a lack of attachment to the parent

Does the parent or adult caregiver . . . ?
- constantly blame, belittle, or berate the child
- appear unconcerned about the child or refuse to consider offers of help for the child's school problems
- overtly reject the child

Note. From Broadhurst (1994). Copyright 1994 by Broadhurst. Adapted by permission.

that abuse or neglect has occurred. There is no single test, single item, or combination of tests and items that conclusively indicate maltreatment. It is crucial to remember that although many of the items will appear to have face validity, a caregiver or child may minimize or exaggerate their responses. An interdisciplinary and interagency investigation is necessary to substantiate child abuse or neglect.

It is also very important to remember that, when using instruments that depend upon client self-disclosure of symptoms, you must take into account individual and cultural reporting styles (Olafson, 1999). When abuse and violence are chronic in a family, denial or minimization often becomes a predominant coping style. In addition, different cultures have different norms for expressing emotions. For example, although members of mainstream U.S. culture may have few prohibitions in reporting psychological symptoms, members of Asian cultures may be more likely to report headaches and stomachaches (somatic symptoms) than sadness or anger (Carlson, 1997; Lee & Lu, 1989).

Diagnoses may mask trauma symptoms. For example, Perry and colleagues point out that children who are suffering from PTSD often are misdiagnosed with attention-deficit/hyperactivity disorder (ADHD). These children may be hypervigilant rather than inattentive and experiencing physiological hyperarousal, hyperreactivity, sleep disturbances, hypertension, increased heart rate, startle reactions, and muscle tension (Perry, 1994; Perry, Pollard, Blakely, Baker, & Vigilante, 1996).

Another important consideration is how to screen parents and children for histories of domestic violence. We know that children exposed to partner violence are at increased risk for physical, sexual, and, especially, emotional maltreatment (see Wolak & Finkelhor, 1998, for a review). Domestic abuse histories should be a routine part of medical and mental health intakes (Olafson & Boat, 2000). Family members must be separated for questioning . Questions for adults should be clear and focused without being leading and should cover specific acts, such as being hit or touched against one's will, verbally berated, or physically isolated.

Review of Screening Measures and Assessment Tools

This section reviews eight screening measures and assessment tools: the Childhood Trust Events Survey, Achenbach Child Behavior Checklist (CBCL), Child Sexual Behavior Inventory (CSBI), Trauma Symptom Checklist for Children (TSCC), Adolescent Sexual Concerns Questionnaire, Parenting Stress Index (PSI), Interview Questions for Alternative Caregivers, and Questions About Animal-Related Experiences. Assessment approaches range from asking the child directly about exposure to possible traumatic events to asking parents to respond to specific questions about the child's sexual behaviors.

Childhood Trust Events Survey: Exposure to Possible Trauma Experiences

Although the protection of the child is paramount in screening for trauma and maltreatment, it is also important to assess for traumatic experiences that may not be abusive or neglectful, such as natural disasters, exposure to violence, or sudden death of a sibling, as these experiences can affect the performance and resources of both children and their parents. The Childhood Trust Events Survey (Boat, Baker, & Abrahamson, 1994) provides a set of screening questions that can be asked of the child, if appropriate, and the parent. A number of topics, as shown in Table 8.3, can be introduced in the interview. If the child

TABLE 8.3. The Childhood Trust Events Survey

1. Child experienced a natural disaster such as a tornado, hurricane, fire, or flood ----------- Y N

   Age of child when event occurred (circle all that apply):
       1) Under age 6   2) 6–12 years   3) Teenager
   How bad was the *worst* event for child?
       1) Not bad   2) Somewhat bad   3) Very bad
   How much does the event bother child now?
       1) Not at all   2) Somewhat   3) A lot

2. Child experienced serious car/motorcycle/bike, etc., accident ---------------------------------- Y N

   Age of child when event occurred (circle all that apply):
       1) Under age 6   2) 6–12 years   3) Teenager
   How bad was the *worst* event for child?
       1) Not bad   2) Somewhat bad   3) Very bad
   How much does the event bother child now?
       1) Not at all   2) Somewhat   3) A lot

3. Child had a serious injury or illness that required hospitalization and/or surgery ---------- Y N

   Age of child when event occurred (circle all that apply):
       1) Under age 6   2) 6–12 years   3) Teenager
   How bad was the *worst* event for child?
       1) Not bad   2) Somewhat bad   3) Very bad
   How much does the event bother child now?
       1) Not at all   2) Somewhat   3) A lot

4. Child or family was robbed --- Y N

   Age of child when event occurred (circle all that apply):
       1) Under age 6   2) 6–12 years   3) Teenager
   How bad was the *worst* event for child?
       1) Not bad   2) Somewhat bad   3) Very bad
   How much does the event bother child now?
       1) Not at all   2) Somewhat   3) A lot

5. Child had a girl/boyfriend who was physically violent toward him/her
   (e.g., punching, slapping) --- Y N

   Age of child when event occurred (circle all that apply):
       1) Under age 6   2) 6–12 years   3) Teenager
   How bad was the *worst* event for child?
       1) Not bad   2) Somewhat bad   3) Very bad
   How much does the event bother child now?
       1) Not at all   2) Somewhat   3) A lot

6. Someone, including family members or other kids, came after child with a weapon
   (e.g., chair, bat, gun) -- Y N

   Age of child when event occurred (circle all that apply):
       1) Under age 6   2) 6–12 years   3) Teenager
   How bad was the *worst* event for child?
       1) Not bad   2) Somewhat bad   3) Very bad
   How much does the event bother child now?
       1) Not at all   2) Somewhat   3) A lot

7. A close friend or family member died or was killed --- Y N
   Age of child when event occurred (circle all that apply):

       1) Under age 6   2) 6–12 years   3) Teenager
   How bad was the *worst* event for child?
       1) Not bad   2) Somewhat bad   3) Very bad
   How much does the event bother child now?
       1) Not at all   2) Somewhat   3) A lot

(continued)

TABLE 8.3. *continued*

8. Child lost a pet that he/she really cared about (e.g., died, was killed or taken away) ----- Y N NA

Age of child when event occurred (circle all that apply):
   1) Under age 6   2) 6–12 years   3) Teenager
How bad was the *worst* event for child?
   1) Not bad   2) Somewhat bad   3) Very bad
How much does the event bother child now?
   1) Not at all   2) Somewhat   3) A lot

9. Someone was violent or abusive toward child's pet -- Y N NA

Age of child when event occurred (circle all that apply):
   1) Under age 6   2) 6–12 years   3) Teenager
How bad was the *worst* event for child?
   1) Not bad   2) Somewhat bad   3) Very bad
How much does the event bother child now?
   1) Not at all   2) Somewhat   3) A lot

10. Child saw someone get badly hurt or die suddenly -- Y N

Age of child when event occurred (circle all that apply):
   1) Under age 6   2) 6–12 years   3) Teenager
How bad was the *worst* event for child?
   1) Not bad   2) Somewhat bad   3) Very bad
How much does the event bother child now?
   1) Not at all   2) Somewhat   3) A lot

11. Child was verbally and/or emotionally abused (e.g., called names, put down,
threatened) by parent(s) or caretaker(s) or other kids -- Y N

Age of child when event occurred (circle all that apply):
   1) Under age 6   2) 6–12 years   3) Teenager
How bad was the *worst* event for child?
   1) Not bad   2) Somewhat bad   3) Very bad
How much does the event bother child now?
   1) Not at all   2) Somewhat   3) A lot

12. Child saw or heard violence take place between members of family
(e.g., saw brothers or sisters get hit hard or saw parent hit or get hit) -------------------------- Y N

Age of child when event occurred (circle all that apply):
   1) Under age 6   2) 6–12 years   3) Teenager
How bad was the *worst* event for child?
   1) Not bad   2) Somewhat bad   3) Very bad
How much does the event bother child now?
   1) Not at all   2) Somewhat   3) A lot

13. A parent or caretaker was physically violent toward child
(e.g., whipping or pushing hard enough to leave marks) -- Y N

Age of child when event occurred (circle all that apply):
   1) Under age 6   2) 6–12 years   3) Teenage
How bad was the *worst* event for child?
   1) Not bad   2) Somewhat bad   3) Very bad
How much does the event bother child now?
   1) Not at all   2) Somewhat   3) A lot

14. Child was separated from a parent or caretaker or brothers/sisters
(e.g., child or others had to live or stay somewhere else) -- Y N

Age of child when event occurred (circle all that apply):
   1) Under age 6   2) 6–12 years   3) Teenager
How bad was the *worst* event for child?
   1) Not bad   2) Somewhat bad   3) Very bad

TABLE 8.3. *continued*

> How much does the event bother child now?
> 1) Not at all   2) Somewhat   3) A lot

15. Someone, including a friend, family member, teacher, or babysitter, touched child— or had child touch them—in a sexual way or performed sex acts -------------------------------- Y N

Age of child when event occurred (circle all that apply):
    1) Under age 6   2) 6–12 years   3) Teenager
How bad was the *worst* event for child?
    1) Not bad   2) Somewhat bad   3) Very bad
How much does the event bother child now?
    1) Not at all   2) Somewhat   3) A lot

16. Child was badly frightened or attacked by an animal -- Y N

Age of child when event occurred (circle all that apply):
    1) Under age 6   2) 6–12 years   3) Teenager
How bad was the *worst* event for child?
    1) Not bad   2) Somewhat bad   3) Very bad
How much does the event bother child now?
    1) Not at all   2) Somewhat   3) A lot

Note. From Boat, Baker, & Abrahamson (1994). Copyright 1994 by Boat. Adapted by permission.

endorses a particular experience, follow-up questions can be asked, including: (1) age or ages of the child when the event occurred (the event may have been ongoing); (2) details of the event; (3) how bad the event was for the child when it occurred; and (4) how much the event bothers the child now. The list of stressors in Table 8.3 is not exhaustive, and you may want to include others.

Achenbach Child Behavior Checklist

The CBCL provides an initial screening of the child's behaviors. Endorsement of particular problematic behaviors provides the evaluator with an opportunity to follow up and gain additional information on possible maltreatment or trauma in the child's history. One advantage to using the CBCL is that it is a common, widely administered instrument, and parent, teacher, and child self-reports can be obtained. (Achenbach, 1991a, 1991b, 1991c). The CBCL is also normed for children aged 2–18. We suggest that parents or teachers who endorse any of the items in Table 8.4 be questioned in greater detail, using prompts such as, "Tell me more about that," "How long have you been aware of such behavior?" "What do you think might be going on?" or "Does this behavior happen at certain times or places?" The purpose of the follow-up questions is to determine that the basis of the behavior is not maltreatment or previously unidentified trauma in the child's life. If you are concerned about possible maltreatment, read the questions to the parent and record the responses. This allows for spontaneous discussion of any concerns noted by the parent.

The evaluator working on Brianna's case supported the teacher's concerns about possible emotional and physical abuse and decided to call the mother at work when she was on her lunch break and verbally administer the CBCL. Brianna's mother rated the following behaviors as "very true or often true" (score of 2): confused or seems in a fog; daydreams or gets lost in his or her own thoughts; fears certain situations; nightmares; secretive; sleeps less than most kids; strange behaviors; strange ideas; use of obscene language; un-

TABLE 8.4. CBCL Questions That May Be Related to Child Maltreatment or Trauma for Children Ages 4–17 and 2–3

Ages 4–17

Behaves like opposite sex	Plays with own sex parts too much
Bowel movements outside toilet	Runs away from home
Can't get his/her mind off certain thoughts; obsessions (describe)	Secretive, keeps things to self
	Sexual problems
Confused or seems to be in a fog	Sleeps less than most kids
Cruel to animals	Smears or plays with bowel movements
Daydreams or gets lost in his/her thoughts	Strange behavior
Deliberately harms self or attempts suicide	Strange ideas
Doesn't eat well	Swearing or obscene language
Fears certain animals, situations, or places, other than school	Talks about killing self
	Thinks about sex too much
Nightmares	Unhappy, sad, or depressed
Overeating	Wets self during the day
Physical problems without known medical cause	Wets the bed
Plays with own sex parts in public	

Ages 2–3

Clings to adults or too dependent/gets too upset when separated from parents	Overeating/overweight
	Plays with own sex parts too much
Constipated, doesn't move bowels/painful bowel movements	Smears or plays with bowel movements/too concerned with neatness or cleanliness
Doesn't want to sleep alone/has trouble getting to sleep	
	Stares into space or seems preoccupied/ strange behavior/angry moods
Fears certain animals, situations, or places/cruel to animals	Unhappy, sad, or depressed/cries a lot
Headaches, stomachaches or cramps, aches or pains/ vomiting	Wakes up often at night/talks or cries out in sleep, has nightmares

happy, sad or depressed; and wets self during the day. When the evaluator asked for specific examples of Brianna's behaviors, it was apparent that the mother shared the developmental and behavioral concerns that the teacher had but believed that Brianna really could perform better, especially if the adults around her would "Make her shape up!" This information was very useful in developing the treatment and parent education intervention strategies for the mother and child.

Child Sexual Behavior Inventory

If a child's reported or observed behaviors are sexualized, the evaluator may want to further explore the range of behaviors by using the CSBI (Friedrich, 1997). The CSBI was specifically developed to assess sexual behavior in children. Empirical findings with sexually abused children indicate that sexualized behavior is one of the more reliable and valid markers of sexual abuse (Friedrich, 1993; Kendall-Tackett, Williams, & Finkelhor, 1993). The original 36-item CSBI has been researched extensively and found to significantly differentiate between a sample of 880 nonabused children with no history of psychiatric disturbance and 276 children with a history of sexual abuse (Friedrich et al., 1992). The CSBI has been revised twice and is designed for use with children aged 2–12. The child's primary caregiver is asked to complete a 36-item measure that rates the numerical frequency of each behavior over the previous 6-month period. The clinican must use the CSBI with interviews and other forms of assessment in order to understand the child and intervene, particularly for the sexually abused child. Items range from standing too close to people to asking others to engage in sexual acts. Friedrich (1995) notes that the CSBI can also be used to guide treatment or to reassure parents that their children are displaying normative behaviors (for example, a 5-year-old boy touching his penis). Scores range from 0 to 3, representing frequency of observed behavior from "never" to "always." Scores are totaled for the instrument. On the CSBI-R, children with no history of behavior problems and no history of sexual abuse rarely receive a total score of more than 5. The mean score for sexually abused children ranges from 7 to 15, with sexually abused girls typically scoring lower than same-age, sexually abused boys.

Trauma Symptom Checklist for Children

The Trauma Symptom Checklist for Children (TSCC) is a 54-item self-report measure for children targeted to assess the impact of interpersonal victimization (Briere, 1996). The measure yields profiles for males and females aged 8–12 and 13–16. If sexual abuse is not suspected, the TSCC-A, which contains no references to sexual issues, is available. However, as children may have never disclosed prior sexual experiences, the full TSCC is recommended. The TSCC has two validity scales and six clinical scales that measure anxiety, depression, anger, posttraumatic stress, dissociation, and sexual concerns. The TSCC contains critical items that may need immediate attention, such as suicidal ideation or the fear of being killed, and can be administered at intervals to assess treatment progress.

Adolescent Sexual Concerns Questionnaire

The Adolescent Sexual Concerns Questionnaire (Hussey & Singer, 1988) can be read aloud or completed individually by the adolescent. The questionnaire is used to screen for general concerns that adolescents have and asks about health, relationship and sexual issues, and thoughts and feelings, and it provides the adolescent with an opportunity to share possible maltreatment experiences. Our hope is to circumvent the fate of 26-year-old Jennie, whose current disabilities are the result of her long-term abuse:

> I was raped repeatedly by my stepfather from the time I was 9 until I was 17. Every night I prayed that someone would ask me if anyone was touching me, but no one ever did. When I was 12, my sister brought rape charges against my stepfather. I remember that the policeman asked me if I had *seen* anything happen with my sister. But he never asked if anything had happened to *me*! The charges against my stepfather were dismissed. Finally, when I left home, I brought charges against my stepfather. He confessed and now is in prison. But it is too late. He has done his damage to me.

Parenting Stress Index

The PSI (Abidin, 1983) is another measure by which detailed follow-up questions can be asked when a parent endorses items that may signal a concern about maltreatment, either by a parent or by another caregiver. These items are listed in Table 8.5.

TABLE 8.5. Parenting Stress Index: Items Warranting Follow-Up Questions

I feel trapped by my responsibilities as a parent.

Having a child has caused more problems than I expected in my relationship with my spouse (male/female friend).

I feel alone without friends.

My child rarely does things for me that make me feel good.

Most times I feel that my child does not like me and does not want to be close to me.

I expected to have closer and warmer feelings for my child than I do and this bothers me.

My child's sleeping or eating schedule was much harder to establish than I expected.

There are some things my child does that really bother me a lot.

Note. From Abidin (1983). Copyright 1983 by Abidin. Adapted by permission.

Interview Questions for Alternative Caregivers

Many children with special needs are in out-of-home placements, and their caregivers can provide important information that may raise or support a suspicion of maltreatment. As noted in the introductory vignette, Brianna's teacher served as a resource for information about possible maltreatment. The child's alternative caregiver can be asked to comment on the issues raised in Table 8.6.

TABLE 8.6. Interview Questions for Alternative Caregivers

Demographics

What children live in the home?
  Ages
  Gender
Did you have this child previously?
Are you keeping notes?

Child characteristics

Response to discipline
Ability to follow directions, conform to rules
Truthfulness, credibility (get examples)
Dissociative symptoms

Placement

Why was child placed with you?
How long been with you?
What is your understanding of the plan for the
  child (permanent foster care, etc.)?

Ongoing adjustment

Relationship with foster mother/caregiver
Relationship with foster father/caregiver
Relationship with natural sibs
Relationship with foster sibs
Relationship with birth parents
Relationship with pets
What is visitation schedule?
Reactions before and after visitation
Does child talk about previous home life?
  What say?
How does child feel about returning home?
How do *you* feel about child returning
  home?

Initial adjustment

Angry, relieved, fearful, etc.
Any behaviors, habits notable in:
  Sleeping
  Eating
  Toileting/bathing
  Physical interactions
  Language
  Sexualized behaviors
  Aggressive behaviors
Too loveable, instantly attached

Questions about Animal-Related Experiences

Finally, one overlooked possible source of trauma for children may be related to violence to animals. The links between violence to children and violence to animals have received implicit acknowledgment throughout history. However, the practical utilization of these links has been largely ignored in the field of child abuse and neglect (Boat, 1995, 1999). Companion animals are an integral part of the lives of children in the United States. In 1997, 6 out of 10 homes in the United States had some type of pet (APPMA, 1998). Despite the fact that research on this topic is in its infancy, evidence continues to mount that when animals are abused, people are abused, and visa versa (Arkow, 1996). Higher rates of animal abuse by parental figures have been found in substantiated cases of child abuse and neglect than in the general population. In one study, abused animals were found in 88% of the homes of 57 families with pets in which child physical abuse had been substantiated. Animal abuse was perpetrated both by fathers and children. Persons living in homes in which pets were abused were 10 times more likely to be bitten or attacked by the abused pet (Deviney, Dickert, & Lockwood, 1983).

Awareness of the child abuse–animal abuse connection is increasing in domestic violence settings. Recent surveys of women who own pets and are in battered women's shelters revealed that almost 75% reported that their violent partners had threatened or actually harmed their pets. For some women, concern over their pets' safety precluded seeking shelter sooner for themselves and their children (Ascione, 1998).

Case studies of sexually abused children contain reports of forcing children to interact sexually with animals and ensuring children's silence by threatening to hurt their pets, or actually killing or maiming the pets and other animals (Boat, 1992; Faller, 1990; Finkelhor, Williams, & Burns, 1988; Kelley, 1989). Rapid turnover of pets in a household may indicate a chaotic environment in which care is compromised for all family members. Frequently, children are willing to describe concerns about pets before they can voice worries about their own safety. Trauma, stress, or violence that involve animals may contribute to symptoms of PTSD, as well as raise concerns about other aspects of a child's functioning. The questions listed in Table 8.7 are useful in gathering information about the child's experiences with pets.

TABLE 8.7. Questions about Animal-Related Experiences

1. Do you have pets in your home? How many?
2. What kind?
3. Who takes care of _____ ?
4. What happens if _____ is naughty, bad, etc.?
5. Have you ever lost a pet you really cared about? What happened?
6. Do you worry about something bad happening to _____ ?
7. Has anyone ever hurt or threatened to hurt your pet? Who? What happened?

CONCLUSION

Child maltreatment is one of the most complex problems in clinical assessment. We know that we are failing to detect most cases in our standard evaluations, and there are several reasons why this is so. First, child maltreatment is seldom designated as the referral problem when we are assessing children. Second, because abuse and trauma experienced by children is frequently obscured by secrecy, spontaneous disclosure will rarely occur during a standard assessment. Concerns about confidentiality may inhibit professionals from asking questions that appear intrusive, and social and family taboos may prevent the child or family from responding to such questions. Third, adequate knowledge of normal and deviant behaviors, especially sexually aggressive behaviors in children, is relatively recent and is not commonly taught to professionals. Fourth, evaluators may have personal barriers to recognizing possible child maltreatment indicators or may be cognizant of the potential conflicts with clients if suspicions about maltreatment are present. Fifth and finally, the complexity of assessing abuse and maltreatment is reflected in the lack of useful standardized and normed instruments. Despite these obstacles, it is essential that clinical assessments of children are sensitive to indicators of trauma and maltreatment.

We must emphasize that clinical assessment of trauma and maltreatment involves a comprehensive approach, including observation and consultation. None of the assessment and screening tools listed in this chapter should be used as the sole basis for a determination of child abuse or neglect. The proper investigation of child abuse and neglect allegations requires a community-based, interdisciplinary, professionally trained team. Ideally, the team would include a lead prosecutor, a children's service worker, a police officer, a physician, and a trained forensic interviewer (psychologist or social worker).

The focus of this chapter is to address trauma and maltreatment in children with special needs and to describe specific approaches to assessing for possible abuse and neglect. The goal of thorough clinical assessment is to protect Brianna and other children like her from the lasting consequences of trauma and maltreatment so that they can realize their true developmental potential. Interagency involvement, parent education classes, and monitoring of Brianna's mother led to the cessation of the physical and psychological abuse of the child. Brianna became more responsive and tolerant of adult interactions, thereby enabling more productive educational and language therapy sessions. Confidence in one's ability to explore suspicions of child maltreatment or trauma can make the difference in reporting or not reporting to the mandated agencies. The first important steps to effecting change are recognition and reporting.

REFERENCES

Abidin, R. R. (1983). *Parenting Stress Index*. Charlotte: University of Virginia, Institute of Clinical Psychology.

Achenbach, T. M. (1991a). *Manual for the Child Behavior Checklist 4–18 and 1991 Profile*. Burlington: University of Vermont, Department of Psychiatry.

Achenbach, T. M. (1991b). *Manual for the Teacher's Report Form and 1991 Profile*. Burlington: University of Vermont, Department of Psychiatry.

Achenbach, T. M. (1991c). *Manual for the Youth Self-Report Form and 1991 Profile*. Burlington: University of Vermont, Department of Psychiatry.

Allen, R. E., & Oliver, J. M. (1982). The effects of child maltreatment on language development. *Child Abuse and Neglect, 6*, 299–305.

American Pet Products Manufacturers Association (1998). *National Pet Owners Survey*. Greenwich, CT: Author.

Ammerman, R. T., Hersen, M., & Van Hasselt, V. B. (1989). Abuse and neglect in psychiatrically hospitalized multihandicapped children. *Child Abuse and Neglect, 13,* 335–343.

Ammerman, R. T., Van Hasselt, V. B., & Hersen, M. (1988). Maltreatment of handicapped children: A critical review. *Journal of Family Violence, 3*(1), 53–72.

Arkow, P. (1996). The relationships between animal abuse and other forms of family violence. *Family Violence Sexual Assault Bulletin, 12*(1–2), 29–34.

Ascione, F. R. (1998). Battered women's reports of their partners' and their children's cruelty to animals. *Journal of Emotional Abuse 1*(1), 119–133.

Beeghly, M., & Cicchetti, D. (1994). Child maltreatment attachment and the self system: Emergence of an internal state lexicon in toddlers at high social risk. *Development and Psychopathology, 6,* 5–30.

Berge, H. G. (1972). Malnutrition learning and intelligence. *American Journal of Public Health, 6*(2), 773–784.

Bladger, F., & Martin, H. P. (1976). Speech and language of abused children. In H. P. Martin (Ed.), *The abused child: A multidisciplinary approach to developmental issues and treatment* (pp. 83–92) Cambridge, MA: Ballinger.

Briere, J. (1996). *TSCC: Trauma Symptom Checklist for Children: Professional Manual.* Odessa, FL: Psychological Assessment Resources.

Boat, B. W. (1992). Caregivers as surrogate therapists in treatment of a ritualistically abused child. In W. N. Friedrich (Ed.), *Casebook of sexual abuse treatment* (pp. 1–26) New York: Norton.

Boat, B. W. (1995). The relationship between violence to children and violence to animals: An ignored link? *Journal of Interpersonal Violence, 10,* 229–235.

Boat, B. W. (1999). Abuse of children and abuse of animals: Using the links to inform child assessment and protection. In P. Arkow & F. Ascione (Eds.), *Child abuse, domestic violence and animal abuse: Linking the circles of compassion for prevention and intervention* (pp. 83–100) West Lafayette, IN: Purdue University Press.

Boat, B. W., Baker, D., & Abrahamson, S. (1994). *The Childhood Trust Events Survey.* Cincinnati, OH: University of Cincinnati, Children's Hospital Medical Center and Department of Psychiatry.

Brandwein, H. (1973). The battered child: A definite and significant factor in mental retardation. *Mental Retardation, 11,* 50–51.

Broadhurst, D. D. (1994). *Educators, schools, and child abuse.* Chicago: National Committee to Prevent Child Abuse.

Carlson, E. B. (1997). *Trauma assessments: A clinician's guide.* New York: Guilford Press.

Chase, P. H., & Martin, H. P. (1970). Undernutrition and child development. *New England Journal of Medicine, 282,* 993–999.

Cicchetti, D. (1984). The emergence of developmental psychopathology. *Child Development, 55,* 1–7.

Cohen, S., & Warren, R. D. (1990). The intersection of disability and child abuse in England and the United States. *Child Welfare, 3,* 253–263.

Coster, W., & Cicchetti, D. (1993). Research on the communicative development of maltreated children: Clinical implications. *Topics in Language Disorders, 1*(3), 25–38.

DeBellis, M. D. (1999). Biological stress systems and brain development in maltreated children. *Traumatic Stress Points, ISTSS, 13*(2), 1–5.

Deviney, E., Dickert, J., & Lockwood, R. (1983). The care of pets within child abusing families. *International Journal for the Study of Animal Problems, 4,* 321–329.

Doren, B., Bullis, M., & Benz, M. (1996). Predictors of victimization experiences of adolescents with disabilities in transition. *Exceptional Children, 63,* 7–18.

Eckenrode, J., Laird, M., & Doris, J. (1993). School performance and disciplinary problems among abused and neglected children. *Developmental Psychology, 29,* 53–62.

Elmer, E., & Gregg, G. S. (1967). Developmental characteristics of abused children. *Pediatrics, 40,* 596–602.

Elmer, E., & Gregg, G. S. (1979). Developmental characteristics of "abused" children. In D. Gill (Ed.), *Child abuse and violence* (pp. 295–308). New York: American Press.

Faller, K. C. (1990). *Understanding child sexual maltreatment.* Newbury Park, CA: Sage.

Finkelhor, D., Hotaling, G., Lewis, I. A., & Smith, C. (1990). Sexual abuse in a national survey of adult men and women: Prevalence, characteristics, and risk factors. *Child Abuse and Neglect, 14,* 19–28.

Finkelhor, D., Williams, L. M., & Burns, N. (1988). *Nursery crimes: Sexual abuse in day care.* Newbury Park, CA: Sage.

Freidrich, W. N. (1993). Sexual victimization and sexual behavior in children: A review of recent literature. *Child Abuse and Neglect, 17,* 59–66.

Freidrich, W. N. (1995). The clinical use of the Child Sexual Behavior Inventory: Commonly asked questions. *APSAC Advisor, 8*(1), 17–20.

Freidrich, W. N. (1997). *CSBI: Child Sexual Behavior Inventory: Professional manual.* Odessa, FL: Psychological Assessment Resources.

Freidrich, W. N., & Boriskin, J. A. (1976). The role of the child in abuse: A review of the literature. *American Journal of Orthopsychiatry, 46*(4), 580–590.

Freidrich, W. N., Grambsch, P., Damon, L., Hewitt, S. C., Koverola, C., Lang, R. A., Wolfe, V., & Broughton, D. (1992). Child Sexual Behavior Inventory: Normative and clinical comparisons. *Psychological Assessment, 4,* 303–311.

Garbarino, J., Brookhauser, P. E., & Authier, J. (Eds.). (1987). *Special children—special risks: The maltreatment of children with disabilities.* New York: De Gruyter.

George, C., & Main, M. (1979). Social interactions of young abused children: Approach, avoidance and aggression. *Child Development, 50,* 306–318.

Gil, D. G. (1970). *Violence against children: Physical child abuse.* Cambridge, MA: Harvard University Press.

Gray, J., & Kempe, R. (1976). The abused child at the time of injury. In H. P. Martin (Ed.), *The abused child: A multidisciplinary approach to developmental issues and treatment* (pp. 57–65). Cambridge, MA: Ballinger.

Greene, A. H., Voeller, K., Gaines, R., & Kubic, J. (1981). Neurological impairment in maltreated children. *Child Abuse and Neglect, 5,* 129–134.

Groce, N. E. (1997). Women with disabilities in the developing world: Arenas for policy revision and programmatic change. *Journal of Disability Policy Studies, 8*(1&2), 177–191.

Horton, C. B., & Kochurka, K. A. (1995). The assessment of children with disabilities who report sexual abuse: A special look at those most vulnerable. In T. Ney (Ed.), *True and false allegations of child sexual abuse* (pp. 275–289), New York: Brunner/Mazel.

Hussey, D., & Singer, M. (1988). Innovations in the assessment and treatment of sexually abused adolescents: An inpatient model. In S. Sgroi (Ed.), *Vulnerable populations* (pp. 43–64). Lexington, MA: Lexington Press.

Jaudes, P. K., & Diamond, L. J. (1985). The handicapped child and child abuse. *Child Abuse and Neglect, 9,* 341–347.

Kelley, S. J. (1989). Stress responses of children to sexual abuse and ritualistic abuse in day care centers. *Journal of Interpersonal Violence, 4,* 1113–1129.

Kempe, C. H., Silverman, F. N., Steele, B. B., Droegemueller, W., & Silver, H. K. (1962). The battered-child syndrome. *Journal of the American Medical Association, 181,* 17–24.

Kendall-Tackett, K. A., Williams, L., & Finkelhor, D. (1993). The impact of sexual abuse on children: A review of synthesis of recent empirical studies. *Psychological Bulletin, 113,* 164–180.

Kidd, A. H., & Kidd, R. M. (1987). Seeking a theory of the human/companion animal bond. *Anthrozoos, 1,* 140–145.

Lee, E., & Lu, F. (1989). Assessment and treatment of Asian-American survivors of mass violence. *Journal of Traumatic Stress, 2,* 93–100.

Martin, H. P. (1972). The child and his development. In C. H. Kempe & R. E. Helfer (Eds.), *Helping the battered child and his family* (pp. 93–114). Philadelphia: Lippincott.

Martin, H. P. (Ed.). (1976). *The abused child: A multidisciplinary approach to developmental issues and treatment.* Cambridge: Ballinger.

Martin, H. P., & Beezley, P. (1977). Behavioral observations of abused children. *Developmental Medicine and Child Neurology, 19,* 373–387.

Martin, H. P., Beezley, P., Conway, E. F., & Kempe, C. H. (1974). The development of abused children. *Advances in Pediatrics, 21,* 25–73.

Monat-Haller, R. K. (1992). *Understanding and expressing sexuality.* Baltimore: Brookes.

Morgan, S. R. (1987). *Abuse and neglect of handicapped children.* Boston: Little, Brown.

Morse, C. W., Sahler, O. J. Z., & Friedman, S. B. (1970). A three-year follow-up study of abused and neglected children. *American Journal of Disabled Children, 120,* 439–446.

Nosek, M. A., Howland, C. A., & Young, M. E. (1997). Abuse of women with disabilities: Policy implications. *Journal of Disability Policy Studies, 8*(1 & 2), 157–175.

Oates, R. K., & Peacock, A., & Forrest, D. (1984). The development of abused children. *Developmental Medicine and Child Neurology, 26,* 649–656.

Olafson, E. (1999). Using testing when family violence and child abuse are issues. In A. R. Nurse (Ed.), *Psychological testing with families* (pp. 230–256). New York: Wiley.

Olafson, E., & Boat, B. W. (2000). Long-term management of the sexually abused child: Considerations and challenges. In R. M. Reece (Ed.), *The treatment of child abuse: Common ground for mental health, medical, and legal practitioners* (pp. 14–35). Baltimore: Johns Hopkins University Press.

Pacer Center. (1988). *A resource manual on child abuse.* Minneapolis, MN: Author.

Perry, B. D. (1994). Neurobiological sequelae of childhood trauma: PTSD in children. In M. M. Murburg (Ed.), *Catecholamine function in posttraumatic stress disorder: Emerging concepts* (pp. 233–255) Washington, DC: American Psychiatric Press.

Perry, B. D., Pollard, R. A., Blakely, T. L., Baker, W., & Vigilante, D. (1996). Childhood trauma, the neurobiology of adaptation and "use-dependent" development of the brain: How "states" become "traits." *Infant Mental Health Journal, 16,* 271–291.

Sandgrund, A., Gaines, R. W., & Green, A. H. (1974). Child abuse and mental retardation: A problem of cause and effect. *American Journal of Mental Deficiency, 79,* 327–330.

Sattler, J. M. (1988). *Assessment of children.* San Diego, CA: Sattler.

Sites, H. J. (1983). *Effects of maltreatment of children on development and learning achievement.* Unpublished doctoral dissertation, University of Cincinnati, Division of Graduate Education.

Sobsey, D. (1994). *Violence and abuse in the lives of people with disabilities.* Baltimore: Brookes.

Sobsey, D., & Varnhagen O. (1989). Sexual abuse of people with disabilities. In M. Csapo & L. Gougen (Eds.), *Special education across Canada: Challenges for the 90's* (pp. 199–218). Vancouver, British Columbia, Canada: Centre for Human Development and Research.

Sobsey, D., Wells, D., Lucardie, R., & Marsell, S. (1995). *Violence and disability: An annotated bibliography.* Baltimore: Brookes.

Sorenson, T., & Snow, B. (1991). How children tell: The process of disclosure in child sexual abuse. *Child Welfare, 22*(1), 3–15.

Stanton, M. P., Seidl, A., Pillitteri, A., & Smith, C. (1994). Nurses' attitudes toward emotional, sexual and physical abusers of children with disabilities. *Rehabilitation Nursing, 19*(4), 214–218.

Sullivan, P. M., Brookhouser, P. E., Knutson, J. F., Scanlan, J. M., & Schulte, L. E. (1991). Patterns of physical and sexual abuse of communicatively handicapped children. *Annals of Otology, Rhinology and Laryngology, 100,* 188–194.

Sullivan, P. M., & Knutson, J. F. (1998). The association between child maltreatment and disabilities in a hospital-based epidemiological study. *Child Abuse and Neglect, 22,* 271–288.

Tharinger, D., Horton, C. B., & Millea, S. (1990). Sexual abuse and exploitation of children and adults with mental retardation and other handicaps. *Child Abuse and Neglect, 14,* 301–312.

U.S. Department of Health and Human Services (1995). *HSS fact sheet: Preliminary finding regarding child abuse and neglect.* Washington, DC: National Center on Child Abuse and Neglect.

U.S. Department of Health and Human Services. (1996). *Child maltreatment 1994: Reports from the states to the National Center on Child Abuse and Neglect.* Washington, DC: National Center on Child Abuse and Neglect.

Wescott, H. L. (1991). The abuse of disabled children: A review of the literature. *Child Care, Health and Development, 17,* 243–258.

Westat, Inc. (1993). *A report on the maltreatment of children with disabilities.* Washington, DC: National Center on Child Abuse and Neglect.

Wolak, J., & Finkelhor, D. (1998). Children exposed to partner violence. In J. L. Jasinski & L. M. Williams (Eds.), *Partner violence: A comprehensive review of 20 years of research* (pp. 73–112). Thousand Oaks, CA: Sage.

Zirpoli, T. J. (1986). Child abuse and children with handicaps, *Remedial and Special Education, 7,* 39–48.

9

INFANT ASSESSMENT

TINA SMITH
REBECCA PRETZEL
KRISTINE LANDRY

Justin is a 6-month-old infant referred for a developmental assessment following his stay in the Neonatal Intensive Care Unit (NICU). Born at 28 weeks' gestation and weighing less than a pound, Justin experienced a number of health problems, mostly related to the immaturity of his lungs, and required hospitalization until he was 2½ months old. Neonatologists warned that Justin remains at risk for health problems, as well as developmental delay. Since being discharged from the NICU, Justin has gained weight well and seems to be gaining strength. Nonetheless, he is much smaller than other babies his age and, developmentally, he seems much younger than his chronological age. Until recently, Justin's parents have been most concerned about his health. However, as Justin has gained strength and his health has stabilized, they've begun to notice that Justin doesn't play with toys or try to sit up the way other babies his age do. They've also expressed frustration that Justin cries more than other infants and often looks away or becomes upset when they try to play with him.

Tamara is a cute, happy 19-month-old who was referred for testing by her pediatrician when she wasn't walking at her 18-month well-child checkup. Physically, Tamara is of average height and weight for her age and has been healthy. The third child born to a single mother, Tamara spends much of her time watching her 3-year-old sister and 4-year-old brother play. Tamara's 20-year-old mother, Ms. Johnson, dropped out of high school when she became pregnant with her first child. Ms. Johnson says that she has tried to tell personnel at the health department that "something's not right" with Tamara, but everyone kept telling her that "all babies develop at their own rates." She thinks it odd that no one listened to her concerns until Tamara still wasn't walking at her 18-month well-child checkup. Although Ms. Johnson continues to acknowledge that Tamara is not developing at the rate of her older children, she says that her primary concern now is finding child care so that she can go to school or find a job—her public assistance is scheduled to end within the year.

Since the mid-1980s, a number of factors have combined to create an emphasis on intervention and assessment during the infancy period. Federal legislation began providing public funds for services for infants and their families (i.e., Part C of Public Law 99-457, 1986). With dramatic improvements in medical technology, more and younger preterm infants are surviving and are eligible for early intervention services because of a number of developmental factors. As exemplified by the case of Justin, infants born prematurely typically are followed closely by a multidisciplinary medical team, including psychologists and other developmental specialists. Further, recent increases in our understanding of the nature and extent of neurological development during infancy have called public attention to the tremendous potential for intervention with these infants. All these factors and others are likely to create demands for infant developmental assessment, as pediatricians and parents become aware of the importance of identifying and addressing developmental problems as early as possible.

This chapter describes common conditions that are likely to result in the referral of infants for assessment. It addresses issues and concerns specific to the infancy period, including legal issues and the role of parents in infant assessment. It also discusses characteristics of and strategies for assessing developmental domains and provides a listing of commonly used instruments, along with analyses of their utility for diagnosis and treatment planning.

CONDITIONS ASSOCIATED WITH REFERRALS FOR INFANT ASSESSMENT

This section reviews selected conditions that frequently result in infants' being referred for developmental or psychological evaluations. For each condition, we give background information (e.g., prevalence, etiology), followed by a discussion of the medical, developmental, and behavioral characteristics associated with the condition, along with assessment-related concerns unique to each. Table 9.1 highlights the assessment considerations we recommend for each of the conditions discussed. Although the section is by no means exhaustive, we have attempted to identify those conditions that most frequently affect infants, as well as those conditions that require special considerations when planning and conducting an assessment.

Prematurity

Background

As technology has improved the life expectancy of infants born prematurely (before 36 weeks' gestation), this condition has become one of the most frequent reasons that infants are assessed. In the United States, about 11% of all newborns are classified as premature (Paneth, 1995). Preterm birth is associated with a number of fetal (e.g., genetic anomalies) and maternal (e.g., age, health status, behaviors, prenatal care) characteristics (Hooper & Edmondson, 1998).

*Developmental and Physical Characteristics
Associated with Prematurity*

The likelihood that premature infants will suffer adverse developmental effects has decreased substantially—from about 40% in 1975 to between 5% and 15% by the mid-1990s (Hack, Klein, & Taylor, 1995). Nonetheless, premature infants remain at increased risk for all types of developmental problems.

TABLE 9.1. Assessment Considerations for Medical Conditions Affecting Infants

Prematurity

The infant's health may affect location of assessment, as well as infant's stamina.
Gestational age should be used for calculating age until at least the first birthday.

Prenatal substance exposure

Family issues, including stability and safety of home environment and social support for care
  providers, should be assessed.
Legal issues (loss of custody, incarceration) may result in parents' reluctance to participate in
  interviews.

Down syndrome

Parents' familiarity with the condition, as well as special education alternatives, may affect their
  expectations for the infant's developmental trajectory.
Infants are generally referred at birth for multidisciplinary team evaluations.

Craniofacial anomalies

The family's needs related to social support, information, etc., should be assessed.
The impact of feeding difficulty on family relationships and routines should be assessed.

HIV/AIDS

Ongoing monitoring of the infants' neurodevelopmental status (including standardized and
  nonstandardized techniques) is recommended.
The psychosocial needs of the family are likely to be complex and must be considered as part of
  assessment and intervention planning.

Predicting outcomes for premature infants is difficult because outcomes vary widely along a number of dimensions related to infant health status, maternal health, and prenatal behaviors. Factors that are generally considered when trying to group premature infants based on their risk status include gestational age, birth weight, and presence, level, and type of medical complications that accompany prematurity. Despite a great deal of research in the area, the variability in prognosis for premature infants remains largely unexplained (Smith, Ulvund, & Lindemann, 1994). Thus gestational age remains the best general predictor of outcome.

Another related yet distinct factor used to group premature infants according to risk status is birth weight. Birth weights are classified into three groups: low birth weight (LBW; 2,500 grams or less); very low birth weight (VLBW; 1,500 grams or less); and extremely low birth weight (ELBW; 1,000 grams or less). As expected, lower birth weight is associated with increased risk for other complications, resulting in poorer developmental prognosis (see, e.g., Smith et al., 1994). In addition to considering total size, it is important also to take into account birth weight in relation to gestational age. Infants who are "small for gestational age" (SGA) may be at greater risk than a baby of similar weight but lower gestational age, particularly if the infant's head size is relatively small.

Two of the most frequently occurring medical complications among premature infants are respiratory problems and intraventricular hemorrhage. Respiratory distress syndrome (RDS) is a term used to describe respiratory problems associated with prematurity; in addition to posing health risks, the chronicity and severity of RDS has been associated with developmental risk (Meisels, Plunkett, Pasick, Stiefel, & Roloff, 1987). Intraventricular hemorrhage (IVH) affects between 13% and 48% of VLBW infants (see, e.g., Goddard-Finegold & Mizrah, 1987; Ross, Liper, & Auld, 1985). Severity of IVH is described in terms of grades, ranging from I (mild) to IV (severe). IVH has been associated with a host of developmental problems, including visual and hearing impairments, cerebral palsy, and mental retardation (see, e.g., Ford, Han, Steichen, Babcock, & Fogelson, 1989; Weislaus-Kuperus, Baerts, Fetter, & Sauer, 1992). However, other researchers report that early medical events, including IVH, are not significant predictors of developmental outcome (see, e.g., Aylward, Pfeiffer, Wright, & Verhulst, 1989; Cohen, Parmelee, Sigman, & Beckwith, 1988; Sostek, Smith, Katz, & Grant, 1987).

Assessment Considerations

The health status of premature infants in many ways dictates the nature and content of assessments with premature infants. Many premature infants remain hospitalized or are technology dependent (e.g., respirators) until their first birthday or later, necessitating that the assessment be conducted in the child's home or hospital room. The child's movements may be restricted either by IV tubing or oxygen tanks. Children who have been extremely ill may also have limited stamina, and assessments may have to be scheduled over a series of short intervals.

Another factor in the assessment of preterm infants is the need to consider their gestational age, as opposed to their chronological age, when deciding on test items or calculating scores. For example, a 6-month-old who was born 8 weeks early is likely to demonstrate the behaviors and developmental characteristics of a 4-month-old. There has been some degree of controversy about the age at which children born prematurely should have "caught up." Some experts argue that gestational age ought to be used until the 2nd birthday when calculating norm-referenced scores, but others say only until the 1st birthday. For most referral questions, a standardized test score would not be necessary and is likely to have limited practical utility.

Prenatal Substance Exposure

This section describes characteristics associated with prenatal exposure to alcohol and other drugs. Prevalence and associated developmental and physical characteristics are first discussed for alcohol, then for other drugs. A discussion of assessment considerations for both follows. Because both illegal drugs and alcohol are similar in that they are "drugs," the term "prenatal substance" is intended to mean either illegal drug use or alcohol use.

Background

Despite widespread public awareness campaigns and warnings from pediatricians and children's advocacy groups, alcohol remains the single most frequent cause of mental retardation in industrialized countries (Reece, Hobbins, Mahoney, & Petrie, 1995), affecting as many as 7 in 10,000 infants in the United States every year (Centers for Disease Control, 1995). Although evidence of the problem of alcohol use during pregnancy has been reported since ancient times, most authors agree that illicit drug use has increased dramatically in recent years, including use during pregnancy. Although estimates vary, several studies suggest that the rate is closer to 11% for most cities (Chasnoff, Landress, & Barrett, 1990; McCalla et al., 1991). Drug use may be related to geography: in nonurban areas, estimates have been less than 1% (Burke & Roth, 1993).

Developmental and Physical Characteristics
Associated with Prenatal Substance Use

Fetal alcohol syndrome (FAS) consists of a predictable pattern of characteristics, including low birth weight, poor growth across infancy and childhood, microcephaly, abnormal facial features (wide-set eyes, flat thin upper lip, and flattened bridge of the nose), poor motor coordination, mental retardation, and hyperactivity (Jones & Smith, 1973). A less severe version of FAS, known as fetal alcohol effects (FAE), also has been identified. The effects of FAE are less severe—with FAE, only some of the characteristics of FAS are expressed, and those features that are expressed often are much more subtle (Autti-Ramo et al., 1992).

The effects of drug use during pregnancy are far less well defined and may include numerous physical effects, ranging from dramatic and life-threatening conditions to more subtle neurological differences. Because of the apparent similarities related to effects on infant development and the findings that most women who use illicit drugs during pregnancy also drink alcohol, determining whether, for a given infant, developmental difficulties are the result of drug or alcohol exposure or a combination of the two is likely to be nonproductive. Some of the physical problems associated with prenatal substance exposure include more fetal distress, increased incidence of meconium staining (Chasnoff, Lewis, Griffith, & Willey, 1989), intracranial hemorrhage (Dominquez, Vila-Coro, Slopis, & Bohan, 1991), assorted structural abnormalities (Chasnoff, Chisum, & Kaplan, 1988; Kaye, Elkind, Goldberg, & Tytun, 1989), and a higher incidence of sudden infant death syndrome (SIDS; Chasnoff, Hunt, Kletter, & Kaplan, 1989). Furthermore, significantly lower birth weights (Bandstra & Burkett, 1991; Coles, Platzman, Smith, & James, 1992; Gustavsson, 1992; Phibbs, Bateman, & Schwartz, 1991; Rosenak, Diamant, Yaffe, & Hornstein, 1990; Singer, Garber, & Kliegman, 1991), increased rates of prematurity (Chasnoff, Lewis, Griffith, & Willey, 1989; Mastrogiannis, Decavalas, Verma, & Tejani, 1990; Neerhof, MacGregor, Retzky, & Sullivan, 1989; Phibbs et al., 1991), and small head circumference (Little & Snell, 1991) place substance-exposed infants at risk for the health and developmental problems described in the previous sections.

In addition to placing children at increased medical risk, the effects of drugs on the developing central nervous system may result in cerebral differences in substance-exposed children. Some findings suggest that, depending on the timing of the exposure, in utero substance exposure has the potential for severe cerebral damage (Dominquez et al., 1991; Salamy, Eldredge, Anderson, & Bull, 1990). Motor differences have been identified as well, including increased tremors (Oro & Dixon 1987; Schneider & Chasnoff, 1992), tremulousness and startle reactions (Chasnoff, Burns, Schnoll, & Burns, 1985), and more abnormal reflexes (Coles et al., 1992).

Significant neurobehavioral differences have also been associated with prenatal drug exposure. When compared with nonexposed infants, these infants were more irritable, had poorer feeding (Oro & Dixon, 1987; Sanders-Phillips, 1992; Singer et al., 1991) and more abnormal sleep patterns (Legido, Clancy, Spitzer, & Finnegan, 1992; Oro & Dixon, 1988; Sanders-Phillips, 1992; Singer et al., 1991), and had more trouble with behavioral state control (Chasnoff et al., 1985; Chasnoff et al., 1988; Hume, O'Donnell, Stanger, Killam, & Gringras, 1989; Sanders-Phillips, 1992; Tudehope, 1989).

It is also important to note that the findings with respect to prenatal drug exposure are not entirely pessimistic. A number of researchers report that although exposed infants demonstrated inferior performance during the neonatal period, their performances improve markedly across time (Black, Shuler, & Nair, 1993; Platzman, Coles, & Raskind-Hind,

1992). Nonetheless, taken together, the potential for less than optimal development of drug-exposed children is clear. Although few clinicians are likely to see the rarer and more dramatic effects of in utero drug exposure, some of the milder effects are likely to affect many more children. Characteristics such as irritability, inadequate state control, and motor differences combine to create challenging caregiving responsibilities for parents (Saylor, Lippa, & Lee, 1991). Therefore, the risk of nonoptimal child development should be viewed in relation to the threat posed to the mother–child relationship, and frequent, serial assessments, both of the infant's neurobehavioral status and its effect on the parent–child system, are recommended for this population.

Assessment Considerations

Assessment of infants prenatally exposed to alcohol and other drugs is a complex and sensitive undertaking. Because several states have laws defining prenatal drug use as a form of child abuse, allegations regarding maternal behavior can have serious consequences for the family. As a result, parents may be reluctant to seek evaluations of their infants. Therefore, it is particularly important that clinicians understand the audience for assessment reports and gather and present only information that addresses the referral question and is appropriate for the intended, as well as potential, audiences. For example, if an infant is referred for evaluation for the purpose of program planning, a prenatal history detailing maternal substance use during pregnancy may be unnecessary. In cases in which a clinician suspects continued substance use that may compromise the child's safety, mandatory child abuse reporting laws apply.

In addition to addressing child safety issues related to substance abuse within the home, other family factors should be included in a comprehensive evaluation of a substance-exposed infant. Because substance-exposed infants are at higher risk for difficult behavior and their parents at higher risk for an assortment of psychosocial stressors, the extent to which the infant "fits" within the family is an important consideration. Identifying social and parenting supports for the family also is an important component of the evaluation.

Down Syndrome

Background

Down syndrome is the most common chromosomal abnormality in humans (Kozma, 1986). It occurs in all races and countries and appears to affect boys and girls evenly. Recent prevalence figures indicate the frequency in North America to be approximately 1 in 800 to 1 in 1,000 births. Down syndrome, also called trisomy-21, is a genetic condition that occurs when a child has three 21st chromosomes. Although the exact cause of Down syndrome is yet unknown and the occurrence appears to be random, there does seem to be a correlation between advanced maternal age and incidence of Down syndrome. Prenatal testing has made it possible for early detection of Down syndrome. The most common source of detection is through amniocentesis, often done between the 13th and 18th week of pregnancy.

Developmental and Physical Characteristics
Associated with Down Syndrome

Even without prenatal testing, children with Down syndrome are usually identified within the first hours of life. Distinctive facial features involve the nose, eyes, mouth, teeth, and ears. Often, low muscle tone is evident and affects the baby's movement and strength. The most common features seen include low muscle tone, upwardly slanting eyes, and small ears (Kozma, 1986).

The growth of children with Down syndrome should be monitored by pediatricians and compared with specific Down syndrome growth charts. In addition, these children should be evaluated for specific medical disorders, including congenital heart disease, congenital hyperthyroidism, gastrointestinal malformations, and diabetes mellitus (Roizen, 1997). Sixty-eight percent of children with Down syndrome have a hearing loss (Roizen, Wolters, Nicol, & Blondis, 1993); 60% have ophthalmic disorders that can require treatment (Roizen, Mets, & Blondis, 1994). Children with Down syndrome also are affected with some degree of mental retardation, ranging from mild to severe.

Assessment Considerations

As soon as they are identified, children with Down syndrome are usually given a multidisciplinary evaluation to assess their skills across domains and subsequently referred to early intervention programs. Unlike many other disabilities, Down syndrome is generally readily identifiable at birth, and its effects are familiar to the general population. Therefore, families may have a number of preconceptions, and in some instances misconceptions, about the long-term impact of the disorder for the infant and family. Early assessment efforts should address these beliefs and expectations and provide appropriate information regarding resources for family support and information.

Cleft Lip and Palate

Background

Cleft lip and cleft palate constitute the fourth most common congenital disability, affecting approximately 1 in 700 children in the United States (Cleft Palate Foundation, 1992). The exact cause of clefting has not been determined; however, research suggests that the majority of clefts are due to a combination of genetic and environmental factors rather than to a single gene inheritance. Between 44% and 64% of all oral cleft patients may have an additional anomaly (Rollnick & Pruzansky, 1981; Sprintzen, Siegel-Sadewitz, Amato, & Goldberg, 1998), and clefts have been associated with multiple syndromes (e.g., Crouzon, Pierre-Robin, Apert, and Goldenhar). (Additional information about the implications of cleft lip and palate for professionals can be found in Edmonson & Reinhartsen, 1998.)

Developmental and Physical Characteristics
Associated with Craniofacial Anomalies

Of immediate concern for children with craniofacial anomalies is their ability to create enough pressure to suck from the breast or bottle. Early adaptive feeding techniques may be critical for the child's health and nourishment, as well as the development of competent sucking, swallowing, and chewing patterns that are precursors to normal speech development. For children affected with cleft lip, repair usually is completed within the first 3 months of life; palatal closure follows repair and is usually conducted between 9 and 18 months of age. In addition, approximately 75% of children with clefts present with defects involving the part of the upper jaw that houses the teeth (El Deeb, Waite, & Curran, 1993). Cleft has been identified as one of seven high-risk factors for hearing loss in infants (Ulvestad & Carlstrom, 1993), with up to 94% of children having continuous fluid in the middle ear, frequently causing conductive hearing loss (Charkins, 1996).

Although the majority of young children with clefts appear to do relatively well during the first 3 years of life, Neiman and Savage (1997) report that developmental data is inconclusive. Their study suggests that 5-month-old infants with clefts may have some developmental lags in motor, self-help, and cognitive domains, although these delays appear to resolve by 13 months of age. School-age children with clefts are more likely to have lower verbal IQ scores and to have language-based disabilities (Richman & Eliason, 1993).

Assessment Considerations

Due to the complex and multiple needs of a child with a craniofacial anomaly, the American Cleft Palate–Craniofacial Association (1993) recommends that these children be managed by an interdisciplinary team of specialists, ideally initiated within the first few days or weeks of life. Because feeding, hearing, speech, and language can all be affected by clefts, early intervention, particularly speech therapy, is likely to be recommended. The assessment should address families' needs for information and support, as they face frequent doctor appointments, surgeries, and hospitalizations and subsequent financial burdens related to the medical care of their child. Because feeding an infant with a cleft palate can take a great deal of time and expertise, parents may experience a violation of their expectations related to this very important caretaking role. The impact of feeding difficulties on mealtimes and family routines, as well as attachment, should be included as part of a complete developmental assessment. Additionally, a child born with a craniofacial anomaly may be at risk for development of psychological problems due to frequent hospitalizations, noticeable differences in speech, and inadequate coping skills.

Human Immunodeficiency Virus

Background

As of the end of 1999, the Centers for Disease Control (CDC) estimated that there were 733,374 reported cases of acquired immune deficiency syndrome (AIDS) in the United States, and 6,753 were children younger than 5 years of age (CDC, 2000). These numbers are alarming given the fact that the CDC estimates that these numbers may be underreported by as much as 20% below actual prevalence (Wolters, Brouwers, & Moss, 1995). Even though AIDS is still fatal, the prognosis for children with human immunodeficiency virus (HIV) continues to improve (Cohen, Papola, & Alvarez, 1994; Meyers, 1994). Large cohort studies of children born infected with HIV report that 50% to 60% of these infants survive beyond age six (Meyers, 1994).

Ninety-one percent of American infants and children under 13 years of age who are infected with HIV acquired it through vertical transmission (i.e., from mother to infant; CDC, 2000). Seven percent of pediatric HIV infections are accounted for by blood transfusions and/or the use of contaminated blood products for the treatment of hemophilia (CDC, 2000). Finally, for approximately 2% of these infections, the risk is not reported or identified (CDC, 2000). Although a small number of cases have been reported in which infection was the result of sexual abuse, vertical transmission is the most common route of transmission for infants and can occur in one of three ways. First, during gestation, HIV may cross the placental barrier into the blood of the fetus. Second, during childbirth, blood may be exchanged between the mother and fetus/newborn. Third, HIV is occasionally transmitted from the mother to the infant through breast-feeding, although this route is much less common than the first two (Friedland & Klein, 1987). Early-intervention professionals need to be aware that not all mothers who are infected with HIV will transmit the virus to their infant, and with improvements in maternal medical care, the rates of transmission are likely to continue to decline. Current estimates of the rate of transmission from an untreated HIV-infected mother to her unborn infant range from 25% to 30% (MacDonald, 1992). Further, one encouraging study reported that the timely administration of zidovudine (AZT) to the mother during pregnancy reduces this rate to 8% (Connor et al., 1994).

Typical Manifestations That Initiate Diagnosis

An "official" diagnosis of HIV infection is rare for infants and young children. Unfortunately, there are no clear medical markers of HIV infection for infants under the age of 12 to 18 months (MacDonald, 1992). Sicklick and Rubenstein (1992) describe a classification system currently being used by the CDC and the medical community to classify infants and young children who may be HIV positive. The system is based on classifying children according to the kind of symptoms they are manifesting and the health of their immune systems (e.g., normal immune system function or cancers). Even though an official diagnosis may come only as the infant ages, medical and social services are organized immediately in order to monitor the newborn's medical and neuropsychological status, to offer financial and social support to the family, and to plan interventions on the child's behalf. Further, experts believe that many infants may benefit from medical protocol that involves administration of antiretroviral drugs (MacDonald, 1992). Often a team that includes medical and psychological personnel is needed to monitor a child's progress or decline.

Developmental and Physical Characteristics Associated with HIV

Providing appropriate services for infants and young children who are infected with HIV is challenging for many reasons. One challenge concerns the extreme variability in the manifestation of the disease. In adults infected with HIV, the effects of the disease are often indirect, compromising the body's immune system and reducing its ability to fight infections, strokes, and cancer. However, the predominant effects of HIV in infants and young children are more direct, affecting the central nervous system (CNS). This direct involvement of the virus in the CNS is called HIV-related encephalopathy, and several levels of CNS involvement have been identified (see Wolters et al., 1995, for a thorough discussion of developmental trajectories resulting from different levels of CNS involvement).

Encephalopathy in HIV-infected children has been characterized according to the level of intrusion of the virus into the CNS. There are different categories of encephalopathy, depending on the gains (or losses) in skills and abilities that the child shows. In some instances, the infant continues to achieve some developmental milestones but from an initially compromised level of development. Some more severe types are characterized by severe deficits in cognitive, motor, socioemotional, linguistic, and adaptive functioning. Cognitive and social functioning may be globally and pervasively impaired. Infants may also be born with HIV without developing encephalopathy. These children are frequently described as having "neuropsychological impairments." This group of children is extremely heterogeneous in terms of health and psychological functioning. Finally, some infants and children infected with HIV appear to demonstrate normal functioning. These children show no impairment upon psychoeducational evaluation and no improvement after medical intervention. Experts believe that children in this group are experiencing HIV infection without CNS involvement (Brouwers, Belman, & Epstein, 1994).

The difficulties in identifying the effects of HIV infection are problematic in evaluations during the neonatal period. Coulter and Chase (1990) report that for neonates exposed in utero to HIV, there is frequently no specific or clear pattern of disturbance. However, a number of warning signs may alert clinicians to the need for continued follow-up. Coulter and Chase (1990) report that HIV infection may affect a number of developmental domains, including social interest (e.g., HIV-exposed neonates have been described as irritable and over- or underresponsive). HIV-infected neonates may also have poor feeding and sleeping patterns and various motor difficulties.

Medical Information

Medical and mental health professionals have joined forces to develop various means of increasing the longevity of infants born with HIV. Infants and children living with HIV are often prescribed antiretroviral drugs (e.g., AZT) in an effort to improve immunological, neurological, and overall health status. Some medications may cause a child's status to improve or decline. One important role of psychologists is to monitor and evaluate development in all domains over time in order to assist medical doctors in decisions about the efficacy of particular drugs for a child.

Assessment Considerations

There are no reports of casual transmission of HIV in school or day-care settings or during contact sports (Wolters et al., 1995). However, all psychologists and personnel who will be working with these children need to be aware of situations that are potentially dangerous (e.g., vomit that may contain blood poses a transmission risk). In order to be prepared for any potentially risky situation, professionals working with (any) children should follow the universal-precautions protocol at all times.

Several features of the HIV itself, as well as its effects on neurocognitive status and the entire family system, suggest the need for a number of special considerations in developing and conducting developmental evaluations with this population. Two specific purposes of assessment are particularly pertinent to infants with HIV: (1) ongoing developmental monitoring to identify the onset of deterioration, document decline, and chart neurocognitive effects of changes in medical treatment; and (2) program planning for families with complex medical and psychosocial needs.

Because of the course of HIV, it is crucial that infants' developmental progress be monitored carefully, initially for the establishment of a baseline. In general, experts suggest that the time interval between longitudinal assessments be determined based on the child's age and neurological status. Several authors recommend that infants be evaluated every 3 to 6 months and preschool children every 6 to 12 months (Rodriguez, Diaz, & Fowler, 1997; Wolters et al., 1995). For the purpose of establishing a baseline, a combination of norm-referenced and competency-based measures is recommended. The use of norm-referenced instruments allows the professional to examine not just current standing in relation to peers but, more important, developmental trajectory in relation to that of typically developing children as well. Care must be taken in using standardized assessment with these infants to insure that the assessment does not miss crucial areas (e.g., adaptive functioning) and to insure that predictions regarding future progress are not based on tests with inadequate reliability and validity data or that are inappropriate for the child being tested. The use of multiple measures over time and across settings can be expected to provide a more complete picture of the child and his or her different environmental supports and risks (Seidel, 1992; Trad, Kentros, Solomon, & Greenblatt, 1994; Wolters et al., 1995). Adaptations, such as the use of multiple sessions and the elimination of redundant items, are likely to be particularly important to avoid lowered scores as the result of attentional problems and limited stamina.

SPECIAL ISSUES AND CONCERNS IN THE DEVELOPMENTAL ASSESSMENT OF INFANTS

Because of the nature of infancy itself, as well as federal legislation governing service provision to infants, the developmental assessment of infants differs in many ways from the assessment of older children. The need to involve the family in meaningful ways and maturational considerations (e.g., rapid, nonlinear neurological development) limit tremendously the utility of traditional psychometric assessment. This section describes those assessment issues that are unique to infancy and strategies to address them.

Federal Law Addressing Services for Infants

In 1986, Congress enacted Public Law 99-457, legislation that mandated services for children aged 3 to 5 who have disabilities and, under Part C, offered incentives for states to provide services to infants with disabilities. In addition to expanding educational services to younger children, this legislation is noteworthy in that it prescribed a significant role for families as partners in the education of their children. Part C goes even further with respect to families by asserting that because families are the most crucial factor in the development of infants, the family—not the infant—is the target of the service delivery system. Thus the needs of the family are as much a focus as the needs of the child, and the family is given the authority to determine which services it will accept and which it will not (Brown, Thurman, & Pearl, 1993). In the 1980s, professionals began a discourse on "family centered" or "family focused" intervention, reflecting the newfound respect for families and their role in the development of their children.

The emphasis on the family, both as a target of intervention and as having the right to determine the nature and extent of services, has profound implications for the assessment and evaluation of infants. For most infants with or at risk for developmental disability, the outcome of the assessment will be an Individualized Family Service Plan (IFSP). The IFSP is similar in some ways to an Individualized Education Plan (IEP). For example, both are legally binding documents that specify the services the child will receive, along with criteria and procedures that will be used to evaluate the services. Both IEPs and IFSPs specify when the services will begin and how long they are expected to last. In addition, although the wording is somewhat different, both IEPs and IFSPs document the environments in which the services will be provided and plans for transitioning into the next service delivery system.

Although there are many similarities between IEPs and IFSPs, there are several important differences as well. Unlike IEPs, which are only required to include statements related to educational functioning, IFSPs require broad statements related to overall development, including specific mention of the following domains of functioning: physical development, cognitive abilities, language development, psychosocial development, and self-help skills. Further, because the family is the target of intervention, the IFSP must also address the family's concerns, resources, and priorities (Individuals with Disabilities Education Act [IDEA], 1986). The implications of this difference for the way services are provided are substantial and reflect fundamental differences in the underlying philosophies of intervention. For example, an IFSP for the Johnson family described in the second vignette at the beginning of this chapter would likely need to address Ms. Johnson's concern about finding appropriate child care for Tamara. (See Chapter 7 for a discussion of the assessment of families' concerns, resources, and priorities.)

The Role of Families in Assessment

The omnipresence of the family in the early intervention process highlights the need for professionals to collaborate effectively with family members, beginning with the initial assessment. Given that families have the right to control the nature of the services they and their infant receive, it is only natural to assume that families also should have the right to determine the nature of the assessment their child receives. A continuum of potential family roles exists and ranges from passive observation of the assessment to identification of the areas assessed and types of instruments utilized. Although within the context of family-centered intervention the goal is to enable families to take leadership roles in all aspects of intervention, including assessment (Dunst, Johanson, Trivette, & Hamby, 1991), this role may not be appealing to all families. A few factors outside the control of the professional (e.g., infants' medical condition, standardization requirements of some instruments) may dictate some aspects of family involvement. For example, attitudes and expectations of the two families described in the chapter-opening vignettes would differ greatly along a number of dimensions. The first task of assessment professionals working with these families is likely to be determining each families' priorities for the assessment itself. As much as possible, the families' wishes should be respected in this regard.

DOMAINS OF ASSESSMENT

Cognitive Functioning

Perhaps more than any other developmental domain, infants' cognitive abilities represent the greatest challenge in assessment and one that has been fraught with controversy. As described earlier in this chapter, a number of behavioral and developmental features characteristic of infancy (e.g., rapid neurological development, temperamental factors, state regulation) make assessment of all developmental domains difficult during this period. However, a number of definitional and theoretical issues, as well as a lack of psychometrically sound instruments, further complicate the assessment of infant cognition.

Theoretical Issues and the Stability of Cognitive Ability

The validity and utility of measures of intelligence for children of any age have long been debated in the fields of psychology and education (Flanagan & Genshaft, 1997), in part because of debates regarding the nature and definition of cognitive abilities. For most practitioners and researchers, the debate over whether cognition represents a stable, genetically predetermined individual difference or a trait that is shaped principally by the environment has been replaced by a more interactionist view, embracing the roles of both nature and nurture behaviors (Hynd & Semrud-Clikeman, 1993). This interaction is particularly pronounced during infancy. Whether due to biological maturation or environmental stimulation, the rapid and often sporadic development of the CNS associated with the first year of life frequently results in dramatic changes in cognitive ability over a very short time. This leaves clinicians attempting to evaluate these abilities with the daunting task of attempting to "hit a moving target."

Sensory–Motor Approach

Because cognitive development during infancy has been assumed to parallel the development of the CNS, cognitive ability traditionally has been inferred from motor behaviors (Hynd & Semrud-Clikeman, 1993). This orientation is supported by Piagetian theories of cognitive development that describe the infancy period as the sensory–motor stage, the primary developmental tasks being gaining control and understanding of motor and sensory functions. Further, because of the limited response repertoires available to infants, our windows into their thought processes largely have been restricted to motor tasks. Thus traditional measures of infant development (e.g., Bayley Scales of Infant Development; Bayley, 1993) have relied almost exclusively on motor and sensory responses. Specific items on traditional Piagetian-based measures are targeted at substages within the sensory–motor stage. (See Table 9.2 for a description of sensory–motor substages and examples of corresponding test items and Chapter 5 for discussion of sensorimotor developments.)

The limitations of equating motor ability or neurological development with cognition are obvious for infants with documented or potential motor or sensory impairments. However, this approach to the assessment of infant cognition has not resulted in the development of stable measures of cognitive ability for any infants. In fact, after examining the performance of infants on a number of sensory–motor tasks over a period of time, Bayley (1993) stated that "behavior growth of the early months of infant development has little predictive relation to the later development of intelligence" (p. 74). Within a Piagetian framework, infants develop representational speech as they move away from the sensory–motor stage. Thus, language takes on an increasingly important role in the assessment of cognitive ability, and the stability of the cognitive measures improves.

At this point, it is important to note that, although measures relying on sensory–motor abilities do not predict later cognitive ability for most children, these measures are more accurate in their predictions for infants with or at significant risk for disability. For example, scores on the Bayley Scales of Infant Development (BSID) of 12-month-old infants at biological risk correlated significantly with measures of verbal and motor abilities administered at 54 months of age (Crowe, Dietz, & Bennett, 1987, cited in Bayley, 1993). Similarly, in the absence of intervention, BSID scores of 6-month-old infants at risk because of environmental factors were significantly related to Stanford–Binet IQ scores at 24 and 48 months (Farran & Harber, 1989, cited in Bayley, 1993). Thus, although far from perfect in terms of predictive validity, the BSID can provide meaningful information in the diagnosis of developmental delay.

Information-Processing Approach

Arguably, the Piagetian view of infancy as the sensory–motor stage has been the most important influence in the conceptualization of infant assessment. However, within the

TABLE 9.2. Sensory–Motor Substages and Corresponding Behaviors

Substage	Definition	Examples
Reflexive activity (Birth–1 month)	Simple, involuntary reflexes lead to the development of motor patterns that allow exploration.	Sucking, grasping, visual following
Primary circular reactions (1–4 months)	Infants repeat behaviors that produce pleasurable or interesting results, centered on their own bodies.	Looking at and manipulating own fingers and hands
Secondary circular reactions (4–8 months)	Infants repeat behaviors that produce interesting results external to their own bodies. Beginning of object permanence occurs as infants begin to search for objects dropped from view or partially hidden.	Plays with a rattle
Coordination of secondary schemes (8–12 months)	Actions, such as shaking or banging, are combined to achieve a goal ("means–ends" behaviors). Continued sophistication of object permanence occurs as infants begin to search for completely hidden objects.	Pulls string to obtain a toy
Tertiary circular reactions (12–18 months)	Infants experiment with different actions to achieve the same goal or observe the outcomes.	Uses of trial and error to obtain an inaccessible toy
Invention of new means through mental combinations	Infants use mental images to think through or solve problems. Deferred imitation occurs as infants observe others and remember the behavior for later experimentation. Object permanence is firmly established as infant maintains a mental image of the absent object.	Uses rudimentary words to label objects Has a tantrum after witnessing a playmate's tantrum

past 20 years, information-processing theories have been applied to infant assessment. The underlying premises of most of these techniques is that of novelty preference—that all other features being equal, infants prefer to look at unfamiliar objects. This preference is then used to infer an infant's cognitive abilities—particularly memory and attention.

The most widely used clinical instrument based on novelty preference is the Fagan Test of Infant Intelligence (FTII; Fagan & Shepherd, 1985). Designed for infants aged 5, 7, 9, and 12 months, the FTII uses photographs of faces. During the habituation phase, the infant is shown two identical photographs. Once the infant has looked for a specified period of time at these photographs, the familiar photograph is paired with a new photograph. The infant's score on the FTII is based on the extent to which the new photograph is viewed to the exclusion of the familiar one. Research examining the relationships between the FTII and later IQ scores suggests that novelty preference is related to IQ. Interestingly, correlations between FTII scores at 12 months and BSID scores at 12 months were not significant. However, significant correlations were obtained between FTII scores at 12 months, BSID scores at 24 months, and Stanford–Binet IQ scores at 36 months. These findings have important implications from a theoretical perspective—in fact, when the BSID was revised in the early 1990s, a number of items were added to provide more of an emphasis on language and novelty preference. However, despite their statistical significance, the correlation coefficients were so low that the clinical significance of the relationships between novelty preference and later cognitive ability is questionable: $r = .21$ between the FTII at 12 months and the BSID at 24 months; $r = .58$ between the FTII at 12 months and the Stanford–Binet IQ at 36 months (Thompson, Fagan, & Fulker, 1991).

Specific Abilities Approach

A more recent measure of infant development, the Mullen Scales of Early Learning (MSEL; Mullen, 1989), embraces yet another theoretical perspective of the nature of cognitive abilities. Mullen suggests that "early cognitive development is best measured by a group of cognitive abilities that are distinct and well-defined in content" (p. 9). Thus, the MSEL consists of a Gross Motor scale and four cognitive scales: Visual Reception, Fine Motor, Receptive Language, and Expressive Language. The cognitive scales can be summed to derive a composite score, the Early Learning Composite. However, the interesting and clinically useful aspect of the scale is that, unlike other standardized measures of infant cognitive development, it provides a means for deriving a profile of strengths and weaknesses.

Clinical Recommendations for the Use of Standardized Cognitive Assessment

Given the theoretical and psychometric problems associated with cognitive assessment of infants, careful interpretation of test results is crucial. Clinicians must recognize that tests are valid only for their intended purpose in order to understand and use the results. In particular, instruments such as the BSID clearly are intended as measures of current development and are in no way intended to be an early measure of IQ. Further, clinicians must be aware of the theoretical foundations and psychometric properties of the instruments they choose, particularly because two instruments, both purporting to measure infant cognitive ability, may in fact be measuring very different skills and abilities. For example, Gerken, Eliason, and Arthur (1994) reported a correlation of –.03 between the BSID Mental Development Index and the Battelle Developmental Inventory Total Score. Depending on the theoretical foundation of the instrument and the nature of the items administered, as well as a host of child behaviors and characteristics, a given cognitive measure may reflect any number of skills and abilities, many of which are unrelated to later cognition.

Finally, although occasions arise when a standard score of infant cognitive ability is needed (e.g., for program eligibility), the functional utility of these instruments and of the resulting scores is likely to be significantly limited. A number of authors have criticized traditional early childhood cognitive measures for their lack of treatment utility, pointing out that many features of this type of assessment are incompatible with the spirit and letter of IDEA (Bagnato & Neisworth, 1994). Therefore, we recommend that standardized assessments of infant cognition be used only as part of an assessment package. Other techniques described in this chapter (e.g., play assessment) are more likely to yield functional information that can be used for program and treatment planning.

Use of Play for Assessing Cognitive Abilities

Play has been defined as active engagement with objects or activities that are "intrinsically motivated, spontaneously performed, flexible, and accomplished with positive affect" (Wolery, 1989, p. 431). Because play is the natural activity for infants and young children, it provides an obvious arena for observing children's functional abilities in all developmental domains, including cognitive ability. Within the context of assessment, play can be structured in order to elicit behaviors most likely to address areas of greatest relevance to program planning. However, the use of play in assessment requires abandoning much of the structure required for traditional standardized assessment. With the types of assessments described earlier in this chapter, the examiner attempts to control the interactions and activities, with the infant assuming the role of passive responder. However, within a play-based approach, the examiner attempts to structure the environment in such a way that the infant actively and spontaneously engages in activities of his or her own choosing. Although the beginning clinician may find the interpretation of such behaviors somewhat daunting, play provides a rich opportunity to examine the infant's unique capabilities and interests.

Play can be used both as an assessment in its own right and as a tool for identifying developmental capabilities and needs. A large number of systems for categorizing play have been developed, some of which correspond to developmental levels. However, this chapter focuses on the use of play skills to infer other abilities. Examiners familiar with infant behavior and developmental stages of infancy can determine a great deal about infants' developmental levels through simple observation of their manipulation of and play with objects. In order to use play effectively as an assessment technique, examiners will need an array of toys to accommodate a wide range of abilities and interests. Table 9.3 provides a list of recommended objects. Another useful strategy is to ask parents or care providers to suggest toys or to bring a few of their child's favorite toys.

One structured approach to the use of play for assessment of development is the Transdisciplinary Play-Based Assessment (TPBA; Linder, 1990). A curriculum-embedded assessment, TPBA utilizes a team approach, with parents playing key roles, to examine young children's development across four domains: cognitive, social-emotional, communication and language, and sensory–motor.

Communication

Communication refers to the process of exchanging ideas, information, and feelings between individuals. It is the basis on which children gain knowledge about the world around them, form social relationships, and participate in everyday activities. Assessment of com-

TABLE 9.3. Recommended Toys

Manipulatives	Large and small blocks, stacking rings, sorting cups, simple and colorful puzzles
Toys that make sounds	Rattles of various sizes and shapes, bells
Dramatic or functional play	Dolls, cups, bottles, toy cars
Cause-and-effect toys	Switch toys, pull toys, "pop-up" toys

munication skills in early childhood must be considered within a developmental context, as communication develops in accordance with a child's social, cognitive, and motor skills. Communication encompasses more than spoken language; it includes gestures, signed or written language, and a variety of other representational systems.

A thorough evaluation of a child's communication abilities should include several components: speech, syntax, and pragmatics. Speech can be defined as the auditory–articulatory code by which we represent spoken languages. This includes phonation and articulation of phonemes. During the first year of life it is expected that children will produce many different vocalizations, including speech and nonspeech sounds. At approximately 6 months, young children are expected to babble and begin repeating consonant–vowel combinations such as ma-ma and ba-ba. Prior to this, infants will have made a variety of vowel-like and cooing sounds and varied their crying to indicate different needs. As children grow, so should their vocabulary, with general estimates that at age 1 a child would have some single words. At age 2, a larger vocabulary of single words is expected, and some two-word combinations such as "more juice" or "where doggie" may be present. By age 3, it is expected that children understand and use two to three hundred words, and they may be asking "why" and "what" questions. The MacArthur Communicative Development Inventories (Fenson et al., 1991) are instruments that yield information about language development from the first nonverbal gestural signals through the expansion of early vocabulary to the beginnings of grammar. There are two separate forms completed by parents, one for infants 8–16 months and one for toddlers 16–30 months.

During early childhood, children still make many articulation errors that are developmental in nature. It will be important to attend to a child's articulation, as well as the ability to imitate sounds correctly and in proper sequence. Standardized measures of articulation typically are not used prior to age 2.

Syntax refers to the organizational rules we use for combining words into phrases and sentences and includes parts of speech, word order, and basic sentence patterns. These rules are acquired gradually by children as they listen to role models in their environments and learn to put words together. As early as 18 months, children are using two-word combinations, and as their sentences increase in length, they begin to learn complex sentence structure. Morphemes are often used in assessing children's grammatical competence. A morpheme is the smallest meaningful element of language, for example, adding an "s" to the word "girl," increasing that word from one to two morphemes. Brown identified 14 grammatical morphemes that children begin to acquire between 24 and 30 months. To estimate their syntactical complexity, the mean length of utterance (MLU) can be calculated after taking a language sample. The MLU is considered to be a good indicator of potential language problems and language growth (Brown, 1973a, 1973b; Miller, 1981).

Pragmatics refers to the use of language in a psychosocial context and includes the rules that govern how language is used for the purpose of communication (Roberts & Crais, 1989). The speech act is considered to be the basic unit of pragmatics; this may be extended to include preverbal communicative acts (Austin, 1962; Easterbrooks, 1998). In infancy, children are communicating, although it may be unintentional and some of the signals may be reflexive or involuntary. For example, infants can communicate feelings of displeasure by crying or physically turning away; they use other nonvocal signals such as yawning, finger splaying, or grimacing. Although the child may not be intentionally communicating a need, listeners in the environment often respond to these signals. When a child's caregivers learn to identify these communication signals and respond to them quickly and consistently, it helps the baby learn that he or she can have an effect on the world (Dunst, Lowe, & Bartholomew, 1990; Wilcox, 1992). By 8–12 months of age, children typically began using some intentional communication; that is, they have some realization that their communicative act, whether verbal, nonverbal, or gestural, will lead to a desired response by the listener. Gestures and gestures combined with vocalizations are frequently seen in this stage and subsequently progress to word-like vocalizations between 12 and 18 months (Chapman, 1981).

Wetherby, Cain, Yonclas, and Walker (1988) elaborate on three broad categories of intentional communication. These include behavioral regulation, social interaction, and joint attention. Behavioral regulation refers to a child's ability to control or regulate another's behavior for a desired outcome. For example, a child may be requesting objects by pointing and/or through vocalizations or protesting. Social interaction refers to the use of intentional communication to initiate or prolong a social exchange. This may include the use of greetings, calling out to gain attention, requesting permission, and requesting a social routine. The third area, joint attention, refers to a child's ability to focus on something and then draw someone else's attention to this object so that it can be shared by the two of them. This usually includes the use of eye gaze, commenting on an object or action, or requesting information about something. The Communication and Symbolic Behavior Scales (Wetherby & Prizant, 1993) is designed to examine communicative, social-affective, and symbolic abilities of children at ages 8 months and 2 years.

Two commonly used measures of language development during infancy and toddlerhood include the Receptive–Expressive Emergent Language Scale—Second Edition (REEL-2; Bzoch & League, 1991) and the Rossetti Infant–Toddler Language Scale (Rossetti, 1990). The REEL-2 examines skills in terms of stages of emergent language development: phonemic level, morphemic level, syntactic level, and semantic level. The Rossetti is a criterion-referenced instrument designed to assess the following areas of communication and interaction: interaction–attachment, pragmatics, gesture, play, language comprehension, and language expression.

In addition to evaluating expressive language and communication skills, it is also important to assess what a child understands and comprehends. The Preschool Language Scale–3 is one measure that provides standard scores in Auditory Comprehension, Expressive Communication, and Total Language (Zimmerman, Steiner, & Pond, 1992).

Motor Skills

Movement is a primary avenue through which children explore and learn about their environment. As sensory motor skills develop, a child gains mastery over the world around him or her and feels increasing competence in his or her own skills. The development of motor skills supports development in other areas such as cognition (banging, shaking, and manipulating objects) and communication (reaching, pointing, and production of oral speech). Additionally, motor skills are crucial components of a child's growth and nutritional status in that children need sucking, swallowing, and chewing skills.

Delayed motor skills may be one of the first indicators that a child is experiencing some sort of delay or possible disability. For example, in the second vignette at the beginning of this chapter, it is Tamara's delayed motor development that concerns her health care provider. A thorough discussion of normal sensory–motor development is beyond the scope of this chapter, although several areas can be highlighted. Prenatally, the movement of the baby is one indicator of normal development. Primitive movements of the fetus are refined and developed to prepare the fetus to find the correct presentation for birth and to actively move itself through the birth canal. After birth, the neonate continues to develop motor patterns that began in the intrauterine environment and to demonstrate maturation of reflex behaviors (Case-Smith & Short Ridge, 1996). The Brazelton Neonatal Behavioral Assessment Scale (BNBAS; Brazelton, 1984) is one measure that is often used to examine the behavioral and motor activity within the first month of life. The BNBAS focuses on a variety of reflexes, the amount and type of motor activity exhibited, and the neonate's tonicity, orientation, and habituation to stimuli. The assessment of muscle tone is critical, as abnormal tone can result in delays in attainment of milestones and atypical postures and movement patterns (Smith, 1989). Terms such as "hypotonia" (low muscle tone) or "hypertonia," or "spasticity" (increased muscle tone), are often used to describe a child. In addition, the child's range of motion and posture is important.

After the first month of life, the infancy period begins, and motor skills begin to develop rapidly and dramatically. Infants gain head control and learn to roll, sit, cruise, and eventually walk independently. It is important not only to consider the age at which a child masters these skills but also to observe the developmental sequence of skill acquisition. As a child's strength, balance, endurance, and coordination increase, his or her motor skills become smoother and more controlled, so that he or she can master more difficult motor skills such as climbing stairs, jumping, hopping, and running (Patz & Dennis, 1998). Assessment measures such as the Psychomotor Scale of the Bayley Scales of Infant Development—Second Edition (Bayley, 1993) and the Gross Motor Scale of the Peabody Developmental Scales are frequently used to determine the developmental skill level.

Fine motor skills are the more refined and precise movements of the hands and fingers that allow a child to functionally reach, grasp, and release objects for purposeful manipulation (Patz & Dennis, 1998). Fine motor skills also appear in a developmental sequence, beginning with a simple reach and subsequent grasp of an object with the hand. Children typically learn to transfer objects from hand to hand, to actively release objects, and to develop a pincer grasp within the first year of life. As they mature, their grasp on writing tools becomes more refined; they begin to show hand preference and can stack blocks, work simple puzzles and pegboards, string beads, and explore their environment in more detail. It is also important to consider the quality of a child's fine motor abilities and to look for tremors, overshooting, and eye–hand coordination. The Fine Motor Scale of the Peabody Developmental Scales can be used to examine a child's fine motor development.

Self-Help Skills

Self-help or adaptive skills are those abilities needed for independent functioning in meeting daily needs such as feeding, toileting, and dressing. Understanding a young child's needs for assistance during such daily caretaking activities can help interventionists in planning the ISFP. Tools such as the Vineland Adaptive Behavior Scales (Sparrow, Balla, & Cicchetti, 1984) and the Scales of Independent Behavior—Revised (Bruininks, Woodcock, Weatherman, & Hill, 1996) can be used to assess a young child's adaptive behavior and determine areas of strengths and weaknesses. The attainment of self-help skills is obviously directly related to a child's motor abilities. For example, a child with poor oral–motor skills may have difficulty sucking from a bottle or breast, or a child with low muscle tone may be delayed in learning to hold his own bottle. During the first year of life a child is expected to have developed eye–hand coordination and the ability to grasp an object to bring it to his or her mouth for finger feeding. Feeding skills continue to develop as a child learns to hold a spoon, control drooling, chew appropriately, drink from a cup, suck from a straw, use a fork, and eventually gain mastery of all eating utensils.

In terms of dressing and grooming, a child's cooperation and beginning assistance in dressing himself or herself can be seen in the first year, as a child will stick out an arm or leg while being dressed. During the second year of life, children may learn to take off shoes and socks and begin to try to put on their own clothes. They may also attempt to brush their teeth and participate in bathing activities on their own. Between 2 and 3 years children may begin to attempt buttons and snaps, use better toothbrushing movements, and show the desire to do things independently (Langone, 1998).

Another area of importance during the first 3 years of life is toileting skills. Again, this is a gradual progression of skills, beginning with a child's awareness of having wet or dirty diapers, becoming comfortable with sitting on a potty chair, communicating a need to go to the toilet, and gaining control over bowels and bladder functions (Langone, 1998).

Social and Emotional Functioning

As is always the case in early childhood assessment, infants' social and emotional functioning must be understood in the context of their overall development. Within this context, the nature of the assessment will vary according to a number of factors, including the referral question, the health and developmental level of the infant, and the composition and preferences of the family. For young, preverbal children, ecobehavioral techniques such as informal observations and unstructured interviews offer clinicians a flexible and efficient means of collecting information for program planning. Although structured and standardized measures are available and may provide information allowing for normative comparisons, such measures are unlikely to provide the amount and quality of information that can be gleaned from naturalistic observations of the infant in a social context. Therefore, we suggest that a thorough evaluation of an infant's social and emotional functioning consist of a number of differing strategies, including observations, interviews, and examiner interactions with the infant.

Attachment

The concept of attachment is regarded as one of the most prominent theories related to human social and emotional development. Defined by Bowlby (1969) as a bidirectional process in which infants and their primary caregivers establish emotional bonds, attachment has long been emphasized by developmental theorists as crucial for children's later social and emotional development. For most infants, the interactions resulting in attachment begin at or shortly after birth and are believed to be the "well-spring for all the infant's subsequent attachments" (Klaus & Kennell, 1976, p. 1). Hanson (1996) points out that for many of the infants and families referred for assessment, opportunities to engage in early bonding experiences may have been lost or diminished due to medical interventions necessary to save the child's life. Further, other events surrounding the infant's birth, such as diagnosis of developmental disability, may affect parents' earliest interactions. Despite the real potential for perinatal complications to affect later interactions, Hanson points out that these effects likely are not irreversible and that by overemphasizing them clinicians run the risk of exacerbating any negative emotions parents may already be experiencing. Consequently, it is important for clinicians to ask about the circumstances that surrounded parents' first interactions with their infants in order to understand the possible effects these may have had on present interactions so that they can provide appropriate support and information. However, equally important is the knowledge that in time, most parents and children with complicated birth histories develop normal healthy inter-actional patterns (Goldberg, 1990).

The most well-known means of assessing attachment is known as the Strange Situa-tion paradigm (Ainsworth, Blehar, Waters, & Wall, 1978). In this procedure, infants are subjected to a series of social situations involving the presence of their mothers, the pres-ence of their mothers and a stranger, and finally the absence of their mothers. Based on responses to the mothers' return, infants are categorized as securely attached, insecure–avoidant, and insecure–ambivalent. Despite its widespread use in the research literature, the Strange Situation is unlikely to be relevant to the clinical assessment of infant social and emotional functioning. Not only is the paradigm unnatural and nonfunctional, but also many infants with healthy attachments become extremely distressed when their mothers leave them. Further, the relevance of the information obtained may vary depending on the families' parenting practices and cultural values (Trawick-Smith, 1997). Unfortunately, although a number of techniques (e.g., Q-sorts, surveys) have been developed to assess attachment in a research context, for the most part, they have not been developed or widely used for clinical purposes. Clinically useful information regarding attachment relationships is perhaps best obtained through observation or interview regarding naturally occurring separations (e.g., parents leaving their infants at day care).

Social Interaction

A transactional model (Sameroff & Chandler, 1975) in which infant and caregiver inter-actions are viewed as dynamic, ongoing, and reciprocal offers a helpful framework for assessing the interactional patterns of infants and their parents. In conceptualizing the assessment of social interactions, it is helpful to consider the characteristics that individu-als involved in the ongoing transactions (parents, caregivers, infants) bring to the relation-ship, as well as a number of social and environmental factors (e.g., cultural expectations). Thus we recommend a three-step process when assessing social interactions that involves examining: (1) relevant caregiver characteristics; (2) relevant infant characteristics; and (3) the nature of the interactions themselves.

CAREGIVER CHARACTERISTICS

A long history of research has examined the maternal characteristics associated with parent–child interaction and its impact on child developmental outcome. Although a complete re-view of this literature is beyond the scope of this chapter, parent and caregiver characteristics that warrant consideration include: knowledge and attitudes (see, e.g., Miller, 1996; Osofsky & Connors, 1979), responsiveness to infant behaviors (see, e.g., Lewis & Goldberg, 1969; Pederson, 1990), depression and overall mental health (see, e.g., Lyons-Ruth, 1996), and stress related to parenting and social support (Hadadian & Merbler, 1996; Miyuki, 1992).

INFANT CHARACTERISTICS

Infants with or at risk for disabilities may have characteristics that can potentially inter-fere with their social interactions. For example, a number of cognitive skills—such as memory, object permanence, and imitation—are prerequisite for social interactions. De-velopmental delays often also manifest as social delays. For example, research suggests that infants with Down syndrome differ from typically developing infants in terms of both the timing and the quality of their social smiles. Further, infant behavioral characteristics such as irritability, responsivity, ability to maintain alert states, and so forth consistently have been demonstrated to influence parent–child interactions. Among typically developing infants, social abilities develop along a predictable continuum, beginning at or shortly after birth. Although rigid adherence to timelines tends to be counterproductive, an understanding of the order in which social behaviors generally appear may help parents know what to expect and encourage. Further, clinicians may gain insight into interactional patterns and potential problems if they determine that parents are concerned that their 6-month-old does not demonstrate the social behaviors they expect.

SOCIAL INTERACTIONS

In considering social interactions, reciprocity becomes a key concept. Several factors should be considered, including affective quality of the interaction, duration of the interaction, responsiveness of both partners, and whether one partner (either the parent or the infant) serves exclusively as the initiator of interactions. A number of observational techniques have been developed to evaluate parent–child interactions. Some observational systems, most often used in research settings, require a prescribed set of toys and a laboratory environment and are less likely to be clinically useful. Others (e.g., the Transdisciplinary Play-Based Assessment: Social Domain; Linder, 1986) are more flexible and can be adapted to a number of clinical settings.

CONCLUSION

Clearly, infant assessment presents a number of unique challenges. Because infancy is a period of rapid neurological development, evaluations during this period can, at best, provide clinicians and families with a "snapshot" of the infant's current development. The limited response repertoire of infants necessitates an assessment package that encompasses a number of developmental domains, including cognitive, motor, language, social, and emotional abilities. Additionally, although standardized formal assessment instruments can provide valuable information, a complete assessment calls for informal strategies as well. (See Table 9.4 for a list of instruments frequently used with infants.) Given these issues, in order to obtain a valid picture of an infant's overall abilities, clinicians will need to work with a team that includes the parents and represents a wide range of expertise.

REFERENCES

Ainsworth, M. D. S., Blehar, M. C., Waters, E., & Walls, S. (1978). *Patterns of attachment: A psychological study of the strange situation.* Hillsdale, NJ: Erlbaum.

Als, H., Lester, B., Tronick, B., & Brazelton, T. B. (1982). Toward a syntactive theory of development: Promise for the assessment and support of infant individuality. *Infant Mental Health Journal, 3,* 229–243.

American Cleft Palate–Craniofacial Association. (1993). *Parameters for evaluation and treatment of patients with cleft lip/palate or other craniofacial anomalies* [Brochure]. Pittsburgh: Author.

Austin, J. (1962). *How to do things with words.* Cambridge, MA: Harvard University Press.

Autti-Ramo, I., Korkman, M., Hilvakivi-Clarke, L., Lehtonen, M., Halmesmaki, E., & Granstrom, M. (1992). Mental development of 2-year-old children exposed to alcohol in utero. *Journal of Pediatrics, 120,* 740–746.

Aylward, G. P. (1992). The relationship between environmental risk and developmental outcome. *Journal of Developmental and Behavioral Pediatrics, 13,* 222–229.

TABLE 9.4. Selected Measures for Infant Assessment

Measure	Age range	Domains measured	Psychometric properties
Battelle Developmental Inventory (Newborg, Stock, & Wnek, 1988)	Birth to 8 years	Personal-Social, Adaptive, Motor, Communication, Cognitive	
Fagan Test of Infant Intelligence (Fagan & Shepherd, 1985)	3 and 7 months	Visual discrimination	
Kent Infant Development Scale (Katoff, Reuter, & Dunn, 1980)	Birth to 12 months	Cognitive, Language, Motor, Self-help, Social	Correlates well with Bayley
Denver Developmental Screening Test—II (Frankenburg & Dodds, 1990)	0–6 years	Cognitive, Motor, Language, Adaptive Behavior	Examiner–observer agreement .99 Test–retest reliability .90
Bayley Scales of Infant Development—II (Bayley, 1993)	1–42 months	Cognitive, Motor, Language, Behavior Rating Scale	
Bayley Infant Neurodevelopmental Screen (Aylward, 1992)	3–24 months	Neurological function, receptive functions, expressive functions, processing, mental activity	
Assessment of the Preterm Infant's Behavior (Als, Lester, Tronick, & Brazelton, 1982)	Preterm–44 weeks gestational age	Differentiation and modulation in physiological, motor, state, regulatory, attention–interaction subsystems	Interrater agreement .90 Can predict 9- and 18-month child outcomes

Instrument	Age range	Domains	Reliability/Validity
Neonatal Behavioral Assessment Scale (Brazelton, 1984)	37–44 weeks gestational age	Physiological, Motor, State Regulation and Organization, Habituation, Reflexes, Social Interaction	Interrater reliability above .90. Strong predictive validity between NBAS and Bayley at 18 months
Gesell Developmental Scales (Gesell & Amatruda, 1947)	Birth to 60 months	Adaptive Behavior, Gross and Fine Motor Behavior, Language, Personal–Social Behavior	
Infant Psychological Development Scales (Uzgiriz & Hunt, 1975)	Birth to 24 months	Piagetian-based scales: visual pursuit and permanence, means–ends, vocal imitations, gestural imitation, operational causality, object relations in space, schemes for relating to objects	Mean test–retest .80. Subscales significantly correlate with Binet scores and Bayley cognitive scores at 2 years
Home Observation for Measurement of the Environment for Infants and Toddlers (HOME; Caldwell & Bradley, 1978)	Birth to 36 months	Caregiver emotional and verbal responsivity, avoidance of restrictive punishment, organization of environment, provision of appropriate play materials, caregiver involvement with child, variety of daily stimulation	Internal consistency .89
Assessment, Evaluation, and Programming System for Infants and Children (Bricker, 1993)	Birth to 3 years	Fine and Gross Motor, Adaptive, Cognitive, Social-Communication, Social	

Aylward, G. P., Pfeiffer, S. I., Wright, A., & Verhulst, S. J. (1989). Outcome studies of low birth weight infants published in the last decade: A meta-analysis. *Journal of Pediatrics, 115*, 515–520.

Bagnato, S. J., & Neisworth, J. T. (1994). A national study of the social and treatment "invalidity" of intelligence testing for early intervention. *School Psychology Quarterly, 9*, 81–102.

Bandstra, E. S., & Burkett, G. (1991). Maternal-fetal and neonatal effects of in utero cocaine exposure. *Seminars in Perinatology, 15*(4), 288–301.

Bayley, N. (1993). *Bayley Scales of Infant Development (BSID-II)—Second Edition.* San Antonio, TX: Psychological Corporation.

Black, M., Schuler, M., & Nair, P. (1993). Prenatal drug exposure: Neurodevelopmental outcome and parenting environment. *Journal of Pediatric Psychology, 18*, 605–620.

Bowlby, J. (1969). *Attachment and loss: Volume 1. Attachment.* New York: Basic Books.

Brazelton, T. B. (1984). *Neonatal Behavioral Assessment Scale.* Philadelphia: Lippincott.

Bricker, D. (1993). *Assessment, Evaluation, and Programming System for infants and children: Volume 1. AEPS measurement for birth to three years.* Baltimore: Brookes.

Brouwers, P., Belman, A., & Epstein, L. (1994). Organ specific complications: Central nervous system involvement: Manifestations, evaluation, and pathogenesis. In P. A. Pizzo & C. M. Wilfert (Eds.), *Pediatric AIDS: The challenge of HIV infection in infants, children, and adolescents* (pp. 433–455). Baltimore: Williams & Wilkins.

Brown, R. (1973a). *A first language: The early stages.* Cambridge, MA: Harvard University Press.

Brown, R. (1973b). Some relationships between measures of early language development. *Journal of Speech and Hearing Disorders, 37*, 64–74.

Brown, W., Thurman, S. K., & Pearl, L. F. (1993). *Family-centered early intervention with infants and toddlers: Innovative cross-disciplinary approaches.* Baltimore: Brookes.

Bruininks, R. H., Woodcock, R. W., Weatherman, R. F., & Hill, B. K. (1996). *SIB-R: Scales of Independent Behavior—Revised.* Chicago: Riverside.

Burke, M. S., & Roth, D. (1993). Anonymous cocaine screening in a private obstetric population. *Obstetrics and Gynecology, 81*(3), 354–355.

Bzoch, K. R., & League, R. (1991). *Receptive-Expressive Emergent Language Test—Second Edition.* Austin, TX: Pro-Ed.

Caldwell, B., & Bradley, R. A. (1978). *Home Observation for Measurement of the Environment (HOME).* Little Rock: University of Arkansas.

Case-Smith, J., & Short Ridge, S. D. (1996). The developmental process, prenatal to adolescence. In J. Case-Smith, A. S. Allen, & P. N. Pratt (Eds.), *Occupational therapy for children* (3rd ed., pp. 46–60). St. Louis, MO: Mosby.

Centers for Disease Control. (1995). Update: Trends in fetal alcohol syndrome—United States, 1979–1993. *Morbidity and Mortality Weekly Report, 44*, 249–251.

Centers for Disease Control. (2000). *The HIV/AIDS Surveillance Report.* Atlanta, GA: U.S. Department of Health and Human Services.

Chapman, R. (1981). Exploring children's communicative intents. In J. Miller (Ed.), *Assessing language production in children* (pp. 111–138). Baltimore: University Park Press.

Charkins, H. (1996). *Children with facial difference: A parent's guide.* Bethesda, MD: Woodbine House.

Chasnoff, I. J., Burns, W. J., Schnoll, S. H., & Burns, K. A. (1985). Cocaine use in pregnancy. *New England Journal of Medicine, 313*(11), 666–669.

Chasnoff, I. J., Chisum, G. M., & Kaplan, W. E. (1988). Maternal cocaine use and genitourinary tract malformations. *Teratology, 37*, 201–204.

Chasnoff, I. J., Hunt, C. E., Kletter, R., & Kaplan, D. (1989). Prenatal cocaine exposure is associated with respiratory pattern abnormalities. *American Journal of Diseases in Childhood, 143*, 583–587.

Chasnoff, I. J., Landress, H. J., & Barrett, M. E. (1990). The prevalence of illicit-drug or alcohol use during pregnancy and discrepancies in mandatory reporting in Pinellas County, Florida. *New England Journal of Medicine, 322*, 1202–1206.

Chasnoff, I. J., Lewis, D. E., Griffith, D. R., & Willey, S. (1989). Cocaine and pregnancy: Clinical and toxicological implications for the neonate. *Clinical Chemistry, 35*(7), 1276–1278.

Cleft Palate Foundation. (1992). *Do you know fact sheet* [Brochure]. Chapel Hill, NC: Author.

Cohen, H. J., Papola, P., & Alvarez, M. (1994). Neurodevelopmental abnormalities in school-aged children with HIV-infection. *Journal of School Health, 64*, 11–13.

Cohen, S. E., Parmelee, A. H., Sigman, M., & Beckwith, L. (1988). Antecedents of school problems in children born preterm. *Journal of Pediatric Psychology, 13*, 493–508.

Coles, C. D., Platzman, K. A., Smith, I., & James, M. E. (1992). Effects of cocaine and alcohol use in pregnancy on neonatal growth and neurobehavioral status. *Neurotoxicology and Teratology, 14*, 23–33.

Connor, E. M., Sperling, R. S., Gelber, R., Kiselev, P., Scott, G., O'Sullivan, M. J., VanDyke, R., Bey, M., Shearer, W., Jacobson, R. L., Jimenez, E., O'Neill, E., Bazin, B., Delfraissy, J. F., Culnane, M., Coombs, R., Elkins, M., Moye, J., Stratton, P., & Balsley, J. (1994). Reduction of maternal-infant transmission of human immunodeficiency virus type 1 with zidovudine treatment. *New England Journal of Medicine, 331*, 1173–1180.

Coulter, D. L., & Chase, C. (1990). Neurological assessment of infants and young children with HIV infection. In P. B. Kozlowski, D. A. Snider, P. M. Vietze, & H. M. Wisniewski (Eds.), *Brain in pediatric AIDS* (pp. 80–90). New York: Karger.

Dominquez, R., Vila-Coro, A. A., Slopis, J. M., & Bohan, T. P. (1991). Brain and ocular abnormalities in infants with in utero exposure to cocaine and other street drugs. *American Journal of Diseases in Childhood, 145*, 688–695.

Dunst, C., Johanson, C., Trivette, C. M., & Hamby, D. (1991). Family-oriented early intervention policies and practices: Family-centered or not? *Exceptional Children, 58*, 115–126.

Dunst, C., Lowe, L., & Bartholomew, P. (1990). Contigent social responsiveness, family ecology and infant communicative competence. *National Students Speech, Language, and Hearing Association Journal, 17*, 39–49.

Easterbrooks, S. R. (1998). Communication. In W. Umansky & S. R. Hooper (Eds.), *Young children with special needs* (3rd ed., pp. 230–275). Upper Saddle River, NJ: Merrill.

Edmondson, R., & Reinhartsen, D. (1998). The young child with cleft lip and palate: Intervention needs in the first three years. *Infants and Young Children, 11*, 12–20.

El Deeb, M., Waite, D. E., & Curran, J. (1993). Oral-maxillofacial Surgery and the management of cleft lip and palate. In K. T. Moller & C. D. Starr (Eds.), *Cleft palate: Interdisciplinary issues and treatment* (pp. 79–120). Austin, TX: Pro-Ed.

Fagan, J., & Shepherd, P. A. (1985). *The Fagan Test of Infant Intelligence.* Cleveland, OH: Infantest Corporation.

Fenson, L., Dale, P. S., Reznick, S., Thal, D., Bates, E., Hartung, J. P., Pethick, S., & Reilly, J. S. (1991). *Technical manual for the MacArthur Communicative Development Inventories.* San Diego, CA: San Diego State University Press.

Flanagan, D. P., & Genshaft, J. L. (1997). Issues in the use and interpretation of intelligence tests in the schools. *School Psychology Review, 26*, 146–149.

Ford, L. M., Han, B. K., Steichen, J., Babcock, D., & Fogelson, H. (1988). Very low birth weight, preterm infants with or without intracranial hemorrhage. *Clinical Pediatrics, 28*, 302–310.

Frankenburg, W. K., & Dodds, J. B. (1990). *Denver II Screening Manual.* Denver, CO: Denver Developmental Materials.

Friedland, G., & Klein, R. (1987). Transmission of the human immunodeficiency virus. *New England Journal of Medicine, 317*, 1125–1135.

Gerken, K. C., Eliason, M. J., & Arthur, C. R. (1994). The assessment of at-risk infants and toddlers with the Bayley Mental Scale and the Battelle Developmental Inventory: Beyond the data. *Psychology in the Schools, 31*, 181–187.

Gesell, A. L., & Armatruda, C. S. (1947). *Developmental diagnosis; normal and abnormal child development: Clinical methods and pediatric applications* (2nd ed.; Rev. ed.). Hagerstown, MD: Harper & Row.

Goddard-Finegold, J., & Mizrah, E. (1987). Understanding and preventing perinatal, intracerebral, peri- and intraventricular hemorrhage. *Journal of Child Neurology, 2*, 170–185.

Goldberg, S. (1990). Attachment in infants at risk: Theory, research, and practice. *Infants and Young Children, 2*, 11–20.

Gustavsson, N. S. (1992). Drug exposed infants and their mothers: Facts, myths, and needs. *Social Work in Health Care, 16*, 87–100.

Hack, M., Klein, N. K., & Taylor, H. G. (1995). Long-term developmental outcomes of low birthweight infants. *Future of Children, 5*, 176–196.

Hadadian, A., & Merbler, J. (1996). Mothers' stress: Implications for attachment relationships. *Early Child Development and Care, 125*, 59–66.

Hanson, M. J. (1996). *Atypical infant development* (2nd ed.). Austin, TX: Pro-Ed.

Hooper, S. R., & Edmondson, R. (1998). Developmental stages and factors affecting development. In W. Umansky & S. R. Hooper (Eds.), *Young children with special needs* (pp. 340–371). Upper Saddle River, NJ: Merrill.

Hume, R. F., O'Donnell, K. J., Stanger, C. L., Killam, A. P., & Gingras, J. L. (1989). In utero cocaine exposure: Observations of fetal behavioral state may predict neonatal outcome. *American Journal of Obstetric Gynecology, 3,* 685–690.

Hynd, G. W., & Semrud-Clikeman, M. (1993). Developmental considerations in cognitive assessment of young children. In J. L. Culbertson & D. J. Willis (Eds.), *Testing young children: A reference guide for developmental, psychoeducational, and psychosocial assessments* (pp. 11–28). Austin, TX: Pro-Ed.

Jones, K. L., & Smith, D. W. (1973). Recognition of fetal alcohol syndrome in early infancy. *Lancet, 2,* 999–1001.

Katoff, L. S., Reuter, J., & Dunn, V. (1980). *The Kent Infant Development Scale manual.* Kent, OH: Kent Developmental Metrics.

Kaye, K., Elkind, L., Goldberg, D., & Tytun, A. (1989). Birth outcomes for infants of drug abusing mothers. *New York State Journal of Medicine, 89,* 256–261.

Klaus, M. H., & Kennell, J. H. (Eds.). (1976). *Maternal-infant bonding: The impact of early separation or loss on family development.* St. Louis, MO: Mosby.

Kozma, C. (1986). What is Down syndrome? In K. Stray-Gundersen (Ed.), *Babies with Down syndrome: A new parent's guide* (pp. 1–25). Rockville, MD: Woodbine House.

Langone, J. (1998). Teaching self-help skills. In W. Umansky & S. R. Hooper (Eds.), *Young children with special needs* (3rd ed., pp. 156–187). Upper Saddle River, NJ: Merrill.

Legido, A., Clancy, R. R., Spitzer, A. R., & Finnegan, L. P. (1992). Electroencephalographic and behavioral state studies in infants of cocaine-addicted mothers. *American Journal of Diseases in Childhood, 146,* 748–752.

Lewis, M., & Goldberg, S. (1969). Perceptual-cognitive development in infancy: A generalized expectancy model as a function of the mother–infant interaction. *Merrill-Palmer Quarterly, 15,* 81–100.

Linder, T. (1990). *Transdisciplinary Play-based Assessment: A functional approach to working with young children.* Baltimore: Brookes.

Little, B. B., & Snell, L. M. (1991). Brain growth among fetuses exposed to cocaine in utero: Asymmetrical growth retardation. *Obstetrics and Gynecology, 77*(3), 361–364.

Lyons-Ruth, K. (1996). Attachment relationships among children with aggressive behavior problems: The role of disorganized early attachment relationships. *Journal of Consulting and Clinical Psychology, 64,* 64–73.

MacDonald, M. (1992). Vertical transmission of HIV: Management of the pregnant mother and her infant. In M. L. Stuber (Ed.), *Children and AIDS* (pp. 3–19). Washington, DC: American Psychiatric Press.

Mastrogiannis, D. S., Decavalas, G. O., Verma, U., & Tejani, N. (1990). Perinatal outcome after recent cocaine usage. *Obstetrics and Gynecology, 76,* 8–11.

McCalla, S. Minkoff, H. L., Feldman, J., Delke, I., Salwin, M., Valencia, G., & Glass, L. (1991). The biologic and social consequences of perinatal cocaine use in an inner-city population: Results of an anonymous cross-sectional study. *American Journal of Obstetrics and Gynecology, 164,* 625–630.

Meisels, S. J., Plunkett, J. W., Pasick, P. L., Stiefel, G. S., & Roloff, D. W. (1987). Effects of severity and chronicity of respiratory illness on the cognitive decelopment of preterm infants. *Journal of Pediatric Psychology, 12,* 117–132.

Meyers, A. (1994). Natural history of congenital HIV infection. *Journal of School Health, 64,* 9–10.

Miller, C. L. (1996). Cognitive readiness to parent and intellectual-emotional development in children of adolescent mothers. *Developmental Psychology, 32,* 533–541.

Miller, J. (1981). *Assessing language production in children: Experimental procedures.* Baltimore: University Park Press.

Miyuki, N. (1992). An ecological study of child-mother attachments among Japanese sojourners in the United States. *Developmental Psychology, 28,* 584–592.

Mullen, E. M. (1989). *Mullen Scales of Early Learning.* Circle Pines, MN: American Guidance Service.

Neerhof, M. G., MacGregor, S. N., Retzky, S. S., & Sullivan, T. P. (1989). Cocaine abuse during pregnancy: Peripartum prevalence and perinatal outcome. *American Journal of Obstetrics and Gynecology, 161,* 633–638.

Neiman, G. S., & Savage, H. E. (1997). Development of infants and toddlers with clefts from birth to three years of age. *Cleft Palate–Craniofacial Journal, 34,* 218–225.

Newborg, J., Stock, J. R., & Wnek, L. (1988). *The Battelle Developmental Inventory.* Allen, TX: DLM.

Oro, A. S., & Dixon, S. D. (1987). Perinatal cocaine and methamphetamine exposure: Maternal and neonatal correlates. *Journal of Pediatrics, 111,* 571–578.

Osofsky, J. D., & Connors, K. (1979). Mother-infant interaction: An integrative view of a complex system. In J. D. Osofsky (Ed.), *Handbook of infant development* (pp. 519–548). New York: Wiley.

Paneth, N. S. (1995). The problem of low birth weight. *Future of Children, 5,* 19–34.

Patz, J. A., & Dennis, B. W. (1998). Sensory motor development. In W. Umansky & S. R. Hooper (Eds.), *Young children with special needs* (3rd ed., pp. 94–155). Upper Saddle River, NJ: Merrill.

Pederson, D. R. (1990). Maternal sensitivity and the security of infant-mother attachment: A Q-sort study. *Child Development, 61,* 1974–1983.

Phibbs, C. S., Bateman, D. A., & Schwartz, R. M. (1991). The neonatal costs of maternal cocaine use. *Journal of the American Medical Association, 266*(11), 1521–1526.

Platzman, K., Coles, C., & Raskind-Hind, C. (1992, May). *State organization in neonates prenatally exposed to cocaine.* Paper presented at the meeting of the International Conference on Infant Studies, Miami, FL.

Reece, E. A., Hobbins, J. C., Mahoney, M. J., & Petrie, R. H. (1995). *Handbook of medicine of the fetus and the mother.* Philadelphia: Lippincott.

Richman, L. C., & Eliason, M. J. (1993). Psychological characteristics associated with cleft palate. In K. T. Moller & C. D. Starr (Eds.), *Cleft palate: Interdisciplinary issues and treatment* (pp. 357–380). Austin, TX: Pro-Ed.

Roberts, J. E., & Crais, E. (1989). Assessing communication skills. In D. B. Bailey & M. Wolery (Eds.), *Assessing infants and preschoolers with handicaps* (pp. 339–389). Columbus, OH: Merrill.

Rodriguez, E. M., Diaz, C., & Fowler, M. G. (1997). The clinical management of children perinatally exposed to HIV. *Primary Care, 24,* 643–666.

Roizen, N. J. (1997). New advances in medical treatment of young children with Down syndrome: Implications for early intervention. *Infants and Young Children, 9,* 36–42.

Roizen, N. J., Mets, M. B., & Blondis, T. A. (1994). Ophthalmic disorders in children with Down syndrome. *Developmental Medicine and Child Neurology, 36,* 594–600.

Roizen, N. J., Wolters, C., Nicol, T., & Blondis, T. A. (1993). Hearing loss in children with Down syndrome. *Journal of Pediatrics, 123*(1), S9–S12.

Rollnick, B. R., & Pruzansky, S. (1981). Genetic services at a center for craniofacial anomalies. *Cleft Palate Journal, 18,* 304–313.

Rosenak, D., Diamant, Y. Z., Yaffe, H., & Hornstein, E. (1990). Cocaine: Maternal use during pregnancy and its effect on the mother, the fetus, and the infant. *Obstetrical and Gynecological Survey, 45*(6), 348–359.

Ross, G., Liper, E., & Auld, P. (1985). Consistency and change in the development of premature infants weighing less than 1501 grams at birth. *Pediatrics, 76,* 885–886.

Rossetti, L. (1990). *The Rossetti Infant–Toddler Language Scale: A measure of communication and interaction.* East Moline, IL: LinguiSystems.

Salamy, A., Eldredge, L., Anderson, J., & Bull, D. (1990). Clinical and laboratory observations: Brainstem transmission time in infants exposed to cocaine in utero. *Journal of Pediatrics, 117*(4), 627–629.

Sameroff, A. J., & Chandler, M. J. (1975). Clinical and laboratory caretaking casualty. In F. D. Horowitz, M. Hetherington, S. Scarr-Salapatek, & G. Siegel (Eds.), *Review of child development research* (Vol. 4, pp. 187–244). Chicago: University of Chicago Press.

Sanders-Phillips, K. (1992, May). *Sucking behavior in infants prenatally exposed to cocaine.* Paper presented at the International Conference on Infant Studies, Miami, FL.

Saylor, C., Lippa, B., & Lee, G. (1991). Drug-exposed infants at home: Strategies and supports. *Public Health Nursing, 8*(1), 33–38.

Schneider, J. W., & Chasnoff, I. J. (1992). Motor assessment of cocaine/polydrug exposed infants at age four months. *Neurotoxicology and Teratology, 14,* 97–101.

Seidel, J. F. (1992, May). *Pediatric HIV infection and developmental disabilities.* Paper presented at the meeting of the American Association on Mental Retardation, New Orleans, LA.

Sicklick, M. J., & Rubenstein, A. (1992). Types of HIV infection and the course of the disease. In A. C. Crocker, H. J. Cohen, & T. A. Kastner (Eds.), *HIV infection and developmental disabilites: A resource for service providers* (pp. 33–42). Baltimore: Brookes.

Singer, L. T., Garber, R., & Kliegman, R. (1991). Neurobehavioral sequelaeof fetal cocaine exposure. *Journal of Pediatrics, 119*(4), 667–672.

Smith, L., Ulvund, S. E., & Lindemann, R. (1994). Very low birth weight infants at double risk. *Developmental and Behavioral Pediatrics, 15*, 7–13.

Smith, P. D. (1989). Assessing motor skills. In D. B. Bailey & M. Wolery (Eds.), *Assessing infants and preschoolers with handicaps* (pp. 301–338). Columbus, OH: Merrill.

Sostek, A. M., Smith, Y. F., Katz, K. S., & Grant, E. G. (1987). Developmental outcome of preterm infants with intraventricular hemorrhage at one and two years of age. *Child Development, 58*, 779–786.

Sparrow, S. S., Balla, D. A., & Cicchetti, D. V. (1984). *Vineland Adaptive Behavior Scales.* Circle Pines, MN: American Guidance Service.

Sprintzen, R. S., Siegel-Sadewitz, V. L., Amato, J., & Goldberg, R. B. (1998). Anomalies associated with cleft lip, cleft palate, or both. *American Journal of Medical Genetics, 20*, 585–595.

Thompson, L. A., Fagan, J. F., & Fulker, D. W. (1991). Longitudinal prediction of specific cognitive abilities from infant novelty preference. *Child Development, 62*, 530–538.

Trad, P. V., Kentros, M., Solomon, G. E., & Greenblatt, E. R. (1994). Assessment of psychotherapeutic intervention for an HIV-infected preschool child. *Journal of the American Academy of Child and Adolescent Psychiatry, 33*, 1338–1345.

Trawick-Smith, J. (1997). *Early child development: A multicultural perspective.* Columbus, OH: Merrill.

Tudehope, D. I. (1989). Perinatal cocaine intoxication: A precaution. *Medical Journal of Australia, 150*, 290–291.

Ulvestad, R. S., & Carlstrom, J. E. (1993). Otologic and audiologic concerns and treatments. In K. T. Moller & C. D. Starr (Eds.), *Cleft palate: Interdisciplinary issues and treatment.* Austin, TX: Pro-Ed.

Uzgiris, I. C., & Hunt, J. M. (1975). *Assessment in infancy: Ordinal scales of psychological development.* Chicago: University of Illinois Press.

Wetherby, A. M., Cain, D. H., Yonclas, D. G., & Walker, V. G. (1988). Analysis of intentional communication of normal children from the prelinguistic to the multiword stage. *Journal of Speech and Hearing Research, 31*, 240–252.

Wetherby, A. M., & Prizant, B. M. (1993). *Communication and Symbolic Behavior Scales.* Chicago: Riverside.

Weislaus-Kuperus, N., Baerts, W., Fetter, W. P. F., & Sauer, P. J. J. (1992). Neonatal cerebral ultrasound, neonatal neurology and perinatal conditions as predictors of neurodevelopmental outcome in very low birth weight infants. *Early Human Development, 31*, 131–148.

Wilcox, J. (1992). Enhancing initial communication skills in young children with development disabilities through partner programming. *Seminars in Speech and Language, 13*, 194–212.

Wolery, M. (1989). Assessing play skills. In D. B. Bailey & M. Wolery (Eds.), *Assessment of infants and preschoolers with handicaps* (pp. 428–446). Columbus, OH: Merrill.

Wolters, P. L., Brouwers, P., & Moss, H. A. (1995). Pediatric HIV disease: Effect on cognition, learning, and behavior. *School Psychology Quarterly, 10*, 305–328.

Zimmerman, I. L., Steiner, V. G., & Pond, R. E. (1992) *Preschool Language Scale—3.* San Antonio, TX: Psychological Corporation.

10

ASSESSMENT OF CHILDREN WITH MOTOR IMPAIRMENTS

MELISSA R. JOHNSON
CYNTHIA WILHELM
DEBORAH EISERT
DEBORAH L. HALPERIN-PHILLIPS

Hannah was born 8 weeks early, by cesarean delivery, after a prenatal diagnosis of hydrocephalus. This condition results from poor functioning of the drainage system in the ventricles of the brain, leading to an accumulation of fluid in the ventricles. During her first 2 years of life, she experienced 11 surgical procedures to try to relieve the pressure on her brain created by the excess fluid. She exhibited recurrent seizures, as well as motor delays. At around her 1st birthday, her parents were told that Hannah had cerebral palsy as a result of damage to her brain from the hydrocephalus and its complications, and she began to receive physical therapy in addition to the early childhood intervention services. Hannah was assessed with the Bayley Scales of Infant Development—Second Edition several times before she turned 3, and she received scores in the low average and borderline range. Now she is 6 years old and getting ready to move from an inclusive preschool program to a public school classroom. She is very verbal and walks independently with braces on her ankles and a noticeably abnormal gait. What questions must the psychologist address in preparing to do her evaluation so that all of her needs are met? What information, and which other professionals, might be helpful or essential?

The term "motor impairment" refers to conditions that restrict or interfere with normal functioning of the motor or musculoskeletal system. The psychologist evaluating a child with a motor impairment must ask two key questions:

1. How can I best determine this child's current functioning and future potential in the areas of cognitive, communicative, emotional and adaptive functioning, given the interference presented by his or her motor challenge?
2. What issues are likely to be particularly salient, given the neurodevelopmental and emotional implications of the child's particular disorder, as well as his or her developmental stage?

These tasks are assisted by an understanding of the most common conditions leading to specific disabilities. These conditions include cerebral palsy (also called static encephalopathy), neural tube defects, neuromuscular diseases, congenital limb anomalies, rheumatoid diseases, and diverse forms of injury to the head, spinal column, or limbs. These and other less common conditions clearly share little medically beyond the fact that they affect motor functioning. The degree of motor impairment can range from mild weakness in one limb to a total lack of motor control accompanied by complete dependence in daily care; however, it is reasonable to consider this heterogeneous group together when discussing psychological assessment because of the similarities in the questions that the assessor must consider.

The assessment of children with motor impairments shares a number of common objectives with assessment of other children. Generally, the purpose of assessment is to provide children, parents, educators, and other professionals with information to assist them in making decisions that will enhance the child's educational and emotional development. There are at least five objectives for evaluation of the motor-impaired child that are common to all children: screening, placement, program planning, program evaluation, and assessment of individual progress. Most of the domains of assessment are also not unique to the child with a motor impairment. For example, assessment of intelligence and related psychoeducational abilities is important for all children. Medical caregivers of children with motor impairments frequently use intellectual assessment as part of planning short- and long-term medical care and independence goals, because the ability to participate in self-care and to use intellectual strengths to compensate for motor challenges can be key variables in planning for a child's future. Teachers and parents use this information to form appropriate expectations concerning the child's development and to plan educational programs. The assessment of a child with a motor impairment must also incorporate measures of communication skills, perceptual–motor skills, adaptive behavior, and psychosocial adjustment. The examiner should address each of these five areas while assessing a child with a motor impairment. Issues related to communication, perceptual–motor, and adaptive domains are briefly considered below. Cognitive issues, because of their central importance for the psychologist, are considered in more detail in the discussion of some of the most common causes of motor impairment in children. Finally, the complex issue of social-emotional functioning is considered after this discussion, in light of the broad concerns inherent in each of the disorders affecting children's motor functioning.

COMMUNICATION

The study of communication in the child with a motor impairment has burgeoned in the last few years to become a discipline in its own right. Speech therapists and other professionals have taken advantage of computer technology to develop augmentative communication systems for individuals with a variety of disabilities. Assessment for augmentative communication is complex, particularly because of the fast growth of the field, the need to keep up with advances in technology, and the opportunities it provides for the individual (Beigel, 2000). The psychologist's role in these evaluations is almost always as part of a multidisciplinary team in which all members work together using computer and other technologies to facilitate the child's ability to express his or her understanding of the world. Receptive language, of course, may be far less affected than expressive language, and finding ways for the child to indicate what he or she understands can be the key that unlocks the team's understanding of the child's potential.

Tiffany suffered an anoxic (oxygen deprivation) injury at birth. She was thought to be profoundly disabled and placed in a residential facility for infants. Her diagnosis was severe athetoid cerebral palsy. When she was 18 months old, a caregiver was "reading" her a Richard Scarry book and noticed that Tiffany was moving her eyes consistently toward the correct picture whenever a particular item was named. This observation led to a detailed assessment and a complete change in her life circumstances, including a return to her own home and intensive intervention. With the help of a communication board and head-pointing device, she attended school with typically developing children, accompanied by an aide. Tiffany graduated from college last month, after using her power wheelchair and laptop computer to work her way through her studies, two courses at a time.

PERCEPTUAL–MOTOR SKILLS

The perceptual–motor development of a child with a motor impairment may vary from that of typically developing children, both because of brain injury and because the child may have very different sensory-motor experiences.

Assessment of perceptual–motor skills, often in collaboration with an occupational therapist, can help to clarify how the child processes information. The challenge for the evaluator is to determine whether the difficulty is one of the output (motor) or input (perceptual) process (Palmer, 1970; Stellern, Vasa, & Little, 1976). This differentiation is not simple in a typically developing child, but in children with motor impairments, it is even more complex. Sattler (1982) has related perceptual–motor difficulties in children with motor impairments to (1) misperception, (2) execution difficulties, and (3) integrative or central processing difficulties. Although assessment of performance in the perceptual–motor area is probably the most challenging, it remains one of the most important domains to document in children with motor impairments.

ADAPTIVE BEHAVIOR

The definition of adaptive behavior usually includes the degree of independent functioning in self-care and daily living that the child can accomplish and his or her ability to engage in social relationships. It is a more recent concept than IQ but has become increasingly important as those working with people who have disabilities have focused on competent function in a broader range of arenas than just the academic. Unfortunately, most standardized assessments of adaptive behavior have been normed on children whose primary disability is cognitive rather than motor, making the scores difficult to interpret and potentially quite inappropriate for children with motor impairments. An alternate approach is to address this important area by teaming with an occupational therapist with whom the psychologist can collaboratively describe the child's strengths and needs in the areas of self-care and other aspects of independent personal and social functioning within the framework of existing motor limitations. This kind of analysis can approach one of the most important questions: whether the child is currently functioning at his or her highest potential, given his or her medical condition, in nonacademic as well as academic spheres. Although closely related to the questions of adaptive behavior, the emotional and social implications of the various motor disorders have their own literature and are considered together later in the chapter.

OVERVIEW OF CONDITIONS CAUSING MOTOR IMPAIRMENTS IN CHILDREN AND THEIR CONSEQUENCES

To set the stage for considering these issues, we briefly review the nature and characteristics of the most prevalent motor impairments that occur in childhood and describe the features that are most likely to concern the psychological assessor. No attempt will be made to review the vast literature on physical impairment.

Cerebral Palsy

Medical Issues

Authors defining cerebral palsy (CP), or static encephalopathy, tend to be cautious in their definitions, no doubt because of the complex and multifaceted nature of the disorder. For example, Pelligrino and Dormans (1998) state that "regardless of the specific cause, or *etiology*, all people with cerebral palsy have a significant problem with controlling *movement* and *posture*" (p. 6), while emphasizing the nonprogressive nature and variable expression of the condition. Because damage to the brain itself is at the root of the problem, many children with CP also have difficulties in sensory and cognitive functions. This definition implies that the assessor must be concerned not only with the consequences of motor impairment for the assessment but also with the concomitants of brain damage, such as attention and perceptual deficits. In addition, there are often emotional consequences of facing ongoing challenges and feeling different from other children; these are discussed in the context of all of the motor disorders later in this chapter.

Many factors can cause cerebral palsy, but most involve an insult to the brain early in life, interfering with normal developmental progress. Most writers consider both *prenatal causes,* such as intrauterine infection, genetic malformation, toxins, metabolic diseases, hemorrhages, or physical trauma; *perinatal causes,* such as oxygen deprivation during the birth process; and *postnatal causes,* including traumatic injuries and infections such as meningitis. For children born prematurely and weighing less than 1,000 grams, the incidence of cerebral palsy has recently been reported to be about 7%, with the earlier-born infants having the greatest chance of motor disability (Finnstrom et al., 1998). These considerations are important to the assessor, because the evaluation of a child who experienced brain damage pre- or perinatally presents a different set of questions from the child who has developed normally prior to experiencing a traumatic insult or acquiring a disability.

The term "cerebral palsy" refers to several forms of movement disorder, which can range from very mild to severe. Although a complete description of all the subtypes of cerebral palsy is beyond the scope of this chapter, the assessor should be aware of the most common terms and should also understand that different authors may use differing classification schemes and labels. Spasticity, the most common type, refers to disharmony of muscle movement accompanied by abnormal reflexes, tight muscles, and jerky motor movements. Dyskinetic, athetoid, ataxic, and mixed types are also described (Pellegrino & Dormans, 1998) and the type depends on the particular motor patterns and also the location of the brain lesion.

Cerebral palsy is also classified according to the sites of neuromotor impairment. Children who are affected on one side of the body are referred to as having hemiplegia. In diplegia, all four extremities are involved, but the arms are significantly less impaired than the legs. Quadriplegia is the type that affects all four limbs, and paraplegia involves only the legs. Direct collaboration with a knowledgeable pediatric physical therapist is the best way to develop a sense of what these items refer to and how a particular child is likely to be affected.

The child with cerebral palsy probably presents more issues for the assessor than do children with other forms of motor impairment because problems such as poor coordination and abnormal muscle tone make it difficult for the child to respond to timed tests in a meaningful way and interfere with their manipulation of materials. Prior to beginning the assessment, the evaluator must ascertain how the child's mobility, manipulative skills, oral–motor functioning, and trunk and head control are affected and plan the assessment to compensate for or adapt to these needs.

Intellectual and Developmental Issues

The difficulties confronted by a child with cerebral palsy are not limited to motor function. They are also at risk for sensory and perceptual dysfunction, seizures, cognitive deficits, and primary or secondary difficulties in the areas of behavior, learning, and emotion.

Estimates of intellectual functioning and the prevalence of mental retardation in individuals with cerebral palsy vary widely based on the population studied and measures used, but based on a literature review, Molnar (1992) estimates that about 50% of children with cerebral palsy also have mental retardation, with about half of those individuals functioning in the severe to profound range. On the other hand, the range of intellect includes not only normal but also superior functioning. The issue is both sensitive and important, because the individual with cerebral palsy may be unjustifiably stereotyped as retarded based on unusual appearance, gait, or speech. Each child should be approached without preconceptions regarding intelligence, because there are many cases of individuals with severe motor and language impairments and normal intelligence. Clearly, the ability to identify a child's level of intellectual functioning despite substantial physical impairment is one of the most challenging and important functions of the psychologist.

In addition to the risk of lowered intelligence, children with cerebral palsy have a high incidence of visual–perceptual and visual–motor problems (Cruickshank, 1976) and may require services for learning disabilities. Depending on the degree of oral–motor dysfunction, speech may be mildly or significantly affected (Solot, 1998), requiring collaboration with a speech–language pathologist to ensure that intelligibility is sufficient for traditional assessment or that alternative communication strategies or assessment approaches are available. Sensory deficits, both visual and auditory, are more common in children with cerebral palsy (Pellegrino & Dormans, 1998) and should be considered in planning assessments.

Neural Tube Defects

Medical Issues

The broad term "neural tube defect" refers to several related conditions involving a failure in development of the structures of the spinal column early in gestation (Baron, Fennell, & Voeller, 1995). The most common neural tube defect is called "spina bifida cystica," or one of two interchangeable terms, "myelomeningocele" and "meningomyelocele." In this condition the incomplete closure of the spinal cord results in a lesion on the back containing exposed elements of neural tissue, evident at birth. A saclike mass covered by skin and containing meninges may protrude at the site of the spina bifida and is called a "meningocele." If the mass contains neural elements of spinal cord, it is called a "myelomeningocele." Although the lesion itself can be surgically closed, the child is invariably left with some degree of neurological impairment (Menkes & Till, 1995). Physicians specify the level at which the lesion begins to affect functioning by identifying the point on the spine below which the nerves are affected. The higher the lesion, the more severe the child's deficits will be. The level of lesion may affect the child's bladder and bowel control, ambulation, sensation, and eventual sexual functioning (Shaer, 1997).

In addition to the medical problems associated with the level of lesion, hydrocephalus affects the majority of children with this diagnosis. Hydrocephalus refers to an enlargement of the ventricles, and potentially of the head, caused by abnormal accumulation of cerebrospinal fluid. It occurs when there is a blockage in the normal pathway by which cerebrospinal fluid moves and is absorbed. Neurosurgeons treat this condition by implanting a small tube, known as a shunt, which drains fluid from the ventricles to the other parts of the body to reduce intracranial pressure and prevent the displacement of the brain within the skull.

Intellectual and Developmental Issues

Children with spina bifida as a group often function in the low normal range of intelligence but display a range of abilities from developmentally disabled to well above average (Friedrich, Lovejoy, Shaffer, Shurtleff, & Beilke, 1991; Wills, Holmbeck, Dillon, & McLone, 1990). The picture for each individual child is complex because eventual cognitive function is affected by medical complications as well as by the treatment options chosen; in addition, the incidence of a variety of learning disabilities (Barnes & Dennis, 1992; Dise & Lohr, 1998) is high. It is clear that children who have spina bifida with hydrocephalus are at increased risk of lower IQs and poorer perceptual–motor functioning compared with those without hydrocephalus (Donders, Rourke, & Canady, 1991; Soare & Raimondi, 1977).

Hydrocephalus is also associated with a number of other difficulties. Behavior, attention, concentration, and perseverance may be affected (Fletcher et al., 1995; Hagberg, 1962). Some children with hydrocephalus appear quite fluent verbally, but on closer examination they are found to have significant deficits in "pragmatic use and understanding of language in discourse" (Dennis & Barnes, 1993, p. 639). These deficits, sometimes called "cocktail party syndrome," can have a significant impact on both academic and social functioning (Byrne, Abbeduto, & Brooks, 1990). Thus the assessor approaching a child with spina bifida needs to maintain a high degree of suspicion of both verbal and perceptual difficulties even in a child who appears to be communicating easily and fluently (Fletcher et al., 1992). Additionally, the child with shunted hydrocephalus may suffer developmental setbacks related to shunt malfunction and needs close follow-up neurodevelopmentally, as well as medically.

Muscular Dystrophy

Medical Issues

Muscular dystrophies involve clinical symptoms of muscle weakness and are differentiated by age of onset, muscle groups involved, progressiveness of muscle degeneration, and genetic factors. Duchenne, or pseudohypertrophic, muscular dystrophy (DMD) is the most common form, although there are a number of other forms of related neuromuscular diseases (Menkes, 1995). In DMD, muscle weakness often appears in the first few years of life, along with related muscular, skeletal, and gait changes that follow a characteristic pattern as the child develops and the muscle weakness progresses. A detailed description of the diagnosis and progression of DMD may be found in Brook (1977). Key issues for the psychological evaluator are the progression of weakness, which eventually affects the child's ability to manipulate objects, and progressive compromise of respiratory status, accelerated in many cases by scoliosis, which can affect endurance and energy levels and interfere with daily function.

Terminal stages of DMD occur in adolescence or young adulthood. Muscle movement becomes negligible, resulting in increasingly poor pulmonary functioning. Most patients eventually die of pneumonia or cardiac failure, some after a period of mechanical ventilation.

Intellectual and Developmental Issues

Reports of decreased intellectual functioning in individuals with DMD as compared with the general population have been noted in the medical literature since the earliest clinical description of the disease by Duchenne in 1886 (Prosser, Murphy, & Thompson, 1969). Various publications prior to 1960 published mixed reports of intellectual functioning in individuals with DMD (Morrow & Cohen, 1954; Truitt, 1955; Zellweger, 1946). More recent research, comparing the cognitive functioning and reading skills of children with DMD to those of children with spinal muscular atrophy, has documented a clear pattern of increased incidence of learning disabilities and in particular, specific reading disabilities (Billard et al., 1992; Billard, Gillet, Barthez, Hommet, & Bertrand, 1998). These data indicate that every child with DMD should receive psychoeducational evaluations as part of routine care.

Regardless of the etiology or psychometric evidence of cognitive difficulties, students with DMD often encounter multiple obstacles in academic development. Hall and Porter (1980) presented case studies that exemplify an array of potential difficulties in school settings. Factors within a school system have in the past added to the difficulties faced by some children with DMD. Misdiagnosis and inadequate information regarding a child's disease, inappropriate academic evaluation, and lack of appropriate placement may critically affect a child's progress in school. Once appropriate educational opportunities are provided, emotional, social, and medical aspects of the disease can be more effectively dealt with.

By adolescence, cognitive abilities are one factor an individual with DMD has to rely on. Constant adaptation to rapid muscle degeneration is the issue at this stage. As adolescents compete with one another and strive to test and prove their abilities, academic performance in school becomes of paramount importance to those who are unable to perform physically like their peers.

Connective Tissue Disease

Medical Issues

Arthritic diseases, involving swelling and inflammation of the joints or connective tissue, include juvenile rheumatoid arthritis (JRA), scleroderma, systemic lupus erythematosus, and ankylosing spondylitis. JRA, the most common of these conditions, is an important cause of motoric limitations in children.

About 1 in 1,000 children will develop arthritis. Most children with JRA have an excellent prognosis, and, with proper therapy, 80% will grow up without deformity and without arthritis in adult life. Children with JRA usually develop a fever and rash and can fatigue easily when the disease is active. The severity and course of JRA vary greatly from child to child. Three varieties have been identified (Gregg, 1971). These types, labeled "acute onset," "polyarticular" or "adult onset," and "monoarticular," vary according to how they first reveal themselves and how the joints are later affected. The results can range from relatively mild inflammatory symptoms and stiffness that pass fairly quickly to complete joint destruction and severe crippling, accompanied by significant amounts of pain. Some children with JRA suffer from an inflammation inside the eye called chronic iridocyclitis, which can damage vision.

Another important issue in this class of illness is its often erratic and unpredictable course. JRA often waxes and wanes, and except for children who have suffered irreversible joint damage, there is always hope that a particular episode of joint inflammation will relent either under treatment or spontaneously. Although some children have only a brief episode, most children have an "up and down" course for 3 to 10 years or longer. The longer the disease remains active, the greater the risk of joint damage. Treatment usually entails physical therapy and drug therapy. Nonsteroidal anti-inflammatory drugs are most commonly prescribed for JRA; however, other, stronger drugs may be necessary in more severe cases (Cassidy & Petty, 1995).

Because of the unpredictability associated with JRA, the task of coping emotionally and in practical terms is complicated for children and their caretakers. Children's abilities and limitations may vary greatly from time to time. For example, a child who is having a severe flare-up of wrist and hand inflammation may be completely unable to carry out the performance tasks on the Wechsler Intelligence Scale for Children (WISC-III; Wechsler, 1991) and may require alternative techniques but may regain his or her full abilities later on. Also, a child who had been unable to use his or her hands might regain these abilities but be reluctant to use them because of fear of recurrent pain. Because the child's anxiety may be a difficult factor to identify, close collaboration with the physicians and physical therapists who are most familiar with the child is important.

Intellectual and Developmental Issues

Several issues are important in evaluating children with connective tissue diseases. First, unlike the previous conditions discussed, there is no correlation between the arthritic and cerebral processes (with the exception of lupus, which does not have nearly the impact on motor function in children as does JRA). Therefore, there is no a priori reason to expect that children with JRA will have low intellectual functioning; however, the impact of continued pain and intermittent motor restriction on achievement, ability to concentrate, and intellectual development should not be underestimated. Very concretely, helping the family and school to work with such issues as stiffness and pain early in the morning in order to help the start of the school day go more smoothly may be crucial. Helping parents and children to develop realistic expectations for themselves and to make appropriate plans for future education and vocational training and assisting school personnel in designing flexible and adaptive programs for these children may require careful evaluation of both intellectual ability and academic achievement, with special attention to discrepancies between various areas.

Adjustment to Motor Impairment

Assessment of the child's adaptation to his or her impairment, as well as to the complexities of family and social life faced by all individuals, is often overlooked in favor of the assessment of intellectual and physical abilities. However, the child's emotional status, including adaptation to the physical challenges he or she faces, as well as self-image and ability to form positive relationships, may be among the most important determinants of function.

The process of adapting to a motor impairment can be viewed from a number of different perspectives. Available research shows that children with motor impairments are not characterized by any particular personality type (Blumberg, 1975; Kirk, 1972; Podietz, 1971), and in general research focusing on determinants of positive or negative adaptation has been more productive than global comparisons of children with and without disabilities (Lavigne & Faier-Routman, 1992). Children with motor impairments pass through the same stages of development as typically developing children and must solve typical developmental tasks, as well as challenges presented by the condition. The developmental crises, however, may be more intense and delayed chronologically (Schlenoff, 1974). Several authors have argued that chronic illness interferes with normal developmental tasks (Travis, 1976; Willis, Elliott, & Jay, 1982). From Erikson's (1963) perspective, for example, chronic illness may interfere with the toddler's quest for autonomy because of reduced physical activity. Similarly, during Erikson's initiative stage, surgical procedures may magnify fears of bodily mutilation and result in a sense of inadequacy because of a poorly functioning body. School entry is often a crisis point because it may trigger the realization that the disability is permanent and highlight differences with peers and because illness may restrict the skill acquisition that is so vital to the stage of industry. Adolescence is typically also a difficult period because of the normal developmental tasks presented at that time. Although typically developing teens may or may not undergo periods of major crisis, those with disabilities face even greater challenges because of the roadblocks likely to be placed in the way of their ability to resolve issues of independence from parents, to form strong connections with the peer group, and to master romantic and sexual feelings. Forming realistic goals and dealing with a changing body may be particularly difficult for these adolescents (Gerring & McCarthy, 1988; Hill, 1993).

Many variables may influence the success of adaptation to disability (Lewandowski & Cruickshank, 1980), including degree of disability, age of onset of disability, visibility of condition, family and social support, attitudes toward the child, and social status with peers. Wright, Schaefer, and Solomons (1979) also added variables such as interpretation of the disability, gender and intelligence of the child, and external trauma (pain, restricted motion, surgery). It should also be remembered that the child with an acquired disability, such as spinal cord injury, may develop a different set of coping tasks from the child with a congenital condition. Acquired disability is often responded to with shock and denial, followed by anger and powerlessness over the loss of a specific function. This loss may be experienced as rage and frustration or as regression to earlier stages of development. Finally, some form of adaptation, either positive or negative, occurs. The final outcome depends on a number of variables, including premorbid personality and body image, family responses, degree of loss, and stage of development (Maddison & Raphael, 1971; Rubinstein, 1982). The psychologist should be familiar with the literature on coping prior to evaluating an individual with an acquired disability.

Although most adaptation issues are not disease specific but rather involve individual and ecological factors (King, Shultz, Steel, Gilpin, & Cathers, 1993), there are special issues involved in some of the conditions that cause motor impairments that do have important implications for the adaptation process. We briefly consider these to highlight the importance of considering both disease-related factors and factors unique to each child.

Cerebral palsy is one of the most difficult conditions for which to offer generalizations or to conduct meaningful research on emotional concerns, because both the physical effects and the level of cognitive, perceptual, and communicative functioning are so very different from child to child. Case studies (Trachtenberg & Rouse, 1998) highlight how important the family's approach to the child's strengths, as well as to the disorder, can be but also how much change can occur as children progress through developmental stages.

Research into spina bifida also is complicated by variation in function; again the research indicates that very different issues are encountered at different ages and different degrees of disability (Holmbeck, Faier-Routman, 1995). For example, several studies of preschoolers have found self-perceptions and social-behavioral adjustment that are very similar to those of peers (Mobley, Harless, & Miller, 1996; Van Hasselt, Ammerman, Hersen, Reigel, & Rowley, 1991), whereas studies of adolescents have noted decreased mood and lower feelings of self-worth, particularly in girls (Appleton et al., 1997).

Because DMD is characterized by such a relentless debilitating and ultimately fatal course, it is not surprising that studies, particularly of older boys, often find reports of poor adjustment and parent-reported behavior problems (Thompson, Zeman, Fanurik, & Sirotkin-Roses, 1992), but even in this disease, these findings are not universal, and resiliency can be as striking as pathology. One of us (M. R. J.) recently learned several new jokes from a late adolescent who breathed with a ventilator and who could also comment wryly, "Prozac is great stuff—everyone should try it."

In the case of JRA, it is obvious that the stress of coping with a disease of uncertain prognosis and etiology that may strike a healthy and active child unexpectedly should be carefully examined, with the understanding that the effects may differ from those found in children with a congenital condition. There is a fairly large literature on psychological issues in this disorder, perhaps in part because past theoretical models included internal conflicts as a causative factor, although data to support this has been unclear. Perhaps the most important conclusion to be drawn from reviewing this literature (Kewman, Warschausky, & Engel, 1995) is that multiple sources of data are crucial, because reports from behavior checklists, parent interviews, teachers, and the children themselves may give very different results. This, along with the need to consider developmental variables, may in fact be the most important conclusion that the clinician can draw in evaluating these children.

One other important factor in considering adjustment issues that may directly affect assessment is the question of motivation in children who have motor impairments. Scarr (1981) argued that intellectual competence is closely intertwined with motivation and adjustment. "Whenever one measures a child's cognitive functioning, one is also measuring cooperation, attention, persistence, ability to sit still, and social responsiveness to an assessment situation" (p. 1161). The same idea is expressed in White's (1959) concept of competence motivation, in that the human being is an active organism with internal motivation to learn and to seek out new experiences. In contrast, children with motor impairments, particularly children with cerebral palsy, are frequently characterized as passive, withdrawn, and failing to initiate responses in the environment. For children with this issue, the psychologist must take the time to identify motivating variables in the child's natural environment that can be incorporated during the evaluation. The clinician can use this information to document the ways in which the child's performance may be motivated to enhance learning and development of new skills.

SPECIAL ISSUES AND CONCERNS IN ASSESSMENT

Accurate assessment of a child with a motor impairment requires a well-designed assessment strategy. A strategy developed specifically for a child with motor impairments must take into consideration a multitude of factors particular to each individual child to iden-tify strengths and limitations accurately (Simeonsson, 1977). In this regard, we provide a brief review of examiner and setting requirements and considerations in the selection of an assessment battery.

Examiner Requirements

1. Prior experience with children with motor impairments and ongoing collaboration with a physical therapist in the assessment of a particular child.
2. Awareness of the medical management issues that may interfere with the test re-sults (for example, recent surgery, medications, and impact of the child's medical experiences on test responses).
3. Consulting skills and an appreciation of one's limitations. Examiners should re-quest consultations from other professionals, including physical, occupational, and speech therapists, when needed.
4. Maintaining an attitude of openness and an avoidance of positive or negative pre-conceptions.
5. Knowledge of particular age groups, particularly the 0–5 population, which pre-sents very different issues from older children
6. Avoiding the *halo effect,* that is, becoming overly invested in a child's performance. Special precautions might include the following:
   a. When using testing adaptations, the evaluator should avoid providing cues about the correct response. For example, when using eye pointing as a response, the examiner should stand behind the pictures to avoid knowing if the response is correct. The position of the eye point should be recorded and scored later. Also, insuring that the child's caretakers are not sitting in the child's line of vision avoids distractions.
   b. Using two persons in the testing situations previously described can increase the reliability of assessment.
   c. The person most familiar with the child may not be the best person to do the testing. Field (1981) found that familiar examiners tend to deflate scores on tests, perhaps via lower expectations.
7. Patience and awareness of the need for sufficient response time.
8. Awareness of fatigue and endurance issues in standardized test conditions (Fair & Birch, 1971; Sattler, 1982). The examiner may need to provide rest periods or sched-ule shorter test sessions spaced over several days.

Setting Requirements

1. Positioning of the child to facilitate support of the trunk and independent use of the arms and hands. If the child is incorrectly positioned, performance will be affected, because the child will expend effort on motor challenges rather than on cognitive tasks. Appropriate positioning can permit better fine motor function, facilitate attention, reduce fatigue, promote improved social interaction, and help to structure the child, thereby op-timizing performance. The evaluator should consult a physical therapist on positioning the child for testing, because this is a complex task requiring specialized knowledge and at times creative solutions. There are a number of positioning procedures and equipment that

may be helpful for the individual child, and a prescriptive checklist is available (Stephens & Lattimore, 1983).

2. Because of the elevated incidence of attention and concentration problems in children with some motor disorders, a testing environment with minimal auditory and visual distractions is especially important.

Test Selection and Adaptation

The selection of an appropriate test battery is a crucial task for the evaluator. Evaluation of the child with motor impairment has been accomplished in several ways: by adapting existing instruments (Sattler & Tozier, 1970); by designing new instruments (Burgemeister, Blum, & Lorge, 1972; French, 1964); by combining a mixture of methods or instruments (Mercer & Lewis, 1977); or by applying clinical, developmental, and naturalistic measures (Linder, 1993). At present no single instrument encompasses all of the necessary components essential to measuring cognitive, emotional-social, adaptive, and communicative aspects of children with multiple disabilities (Langley, 1979). In addition, most commercially available standardized tests were designed for use with typically developing children. It is important to consider some of the issues complicating the testing of children with physical disabilities and some of the strategies that have been employed to adapt existing tests. Salvia and Ysseldyke (1978) describe two kinds of test modifications regularly made in assessment of children with disabilities: (1) modification of stimulus demands and (2) modification of the response requirements. Examples of these modifications include eliminating time requirements, using multiple-choice formats and choice-pointing responses, pantomiming responses, stabilizing the child's hand, and enlarging objects (Bice & Cruickshank, 1966; Keats, 1965; Neuhaus, 1967; Newland, 1971). Several specific test modification suggestions are offered by Sattler (1982). Alternatives to modifying individual test items are to select tests that allow the child to respond with minimal difficulty or to employ subscales of commonly used tests whose demands are more appropriate for the individual child.

The extent to which modifying tests for children who have motor impairments invalidates standardized norms is inconclusive (Maisel, Allen, & Tallarico, 1962). In spite of the problems in comparing children with motor impairments with norms obtained from populations without these impairments, it may be necessary to do so for educational and vocational planning until meaningful norms are developed for children with motor challenges of varying degrees. Supplementing normed instruments with the highly individualized, functional, and naturalistic approach described by Linder (1993) as play-based assessment may provide rich information for planning programming and delineating potential and strengths.

Keeping these considerations in mind, it still may be possible to gather much information about cognitive function from conventional assessment instruments. For example, Cruickshank, Hallahan, and Bice (1976) point out that many children with cerebral palsy can be assessed with standard batteries because most children with this disability can see, hear, and speak adequately and have at least one functional arm and hand. For the assessment of intelligence, then, the examiner may have the option of using the Stanford–Binet IV, the K-ABC (Kaufman & Kaufman, 1983), or the Wechsler series (Wechsler, 1989, 1991). The Stanford–Binet IV offers some guidelines for assessing children with disabilities and also allows the calculation of standard scores along dimensions often very relevant to children with motor impairments (verbal, abstract/visual, quantitative, and short-term memory). Ironically, the older version offered some advantages for assessing children with motor impairments because of its wide age range and wealth of verbal items, but the norms are so old that it should be used only to enrich another, more standard battery, if at all. The K-ABC included exceptional children in the standardization population, and its focus on process variables and problem-solving styles makes it a valuable alternative in many cases. It also offers the opportunity to assess some aspects of nonverbal reasoning through purely visual and verbal responses.

The Wechsler Preschool and Primary Scale of Intelligence—Revised (WPPSI-R) and the WISC-III have a number of advantages for children who have motor impairments without severe arm and hand involvement. They permit an examination of perceptual–performance skills, which are particularly important in the early elementary years as early reading and writing skills are acquired. In addition, the WISC-III gives separate scores for verbal and performance scales, assisting in identification of difficulties with information processing and attention. Furthermore, the Wechsler scales are helpful in understanding strengths and weaknesses in cognitive skills through subtest analysis. Finally, Kaufman (1979) studied the contribution of speed of correct response to scores on the perceptual performance subtests of the WISC-R. He found that speed contributes very little to earning bonus points for children below 10 years of age and suggests that the WISC-R can be administered to motor-impaired children between ages 6 and 10, as they are not unduly penalized.

Despite the usefulness of this group of instruments, they have obvious disadvantages for the severely motor impaired. The psychomotor difficulties and associated disabilities of some children with cerebral palsy make it difficult for them to respond to timed tests or tests requiring manipulation of objects. For this reason, alternative tests such as the Columbia Mental Maturity Scale (CMMS; Burgemeister, Blum, & Lorge, 1972), the Peabody Picture Vocabulary Test—Third Edition (PPVT-III; Dunn & Dunn, 1981), or the Pictorial Test of Intelligence (PTI; French, 1964) are usually recommended for assessment of motor-impaired children who cannot respond to the typical tests. Given the nature of the response requirements of these measures, they may also be defined as tests of receptive communication skills. It is useful to examine the research that compares the effectiveness of these instruments so that guidelines for test selection can be established. One study (Coop, Eckel, & Stuck, 1975) examined the use of the PTI (French, 1964) with 46 young children with cerebral palsy, aged 4–7 years. Results indicated that the PTI was highly correlated with the CMMS and PPVT, showing good concurrent validity, and its six subtests were significantly related to achievement, indicating the possibility of using the subtest scores diagnostically. There were no significant increases in explained variance resulting from adding CMMS and PPVT scores to the PTI. The PTI offers a number of advantages, including ease of administration, moderate testing time, and subtest scores that can be used diagnostically. It assesses more areas of reasoning than either the PPVT or the CMMS. Limitations include its restricted age range and the age of the instrument.

In summary, evaluators should keep in mind two key factors in the selection of tests for individuals with physical disabilities: (1) the response requirements should be fair and reasonable, and (2) caution must be exercised in the use of norms (Anastasi, 1982; Salvia & Ysseldyke, 1978; Schlenoff, 1974).

Obtaining Background Information and Observing Behavior

To complete a full assessment, the evaluator should ask specific referral questions of both the formal referral source and the significant caretakers who are involved with the child, including classroom teachers, therapists, day care providers, and others who know the child well. The next step in most evaluations is an interview of parent and child, including an explanation of the goals of the assessment and clarifications of questions and concerns. The nature of the interview depends, of course, on its purpose (Lindemann, 1981), the age of the child, and the child's ability to communicate verbally. For example, Lindemann and Boyd (1981, p. 259) suggest the following types of questions when evaluating the adolescent with spina bifida:

> The interview should probe perceptions of the past ("What were your major strengths?" "What brought you the greatest recognition?" "How did you feel about your relationship with your peers?"), perceptions of the present ("What do you most enjoy doing now?" "What causes you the most difficulty at the present time?" "What kind of people do you most enjoy being with?"), and hopes and expectations for the future ("What do you expect to be doing ten years from now?" "What occupational choices have you been considering?" "How do you feel about marrying and having children?").

Most of these questions are relevant to evaluation of many motor-impaired adolescents, although judgment and consideration of trust development should precede discussion of issues such as marriage and reproduction.

Assessment of members of the child's family or of issues broadly affecting the family may also be important, as is discussed in Chapter 7. Although in the past much attention was often given to parental psychopathology, trends in family-centered care and parent advocacy have led to a current emphasis on resilience and strength in families and on the need for parents and professionals to collaborate on behalf of the child (Brazelton, 1992; Geralis, 1991; Leff & Walizer, 1992; McConkey, 1985; Miezio, 1983; Thompson, 1986). Keeping this in mind, and with openness and respect, the clinician may find it productive to assess both parental and child perceptions of the disability, its effect on the child and family, the cause of the impairment, and its impact on the future.

As with all children, the evaluator should carefully observe the child's behavior in both informal interactions and formal testing. The examiner should be alert for changes in responsiveness that may reflect auditory inattention, problems with vision or speech fluency, or petit mal seizures. In verbal children, speech dysfluencies should be noted and pursued in more depth in collaboration with a speech pathologist, as a motor, cognitive, or primary communication disorder may be present and unrecognized. The child's reading and writing should be carefully observed when appropriate because difficulties with visual–motor coordination may be reflected in the individual's performance. Finally, if performance tasks such as Block Design are administered, the examiner should carefully consider whether difficulties in performing the task are due to slow motor speed, perceptual problems, or difficulty manipulating the materials.

Assessing Social-Emotional Functioning

The social-emotional domain is an extremely important yet often neglected area of psychological assessment with children who have disabilities. As is apparent from the earlier discussion of issues related to adaptation to motor impairment, it is inappropriate to make assumptions about each individual child's adaptation and subsequent social-emotional functioning but equally hazardous to overlook its assessment. Though most instruments were developed for nondisabled children, many common approaches and instruments can be applied with motor-impaired children who can talk understandably and have the mental ability to understand task demands.

Assessment of the social-emotional area should include an interview with the child and may include the administration of selected projective and/or objective tests. Koppitz (1980) reviewed the available techniques in personality assessment and made recommendations that can be applied to the motor-impaired child with verbal skills. Her review included verbal, visual, drawing, manipulative, and objective techniques. For verbal children, conversation is the most direct and normalized place to start. Drawing techniques may be very useful if the child has good hand functioning, but interpretation can be difficult if the child's psychomotor deficits result in unusual features that could be misinterpreted as emotionally based. In the interview, the evaluator should gather information on the child's perception of his or her disability, on the perception of how others respond to it, and on strategies for adapting to the disability. A number of useful approaches to interviewing the child have been developed and are described elsewhere (Greenspan, 1981; Herjanic, Herjanic, Brown, & Wheatt, 1975; Palmer, 1970).

Personality assessment using objective standardized instruments has not always been regarded as an integral part of the evaluation of children with disabilities and chronic conditions (Magrab & Lehr, 1982). Issues such as social desirability responses and the limited ability of standardized instruments to differentiate between normal and ill children have limited their use. Magrab and Lehr suggest that this circumstance may be due to the population utilized in the research rather than to the techniques themselves. However, there does not appear to be consensus on a specific test or battery of tests best suited to this group of children.

Many authors have recommended measurement of the self-concept because of the assumption that a positive self-concept is fundamental to adjustment; however, the research on self-concept is controversial, with studies finding both positive and negative self-concept in children with disabilities. Clinically, many motor-impaired children appear to have low self-esteem, manifested as poor persistence and motivation on tasks, poor frustration tolerance, difficulty with risk taking, and frequent negative self-statements. One reason for the discrepancy between clinical observations and objective results may be the well-known problem of responses that are based on social desirability. Magrab and Lehr (1982) recommend that self-concept measures such as the Piers-Harris Self-Concept Scale (Piers & Harris, 1969), the Self-Esteem Inventory (Coopersmith, 1959), and the Tennessee Self-Concept Scale (Fitts, 1965) should be used in conjunction with other measures to assessment psychosocial issues.

Assessment of behavioral concerns should be included in the personal-social-emotional domain. Direct observation, interviews with caregivers, and behavioral checklists (Achenbach, 1991; Sattler, 1992) should all be considered as strategies for assessing behavior problems commonly found in children with motor impairments. These may include distractibility, impulsivity, passivity, lack of motivation, fears, and anxieties (Anderson, 1979). All motor-impaired children must deal with the issue of independence versus dependence and face challenges in their effort to establish and maintain a social network. With careful selection and modification, one of the many available behavioral checklists may help increase the completeness and objectivity of the assessment of these issues.

Reporting and Interpreting Results

The interpretation of test scores for the motor-impaired child can be complex, and great caution should be exercised in this area (Bice & Cruickshank, 1966). Interpretation should begin by comparing obtained scores with any previous test results. Motor-impaired children frequently acquire a host of test scores during their school years, but assessors fail to integrate past with present data. Because most standardized assessments have good test–retest reliability, the examiner should closely study variation over time. We have seen case histories in which intelligence quotients varied from the mid-50s to the low 120s. The psychologist must conduct a careful evaluation of the effects of the particular test administered, the age of the child, and the impact of specific disabilities on the results; such an evaluation may reveal important issues in the development of the individual child.

In preschool children, test results should be used for planning rather than for prediction. Because most assessment instruments designed for the 0–5 population naturally use more nonverbal tasks, the challenges of working with this group are particularly significant, and the need for multidisciplinary or transdisciplinary teams is most acute. Some authorities on this population maintain that the emphasis of this entire field should shift to collaborative process-oriented performance assessments that avoid the standardized norm-based approach altogether (Meisels & Fenichel, 1996). Although a discussion of this complex area is beyond the scope of this chapter, clinicians need to be aware of ongoing change and development in the subspecialty of infant and preschool assessment.

Many states now require an adaptive behavior measure for placement in special classes. As discussed earlier in this chapter, this is problematic for many motor-impaired children because of the limitations of the instruments available. Thus, although it is important to assess adaptive behavior, the assessment should be used for program planning rather than placement and should be done in collaboration with occupational and physical therapists.

Because of the unique challenges faced by each child who has a motor impairment, the evaluator must consider each child individually, looking at strengths and needs in each of the domains in order to provide a comprehensive evaluation.

SUMMARY AND RECOMMENDATIONS

The importance of a well-designed and comprehensive strategy for the assessment of the motor-impaired child is clear. We stress three points in summarizing the psychologist's approach to the child with a motor impairment: (1) the need for a multidisciplinary team approach, (2) the importance of consultation skills, and (3) the importance of referral and advocacy skills. Often the motor-impaired child has challenges not only with movement but also with other systems, which makes an evaluator's task more complex. It is rarely possible for an evaluator to work alone in the assessment of children with motor impairments. The collaboration of members of a multidisciplinary team—which, depending on the child's needs, may consist of a physician, nurse, social worker, special educator, and physical, speech, and occupational therapists, as well as the psychologist—is crucial to comprehensive assessment. The family should be considered a crucial part of the team and should be consulted and included throughout the process of assessment. The team concept allows the psychologist not only to consider essential physical problems but also to enlist other professionals in the modification of variables for the child's assessment. It becomes obvious that consulting skills are an extremely important part of an evaluator's repertoire, allowing him or her to gather information and assistance in planning for and carrying out the assessment of the motor-impaired child. Finally, the recommendations resulting from the assessment will be most helpful if they are generated using the same collaborative approach. The psychologist who is familiar with the resources available in the community for children with motor impairments, who can communicate well with these resources, and who is willing to engage in creative solution building and problem solving with those who care for, teach, and support these children and their families will produce the most useful and satisfying assessments.

REFERENCES

Achenbach, T. M. (1991). *Manual for the Child Behavior Checklist/4–18 and 1991 Profile.* Burlington: University of Vermont, Department of Psychiatry.

Anastasi, A. (1982). *Psychological testing.* New York: Macmillan.

Anderson, E. M. (1979). The psychological and social adjustment of adolescents with cerebral palsy or spina bifida and hydrocephalus. *International Journal of Rehabilitation Research, 2,* 245–247.

Appleton, P. L., Ellis, N. C., Minchom, P. E., Lawson, V., Boll, V., & Jones, P. (1997). Depressive symptoms and self-concept in young people with spina bifida. *Journal of Pediatric Psychology, 22*(5), 707–722.

Barnes, M. A., & Dennis, M. (1992). Reading in children and adolescents after early onset hydrocephalus and in normally developing age peers: Phonological analysis, word recognition, word comprehension, and passage comprehension skill. *Journal of Pediatric Psychology, 17*(4), 445–466.

Baron, I. S., Fennell, E. B., & Voeller, K. K. S. (1995). Hydrocephalus and myelomeningocele. In *Pediatric neuropsychology in the medical setting* (pp. 221–243). New York: Oxford University Press.

Beigel, A. R. (2000). Assistive technology assessment: More than the device. *Intervention in School and Clinic, 35*(4), 237–243.

Bice, H. V., & Cruickshank, W. M. (1966). The evaluation of intelligence. In W. M. Cruickshank (Ed.), *Cerebral palsy: Its individual and community problems* (pp. 101–134). Syracuse, NY: Syracuse University Press.

Billard, C., Gillet, P., Barthez, M., Hommet, C., & Bertrand, P. (1998). Reading ability and processing in Duchenne muscular dystrophy and spinal muscular atrophy. *Developmental Medicine and Child Neurology, 40,* 12–20.

Billard, C., Gillet, P., Signoret, J. L., Uicaut, E., Bertrand, P., Fardeau, M., Barthez-Carpentier, M. A., & Santini, J. J. (1992). Cognitive functions in Duchenne muscular dystrophy: A reappraisal and comparison with spinal muscular atrophy. *Neuromuscular Disorders, 2,* 371–377.

Blumberg, M. L. (1975). Psychodynamics of the young handicapped person. *American Journal of Psychotherapy, 29,* 466–476.

Brazelton, T. B. (1992). *Touchpoints: Your child's emotional and behavioral development.* Reading, MA: Addison-Wesley.

Brook, M. H. (1977). *Clinicians' view of neuromuscular disease.* Baltimore: Waverly Press.

Burgemeister, B. B., Blum, L. H., & Lorge, I. (1972). *Columbia Mental Maturity Scale* (3rd ed.). San Antonio, TX: Psychological Corporation.

Byrne, K., Abbeduto, L., & Brooks, P. (1990). The language of children with spina bifida and hydrocephalus: Meeting task demands and mastering syntax. *Journal of Speech and Hearing Disorders, 55,* 118–123.

Cassidy, J. T., & Petty, R. E. (1995). *Textbook of Pediatric Rheumatology* (3rd ed.). Philadelphia: Saunders.

Coop, R. H., Eckel, E., & Stuck, G. B. (1975). An assessment of the Pictorial Test of Intelligence for use with young cerebral-palsied children. *Developmental Medicine and Child Neurology, 17,* 287–292.

Coopersmith, S. (1959). A method of determining types of self-esteem. *Journal of Abnormal Psychology, 59,* 87–94.

Cruickshank, W. M. (Ed.). (1976). *Cerebral palsy: A developmental disability.* Syracuse, NY: Syracuse University Press.

Cruickshank, W. M., Hallahan, D. P., & Bice, H. (1976). The evaluation of intelligence. In W. M. Cruickshank (Ed.), *Cerebral palsy: A developmental disability* (pp. 95–122). Syracuse, NY: Syracuse University Press.

Dennis, M., & Barnes, M. A. (1993). Oral discourse after early-onset hydrocephalus: Linguistic ambiguity, figurative language, speech acts, and script-based inferences. *Journal of Pediatric Psychology, 18*(5), 639–652.

Dise, J. E., & Lohr, M. E. (1998). Examination of deficits in conceptual reasoning abilities associated with spina bifida. *American Journal of Physical Medicine and Rehabilitation, 8,* 247–251.

Donders, J., Rourke, B. P., & Canady, A. I. (1991). Neuropsychological functioning of hydrocephalic children. *Journal of Clinical and Experimental Neurology, 13*(4), 607–613.

Dunn, L. M., & Dunn, L. M. (1981). *Peabody Picture Vocabulary Test—Revised.* Circle Pines, MN: American Guidance Service.

Erikson, E. H. (1963). *Childhood and society* (2nd ed.). New York: Norton.

Fair, D. T., & Birch, J. W. (1971). Effect of rest on test scores of physically handicapped and non-handicapped children. *Exceptional Children, 37,* 335–336.

Field, T. (1981). Ecological variables and examiner biases in assessing handicapped preschool children. *Journal of Pediatric Psychology, 16,* 155–163.

Finnstrom, O., Olausson, P. O., Sedin, G., Serenius, F., Svenningsen, N., Thiringer, K., Tunnell, R., & Wesstrom, G. (1998). Neurosensory outcome and growth at three years in extremely low birth weight infants: Follow-up results from the Swedish national prospective study. *Acta Paediatrica, 87,* 1055–1060.

Fitts, W. H. (1965). *Tennessee Self-Concept Scale.* Nashville, TN: Counselor Recordings and Tests.

Fletcher, J. M., Brookshire, B. L., Landry, S. H., Bohan, T. P., Davidson, K. C., Francis, D. J., Thompson, N. M., & Miner, M. E. (1995). Behavioral adjustment of children with hydrocephalus: Relationships with etiology, neurological, and family status. *Journal of Pediatric Psychology, 20*(1), 109–125.

Fletcher, J. M., Francis, D. J., Thompson, N. M., Brookshire, B. L., Bohan, T. P., Landry, S. H., Davidson, K. C., & Miner, M. E. (1992). Verbal and nonverbal skills discrepancies in hydrocephalic children. *Journal of Clinical and Experimental Neuropsychology, 14*(4), 593–609.

French, J. L. (1964). *Manual: Pictorial Test of Intelligence.* Boston: Houghton Mifflin.

Friedrich, W. N., Lovejoy, M. C., Shaffer, J., Shurtleff, D. B., & Beilke, R. L. (1991). Cognitive abilities and achievement status of children with myelomeningocele: A contemporary sample. *Journal of Pediatric Psychology, 16*(4), 423–428.

Geralis, E. (Ed.). (1991). *Children with cerebral palsy: A parents' guide.* Rockville, MD: Woodbine House.

Gerring, J. P., & McCarthy, L. P. (1988). *The psychiatry of handicapped children and adolescents: Managing emotional and behavioral problems.* Boston, MA: Little, Brown.

Greenspan, S. I. (1981). *The clinical interview of the child.* New York: McGraw-Hill.

Gregg, S. (1971). Rheumatoid arthritis in childhood. *Arizona Medicine, 28,* 577–585.

Hagberg, B. (1962). The sequelae of spontaneously arrested infantile hydrocephalus. *Developmental Medicine and Child Neurology, 4,* 583–587.

Hall, C. D., & Porter, P. B. (1980). *School intervention for the neuromuscularly handicapped child.* Unpublished manuscript, University of North Carolina at Chapel Hill.

Herjanic, B., Herjanic, M., Brown, F., & Wheatt, T. (1975). Are children reliable reporters? *Journal of Abnormal Child Psychology, 3,* 41–48.

Hill, A. E. (1993). Problems in relation to independent living: A retrospective study of physically disabled school leavers. *Developmental Medicine and Child Neurology, 35*(12), 1111–1115.

Holmbeck, G. N., & Faier-Routman, J. (1995). Spinal lesion level, shunt status, family relationships, and psychosocial adjustment in children and adolescents with spina bifida myelomeningocele. *Journal of Pediatric Psychology, 20*(6), 817–832.

Kaufman, A. S. (1979). The role of speed on WISC-R performance across the age range. *Journal of Consulting and Clinical Psychology, 47,* 595–597.

Kaufman, A. S., & Karfman, N. L. (1983). *Kaufman Assessment Battery for Children (K-ABC).* Circle Pines, MN: American Guidance Service.

Keats, S. (1965). *Cerebral palsy.* Springfield, IL: Thomas.

Kewman, D. G., Warschausky, S. A., & Engel, L. (1995). Juvenile rheumatoid arthritis and neuromuscular conditions: Scoliosis, spinal cord injury, and muscular dystrophy. In M. C. Roberts (Ed.), *Handbook of pediatric psychology* (2nd ed., pp. 384–402). New York: Guilford Press.

King, G. A., Shultz, I. Z., Steel, K., Gilpin, M., & Cathers, T. (1993). Self-evaluation and self-concept of adolescents with physical disorders. *American Journal of Occupational Therapy, 47*(2), 132–140.

Kirk, S. A. (1972). *Educating exceptional children* (2nd ed.). Boston: Houghton Mifflin.

Koppitz, E. M. (1980). Personality assessments in the schools. In C. Reynolds & T. Gutkin (Eds.), *Handbook of school psychology.* New York: Wiley.

Langley, M. B. (1979, Winter). Psychoeducational assessment of the multiply handicapped blind child: Issues and methods. *Education of the Visually Handicapped, 97–114.*

Lavigne, J. V., & Faier-Routman, J. (1992). Psychological adjustment to pediatric disorders: A meta-analytic review. *Journal of Pediatric Psychology, 17(2),* 133–157.

Leff, P. T., & Walizer, E. H. (1992). *Building the healing partnership: Parents, professionals, and children with chronic illnesses and disabilities.* Cambridge, MA: Brookline Books.

Lewandowski, L. J., & Cruickshank, W. M. (1980). Psychological development of crippled children and youth. In W. Cruickshank (Ed.), *Psychology of exceptional children* (4th ed.). Englewood Cliffs, NJ: Prentice-Hall.

Lindemann, J. E. (1981). *Psychological and behavioral aspects of physical disability: A manual for health practitioners.* New York: Plenum Press.

Lindemann, J. E., & Boyd, R. D. (1981). Myelo-meningocele (spina bifida). In J. Lindemann (Ed.), *Psychological and behavioral aspects of physical disability: A manual for health practitioners* (pp. 243–271). New York: Plenum Press.

Linder, T. W. (1993). *Transdisciplinary play-based assessment: A functional approach to working with young children.* Baltimore: Brookes.

Maddison, D., & Raphael, B. (1971). Social and psychological consequences of chronic disease in childhood. *Medical Journal of Australia, 2,* 1265–1270.

Magrab, P. R., & Lehr, E. (1982). Assessment techniques in pediatric psychology. In J. Tuma (Ed.), *Handbook for the practice of pediatric psychology* (pp. 67–109). New York: Wiley.

Maisel, R. N., Allen, R. M., & Tallarico, R. B. (1962). A comparison of the adaptive and standard administration of the Leiter International Performance Scale with normal children. *Cerebral Palsy Review, 22(3–4),* 16.

McConkey, R. (1985). *Working with parents: A practical guide for teachers and therapists.* Cambridge, MA: Brookline Books.

Meisels, S. J., & Fenichel, E. (Eds.). (1996). *New visions for the developmental assessment of infants and young children.* Washington, DC: Zero to Three National Center for Infants, Toddlers, and Families.

Menkes, J. H. (Ed.). (1995). *Textbook of child neurology* (5th ed.). Baltimore: Williams & Wilkins.

Menkes, J. H., & Till, K. (1995). Malformations of the central nervous system. In J. H. Menkes (Ed.), *Textbook of child neurology* (5th ed., pp. 240–324). Baltimore: Williams & Wilkins.

Mercer, J., & Lewis, J. (1977). *System of multicultural pluralistic assessment.* New York: Psychological Corporation.

Miezio, P. M. (1983). *Parenting children with disabilities: A professional source for physicians and guide for parents.* New York: Marcel Dekker.

Mobley, C. E., Harless, L. S., & Miller, K. L. (1996). Self-perceptions of preschool children with spina bifida. *Journal of Pediatric Nursing, 11,* 217–224.

Molnar, G. E. (1992). Cerebral palsy. In G. E. Molnar (Ed.) *Pediatric rehabilitation* (pp. 481–533). Baltimore: Williams & Wilkins.

Morrow, R. S., & Cohen, J. (1954). The psychosocial factors in muscular dystrophy. *Journal of Child Psychiatry, 3,* 70.

Neuhaus, M. (1967). Modifications in the administration of the WISC performance subtests for children with profound hearing losses. *Exceptional Children, 33,* 573–574.

Newland, T. E. (1971). Psychological assessment of exceptional children and youth. In W. M. Cruickshank (Ed.), *Psychology of exceptional children and youth* (pp. 115–172). Englewood Cliffs, NJ: Prentice-Hall.

Palmer, J. O. (1970). *The psychological assessment of children.* New York: Wiley.

Pellegrino, L., & Dormans, J. P. (1998). Definitions, etiology, and epidemiology of cerebral palsy. In J. Dormans & L. Pellegrino (Eds.), *Caring for children with cerebral palsy: A team approach* (pp. 3–30). Baltimore: Brookes.

Piers, E., & Harris, D. (1969). *Manual for the Piers-Harris Children's Self-Concept Scale.* Nashville, TN: Counselor Recordings and Tests.

Podietz, L. (1971). Activity group therapy for adolescents with orthopedic handicaps. *Proceedings of the 79th Annual Convention of the American Psychological Association, 6,* 639–640.

Prosser, V., Murphy, E. G., & Thompson, M. W. (1969). Intelligence and the gene for Duchenne Muscular Dystrophy. *Archives of Disease of Childhood, 44,* 221–229.

Rubinstein, B. (1982). Psychological aspects of chronic handicaps. In A. Downey & N. L. Low (Eds.), *The child with disabling illness: Principles of rehabilitation* (2nd ed., pp. 565–594). New York: Raven Press.

Salvia, J., & Ysseldyke, J. E. (1978). *Assessment in special and remedial education.* Boston: Houghton Mifflin.

Sattler, J. M. (1982). *Assessment of Children's Intelligence and Special Abilities* (2nd ed.). Boston: Allyn & Bacon.

Sattler, J. M. (1992). *Assessment of children* (3rd ed.). San Diego: Sattler.

Sattler, J. M., & Tozier, L. L. (1970). A review of intelligence test modifications used with cerebral palsied and other handicapped groups. *Journal of Special Education, 4,* 391–398.

Scarr, S. (1981). Testing for children: Assessment and the many determinants of intellectual competence. *American Psychologist, 36,* 1159–1166.

Schlenoff, D. (1974). Considerations in administering intelligence tests to the physically disabled. *Rehabilitation Literature, 35*(12), 362–363.

Shaer, C. M. (1997). The infant and young child with spina bifida: Major medical concerns. *Infants and Young Children, 9*(3), 13–25.

Simeonsson, R. J. (1977). Infant assessment. In B. M. Caldwell, D. J. Stedman, & K. W. Goin (Eds.), *Infant education: A guide for helping handicapped children* (pp. 27–44). New York: Walker.

Soare, P. L., & Raimondi, A. J. (1977). Intellectual and perceptual-motor characteristics of treatment of myelomeningocele children. *American Journal of Diseases of Children, 131,* 199–204.

Solot, C. B. (1998). Promoting function: Communication and feeding. In J. P. Dormans & L. Pelligrino (Eds.), *Caring for children with cerebral palsy: A team approach* (pp. 347–370). Baltimore: Brookes.

Stellern, J., Vasa, S. F., & Little, J. (1976). *Introduction to diagnostic-prescriptive teaching and programming.* Glen Ridge, NJ: Exceptional Press.

Stephens, T. E., & Lattimore, J. (1983). Prescriptive checklist for positioning multihandicapped residential clients: A clinical report. *Physical Therapy, 63,* 1113–1115.

Thompson, C. E. (1986). *Raising a handicapped child: A helpful guide for parents of the physically disabled.* New York: Morrow.

Thompson, R. J., Zeman, J. L., Fanurik, D., & Sirotkin-Roses, M. (1992). The role of parent stress and coping and family functioning in parent and child adjustment to Duchenne muscular dystrophy. *Journal of Clinical Psychology, 17*(6), 705–724.

Trachtenberg, S. W., & Rouse, C. F. (1998). The family. In J. P. Dormans & L. Pellegrino (Eds.), *Caring for children with cerebral palsy: A team approach* (pp. 429–445). Baltimore: Brookes.

Travis, G. (1976). *Chronic illness in children: Its impact on child and family.* Stanford, CA: Stanford University Press.

Truitt, C. J. (1955). Personal and social adjustments of children with muscular dystrophy. *American Journal of Physical Medicine, 34,* 124.

Van Hasselt, V. B., Ammerman, R. T., Hersen, M., Reigel, D. H., & Rowley, F. L. (1991). Assessment of social skills and problem behaviors in young children with spina bifida. *Journal of Developmental Disabilities and Physical Disabilities, 3*(1), 69–80.

Wechsler, D. (1989). *Wechsler Preschool and Primary Scales of Intelligence—Revised.* San Antonio, TX: Psychological Corporation.

Wechsler, D. (1991). *Wechsler Intelligence Scale for Children—Third Edition.* San Antonio, TX: Psychological Corporation.

White, R. W. (1959). Motivation considered: The concept of competence. *Psychological Review, 66,* 299–333.

Willis, D. J., Elliott, C. H., & Jay, S. (1982). Psychological effects of physical illness and its concomitants. In J. Tuma (Ed.), *Handbook for the practice of pediatric psychology* (pp. 28–66). New York: Wiley.

Wills, K. E., Holmbeck, G. N., Dillon, K., & McLone, D. G. (1990). Intelligence and achievement in children with myelomeningocele. *Journal of Pediatric Psychology, 15*(2), 161–176.

Wright, L., Schaefer, A., & Solomons, G. (1979). *Encyclopedia of pediatric psychology.* Baltimore: University Park Press.

Zellweger, H. (1946). Uber knochenveranderungen bes dur Dystrophia Musculorum Progressiva. *Annotated Pediatrics, 167,* 287.

11

ASSESSMENT OF CHILDREN WITH VISUAL IMPAIRMENT OR BLINDNESS

NAEELA M. CHAUDRY
PHILIP W. DAVIDSON

P. J. is a 5-year-old child with total blindness secondary to retinopathy of prematurity (ROP). She was born after a gestation period of 26 weeks and was treated for broncho-pulmonary dysplasia for 3 months postdelivery in the Neonatal Intensive Care Nursery. Her early treatment required placement in a high O_2 environment to assist her breathing, causing her to develop ROP.

She showed evidence of delayed motor development as early as 12 months of age. She did not begin to crawl until 24 months but walked at 36 months. Her language development appeared normal, but her skills of daily living were less than age appropriate. She had no evidence of neuromotor disorders such as cerebral palsy.

At the age of 3 years, she refused to tolerate separation from her parents, even for brief periods, screaming and displaying tantrums until one of them touched her. She also showed excessive fear of strangers. Her tantrums were sometimes accompanied by violent outbursts, including aggression and self-injurious behavior.

She had never been successfully tested on a formal psychometric battery, but her IQ, estimated from checklists, was believed to be in the range of mild mental retardation. At last report, she was attending her final year of preschool at a special program for toddlers with visual impairments. Her parents reported concerns about her successful transition to an inclusive primary educational setting while retaining continuity of her specialized services and supports.

There is no single universally accepted definition of visual impairment or blindness. Legal blindness governs eligibility for social services. It is defined by the U.S. Social Security Act as "visual acuity for distant vision of 20/200 or less in the better eye, with best correction; or a visual field of 20° or less" (National Society for the Prevention of Blindness, 1996, p. 10). The term "blindness" is frequently utilized to describe individuals with complete loss of vision. There are few people who are totally blind (Bradley-Johnson, 1994). Between 80% and 90% of all children considered legally blind or severely visually impaired have low vision, indicating that they can perceive light or details and have some useable vision (Buncic, 1987; O'Donnell & Livingston, 1991).

Federal legislation that mandates special education services for children and youth does not limit the definition of visual impairment to legal blindness. According to Scholl (1985), the classification of blindness should be applied only to children who must use senses other than vision in academic activities. A functional definition, more useful for educational purposes in describing visual impairment, is "a student with a visual loss who requires more than glasses to function adequately in the classroom" (Bradley-Johnson, 1994, p. 38). Under the Individuals with Disabilities Education Act (IDEA) reauthorization of 1997, visual disabilities include all impairments from legal blindness to total blindness.

INCIDENCE AND PREVALENCE

Actual incidence and prevalence is difficult to estimate. There are several sources of information about incidence and prevalence of visual impairments, including examination data, population statistics, and counts of persons receiving services or entitlements.

Projections of legal blindness in children by the National Society for the Prevention of Blindness (1980) estimated the number of legally blind children in the United States under age 20 years to be approximately 41,500; 6,900 were under age 5 years (Kirchner, 1989, p. 144). The incidence of severe visual impairments is approximately 1 per 3,000 live births (Batshaw & Perret, 1993; Foster, 1988; Olson, 1987). About 46% of these children are born with total blindness, and another 38% lose vision prior to their first birthdays (Foster, 1988).

According to the U.S. Department of Education (1992), 25,125 students were classified as visually impaired or deaf-blind and served under IDEA, Part B, in the 1990–1991 school year. The American Printing House for the Blind reported data from 1983–1984 indicating a prevalence rate of 0.86 per 1,000 for children from birth to age 24 years who were considered legally blind, were enrolled in educational programs below college level, and were registered for adaptive educational material (Kirchner, 1989).

DISORDERS OF VISION

The etiologies of childhood blindness include (1) prenatal influences, such as inherited conditions; (2) infectious diseases, such as rubella; (3) injuries or poisoning; and (4) exposure to drugs or medical interventions, such as excess O_2 or diseases of the eye (National Society for the Prevention of Blindness, 1980). Most visual losses in the school-age population are associated with congenital factors (Scholl, 1985). However, visual loss may result from traumatic injury or accidents, secondary complications of other diseases or disorders (such as diabetes), biological changes (such as retinal detachment or tumor), secondary effects of surgery (such as lens removal), and inflammatory and progressive disorders (Olson, 1987).

Congenital Cataracts

A cataract is an opacity that clouds the crystalline lens, obstructing vision by preventing passage of light. Although this disorder commonly occurs in older individuals, it has been found in young children as a result of intrauterine infection, genetic inheritance, or trauma (Olson, 1987; Vander Kolk, 1987). Cataracts account for about 15% of blindness in children (Nelson, Calhoun, & Harley, 1991). Small cataracts remain stable and do not need to be removed (Batshaw & Perret, 1992). If the cataract becomes dense enough to be visible in the pupil, it is likely to significantly obscure vision. Surgical removal is necessary to avoid additional visual loss due to amblyopia. Corrective glasses or a contact lens must be used to compensate for the loss of part of the natural lens (Batshaw & Perret, 1993).

Optic Nerve Atrophy

Pressure on the optic nerve may cut off the blood supply, resulting in degeneration of any part of the optic nerve (Bradley-Johnson, 1994; Olson, 1987). Pressure can result from a tumor, hereditary factors, or prenatal trauma. The loss of vision may be irreversible (Bradley-Johnson, 1994). Optic nerve atrophy has been estimated to account for approximately 22% of all blindness in children (Nelson, Calhoun, & Harley, 1991).

Retinopathy of Prematurity

First known as retrolental fibroplasia (RLF), retinopathy of prematurity (ROP) involves the development of an abnormal number of blood vessels in the retina, resulting in its scarring, bleeding, or detachment (Bradley-Johnson, 1994). It occurs primarily in premature infants. Blood vessel formation in the retina during prenatal development progresses outward from the optic nerve. As a result, infants born following less than 28–30 weeks' gestation have an increased likelihood of developing ROP involving greater areas of the retina. Because the formation of blood vessels is completed by 40 weeks' gestation, infants born after this time have little risk of ROP.

The most common cause of ROP prior to the 1960s was the placement of newborns in isolettes with high levels of oxygen to treat respiratory distress syndrome (Batshaw & Perret, 1992; Olson, 1989). Infants are now given the lowest possible concentration of oxygen and treated with Surfactin replacement for respiratory distress syndrome (Batshaw & Perret, 1992). Although the risk of ROP has been reduced, it remains a leading cause of blindness in young children due to the increasing survival rate of very small premature babies (Valentine, Jackson, Kalina, & Woodrum, 1989).

Upon detection of ROP, laser surgery is often conducted to cauterize the affected area of the retina. This reduces the likelihood of traction and retinal detachment and has resulted in a significant reduction in blindness due to ROP (Batshaw & Perret, 1992; Gallo & Lennerstrand, 1991). Some common residual effects of ROP include high myopia (which may be corrected by glasses), macular distortions, glaucoma, and strabismus (Batshaw & Perret, 1992).

Congenital Glaucoma

Glaucoma results from blockage of fluid from the anterior chamber of the eye behind the cornea, increasing intraocular pressure and reducing blood supply to the retina. Visual loss results from nerve cell necrosis. Glaucoma is typically a disease of older persons, but it can occur congenitally.

Cortical Blindness

Degeneration of occipital connections, injury, or a tumor causes a lesion in the occipital lobe of the brain, resulting in vision loss. Cortical blindness may result from congenital infections or traumatic injury to the brain. It is often not diagnosed in a young child because there are usually no noticeable effects on the functions of the eye (e.g., the pupils respond normally to light and fundi indicate no changes). However, the child may have restricted vision and require educational supports (Olson, 1987).

Retinoblastoma

Retinoblastoma results from a tumor in the retina. If the tumor is untreated, this disorder can be fatal (Olson, 1987). The typical treatment for this neoplasm is innunculation, resulting in immediate loss of all vision. Following postsurgical oncology therapies, a prosthetic eyeball is typically inserted, preventing disfigurement secondary to hypoplasia of the area around the socket.

Retinitis Pigmentosa

This hereditary disorder involving degeneration of the rods or cones of the retina results in depletion of the retina pigment and atrophy of the remainder of the retina. Night blindness is an immediate result, followed by generalized visual impairment (Pagon, 1988). Loss of vision is gradual and progresses into adulthood. Its effects can be initially minimized by corrective lenses, but total loss of vision is inevitable.

Albinism

Albinism is a hereditary disease that affects the metabolism of melanin and results in a lack of pigment in all or part of the body. Ocular signs present at birth include white eyebrows and lashes, gray or red irises, and pupils that appear red. The macula is underdeveloped, resulting in loss of acuity and nystagmus (abnormal movement of the eye muscles). Individuals with albinism have limited vision and extreme sensitivity to light (Bradley-Johnson, 1994; Olson, 1987). Although there is no cure for this disease, special lenses can be used to increase vision and decrease the amount of light entering the eye.

ASSESSMENT AND DOMAIN PRIORITIES

Serious visual loss not only affects the visual system itself but may also have either direct or indirect influences on virtually every other developmental domain. The influence may be modulated by the child's interaction with his or her environment. As is the case for any child, the reason for assessment will play a key role in determining the specific domains to be assessed and the type of information required to make various types of decisions. However, because the standard assessment instruments that are appropriate for children with visual impairment may not be available, one may need to obtain data from alternative sources. School and medical records, criterion-referenced tests, curriculum-based measures, interviews, observation, and behavior rating scales should be used in making diagnostic and treatment recommendations. Children with severe visual loss have also been found to have additional disabilities including children who are deaf-blind (Tedder, Warden, & Sikka, 1993). Kirchner (1983) reported that 30% to 50% of children who are visually impaired have one or two additional disabilities. These factors highlight the importance of multiple sources of information, as well as of using an interdisciplinary approach to evaluation. Domains that should be assessed in children with visual impairment or blindness include motor development, language development, cognition, educational needs and academic achievement, social skills, personality, and emotional and behavioral functioning.

Motor Development

Motor development, especially functional hand use, may be delayed in some infants with visual impairment (Fraiberg, 1977). Infants with visual impairments typically display delays in reaching for objects based on auditory cues and in crawling and walking. The emergence of the hands as a major perceptual organ for fingering, grasping, and transferring objects (Van Hasselt & Sisson, 1987) has a significant impact on learning about the environment. Motor development may also be delayed in older children with visual impairments, perhaps due to insufficient physical activity (Warren, 1989).

Language Development

In general, the course of language development in children with visual impairment is similar to the pattern found in sighted children (Vander Kolk, 1987). However, although infants with visual impairment may babble and imitate words sooner than sighted children, they frequently display delays in combining words to make their wants known (Fraiberg, 1977). Furthermore, children with visual impairments have been found to obtain higher expressive than receptive language scores on language tests (Van Hasselt & Sisson, 1987). This may be due to echolalic tendencies and a facility in retrieving rote facts. Severity of the visual impairment may also influence language development: McConachie and Moore (1994) reported that language delays were noted in young children with severe visual impairment. With children who are deaf-blind, play assessment can be a useful way to document communication skills (Finn & Fewell, 1994).

The expressive skills demonstrated by a visually impaired child may not accurately represent understanding of vocabulary and concepts. This situation is typified by "verbalism" in the language of children with visual impairment. For example, a child may describe an object using descriptors derived from the visual context, such as colorful or bright, while lacking comprehension of the functional meaning or the appropriate underlying sensory base. In fact, the object may or may not merit such descriptors to a sighted person. This phenomenon is likely due to lack of sensory experience with objects (Warren, 1989).

Cognition

Vision plays a central role in the identification of objects and events and provides the basis for acquisition of concepts pertaining to the structure of physical space and spatial relationships (Sisson & Van Hasselt, 1987). In addition to acquisition of concepts, reasoning skills, problem solving, and judgment are all learned primarily through sight. As children and adults with visual impairment acquire this information on the basis of other senses, they may use a different cognitive style than sighted individuals (Vander Kolk, 1987).

Educational Needs and Academic Achievement

Assessment of academic skills in reading, mathematics, and language is crucial in determining a child's strengths and areas of difficulty. Such assessment can serve as the basis for identifying instructional needs and in documenting progress in school. Once instructional needs are identified, appropriate adaptive devices or materials can be determined and an instructional plan developed to maximize the student's learning. For children with visual impairments serious enough to require dependence upon touch, it may also be important to assess Braille reading skills in addition to evaluation of the child's skills in other academic areas.

Social Skills

Deficits or delays in adaptive and social behaviors are common in children with visual impairments (Van Hasselt, 1983). In the case of children with congenital blindness, the lack of vision is immediately noticeable in the quality of interaction between infant and caregiver (Fraiberg, 1977). A number of factors may be responsible for inadequate social skills in children with visual impairment, including (1) difficulty acquiring nonverbal, interpersonal skill components, such as physical gestures and facial expressions; (2) inability to acquire social skills by modeling through the use of visual cues; (3) accurate feedback concerning interpersonal effectiveness from the environment; and (4) failure of others to encourage independence or to provide reinforcement contingent on adequate social performance (Van Hasselt & Sisson, 1987).

Personality and Emotional and Behavioral Functioning

Several research studies suggest that children with visual impairments score differently on personality tests than sighted children (Van Hasselt & Sisson, 1987). Visual impairment has also been found to be associated with stereotypical behavior in young children (Brambring & Troester, 1992) and with limited social skill in adolescents (Van Hasselt, Hersen, & Kazdin, 1985). The blind child may prefer to withdraw from social groups that include sighted children rather than to attempt to fit in as a peer (Van Hasselt & Sisson, 1987).

The Family Context

The examiner can obtain pertinent family information from a parent interview, including family history, course of pregnancy and birth, attainment of developmental milestones, time of visual loss, congenital versus later loss of vision, self-care skills, mobility, daily living skills, and the child's level of acceptance of the visual loss. Such information is important in that it provides a framework from which to interpret standardized tests and behavioral assessments (Van Hasselt & Sisson, 1987).

The examiner should also obtain information regarding the parents' and significant others' reactions, feelings, knowledge, and behavior toward the child with visual impairment (Van Hasselt & Sisson, 1987). Equally essential is assessment regarding the family members' beliefs about visual impairment or blindness as a physical and/or psychological disability (Van Hasselt & Sisson, 1987). Appreciation of parents' perceptions of their child's limitations, fears about their child's experiences growing up, and unrealistic demands or overprotectiveness can help the examiner to determine the degree of parental involvement with the educational program and can add information necessary in developing a program to optimize the development of the child with visual impairment (Van Hasselt & Sisson, 1987). Other areas that should be investigated include the availability of adequate learning resources, the degree to which parents and the community are actively providing normative learning experiences, and the parents' hopes and expectations for the evaluation and the child's development in general (Bradley-Johnson, 1994).

A parent interview may be conducted in a number of places. The ideal situation would include a home visit during which the examiner can observe the environment, parent–child interaction, and the child in a familiar setting. In fact, when assessment involves infants, toddlers, or preschool children, more information can usually be obtained from a home interview than from one conducted in a school or office setting (Bradley-Johnson, 1994).

Family needs, critical events, and family resources are areas of particular relevance for infants and toddlers with visual impairment (Bradley-Johnson, 1994). The Family Need Survey (Bailey & Simeonsson, 1988) is a 35-item parent questionnaire that assesses six areas in which the family might have need: information on the child's disability, support from others, help explaining the child's disability, help obtaining services, financial assistance, and help with family functioning. The parent responds to each item on a 3-point scale, with a rating of 3 indicating that help is definitely needed. In addition to completing the individual items, the parents are asked to list their five greatest needs as a family (Bradley-Johnson, 1994).

Bailey, Simeonsson, and their colleagues (1986) also developed the Critical Events Checklist. This instrument consists of eight items (four nondevelopmental and four developmental events) and is usually completed by the examiner as he or she interviews the parents. Situations frequently change, making monitoring and periodic use of the Critical Events Checklist necessary. The Family Resource Scale is a measure developed by Dunst and Leet (1987). This scale consists of 30 items that are completed by the parents and includes seven different factors, from basic nutrition to opportunities for growth (Bradley-Johnson, 1987).

Although the three areas just described are very important in the assessment of families of infant, toddlers, and preschool children, they can also be used with families of school-age children. There are no other general guidelines in the literature concerning developmental considerations for children of school age or older. However, as with typical children, the assessment process usually includes use of a wider variety of assessment tools and areas of assessment.

Elements of an Assessment Approach

The evaluator should recognize the limits of particular assessment tools, especially in the case of young children with severe visual loss (Bradley-Johnson, 1994). Due to such difficulties and rapid development, especially in the first few years of life, assessment at frequent intervals may be useful in tracking the child's progress. Cumulative records and trends in development over time should be used in making conclusions and recommendations.

Interviewing the child is an important complement to assessment with tests and measures. The evaluator can obtain the child's opinion about his or her own performance, areas of difficulty, perceptions of limitations placed on him or her by the environment, the child's attitude toward his or her visual loss, and his or her level of academic motivation.

Observations of the visually impaired child in the classroom are an integral part of the assessment process and can provide information on how the child functions at school, on his or her interactions with teachers and peers, and on the teachers' expectations. Observation of visually impaired children at home and school can then be compared to determine the best approaches to interacting with and teaching the child.

The examiner should review medical records to ascertain the type and extent of visual loss, visual acuity with and without correction, field of vision, degree of light perception, prescriptions, and restrictions on the use of the eye. These data can be useful in determining special lighting requirements or the use of visual aides and other environment modifications that might be useful in the assessment process. The evaluator should also gather data on functioning of other sensory modalities, especially hearing.

A functional visual assessment should be requested from a teacher or a consultant who is certified in working with visually impaired or blind children. The assessment involves observing the visually impaired child perform a variety of activities and routine tests. The scope of the observations depends on various factors, such as the age of the child. For the school-age child, the assessment includes evaluation of the most appropriate means of receiving information and the most efficient means of reading and writing. Information from the functional visual assessment is used in determining the optimal environment, procedures, and materials for classroom use, as well as for psychological evaluation. The functional visual assessment may also include recommendations for appropriate lighting, optimal viewing distance and print size, seating arrangement, and other modifications that facilitate use of functional vision (Bradley-Johnson, 1994).

Special Issues and Concerns

Only a limited number of tests and other assessment procedures are specifically designed for children with visual impairment and blindness. There is also little consensus as to which instruments should be used and how they should be adapted or modified for this population. Furthermore, few guidelines for assessment of children with visual impairments and blindness are commonly accepted by researchers and psychologists working in this field.

A number of factors may be responsible for the lack of consensus in assessing this population. One of the most significant factors may be the paucity of research on the growth and development of blind and visually impaired children. Without knowing developmental and general characteristics of the population for which the test is being developed, it is extremely difficult for researchers to develop and standardize valid and reliable assessment instruments (Scholl & Theodorou, 1989).

The heterogeneity of children with visual impairment also presents a problem. This heterogeneity is reflected in the time of onset of blindness or visual impairment, the degree of blindness or visual impairment, whether the visual loss is progressive or stable, and the frequent presence of additional disabilities that complicate development of test norms (Scholl & Theodorou, 1989).

The process of developing norms specific to this population is problematic (Hull & Mason, 1993). Thus tests standardized on typical children are frequently used, and evaluators should be cautious in interpreting assessment results based on such tests. The environment, learning experience, general life experience, and thus overall development of these children may differ from those of the normative group, making comparisons questionable at best and useless at worst. Comparison of test results of children with visual impairment to those of typical children may promote an assumption that the child with visual impairment is similar to children in the normative group. In addition, modifications such as differences in response styles, instructions, or test forms (such as using braille) violate standardization procedures and thus change interpretations of test results (Van Hasselt & Sisson, 1987).

One approach to circumventing some problems inherent in assessing children with visual impairment and blindness is to use information about the child from numerous sources and to use a variety of instruments to measure a wide range of behaviors. This process may include the use of standardized tests, as well as the use of criterion-referenced tests, curriculum-based tests, behavioral observations, and assessment of functional skills (Sisson & Van Hasselt, 1987). The use of multiple sources and instruments should be standard in assessment in general, but its importance is increased when the results are used to make decisions about treatment and educational recommendations for children with visual impairment and blindness.

The selection of tests and procedures to be utilized may sometimes depend on the referral question. However, it takes a qualified professional to select all of the appropriate instruments, to determine modifications to be made based on the characteristics of the child, and to know how to interpret the results to most accurately describe the child and his or her strengths and deficits. Van Hasselt and Sisson (1987) outline several important qualifications of the examiner. The person conducting the psychological evaluation should have knowledge of the impact of visual disorders across major areas of development. This is a prerequisite for appropriate interpretation of test results, especially in young children. The individual conducting the evaluation should also know how to guide a child with visual impairment and should be able to explain visual material to that child. The professional must formulate clear and specific questions to be addressed by the assessment. This may require clarification from referral sources, as well as from the individual and his or her parents. The examiner should also determine the amount of useful vision the child has and what materials he or she can see and can use functionally. The child should be familiar with tests that are available in braille, large print, or other forms that are appropriate for the individual child.

Hansen, Young, and Ulrey (1982) list six general principles that should be considered when assessing children with special educational needs. These include first evaluating the child over a period of time, perhaps over several weeks rather than in just one session. This permits observation of a wide variety of behaviors. Second, the child should be provided with sufficient time to explore and to adapt to the testing environment and material. Visually impaired children need longer to adapt to new sounds, smells, temperature, and strangers than sighted children. If braille or large print is used, extra time is also required, given that reading in these modes takes 2 to 2½ times longer than reading in normal print type. Children should be given an adequate amount of time to become familiar with each test object before a standardized response is expected. This may be accomplished through tactile exploration and manipulation of the objects. Third, when handing materials to the child, the examiner may find it helpful to explain that he or she will be handing the child something and then to touch the child's hand with the object or put the child's hand on the material and indicate its location. This prevents startling the child (Bradley-Johnson, 1994).

Fourth, the examiner should be aware of normal and dysfunctional behavior exhibited by visually impaired children. In particular, stereotyped responses, such as hand clapping, rocking, or eye poking, should be noted, as they may interfere with the testing situation. Hansen and his colleagues (1982) also recommend that the examiner be flexible in evaluating the child. Fifth, it may be more important to focus on the functional skills that the child has acquired and how he or she solves problems rather than on his or her performance on tests designed to measure abilities in sighted children. And sixth, supplemental use of systematic direct behavioral observations, both within the assessment setting and within the child's natural environment, are important components. Such observations can help the examiner to obtain a more complete picture of the child's strengths and weaknesses in all areas of functioning, as well as in the subsequent development of appropriate interaction and instructional strategies.

Bradley-Johnson (1994) suggests that examiners should consider giving results in terms of range of performance rather than to report single scores because many tests lack technical adequacy and because many other factors may affect the child's test performance. She also suggests that if the examiner has to administer an out-of-date test, it is useful to report the age of the test. This is important because inflated scores may be obtained with old norms.

DESCRIPTION OF SELECTED ASSESSMENT MEASURES

Table 11.1 lists measures that are used in assessing children with visual impairments. These instruments were selected based on age of test, frequency of use, and types of information gained from the measure. Table 11.1 is divided into three sections: tests for infants and toddlers; tests for preschoolers and early childhood; and tests for school-age children and adolescents. Tests with publication dates prior to 1978 were not included because the normative data may no longer be relevant. The reader is referred to Bradley-Johnson (1994) for more detailed information on these tests.

Strengths and Weaknesses of Commonly Used Tests

Although several tests or parts of tests are used with children with visual impairment or blindness, some are more appropriate than others for particular purposes (e.g., diagnosis, treatment, achievement, or educational planning). Selected tests from the table are reviewed below. These tests were selected for review based on the following criteria: popularity (frequency of usage), usefulness (or lack thereof) in obtaining important information, and adherence to standards for good technical accuracy.

The Batelle Developmental Inventory (Newborg, Stock, Wnek, Guidubaldi, & Svinicki, 1984) was designed to provide data to help in making decisions regarding diagnosis and eligibility for special educational services and to plan instructional programs. This test has

TABLE 11.1. Common Tests and Measurement Tools for Assessing Abilities and Achievement in Children with Visual Impairments

Measure author/publisher	Age/stage	Domain assessed	Format	Psychometric properties
		Tests for infants and young children		
Batelle Developmental Inventory (Newborg, Stock, Wnek, Guidubaldi, & Svinicki, 1984; DLM/Teaching Resources)	0–8 yr	Cognitive, communication, motor, adaptive, and personal–social	Scores for total test, domains, and subdomains given as percentiles, standard scores, and age-equivalents	• 4-week test–retest reliability for domains = .76–.99; BDI = .90–.9 • Interrater reliability for domains .85–1.0 • High correlation of BDI with Vineland Social Maturity Scale and Developmental Activities Screening Inventory • Adequate correlation with Stanford–Binet, WISC-R, and PPVT
Bayley Scales of Infant Development—Second Edition (Bayley, 1993; Psychological Corporation)	1–42 mo	Mental, motor, and infant behavior scales	• Item scored pass, fail, or other • Standard score for mental and motor scale	• Stability coefficients (1–2 week test–retest reliability) = .87 on mental scale, .78 on motor scale
Cognitive Abilities Scale (Bradley-Johnson, 1987; Pro-Ed)	2–3 yr	Language, reading, math, handwriting, enabling behaviors	Standard score for subtests, cognitive quotient	• 2 week test–retest for cognitive quotient = .90 for subtests = .69–.98 • Internal consistency r = .75–.94 for subtests, r = .90 or higher for higher cognitive quotient • Concurrent validity with K-ABC mental composite and achievement section of Stanford–Binet and TELD r = .59–.84 • Predictive validity with Stanford–Binet = .50; WISC-R = .52; TERA = .37; TEMA = .42; K-TEA Reading = .42; K-TEA Math = .50

(continued)

TABLE 11.1. *continued*

Measure author/publisher	Age/stage	Domain assessed	Format	Psychometric properties
Tests for infants and young children				
Revised Brigance Diagnostic Inventory of Early Development (Brigance, 1991; Curriculum Associates)	0–6 yr	Motor, self-help, speech/language, general knowledge comprehension, reading, math, social, emotional	Criterion-referenced test	Information not found
Carolina Curriculum for Infants and Toddlers with Special Needs—Second Edition (Johnson-Martin, Jens, & Attermeier, 1991; Brookes)	6 mo–2 yr	Cognition, communication, adaptation, motor	Scoring based on observation of caregiver playing with child for 15–20 minutes, direct talking, parent support	Information not found
Ordinal Scales of Psychological Development (Uzgiris & Hunt, 1989; University of Illinois Press)	0–2 yr	Cognitive development (Piagetian)	Items arranged in hierarchy of development according to sensorimotor period	Interrater reliability r = .85–.99 Test–retest r = .88–.96 Subtest intercorrelations r = .70–.92
Tests for preschoolers and early childhood				
Informal Assessment of Developmental Skills for Visually Handicapped Students: Part 2. Informal Assessment of Developmental Skills for Younger Visually Handicapped and Multihandicapped Children (Swallow, Mangold, & Mangold, 1978; American Foundation for the Blind)	Infants, preschoolers	Self-help psychomotor, social-emotional, language, and cognition	Checklist with 4–9 descriptions per item	None available
Oregon Project for Visually Impaired and Blind Preschool Children (5th ed.; Anderson, Boigon, & Davis, 1986; Jackson County Education Service District)	0–6 yr	Cognitive, language, social, vision, compensatory, self-help, and motor	Results measured in terms of skills and in percent of skills mastered for each area tested	• Reliability: no data available • Validity: items based on review of literature on children in Southern Oregon Program for Visually Impaired and input from preschool teachers

	Age	Domain	Description	Psychometric Properties
Basic School Skills Inventory—Diagnostic (Hammill & Leigh, 1983; Pro-Ed)	4 yr to 6 yr, 11 mo	Daily living skills, language, reading, math, classroom behavior	• Scored by someone who has observed child in class over period of time • Standard score, percentile, and total score	• Reliability: no test–retest data • Internal consistency: $r = .85-.90$ for daily living skills $r = .81-.93$ for spoken language $r = .93-.97$ for classroom behavior • Criterion-related validity with teacher ratings $r = .35$ daily living skills $r = .38$ spoken language $r = .37$ classroom behavior • Construct validity: $r = .34-.83$
Weschler Preschool and Primary Scale of Intelligence (WPPSI; Weschler, 1967; Psychological Corporation)	4 yr–6 yr, 6 mo	Cognition	• 11 subtest • Verbal and Performance Scale • Full Scale • Results in terms of intelligence quotients and scaled scores for subtests	• Test–retest reliability: $r = .60-.89$ for Verbal subtests $r = .86$ Verbal IQ • Internal consistency ranged from .77 to .88 on verbal subtests and from .93 to .95 on Verbal IQ • Intercorrelation of subtests on verbal scale range from .46-.60. Average intercorrelation of Verbal IQ and Verbal subtests range from .62 to .73 • Concurrent validity: Correlation with Stanford–Binet Verbal scale range from .39 to .63 and with Pictorial Test of Intelligence .22-.56

(continued)

TABLE 11.1. *continued*

Measure author/publisher	Age/stage	Domain assessed	Format	Psychometric properties
		Tests for school-age children and adolescents		
Social Skills Rating System (Gresham & Elliott, 1990; American Guidance Service)	Preschool–high school	Social skills, problem behavior, academic competence	• Standard score and percentile rank for each domain • Behavior level for subscore include: fewer, average, or more than average • Items rated on frequency and importance of behavior by rater on scale from 0–2	• 4-week test–retest reliability: Social Skills: $r = .85$ (teacher form); $r = .87$ (parent form); $r = .84$ (student form); Problem Behavior: $r = .84$ (teacher form); $r = .65$ (parent form) Academic Competence: $r = .93$ (teacher form) • Internal Consistency: Parent Form: $r = .65–.90$ Social Skills; $r = .51–.87$ Problem Behavior Teacher Form: $r = .86–.94$ Social Skills; $r = .74–.89$ for Academic Competence Student Form: $r = .68$ Social Skills • Construct validity: all scales correlated satisfactorily • Criterion-related validity with Social Behavior Checklist, Harter Teacher Rating Scale, and Piers-Harris Self-Concept Scale is acceptable
Test of Language Development (TELD)—Primary (2nd ed.; Newcomer & Hammill, 1988; Pro-Ed)	4 yr–6 yr, 11 mo	Receptive and expressive language	• 7 subtests • Results in terms of quotients for overall spoken language and composites of listening, speaking, semantics, syntax, and phonology	• 5-day test–retest reliability ranges from .93 to .98 for subtests • Internal consistency ranges from .82 to .95 • Criterion validity for tests not requiring vision: $r = .67–.76$ WISC with oral vocabulary $r = .55–.66$ Northwestern Syntax Screening Test—Expressive and Sentence Imitation (see Bradley-Johnson, 1994, for more)

Blind Learning Aptitude Test (Newland, 1971; University of Illinois Press)	6–12 yr	Cognition	• Six scales of nonverbal problems (total of 49 items) • Results in form of learning quotient and test age	• Test-retest reliability $r = .87$ • Internal consistency $r = .93$ • Concurrent validity with WISC Verbal scale $r = .71$
Detroit Test of Learning Aptitude (3rd ed.; Hammill, 1991; Pro-Ed)	6 yr–17 yr, 11 mo	Cognition	• 4 of 11 subtests are verbal and do not require vision • Results in form of standard scores, percentiles, and age equivalents	• 2-week test–retest reliability for verbal tests $r = >.89$ • Internal consistency $r = >.85$ • Moderate to high concurrent validity with Kaufman Assessment Battery for Children, Woodcock–Johnson Psycho-Educational Battery and Scholastic Aptitude Scale
Diagnostic Achievement Battery (2nd ed.; Newcomer, 1990; Pro-Ed)	6 yr–14 yr, 11 mo	Educational achievement	Subscales: Reading, math, written expression, and oral language. Oral language only subtest not requiring vision (includes story comprehension and speaking). Results in form of standard scores and percentile for subscales and composite scores	• Test-retest reliability $r = .94$ for listening composite; $r = .95$ for speaking composite • Internal consistency for listening subtests $r = >.85$ • Internal consistency for speaking subtests $r = >.85$ • Concurrent validity for Language Development—Primary and Intermediate • Construct validity: low to moderate correlation with Detroit Test of Learning Aptitude—Primary and WISC-R
Diagnostic Reading Scales (Spache, 1981; CTB/McGraw-Hill)	Mid–1st to mid-7th grade level	Reading skills and listening comprehension	• Braille and large print available • Grade level used to describe results	• Test-retest reliability at 2 to 8 weeks $r = .89$ • Grade levels highly correlated with student's mean grade in school, assigned reading level, and mean grade equivalent on standardized group achievement test results

(continued)

239

TABLE 11.1. *continued*

Measure author/publisher	Age/stage	Domain assessed	Format	Psychometric properties
Tests for school-age children and adolescents				
Test of Language Development—Second Edition (Hammill & Newcomer, 1988; Pro-Ed)	8 yr, 6 mo to 12 yr, 11 mo	Receptive and expressive language	• Six subtests • No vision required • Results described in terms of quotients, composite, and standard score	• 1-week test–retest reliability $r = .83–.92$ • Internal consistency for composite $r = >.91$ • Criterion-related validity moderate to high with Test of Adolescent Language
Test of Adolescent Language (2nd ed.; Hammill, Brown, Larsen, & Wiederholt, 1987; Pro-Ed)	12 yr to 18 yr, 5 mo	Language	• Four sections • Results described in terms of percentile and standard scores	• 2-week test–retest reliability $.85–.99$ • Internal Consistency $r = >.89$ for speaking quotient • Moderate correlation with PPVT
Wechsler Intelligence Scale for Children—Third Edition (Wechsler, 1991; Psychological Corporation)	6 yr–16 yr, 11 mo	Cognition (intelligence)	• Consists of 13 subscales; only verbal scores can be administered because no vision is required • Results described in terms of quotients, scaled scores, percentiles, and age equivalents	• Test–retest reliability: Verbal subscales $r = .80–.89$; Verbal IQ $r = .90–.93$ • Interrater reliability $r = .90$ • High construct validity based on factor analytic studies and correlation of the results with other intelligence tests
Wechsler Adult Intelligence Scale—Revised (Wechsler, 1981; Psychological Corporation)	16–74 yr	Cognition (intelligence)	• Only verbal subtests administered because no vision is required on these subtests • Results described in terms of standard scores, quotients, and percentiles	• No test–retest data for ages 16–25 • Internal consistency for Verbal score for ages 16–19 $r = .70–.96$ • Good correlation with other intelligence tests

Instrument	Population	Format	Reliability/Validity
Basic Reading Rate Scale: Braille Edition (Duckworth & Caton, 1986; American Printing House for the Blind)	Beginning (2nd grade) braille readers to accomplished braille readers	Braille reading rate	• Criterion-referenced	• Correlation with reading achievement levels; $r = .71$
Braille Unit Recognition Battery: Diagnostic Test of Grade 2 Literacy Braille (Caton, Duckworth, & Ranken, 1985; American Printing House for the Blind)	Designed for Grades 3–12, can be used for younger children and adults	Reading braille	• Items presented orally • Multiple-choice format (4–5 choices) • Criterion referenced	• Moderate correlation on various parts of battery
Brigance Diagnostic Comprehensive Inventory of Basic Skills (Brigance, 1983; Curriculum Associates) APH Tactile Supplement (American Printing House for the Blind, 1992)	Kindergarten through 9th grade	• Educational achievement	• Criterion referenced • Results in terms of skills learned and those that need to be taught next • American Printing House for braille readers	Reliability: skills assessed three times • Good content validity in testing skills taught in the classroom
Informal Assessment of Developmental Skills for Visually Handicapped Students (School-Age Section; Swallow, Swallow, & Mangold, 1978; American Foundation for the Blind)	None specified	• Academic performance • Functional skills (i.e., mobility and orientation)	• Series of checklists • Criterion referenced	• No data available

241

TABLE 11.1. continued

Measure author/publisher	Age/stage	Domain assessed	Format	Psychometric properties
		Tests for school-age children and adolescents		
Vineland Adaptive Behavior Scales—Expanded (Sparrow, Balla, & Cicchetti, 1984; American Guidance Service)	0–18 yr	Adaptive behavior	• Domains assessed include communication, daily living skills, socialization, motor skills, and mal-adaptive behavior • Results expressed as standard scores, percentile ranks, standards, adaptive levels, and age equivalents • Caregiver interviews • Items recorded 0–2, Don't know, no opportunity	• 2–4 weeks test–retest reliability across domains; $r = .80$–.98 • Internal consistency $r = .83$–.97 for domains $r = .94$–.99 for Adaptive Behavior Composite • Moderate to high correlation with other adaptive measures
Matson Evaluation of Social Skills with Youngsters (MESSY; Matson, Rotatori, & Helsel, 1983)	9–22	Social skills	• Likert scale • Self-report and teacher report • Large print and audio cassettes as alternate forms	• Internal reliability $r = >.78$ on both forms
Child Behavior Checklist (Achenbach & Edelbrock, 1983; University of Vermont)	0–18 yr	Psychological and social adjustments	• Parent form • Teacher form • Youth self-report form • Items rated on a 3-point scale	

suggestions and supplementary material to be used with children with visual impairment or blindness. Bradley-Johnson (1994) notes that this measure has excellent reliability data. However, due to the small number of items, many subdomains and domain scores may be meaningless, especially for children with little or no vision. The strength of this inventory is in describing how many of the items can be adapted for children with little or no vision, though not all items can be adapted. In addition, the age-referenced items can be used to describe a range of performance for children with little or no vision. This information can be used for instructional planning, and a particular strength is the personal–social domain.

The Bayley Scales of Infant Development—Second Edition (BSID-2; Bayley, 1993) are often used with children because so few tests are available at this young age. The BSID-2 is not particularly useful for describing a performance range for a child with severe visual impairments. It can be very helpful in identifying limited functioning in very young children because some of the items on the Mental scale and many items from the Motor scale demand visual guidance, such as visually directed reaching. This behavior is fully functional in the typical infant by about 6 months of age. Changes in visual-motor functioning has been documented through the longitudinal use of the BSID (Leguire, Fellows, & Bier, 1990).

The Revised Brigance Diagnostic Inventory of Early Development (Brigance, 1991) is a criterion-referenced test designed to provide information for instructional planning. No adaptations are suggested for visually impaired children. The American Printing House for the Blind has developed a tactile supplement for the inventory (Duckworth & Stratton, 1992) that provides alternate procedures and materials for items involving visual stimuli. Alternate directions and suggestions for eliciting behaviors from children with little or no vision are also provided.

The Carolina Curriculum for Infants and Toddlers with Special Needs—Second Edition (Johnson-Martin, Jens, & Attermeier, 1991) is a curriculum-based measure to assess skills that are typically learned by children without disabilities from birth to 2 years of age. This measure is useful in planning intervention programs and monitoring children's progress. In addition, many adaptations for children with little or no vision are presented in the manual. Administration of this test can be quite time-consuming (Bradley-Johnson, 1994).

The Oregon Project for Visually Impaired and Blind Preschool Children (Anderson, Boigon, & Davis, 1986) is a curriculum-based inventory designed for children with special needs that can help in providing information on instructional planning and monitoring for young visually impaired children. This instrument is not as comprehensive as the Revised Brigance Diagnostic Inventory of Early Development. Combining it with administration of the Revised Brigance may provide more detailed information to aid with instructional planning (Bradley-Johnson, 1994).

The Weschler Preschool and Primary Scales of Intelligence (WPPSI; Weschler, 1967) are not particularly useful in assessing youngsters with moderate to severe visual impairments because this test involves the use of many visual stimuli. In addition, there are no norms for visually impaired children.

The Social Skills Rating System (Gresham & Elliott, 1990) has three versions, one for teachers, one for parents, and one that students can complete independently. Only the teacher and parent forms are reliable for use in making decisions pertaining to eligibility for services (Bradley-Johnson, 1994). These measures can provide information for both instructional planning and measuring the social validity of interventions. No adaptations are necessary for children and adolescents who are visually impaired or blind.

The Wechsler Intelligence Scales (Wechsler, 1974, 1981, 1991) are widely used for children with visual impairments (Groenveld & James, 1992; Sisson & Van Hasselt, 1987; Stuart, 1995). It is generally acceptable to administer only the Verbal scale subtests because they do not require vision and yield a separate Verbal IQ score. For children with very limited or no vision, special cards with raised drawings are needed on the arithmetic subtest (Bradley-Johnson, 1994). Although validity data are good on this measure, normative data are not available for children who are visually impaired or blind, and the norms are dated. Variability between subtest scores cannot be interpreted as evidence of a learning disability as it might be in typical children because variability in subtest scores is the rule with visually impaired children (Van Hasselt & Sisson, 1987).

The Blind Learning Aptitude Test (Newland, 1971) was designed to measure learning potential. Designed specifically for children with visual impairments or blindness, it has been found to yield useful information (Mason, 1991) with results associated with braille reading skills and measures of intelligence and achievement (Baker, Koenig, Alan, & Sowell, 1995).

The Diagnostic Reading Scales (Spache, 1981) has a braille transcription and a large-type edition available. This test is the most technically adequate, norm-referenced measure that is currently used for determining reading achievement levels. It assesses actual reading levels by using passages instead of just word lists. The standardization group included no visually impaired students.

The Vineland Adaptive Behavior Scales (Sparrow, Balla, & Cicchetti, 1984) are widely used for planning individual programs for adaptive behavior. Although this measure has very good psychometric properties, problems may arise when it is used with children with visual impairment or blindness. One such problem is that many items require vision, and so the child may be penalized on these items. In addition, as with any interview measure, this test may not yield accurate results because it is based on subjective rather than objective data (Bradley-Johnson, 1994).

As can be seen from the table of selected measures, no personality or emotional assessments are included. The reason for the exclusion of tests such as the Beureuter Personality Inventory (cited in Van Hasselt & Sisson, 1987) is that these tests are quite old, and the norms are not valid. There is a lack of data on the use of the Minnesota Multiphasic Personality Inventory with adolescents with visual impairments. Therefore, further research must be conducted on personality characteristics and emotional development of children and adolescents with visual impairment. Development of a test to measure these characteristics in visually impaired and blind individuals would fill a big gap and provide useful information for diagnosis and treatment of emotional problems.

SUMMARY AND CONCLUSIONS

Children with blindness or visual impairments compose a small but not insubstantial proportion of the population. The disorders that cause visual impairments are numerous and are expected to continue to influence child development for the foreseeable future. It is therefore likely that children with visual disorders will continue to appear for developmental evaluations to determine their psychological, educational, emotional, and social needs.

The evaluation protocol for assessment of children with visual impairments must address the direct and indirect developmental impacts of the visual loss and should represent views of the child in the settings in which he or she must function. Selection of evaluation tools must take into account both the developmental domains relevant to the child's functioning and the applicability of the instruments to children with visual loss.

REFERENCES

Achenbach, T., & Edelbrock, C. (1983). *Child Behavior Checklist and Revised Child Behavior Profile*. Burlington: University of Vermont, Department of Psychiatry.

American Printing House for the Blind. (1992). *Brigance Diagnostic Inventory of Early Development: APH Tactile Supplement*. Louisville, KY: American Printing House.

Anderson, S., Boigon, S., & Davis, K. (1986). *The Oregon Project for Visually Impaired and Blind Preschool Children* (5th ed.). Medford, OR: Jackson County Education Service District.

Bailey, D. B., & Simeonsson, R. J. (1988). *Family assessment in early intervention*. Columbus, OH: Merrill.

Bailey, D. B., Simeonsson, R. J., Winton, P. J., Huntington, G. S., Comfort, M., Isbell, P., O'Donnell, K. L., & Helm, J. M. (1986). Family-focused intervention: A functional model for planning, implementing, and evaluating individualized family services in early intervention. *Journal of the Division of Early Childhood, 10*, 156–171.

Baker, C. P., Koenig, A. J., Alan, J., & Sowell, V. M. (1995). Relationship of the Blind Learning Aptitude Test to braille reading skills. *Journal of Visual Impairment and Blindness, 89*(5), 440-447.

Batshaw, M. L., & Perret, Y. M. (Eds.). (1993). *Children with disabilities: A medical primer*. Baltimore: Brookes.

Bayley, N. (1993). *Bayley Scales of Infant Development—Second Edition*. San Antonio, TX: Psychological Corporation.

Bradley-Johnson, S. (1987). *Cognitive Ability Scale*. Austin, TX: Pro-Ed.

Bradley-Johnson, S. (1994). *Psychoeducational assessment of students who are visually impaired or blind: Infancy through high school*. Austin, TX: Pro-Ed.

Brambring, M., & Troester, H. (1992). On the stability of stereotyped behaviors in infants and preschoolers. *Journal of Visual Impairment and Blindness, 86*(2), 105–110.

Brigance, A. (1983). *Brigance Diagnostic Comprehensive Inventory of Basic Skills*. North Billerica, MA: Curriculum Associates.

Brigance, A. (1991). *Revised Brigance Diagnostic Inventory of Early Development*. North Billerica, MA: Curriculum Associates.

Buncic, J. R. (1987). The blind child. *Pediatric Clinics of North America, 34*, 1403–1414.

Duckworth, B. J., & Caton, H. (1986). *Basic Reading Rate Scale: Braille edition or large type*. Louisville, KY: American Printing House for the Blind.

Dunst, C. J., & Leet, H. E. (1987). Measuring the adequacy of resources in households with young children. *Child Care, Health, and Development, 13*, 111–125.

Finn, D. M., & Fewell, R. R. (1994). The use of play assessment to examine the development of communication skills in children who are deaf-blind. *Journal of Visual Impairment and Blindness, 88*(4), 349–356.

Foster, A. (1988). Childhood blindness. *Eye, 2*(Suppl.), S27–S36.

Fraiberg, S. (1977). *Insights from the blind*. New York: Basic Books.

Gallo, J. E., & Lennerstrand, G. (1991). A population-based study of ocular abnormalities in premature children aged 5 to 10 years. *American Journal of Ophthalmology, 14*, 135–140.

Gresham, F. M., & Elliott, S. N. (1990). *Social Skills Rating System*. Circle Pines, MN: American Guidance Service.

Groenveld, M., & James, J. E. (1992). Intelligence profiles of low vision and blind children. *Journal of Visual Impairment and Blindness, 86*(1), 68–71.

Hammill, D. D. (1991). *Detroit Test of Learning Aptitude* (3rd ed.). Austin, TX: Pro-Ed.

Hammill, D. D., Brown, V. L, Larsen, S. C., & Wiederholt, J. L. (1987). *Test of Adolescent Language* (2nd ed.). Austin, TX: Pro-Ed.

Hammill, D. D., & Leigh, J. F. (1983). *Basic School Skills Inventory—Diagnostic*. Austin, TX: Pro-Ed.

Hammill, D. D., & Newcomer, P. L. (1988). *Test of Language Development—Second Edition: A multidimensional approach to assessment*. Austin, TX: Pro-Ed.

Hansen, R., Young, J., & Ulrey, G. (1982). Assessment considerations with the visually handicapped child. In G. Ulrey & S. Rogers (Eds.), *Psychological assessment of handicapped infants and young children* (pp. 108–114). New York: Thieme-Stratton.

Hull, T., & Mason, H. (1993). Issues in standardizing psychometric tests for children who are blind. *Journal of Visual Impairment and Blindness, 87*(5), 149–150.

Johnson-Martin, N. M., Jens, K. G., & Attermeier, S. M. (1991). *The Carolina Curriculum for Infants and Toddlers with Special Needs.* Baltimore: Brookes.

Kirchner, C. (1983). Special education for visually handicapped children: A critique of data on numbers served and costs. *Journal of Visual Impairment and Blindness, 77*, 219–223.

Kirchner, C. (1989). National estimates of prevalence and demographics of children with visual impairments. In M. Wang, M. Reynolds, & H. Herbert (Eds.), *Handbook of special education, research, and practice* (Vol. 3, pp. 135–154). Oxford, England: Pergamon Press.

Leguire, L. E., Fellows, R. R., & Bier, G. (1990). Bayley Mental Scale of Infant Development and visually impaired children. *Journal of Visual Impairment and Blindness, 84*(8), 400–404.

Mason, H. L. (1991). Use of the Blind Learning Aptitude Test with children in England and Wales and the United States. *Journal of Visual Impairment and Blindness, 85*(8), 335–337.

Matson, J. L., Rotatori, A. F., & Helsel, W. J. (1983). Development of a rating scale to measure social skills in children: The Matson Evaluation of Social Skills with Youngsters (MESSY). *Behavior Research and Therapy, 21*, 335–340.

McConachie, H. R., & Moore, V. (1994). Early Expressive Language of Severely Visually Impaired Children. *Developmental Medicine and Child Neurology, 36*(3), 230–240.

National Society for the Prevention of Blindness. (1980). *Visual problems in the U.S.: Facts and figures.* New York: Author.

National Society for the Prevention of Blindness. (1996). *N.S.P.B. fact book: Estimated statistics on blindness and visual problems.* New York: Author.

Nelson, L. B., Calhoun, J. H., & Harley, R. D. (1991). *Pediatric ophthalmology* (3rd ed.). Philadelphia: Saunders.

Newborg, J., Stock, J. R., Wnek, L., Guidubaldi, J., & Svinicki, J. (1984). *Battelle Developmental Inventory.* Allen, TX: DLM/Teaching Resources.

Newcomer, P. L. (1990). *Diagnostic Achievement Battery* (2nd ed.). Austin, TX: Pro-Ed.

Newcomer, P. L., & Hammill, D. D. (1988). *Test of Language Development—Primary* (2nd ed.). Austin, TX: Pro-Ed.

Newland, T. E. (1971). *Blind Learning Aptitude Test.* Urbana: University of Illinois Press.

O'Donnell, L. M., & Livingston, R. L. (1991). Active exploration of the environment by young children with low vision: A review of the literature. *Journal of Visual Impairment and Blindness, 74*, 142–149.

Olson, M. (1987). Early intervention for children with visual impairment. In M. Guralnick & F. Bennett (Eds.), *The effectiveness of early intervention for at-risk and handicapped children* (pp. 297–324). Orlando, FL: Academic Press.

Pagon, R. A. (1988). Retinitis pigmentosa. *Survey of Ophthalmology, 33*, 137–177.

Scholl, G. T. (1990). Education of visually handicapped children and youth. In M. Wang, M. Reynolds, & H. Walberg (Eds.), *Special education: Research and practice synthesis of findings* (pp. 161–170). Oxford, England: Pergamon Press.

Scholl, G. T, & Theodorou, E. (1989). Assessment of blind and handicapped children and youth. In M. Wang, M. Reynolds, & H. Herbert (Eds.), *Handbook of special education: Research and practice* (Vol. 3, pp. 1189–203). Oxford, England: Pergamon Press.

Sisson, L. A., & Van Hasselt, V. B. (1987). Visual impairment. In V. Van Hasselt & M. Hersen (Eds.), *Psychological evaluation of the developmentally and physically disabled* (pp. 115–153). New York: Plenum Press.

Spache, G. (1981). *Diagnostic Reading Scales.* Monterey, CA: CTB/McGraw-Hill.

Sparrow, S. S., Balla, D. A., & Cicchetti, D. V. (1984). *Vineland Adaptive Behavior Scales—Expanded or Survey Edition.* Circle Pines, MN: American Guidance Service.

Stuart, I. (1995). Spatial orientation and congenital blindness. *Journal of Visual Impairment and Blindness, 89*(2), 129–141.

Swallow, R., Mangold, S., & Mangold, P. (1978). *Informal assessment of skills for visually handicapped students.* New York: American Foundation for the Blind.

Tedder, N. E., Warden, K., & Sikka, A. (1993). Prelanguage communication of students who are deaf-blind and have other severe impairments. *Journal of Visual Impairment and Blindness, 87*(8), 302–307.

U.S. Department of Education. (1992). *14th annual report to Congress on the implementation of the Individuals with Disabilities Education Act*. Washington, DC: Office of Special Education Programs.

Uzgiris, I. C., & Hunt, J. M. (1989). *Assessment in infancy: Ordinal Scales of Psychological Development*. Urbana: University of Illinois Press.

Valentine, P. H., Jackson, J. C., Kalina, R. E., & Woodrum, D. E. (1989). Increased survival of low birth weight infants: Impact on the incidence of retinopathy of prematurity. *Pediatrics, 84*, 442–445.

Vander Kolk, C. J. (1987). Psychosocial assessment of visually impaired persons. In B. Heller, L. Flohr, & L. Zegan (Eds.), *Psychosocial interventions with sensorially disabled persons* (pp. 33–52). Orlando, FL: Grune & Stratton.

Van Hasselt, V. B. (1983). Social adaptations for the blind. *Clinical Psychology Review, 3*, 87–102.

Van Hasselt, V. B., Herson, M., & Kazdin, A. E. (1985). Assessment of social skills in visually-handicapped adolescents. *Behaviour Research and Therapy, 23*(1), 53–63.

Van Hasselt, V. B., & Sisson, L. A. (1987). Visual impairment. In C. Frame & J. Matson (Eds.), *Handbook of assessment in child psychopathology: Applied issues in diagnosis and treatment evaluation* (pp. 593–618). New York: Plenum Press.

Warren, D. H. (1989). Implications of visual impairments for child development. In M. Wang, M. Reynolds, & H. Herbert (Eds.), *Handbook of special education: Research and practice* (Vol. 3, pp. 155–172). Oxford, England: Pergamon Press.

Wechsler, D. (1967). *Manual for the Wechsler Preschool and Primary Scale of Intelligence*. San Antonio, TX: Psychological Corporation.

Wechsler, D. (1974). *Manual for the Wechsler Intelligence Scale for Children—Revised*. San Antonio, TX: Psychological Corporation.

Wechsler, D. (1981). *Manual for the Wechsler Adult Intelligence Scale—Revised*. San Antonio, TX: Psychological Corporation.

Wechsler, D. (1991). *Manual for the Wechsler Intelligence Scale for Children—Third Edition*. San Antonio, TX: Psychological Corporation.

12

ASSESSMENT OF CHILDREN
WHO ARE DEAF OR HARD
OF HEARING

RUNE J. SIMEONSSON
TOVAH M. WAX
KATHLEEN WHITE

Early on, it was obvious that Ann was not hearing sounds, and later, she was found to have a 25- to 35-decibel loss at 18 months of age. She was fitted with hearing aids at age 21 months, and her parents were expecting her to function in a typical auditory speech environment. Ann was administered a developmental assessment when she was 29 months old. The measure revealed her receptive language functioning to be estimated at the 12-month age equivalent and expressive functioning at the 8-month level. At 36 months of age, Ann's expressive and receptive skills were estimated to be the age equivalent of 18–20 months and 20–22 months, respectively. Given that Ann had no exposure to sign language, a follow-up developmental assessment when Ann was 3½ years old focused on the administration of nonverbal portions of the Bayley and McCarthy scales, complemented by systematic observation and an interview with Ann's mother. Ann is now 5 years of age, and further assessment is needed to estimate future educational planning.

Children like Ann who are deaf or hard of hearing present with unique and demanding assessment challenges. Perhaps with the exception of children diagnosed as autistic, there is no other subgroup for which use of auditory/oral communication is limited or not functional. Substantive differences in the experiential backgrounds and linguistic acquisition of deaf and hard-of-hearing children, compared with those of children with normal hearing, provides the basis for considering them a minority group characterized by a bicultural identity (Holcomb, 1997).

In the context of this bicultural identity, English is a second language with about one-half million deaf and hard-of-hearing persons in the United States communicating in American Sign Language (ASL; Anonymous, 1997). In the context of changing demographics, it is important to recognize trilingual or tricultural identities, such as those of Latino students (Walker-Vann, 1998). Clinical assessment of deaf and hard-of-hearing children mandates a thorough understanding of the linguistic and cultural factors that could influence interpretation of findings. The purpose of this chapter is to describe the nature of hearing and to identify issues pertinent to clinical assessment with this population. The philosophy of total communication (TC) stipulates that any and all methods that facilitate communication should be used, including any effective combination of oral/aural and sign language communication. A review of selected measures for various domains of development and the implications of assessment for planning and implementing interventions are also discussed.

OVERVIEW OF HEARING IMPAIRMENT

The nature of hearing impairment can be defined in terms of type, degree, and age at onset. Audiologically, the term "hearing impairment" can be used to define any hearing loss, whereas the term "deaf" usually describes hearing loss profound enough to render unaided speech reception useless. Conductive hearing loss is typically associated with abnormalities in the middle ear, such as structural damage, infections, or excessive fluid, that block transmission of sound vibrations from outer to inner ear. Sensorineural impairment refers to structural damage to the auditory nerve and receptors. The mixed type of hearing impairment implies both a conductive and a sensorineural basis for hearing loss. The degree of hearing loss, measured in decibels, ranges from mild to profound. Almost half (45%) of deaf and hard-of-hearing students enrolled in special education programs are diagnosed with profound hearing loss, and another 21% are diagnosed as having a severe hearing loss (Meadow, 1983). The remaining third have losses from minimal to the moderate/severe range.

In regard to etiological factors, for about 50% of deaf and hard-of-hearing students there is a genetic origin, and for the remaining 50% the cause is unknown (Lindhout, Frets, & Neirmeijer, 1991). According to Meadow (1983), approximately 76.5% of students enrolled in special education programs were reported to have congenital hearing loss, and hearing loss was reportedly acquired within the first year of life for another 8% of these children. Approximately 15% of children sustained hearing loss acquired 1 year or more after birth. Major contributors include genetic factors, infections, ototoxic medications (e.g., the "mycin" family of antibiotics), trauma, and other as yet unknown influences.

Children who are deaf or hard of hearing cannot be considered a homogeneous population, because the development of language, cognition, and thought is so intimately related to the primary method of communication (Quigley & Paul, 1984). For some children educated with oral/aural methods, English becomes internalized as their primary medium for thought, whereas children educated through manual communication methods tend to internalize sign language representations as primary linguistic mediators. Neuropsychological research has shown that deaf participants who use oral/aural communication show lateralization favoring the right hemisphere in perceiving both verbal and nonverbal materials, whereas those who use total communication methods show no such lateralization. Additionally, participants in the former group tended to use auditory codes more frequently in short-term memory tasks; by contrast, those in the latter group tended to rely on finger spelling for short-term memory tasks and also performed better on tests of spatial memory but poorer on tests of sequential memory than children with normal hearing (Rodda, Buranyi, Cumming, & Muendel-Atherstone, 1985).

Families in which a child has been diagnosed deaf or hard of hearing are faced with a multitude of choices regarding methods of communication and education, including oral and aural approaches, cued speech, the Rochester method, ASL, and varieties of contact sign language communication systems, including what have been described as manually coded English (MCE), seeing exact English (SEE), and pidgin signed English (PSE; see, e.g., Lucas & Valli, 1993.)

Most educational programs that subscribe to the philosophy of total communication use some system involving contact signing, such as MCE, which uses a combination of ASL vocabulary, finger spelling, and English grammar structure. Although all MCE systems use primarily ASL signs and appear very similar to the casual observer, there are some differences, particularly in the treatment of complex and compound words. Because MCE conforms to the syntactic structure of spoken and written English, the acquisition of reading and writing skills will presumably be easier for the deaf or hard-of-hearing child (Knell & Klonoff, 1983). The Rochester method uses no signs but combines finger spelling with expressive and receptive speech, with all words spelled and used in English word order.

ASSESSMENT OBJECTIVES

The characteristics of deaf and hard-of-hearing children described previously define major objectives for assessment of cognitive, communicative, and personal characteristics essential for planning instructional and other interventions that promote development. These objectives can be framed as addressing the following three discrepancies that characterize performance and functioning of deaf and hard-of-hearing children.

Cognitive Competency and Achievement Discrepancy

One of the salient issues in the assessment of a deaf or hard-of-hearing child involves the distinction between cognitive ability and competence or achievement. Often, in an apparently paradoxical finding, the measured nonverbal IQ of deaf or hard-of-hearing children may be in the normal range even though their achievement scores reflect substantial deficits when compared with similar score patterns of hearing peers (Tomlinson-Keasey & Kelley, 1978). A central purpose for the assessment of many deaf and hard-of-hearing children should thus be the identification of characteristics associated with discrepancies between ability and effective learning and achievement.

Cognitive and Linguistic Competence Discrepancy

A second major issue pertains to the differentiation of linguistic and cognitive competence in assessment. The distinction between these two domains is important, because the performances of deaf and hard-of-hearing children on tests that are verbal in nature or orientation are likely to be interpreted in terms of language problems rather than intellectual ability (Sullivan & Vernon, 1979).

Cognitive-Linguistic Competency and Personal-Social Functioning Discrepancy

Because responses of deaf and hard-of-hearing children or adolescents on measures of personal and social functioning may often be interpreted as deviant or pathological rather than merely reflecting difficulties with the instruments' linguistic demands, it is also important to untangle the roles of cognitive and linguistic competency and personal and social functioning during assessment with this population. Caution should be exercised in the use of personal-social assessment instruments in that difficulties in reading and other linguistic factors may confound the results from these tests and lead to erroneous attributions. In other cases, findings of behavioral and communicative problems in deaf and hard-of-hearing children may be difficult to distinguish from those in children diagnosed with other developmental disabilities.

SPECIAL ISSUES IN CLINICAL ASSESSMENT OF CHILDREN WITH HEARING IMPAIRMENT

Assessment of deaf and hard-of-hearing children and adolescents requires not only a recognition of characteristics such as etiology, age of onset, and history, but also additional knowledge about cultural identity and preferred mode of communication (Anonymous, 1997), the confounding effects of additional disabilities, and the developmental and psychosocial experiences of the children and their families.

Communication Issues

An essential prerequisite for assessing deaf and hard-of-hearing children is the establishment of a maximally effective communication process between examiner and examinee. Although the communication preference(s) of the child should be taken into account, the receptive language capacity of deaf and hard-of-hearing children trained in oral/aural methods remains limited (Sullivan & Vernon, 1979), and specific cautions should be observed when assessment is being conducted with a child using primarily oral or aural communication methods. The examiner should arrange to sit in front of and within 2 to 3 feet of the child, avoid glare, and secure the child's attention. Speech should be distinct, but the examiner should not exaggerate lip movements. Obstructions of the examiner's face (such as a beard) or mouth (such as gum) should be minimized or eliminated. Children who are fitted for—and habitually use—hearing aids, cochlear implants, or other assistive listening devices (e.g., Phonic Ear) should be encouraged to wear them. Further, it is important to have hearing aids or cochlear implant program devices checked immediately prior to the test administration and to assure they are set to the proper frequency. In situations in which assistive listening devices are being used, the examiner should wear the microphone about 6 inches from the mouth and take care to control extraneous noise in the assessment environment, as it may be distracting to the child (Sullivan & Vernon, 1979).

In addition to facing the challenges presented by oral/aural approaches with deaf and hard-of-hearing children, a clinician may see children who use primarily sign language communication systems (Stanfield & Veltri, 1987). In these cases, consideration must be given to the child's linguistic familiarity with the spoken-written-read English language and the accuracy or faithfulness of translation. Linguistic unfamiliarity with the material and the fact that many language-based test items are essentially impossible to translate are also problems (Brauer, Braden, Pollard, & Hardy-Braz, 1998; Garrison, Tesch, & DeCaro, 1978). In the Garrison and colleagues (1978) study, follow-up interviews of a subsample revealed that a substantial percentage of items were not understood because they involved idiomatic expressions, commonly referred to as "hearing idioms." For example, phrases such as "raining cats and dogs" and "time flies" change meaning completely when transliterated into ASL. Conversely, idiomatic expressions in ASL (e.g., "train gone" or "strong, same, funny zero") are equally difficult to render faithfully into English. Temporal sequencing of events and grammatical construction in ASL are different from those in English: Deaf and hard-of-hearing children tend to comprehend a presented situation better if the setting and antecedent events are established first.

In this regard, findings indicate that modes of administration influence performance of deaf and hard-of-hearing children. Sullivan (1982) points out that the mean WISC-R PIQ scores (mid-90's) reported by Anderson and Sisco (1977) as standardization data for 1,200 deaf or hard-of-hearing children were likely to be underestimates due to the fact that almost 23% of the participants in that study were administered the WISC-R in modes other than total communication.

Of interest are the studies showing that deaf and hard-of-hearing children who were given directions for the WISC-R Performance scale administration using a total communication (TC) approach, for example, scored a mean PIQ of 18 points higher than those who were given the same directions using the standardized verbal directions (Sullivan, 1982). A later similar study found that the mean WISC-III PIQ was about 10 points higher for children given directions using a TC approach (Slate & Fawcett, 1995). In these studies, the TC approach consisted of presenting the directions verbally, accompanied by signed English; the children receiving instructions using this approach obtained a mean WISC-R PIQ of 104, compared with mean PIQs of 88 and 90 for those receiving the instructions in pantomime and visual aids, respectively.

If examiners use sign language interpreters in psychological assessment, they should recognize that the interpreters may influence the assessment process in a number of ways. The accuracy of their translation depends on their own understanding of the material, which may differ from that of the examiner and the examinee. Their presence may distract either the examiner or the examinee. They may project their own interpretations of the material as influenced by their own perceptions or experiences. They may also contaminate the test items (e.g., offering "examples" or "illustrations" or using signs that give away answers). If sign language interpreters are used, the examiner should be aware of and duly note appropriate caveats regarding their participation in the clinical assessment process.

Two important considerations can be derived from the preceding discussion. First, it is of paramount importance for the examiner to establish optimally accessible communication in order to maximize the validity of assessments done with this population. Second, the use of multifaceted approaches to assessment is highly recommended, with at least two different performance IQ measures being obtained.

Additional Disability Factors

The particular etiology of deafness and/or the presence of additional disabilities is an issue of growing importance in psychological assessment of deaf and hard-of-hearing children. Studies of the WISC-R and WISC-III tests used with deaf and hard-of-hearing children (see, e.g., Sullivan & Montoya, 1997; Sullivan & Schulte, 1992) have shown that performance IQ scores of children with known etiologies of deafness (rubella, meningitis, etc.) are significantly lower than those of children with unknown etiologies.

Additional disabilities such as visual problems, cerebral palsy, and deaf–blindness have been reported among preschool children with hearing loss (Scherer, 1983). Children who are deaf–blind present with very complex assessment needs (Mars, 1998; Vernon, 1987).

Another major group of children with multiple disabilities includes those who are deaf or hard of hearing and also have learning disabilities. An added assessment consideration are children who are deaf and hard of hearing with attention deficit disorder (Kelley, Forney, Parker-Fisher, & Jones, 1993). According to the 1997 demographic survey of the deaf and hard of hearing completed by Gallaudet University, the incidence of deaf and hard-of-hearing children with additional learning disabilities is about 8.4%–11% (Samar, 1999; Samar, Parasnis, & Berent, 1998).

Developmental and Psychosocial Issues

Awareness of developmental history and experiences of deaf and hard-of-hearing children is an important aspect of the assessment process. About 90% of deaf and hard-of-hearing children are born to hearing parents, whereas the remaining 10% have deaf parents or families (Schein, 1989). Further, the cognitive, linguistic, and psychosocial skills of deaf and hard-of-hearing children born to deaf parents are generally more similar to those of hearing children than to those of deaf and hard-of-hearing children born to hearing families (Marsharck, 1993; Paul & Jackson, 1993). According to Lane, Hoffmeister, and Bahan (1996), most hearing parents who experience the birth or arrival of a deaf or hard-of-hearing child are initially exposed to a deficit model of medical–audiological interventions. Discomfited by the diagnostic and treatment issues incurred by this perspective, parents may engage in denial about the communication and linguistic needs of their children and consequently contribute to delayed development in these areas. When hearing parents are exposed to a "difference" (that is, cultural or bicultural) model of deafness, the likelihood increases that deaf and hard-of-hearing children will receive more options for communication, language, and social exposure to a variety of both deaf and hearing contexts. This in turn should be reflected in performance scores that are more on target developmentally when compared with either deaf or hearing norms (Lane, Hoffmeister, & Bahan, 1996).

Delgado (1982) has observed that truncation of communication itself has more severe effects than the lack of auditory stimulation, with deaf and hard-of-hearing children essentially barred from access to what deaf educators have described as the "unwritten curriculum" or "incidental learning" (see Lane, 1992). Lowered scores on tests of personality, social skills, language, and even nonverbal intelligence may be a result of fewer opportunities to "absorb" this "mainstream" of continuous auditory environmental input.

SELECTED INSTRUMENTS AND PROCEDURES

The nature of differences in communication for deaf and hard-of-hearing children has prompted the use of at least three major strategies for conducting psychological assessment with this population: (1) modifying standard instruments so as to minimize their communicative demands; (2) using existing nonverbal measures or measures that impose minimal communicative requirements on the child; and (3) using measures specifically designed and/or normed for deaf and hard-of-hearing people. The representative measures identified in this section represent all three approaches, although in some domains there are more of one kind than another. Within each domain, we consider measures in a developmental sequence, from those used during infancy to those used with older children and adolescents.

Cognition

A number of cognitive measures are applicable to assessment of deaf and hard-of-hearing children (Vernon & Andrews, 1990); some are available for general use and others were developed specifically for this population. In assessment of infants with hearing impairment, the Bayley Scales of Infant Development (Bayley, 1993) can be used with the understanding that items involving speech and hearing are likely to yield results different from the norms for hearing infants. In addition, such items can yield anecdotal information about the child's language skills. The Cattell Infant Intelligence Scale (Cattell, 1960; see Chapter 5) has been used selectively with young deaf and hard-of-hearing children (Scherer, 1983), with caveats regarding items involving speech and hearing similar to those indicated for the Bayley Scales. The Infant Psychological Development Scale (Uzgiris & Hunt, 1975), described in Chapter 5, is a qualitative-developmental measure that is appropriate for use with deaf and hard-of-hearing infants given its focus on sensory-motor activities. Its applicability has been demonstrated by Best and Roberts (1976), who found that the performance of deaf and hard-of-hearing children (23 to 38 months of age) was developmentally comparable to that of hearing peers on all subscales except Verbal Imitation, indicating normal progression through sensory-motor stages. Furthermore, areas of causality and motor imitation were found to be correlated with environmental stimulation, as measured by the HOME Inventory (Caldwell, 1972).

The Hiskey–Nebraska Test of Learning Aptitude (HNTLA; Hiskey, 1966) was normed for deaf and hard-of-hearing children, as well as for hearing children. Linguistic demands were reduced or minimized by using a variety of performance items as well as pantomime for administration. A reliability study of a group of 43 children with moderate to profound hearing impairment tested at mean time intervals of 9 months, 34 months, and 62 months yielded test–retest reliability coefficients of .791, .849, and .624 respectively (Watson, 1983). Watson concluded that these reliability figures are similar to those reported for intelligence measures obtained from children with normal hearing. In addition, she noted that among the deaf and hard-of-hearing children tested, scores for one-third of the group differed by 10 points or more and that those for another one-third differed by 15 points or more. She emphasized that these findings demonstrate the importance of obtaining at least two measures of intellectual functioning when assessing deaf and hard-of-hearing children.

Two other measures used with preschool and older children with hearing impairment are the Leiter International Performance Scale (LIPS; Leiter, 1952) and the Arthur Adaptation of the LIPS (AALIPS; Arthur, 1949). The LIPS covers the age range of 2 to 18 years and has some timed tasks, whereas the AALIPS is restricted to the age range of 3 to 8 years and has no timed tasks. Although the nonverbal nature of the tasks and the pantomime form of administration of these measures has made them attractive for assessing deaf and hard-of-hearing children, Ratcliffe and Ratcliffe (1979) cite inadequate psychometric characteristics as a factor limiting their utility. Restandardization of the Leiter International Performance Scale—Revised (LIPS-R; Leiter, 1969) has addressed its psychometric weaknesses and increased its culture fairness from the earlier version (Flemmer & Roid, 1997).

Because a variety of performance items are used and scoring adjustments are possible for items not administered or included, the Merrill–Palmer Scale of Mental Tests (MPSMT; Stutsman, 1948) may have some applicability with young (2- to 3-year-old) deaf and hard-of-hearing children, especially when supplemented by other performance data. Although dated, the test items appeal to deaf and hard-of-hearing children and can serve as screening for developmental function as well (Vernon & Andrews, 1990). The Smith–Johnson

Nonverbal Performance Scale (SJNPS; Smith & Johnson, 1977) is another measure that may be of value in assessing young deaf or hard-of-hearing children. Normed separately for children having normal hearing and for deaf and hard-of-hearing children, the SJNPS consists of 14 subtests and utilizes pantomimed directions.

The Verbal scales of the Wechsler Preschool and Primary Scale of Intelligence (WPPSI; Wechsler, 1967) are not recommended for administration to children who are deaf or hard of hearing. However, the Performance scales of the WPPSI (and, in general, all the Wechsler Performance scales) have been adapted by providing alternate and supplementary instructions to reduce language requirements as well as practice items to be used as needed (Braden & Hannah, 1998; Ray & Ulissi, 1982).

After adapting the WISC-R Performance scale by providing supplemental and alternate instructions for each subtest, Ray (1982) reported a mean WISC-R PIQ of 99.25 and a standard deviation of 19.35 based on the performance of a sample of 127 deaf and hard-of-hearing children. This mean score is somewhat higher than that reported by Sisco and Anderson (1978) and is comparable to that reported by Sullivan (1982) when the TC approach was used. Sullivan (1982) has suggested modifications of instructions for administering the WISC-R to deaf and hard-of-hearing children. The WPPSI-R has not yet been revised in this manner for use with deaf and hearing-impaired children.

The Goodenough–Harris Drawing Test (Harris, 1963) can be used in assessment with deaf and hard-of-hearing children. Studies exploring whether or not deaf and hard-of-hearing children had the same knowledge about the body as hearing children found that the former were not as familiar with anatomy, representations, or names of body parts (Gibbins, 1989; Jones & Badger, 1991). When asked to draw themselves, deaf and hard-of-hearing children drew figures that were larger and richer in detail than they did when asked to draw a person (Gillies, 1968). Myklebust (1964) found differences in size, placement, mood, and details of individual body parts, such as ears, arms, and fingers, between deaf and hearing children. Davis and Hoopers (1975), however, did not find significant differences between hearing and deaf children in the treatment of ears and mouths on the House-Tree-Person Test, but drawings of the tree were more detailed when done by hearing than by deaf children. However, emotional indicators based on the drawings do not perform as predicted (Briccetti, 1994; Cates, 1991).

Prior to the availability of the Wechsler Intelligence Scale for Children—Third Edition (WISC-III; Wechsler, 1991), the assessment measure most widely used with school-age children appeared to be the Performance scale of the Wechsler Intelligence Scale for Children–Revised (PS-WISC-R; Wechsler, 1974). As indicated earlier, the Performance scale has been administered in a variety of ways to deaf and hard-of-hearing children, yielding mean scores within the low normal to normal range. Research using the Wechsler Performance scales with deaf and hearing-impaired children have yielded equivocal results with respect to normative data and correlations with measures of achievement (Paul & Jackson, 1993). Some researchers have found a relationship between performance IQs and achievement scores in language, reading, and mathematics (Kusche, Greenberg, & Garfield, 1983), whereas others have found little or no correlation between these IQ and achievement test scores (Brooks & Riggs, 1980).

Research on WISC-III testing with deaf and hard-of-hearing children revealed no statistically significant differences in Verbal, Performance, or Full Scale IQ scores among children with respect to school program (residential vs. mainstream), communication method (oral vs. signed communication) or severity of hearing loss (Sullivan & Montoya, 1997). Other research illustrates that items on several different subtests of the WISC-III function differently for deaf than for hearing children; for example, items did not retain similar order of difficulty for these two groups (Maller, 1996, 1997). Overall, these findings suggest that Wechsler IQ test performances of deaf and hard-of-hearing children should not be readily compared with those of hearing children and that separate norms for these two populations may have different interpretations for their IQ performance (Braden, 1990).

The Raven Colored Progressive Matrices (CPM; Raven, 1960, 2000) and the Standard Progressive Matrices (SPM; Raven, 1960, 2000), as described in Chapter 4, are useful nonverbal measures of cognition with younger, as well as older, children and adults, respectively. The ease of administration and simplicity of format of these measures have resulted in their frequent use with children who are deaf and hard of hearing. Using the CPM with a group of children with mild to moderate hearing loss, Ritter (1976) found mean IQ scores on the CPM to be significantly higher than WISC PIQ scores but comparable to scores on the AALIPS. Scores from the LIPS and the CPM, however, are not interchangeable, given that less than half of the variance was found in common between these measures (Musgrove & Counts, 1975). The use of these measures to complement more comprehensive intelligence testing is supported by the research of Blennerhassett, Strohmeier, and Hibbett (1994), who noted significant correlations between SPM scores and WISC-R PIQ (for both hearing and deaf norms), as well as scores from the standard achievement tests of reading comprehension, spelling, and language.

The Mental Processing component of the Kaufman Assessment Battery for Children, involving relatively little oral language requirement, has also been widely used with deaf and hard-of-hearing children (K-ABC; Kaufman & Kaufman, 1983). A validity study using a sample of deaf and hard-of-hearing children is reported in the test manual (Courtney, Hayes, Watkins, & Frick, 1983). This and subsequent studies have shown that the Simultaneous Processing and Nonverbal scales seemed appropriate for use with deaf and hard-of-hearing students, with their scores being comparable to those of the normative sample (Ulissi, Brice, & Gibbins, 1989). In the Courtney and colleagues (1983) study, the mean Simultaneous Processing score was 90.5 with a standard deviation of 15.8, and the mean Nonverbal score was 88.6 with a standard deviation of 17.2. The deaf and hard-of-hearing children in the sample scored highest on the Gestalt Closure and Triangles subtests, but they performed relatively poorly on the Matrix Analogies, Photo Series, and Hand Movement subtests. Other studies suggest that the K-ABC Nonverbal scale IQ scores of deaf and hard-of-hearing children are significantly lower than those obtained from the WISC-R (Performance scale), the Hiskey–Nebraska Test of Learning Aptitude, and the Leiter International Performance Scale (Phelps & Branyan, 1988). These findings indicate that the Nonverbal scales of the K-ABC should be used cautiously with deaf and hard-of-hearing children and/or that norms need to be developed separately for this population.

More recent formulations about process- rather than product-oriented intelligence testing present challenges to prevailing views about the relationship between cognition and language (Paul & Jackson, 1993) in testing children who are deaf and hard of hearing. Broesterhuizen (1997), for example, has demonstrated that automatized fine motor movements and specific memory functions, defined as eupraxia, are significant in predicting speech and speech reading skills of deaf preschool children. Of increasing importance is a better understanding of the perceptual and cognitive abilities that exist and that are applied across a range of experiences rather than a focus only or exclusively on unitary constructs of intelligence (Horn, 1989). Illustrating that deaf children lagged behind hearing children by only 1–2 years in certain concrete operational tasks, Furth (1981) has contended that thinking processes of deaf and hearing children are similar, regardless of differences in language acquisition. However, other researchers (Bornstein & Roy, 1973) were not convinced that his work supported or refuted the hypothesis that language is not related to cognitive development. Studies of conservation in deaf and hearing children indicate variability between these two groups. In their research on conservation, Witters-Churchill, Kelly, and Witters (1983) found that deaf and hearing children of junior high school age performed similarly on a task to assess perception of liquid horizontality. Inman and Lian (1991), however, noted that the pattern of conservation emergence among deaf and hard-of-hearing children using either cued speech or oral/aural communication methods was different from the specific developmental sequence suggested by Piaget.

Zweibel and Mertens (1985) reviewed factor analysis research suggesting cognitive structure differences among deaf children at different ages, as well as between deaf and hearing children. In general, deaf children seemed to rely more on visual perceptual skills, whereas their hearing peers showed relatively stronger abstract thinking skills. These findings are corroborated by data collected on cognitive diversity among deaf people and between deaf and hearing people with respect to acquisition and use of sign language (Parasnis, 1998, and from cognitive neuroscience research demonstrating different cortical representation patterns for spoken and signed language acquisition (Neville & Mills, 1997; Peperkamp & Mehler, 1999).

In general, there is increasing support for Furth's (1981) early arguments that cognitive ability and language competence are not unilaterally related; more to the point, the value of process-oriented, or qualitative-developmental, approaches to cognitive assessment lies not only in gaining more accurate reflection of intelligence functioning in deaf and hard-of-hearing children but also in obtaining more detailed understanding of the relationship between reasoning skills and academic accomplishment in individuals.

Communication and Language

Before assessing expressive and receptive language skills of deaf and hard-of-hearing individuals, the clinician should establish their communication preferences and styles, as discussed earlier in this chapter. Generally speaking, the Verbal scales of the Wechsler series (WPPSI, WISC-R and WISC-III, WAIS-R and WAIS-III) are not considered trustworthy measures of intelligence in deaf and hard-of-hearing people. In selected cases, VIQ scores obtained for deaf and hard-of-hearing students can provide some information about how they are performing relative to hearing peers when placed in a mainstreamed setting (Levine, 1971). However, these verbal scores should be treated as verbal achievement scores and discussed in the language section, rather than the intelligence section, of the psychoeducational report (Kretschmer, 1983).

The Peabody Picture Vocabulary Test—Revised (PPVT-R; Dunn & Dunn, 1981), has been used with deaf and hard-of-hearing children (Dodd, Woodhouse, & McIntosh, 1992), but there are difficulties with translating many of the PPVT stimulus words into sign language. The Carolina Picture Vocabulary Test (CPVT; Layton & Holmes, 1985) was developed as a test of receptive sign language vocabulary skills, standardized on a sample of 100 deaf students aged 4 years, 0 months to 11 years, 6 months, and scaled with a mean of 50 and standard deviation of 10. Kline and Sapp (1989) found significant differences between CPVT scores and WISC-R Performance scale IQ scores and minimal correlations with both the Performance IQ and subtest scores. However, the WISC-R Picture Arrangement subtest score did correlate significantly with the CPVT score.

A key measure of communicative competence is referential communication, which is described as the extent to which a speaker (sender) effectively communicates referents to a listener (receiver; see also Chapter 5). The assumption underlying this skill is that the child not only possesses adequate descriptors but also can take into account the informational needs of the receiver. Communicative competence is determined by the receiver's accuracy in correctly identifying the stimulus based on the sender's message.

Breslaw, Griffiths, Wood, and Howarth (1981) compared the referential communication skills of deaf and hearing children using tasks with relatively simple linguistic demands for a younger (about 8 years old) group and those with more complex linguistic demands for an older group (about 10 years old). The results on four performance measures—of a task requiring the sender to communicate the placement of a block described in three dimensions (shape, color, size) into an appropriate hole on a form board—indicated that the deaf children did as well as, if not sometimes better than, their normal-hearing peers. In the second study, using a more complex task that required the sender to describe a picture from a book so that the receiver could locate it in an identical book, the deaf students from one of the three schools for the deaf performed similarly to their hearing cohorts, whereas those from the other two schools for the deaf performed less well. The finding of performance differences as a function of specific schools for deaf students led to the inference that such differences may reflect different teaching philosophies underlying language training. Still other studies showing that deaf and hearing children perform similarly on referential communication tasks suggest that the demands of the task may be addressed in different ways, including through development of message formulation skills (MacKay-Soroka, Trehub, & Thorpe, 1987) or use of a variety of additional communication modes (e.g., gesture, pantomime; Alegria, 1981). Ultimately, the value of process-oriented assessment of intellectual, communication, and linguistic functioning of deaf children is that it yields the kind of data and detail that enables the formulation of individual educational and clinical interventions.

Personal-Social Domain

Psychological assessment related to mental health issues (Blennerhassett, 2000) is an important area with deaf and hard-of-hearing persons. Assessment of personal and social characteristics of children, however, is a particular challenge, given the spoken-language emphasis of most measures in this domain. Although a number of measures of personal, social, and behavioral functions have been used with deaf and hard-of-hearing children, considerable caution must be given to their use with this population. With many cultural and linguistic differences between deaf and hearing people, as briefly discussed earlier, a particular concern must be to avoid erroneous inferences of psychopathology with respect to "unique" responses of deaf and hard-of-hearing individuals (Freeman, 1989).

In a survey of school psychologists, Gibbins (1989) found that human figure drawing tests were among the most popular measures for assessing the social-emotional status of deaf and hard-of-hearing children. There is, however, disagreement among several studies concerning the validity of this procedure with this population (Briccetti, 1994). A comparative study of self-concept among deaf and hard-of-hearing students and other groups of disabled and nondisabled students, using a human figure drawing test and a self-concept scale, found that the students with disabilities in general had more negative self-concepts and more negative attitudes and feelings about their abilities and social relationships (Jones, 1985). Davis and Hoopes (1975) also did not find any differences between the two groups in number of indicators of emotional disturbance. Other studies have found that although the projective drawings of deaf and hearing children were generally similar, the emotional functioning indicators did not perform as predicted in classifying the deaf and hard-of-hearing children (Briccetti, 1994; Cates, 1991).

The Meadow–Kendall Social-Emotional Assessment Inventory for Deaf Students (M/K SEAI; Meadow, 1983) is a measure of social and emotional adjustment of deaf and hard-of-hearing children and adolescents (aged 7 to 21 years). Based on teacher ratings, Cartledge, Paul, Jackson, and Cochran (1991) found no significant differences between deaf and hard-of-hearing adolescent students enrolled in residential and public schools that used different communication philosophies. In another study, self-descriptions by deaf students and teacher ratings on the Meadow–Kendall inventory revealed small but significant positive correlations with reading achievement scores (Chovan & Roberts, 1993). In their study of an adaptation of the ACOPE (Adolescent Coping Orientation for Problem Experiences) instrument for use with deaf and hard-of-hearing adolescents, Kluwin, Blennerhassett, and Sweet (1990) found concurrent validity between this instrument and the teacher-rated Meadow–Kendall inventory for deaf students.

The Matching Familiar Figures Test (MFFT; Kagan, Rosman, Day, & Phillips, 1964) is a measure widely used to assess conceptual tempo in terms of impulsivity and reflectivity, with scores being determined by the amount of time required to select one of six items to match a reference item and the number of errors made. In a multivariate study of 8- to 12-year-old deaf and hard-of-hearing children, Dillon (1980) found that MFFT errors and latency scores were related to performance on cognitive tasks. The Assessment of Developmental Levels by Observation (ADLO) instrument was also found to be of use with deaf children when other psychometric tools could not be applied (Wolf-Schein, 1993).

Common social development measures used with deaf and hard-of-hearing adolescents have included those addressing locus of control and self-concept. Dillon (1980) adapted the Nowicki–Strickland Locus of Control Scale for Children (Nowicki & Strickland, 1973; see Chapter 4) for use with deaf and hard-of-hearing children by rephrasing and truncating some items and shortening the scale from 40 to 19 items. The modified version is reproduced in Dillon's (1980) article. Other studies of locus of control assessment have yielded mixed results with deaf and hard-of-hearing children, revealing unacceptable internal consistency for a videotaped presentation of the Children's Locus of Control Scale (Bodner & Johns, 1977). Another study found that a modified version of Rotter's Internal–External Locus of Control Scale (Rotter, 1966) yielded favorable predictions of academic achievement (Koelle & Convey, 1982). This study (1982) also included a modification of the Piers–Harris Children's Self-Concept Scale (PHCSCS; Piers & Harris, 1969) and yielded satisfactory internal consistency values for both original and modified versions of these scales. Another interesting result was that significant differences were found on achievement, self-concept, and locus of control variables that favored deaf students with deaf parents. This result is consistent with earlier findings pertaining to the hearing status of parents relative to the functioning of their children (Bat-Chava, 1993).

The Tennessee Self-Concept Scale (TSCS; Fitts, 1965) is a widely used written measure of personal characteristics that has also been used with deaf and hard-of-hearing adolescents. Results of a study using the TSCS with newly enrolled students at the National Technical School for the Deaf, Garrison and colleagues (1978) found that deaf students showed lower levels of self-esteem compared with the norm. Further analysis of the results showed also that the deaf students who scored higher on tests of reading comprehension also showed higher self-esteem scores and that many deaf students had "peculiar" responses to test items. These observations suggested that the written form of the TSCS may not provide a valid assessment of self-concept among deaf and hard-of-hearing individuals. Gibson-Harman and Austin (1985) developed a revision of the TSCS by adapting the items in terms of reading and language levels. Their results provided sufficiently good reliability to warrant the development of norms based on a sample of deaf and hard-of-hearing individuals. Using this revised form of the TSCS, Searls (1993) found no differences between deaf and hearing college students who had deaf parents, except on the Behavior and Moral–Ethical scales; he concluded that both deaf and hearing children of deaf parents generally develop comparable self-esteem.

Although caution should be exercised in the use of language-dependent measures of personality with deaf and hard-of-hearing persons, some projective measures have been used. Two of these are the Hand Test (Levine, 1974) and the Lowenthal "World" Technique (Gillies, 1983). Levine (1974) showed that 20 out of 24 Hand Test variables distinguished among four groups of deaf individuals with differing levels of linguistic competence and suggested its diagnostic potential within a larger battery of tests. In a comparative analysis, Gillies (1983) found that deaf children showed higher levels of acting-out and antisocial behaviors than hearing children on the Lowenthal "World" Technique.

Behavior

As the domain of behavior is one in which assessment is less dependent on language use, behavioral measures may be particularly applicable with deaf and hard-of-hearing children. A number of the checklist and rating scales described in Chapter 4 are suitable for use across the range of childhood through adolescence. Research documenting the utility of many of these measures, however, is variable.

The Revised Behavior Problem Checklist (RBPC; Quay, 1983), for example, was used with other measures to identify characteristics of students with minimal sensorineural hearing loss in a prevalence study of third, sixth, and ninth graders (Bess, Dodd-Murphy, & Parker, 1998). It was also used in a study of peer relations and aggression comparing adolescents with and without hearing impairments (Heneggler, Watson, & Whelan, 1990). Providing a dimensional measure of behavior problems for the age range of 3 years to 22 years, the RBPC has also been translated into Spanish (Curtis & Schmidt, 1993). Along with the Child Behavior Checklist (Heneggler et al., 1990; Vostanis, Hayes, Du Feu, & Warren, 1997), it has demonstrated utility with deaf and hard-of-hearing populations.

The assessment of adaptive behavior has been an area of interest with deaf and hard-of-hearing children. The common measures have been the AAMD Adaptive Behavior Scale (ABS) and the Vineland Adaptive Behavior Scale (VABS). Suess, Dickson, Anderson, and Hildman (1981) have generated norms for a sample of 77 deaf–blind children and young adults on the basis of ratings on Part 1 of the ABS (Nihira, Foster, Shellhaas, & Leland, 1974). As a further step to enhance the utility of adaptive behavior measures in deaf–blind individuals, Suess, Cotten, and Sison (1983) revised the instructions for Part 1 of the ABS to allow credit for alternative forms of communication (e.g., sign language, braille), and found no differences in ratings on 9 of the 10 domains for the revised and original forms. On Domain IV (Language Development) of the ABS, however, all item scores were higher in the revised version. The role of additional disabilities in adaptive behavior was also evident in the use of the VABS to assess independent living skills of adolescents and adults with hearing impairments (Dunlap & Sands, 1990). Classification on the basis of the VABS indicated that factors in addition to severity of auditory impairment accounted for behavior problems. These efforts represent important steps in addressing the assessment needs of children with hearing impairment and additional disabilities.

IMPLICATIONS FOR PRACTICE

Given limitations of auditory input, differences in communication and linguistic strategies, and cultural impact of deafness, the importance of selecting appropriate instruments for psychological assessment cannot be overstated. Unless instruments are known to be valid for use with this population, the risks of underestimating the actual cognitive abilities and academic achievement, as well as of misrepresenting the psychosocial development, of deaf and hard-of-hearing children and adolescents is considerably elevated. We summarized recommendations for enhancing the validity of assessment efforts with deaf and hard-of-hearing children.

    1. As effective communication with the deaf or hard-of-hearing child or adolescent is paramount, examiners should be knowledgeable about the variety of communication modes used by deaf and hard-of-hearing individuals. Because it requires years to become fluent in sign language and other visual communication systems, examiners who are not themselves skilled in signing should be familiar with interpreter services. They should keep in mind that total communication approaches tend to yield more effective assessment results. It is also important to remember that students from particular schools may use signs or other visual cues unique to those settings. Further, in some cases even interpreters may have difficulty understanding children or adolescents with minimal language skills or idiosyncratic sign or gesture systems; in these instances, consultation with family members, teachers, or other caregivers familiar with the child is encouraged (Stansfield & Veltri, 1987). A helpful strategy would be simply to allow enough time for casual or "warm-up" conversation with the child or adolescent so as to become accustomed to his or her preferred style of communication and to have him or her become accustomed to the examiner's or interpreter's style as well.

    2. Given the different time and communication demands in assessment of deaf and hard-of-hearing children, including the involvement of an interpreter, fatigue may become an important factor. Frequent breaks and/or shorter testing sessions are often helpful.

    3. As the potential for misunderstanding and misinterpretation is high with deaf and hard-of-hearing persons, every effort should be made to use standardized modifications of test instructions or demonstrations developed for this population and to adapt procedures to maximize comprehension of task demands.

    4. The validity of assessment findings is enhanced by combining results from more than one measure of the same construct. Although this procedure has been advocated most frequently in the area of intellectual assessment, this guideline is appropriate for any area of assessment. The value of assessing emotional functioning using the Child Behavior Checklist in documenting performance outcomes such as productivity and interpersonal skills has been demonstrated by Frustenberg and Doyal (1994) in a study of deaf and hard-of-hearing students.

    5. Demographic and other background information about deaf and hard-of-hearing children should be given consideration in interpretation of assessment findings. Attention to developmental history, for example, is important in that children with parents who are deaf often show different psychosocial developmental characteristics from those of hearing parents (Bat-Chava, 1993; Tomlinson-Keasey & Kelly, 1978). Other mediating factors, such as child personality, cognitive style, temperament, or idiosyncratic characteristics, may also affect performance and confound interpretation of assessment results.

    6. Research has suggested that deaf children show responses on motor-reduced and motor-intensive nonverbal tests that are more reflective of impulsivity than of processing speed difficulties (Braden, Kostrubala, & Reed, 1994). It may be helpful to avoid tests that

involve timed tasks, as deaf children may react by working as quickly as possible without considering accuracy, increasing the likelihood of unfavorable performance.

7. Of central importance is the recognition that assessment results for deaf and hard-of-hearing children and youth may be negatively biased by a "deficit" orientation instead of a competence (Delgado, 1982) or "difference" interpretation of their performance (Lane, 1992). In this regard it is essential that the helping professions are informed of, and sensitive to, the deaf culture in order to effectively assess and support children who are deaf and hard of hearing (Lala, 1998).

Finally, although assessment should be based on a liberal approach of selecting, adapting, and administering measures, the results should be interpreted conservatively with respect to inferences made regarding the child's abilities or characteristics. Recommendations for intervention or implementation for deaf and hard-of-hearing children and adolescents should incorporate not only assessment results but also detailed information about their development and the particular communication, linguistic, educational, and psychosocial context(s) of their lives.

REFERENCES

Alegria, J. (1981). The development of referential communication in deaf and hearing children: Competence and style. *International Journal of Behavioral Development, 4*(3), 295–312.

Anderson, R. J., & Sisco, F. H. (1977). *Standardization of the WISC-R Performance scale for deaf children* (Series T, No. 1). Washington, DC: Gallaudet College, Office of Demographic Studies.

Anonymous. (1997). Issues to consider in deaf and hard-of-hearing patients. *American Family Physician, 56*(8), 2057–2064, 2067–2068.

Arthur, G. (1949). The Arthur adaptation of the Leiter International Performance Scales. *Journal of Clinical Psychology, 5*, 345–349.

Bat-Chava, Y. (1993). Antecedents of self-esteem in deaf people: A meta-analytic review. *Rehabilitation Psychology, 38*(4), 221–234.

Bayley, N. (1993). *Bayley Scales of Infant Development, Second Edition (BSID–II)*. San Antonio, TX: Psychological Corporation.

Bess, F., Dodd-Murphy, J., & Parker, R. (1998). Children with minimal sensorineural hearing loss: Prevalence, educational performance, and functional status. *Ear and Hearing, 19*(5), 339–354.

Best, B., & Roberts, G. (1976). Early cognitive development in hearing impaired children. *American Annals of the Deaf, 121*, 560–564.

Blennerhassett, L. (2000). Psychological assessments. In P. Hindley & N. Kitson (Eds.), *Mental health and deafness* (pp. 185–205). Philadelphia: Whurr.

Blennerhassett, L., Strohmeier, S. J., & Hibbett, C. (1994). Criterion-related validity of Raven's Progressive Matrices with deaf residential school students. *American Annals of the Deaf, 139*(2), 104–110.

Bodner, B., & Johns, J. (1977). Personality and hearing impairment: A study in locus of control. *Volta Review, 79*(6), 362–372.

Bornstein, H., & Roy, H. L. (1973). Comment on "Linguistic deficiency and thinking: Research with deaf subjects 1964–1969." *Psychological Bulletin, 79*(3), 211–214.

Braden, J. (1990). Do deaf persons have a characteristic psychometric profile on the Wechsler Performance scales? *Journal of Psychoeducational Assessment, 8*(4), 518–526.

Braden, J., & Hannah, J. (1998). Assessment of hearing impaired and deaf children with the WISC-III. In D. Saklofske & A. Prifitera (Eds.), *Use of the WISC-III in clinical practice* (pp. 175–201). New York: Houghton-Mifflin.

Braden, J., Kostrubala, C., & Reed, J. (1994). Why do deaf children score differentially on performance vs. motor-reduced nonverbal intelligence tests? *Journal of Psychoeducational Assessment, 12*(4), 357–363.

Brauer, B. A., Braden, J. P., Pollard, R. Q., & Hardy-Braz, S. T. (1998). Deaf and hard of hearing people. In J. H. Sandoval & C. L. Frisby (Eds.), *Test interpretation and diversity: Achieving equity in assessment* (pp. 297–315). Washington, DC: American Psychological Association.

Breslaw, P. I., Griffiths, A. J., Wood, D. J., & Howarth, C. I. (1981). The referential communication skills of deaf children from different educational environments. *Journal of Child Psychology and Psychiatry, 22*, 269–283.

Briccetti, K. A. (1994). Emotional indicators of deaf children on the Draw-A-Person Test. *American Annals of the Deaf, 139*, 500–505.

Broesterhuizen, M. (1997). Psychological assessment of deaf children. *Scandinavian Audiology, 26*, 43–49.

Brooks, C. R., & Riggs, S. T. (1980). WISC-R, WISC, and reading achievement relationships among hearing-impaired children attending public schools. *Volta Review, 82*(2), 96–102.

Caldwell, B. (1972). *HOME Inventory*. Little Rock: University of Arkansas.

Cartledge, G., Paul, P., Jackson, D., & Cochran, L. (1991). Teachers' perceptions of the social skills of adolescents with hearing impairment in residential and public school settings. *RASE: Remedial and Special Education, 12*(2), 34–39, 47.

Cates, J. (1991). Comparison of human figure drawings by hearing and hearing impaired children. *Volta Review, 93*(1), 31–39.

Cattell, P. (1960). *Cattell Infant Intelligence Scale*. New York: Psychological Corporation.

Chovan, W., & Roberts, K. (1993). Deaf students' self-appraisals, achievement outcomes, and teachers' inferences about social-emotional adjustment in academic settings. *Perceptual and Motor Skills, 77*(3, Part 1), 1021–1022.

Courtney, A. S., Hayes, F. B., Watkins, K. M., & Frick, M. (1983). K-ABC validity study No. 11. In A. S. Kaufman & N. L. Kaufman, *Kaufman Assessment Battery for Children: Interpretive manual* (pp. 35, 95, 114–115, 145). Circle Pines, MN: American Guidance Service.

Curtis, P. A., & Schmidt, L. L. (1993). A Spanish translation of the Revised Behavior Problem Checklist. *Child Welfare, 72*(5), 453–460.

Davis, C. J., & Hoopes, J. L. (1975). Comparison of House-Tree-Person drawings of young deaf and hearing children. *Journal of Personality Assessment, 39*, 28–33.

Delgado, G. L. (1982). Beyond the norm. Social maturity and deafness. *American Annals of the Deaf, 127*, 356–360.

Dillon, R. F. (1980). Cognitive style and elaboration of logical abilities in hearing-impaired children. *Journal of Experimental Child Psychology, 30*, 389–400.

Dodd, B., Woodhouse, L., & McIntosh, B. (1992). The linguistic abilities of young children with hearing impairment: First report of a longitudinal study. *Australia and New Zealand Journal of Developmental Disabilities, 18*(1), 17–34.

Dunlap, W. R., & Sands, D. I. (1990). Classification of the hearing impaired for independent living using the Vineland Adaptive Behavior Scale. *American Annals of the Deaf, 135*(5), 384–388.

Dunn, L. M., & Dunn, L. M. (1981). *Peabody Picture Vocabulary Test–Revised*. Circle Pines, MN: American Guidance Service.

Fitts, W. H. (1965). *Tennessee Self-Concept Scale*. Nashville, TN: Counselor Recordings and Tests.

Flemmer, D., & Roid, G. (1997). Nonverbal intelligence assessment of Hispanic and speech-impaired adolescents. *Psychological Reports, 80*(3, Part 2), 1115–1122.

Freeman, S. (1989). Cultural and linguistic bias in mental health evaluations of deaf people. *Rehabilitation Psychology, 34*(1), 51–63.

Frustenberg, K., & Doyal, G. (1994). The relationship between emotional-behavioral functioning and personal characteristics on performance outcomes of hearing impaired students. *American Annals of the Deaf, 139*(4), 411–414.

Furth, H. G. (1981). *Piaget and knowledge: Theoretical foundations*. Chicago: University of Chicago Press.

Garrison, W. M., Tesch, S. C., & DeCaro, P. (1978). An assessment of self-concept levels among postsecondary deaf adolescents. *American Annals of the Deaf, 123*, 968–975.

Gibbins, S. (1989). The provision of school psychological assessment services for the hearing impaired: A national survey. *Volta Review, 91*, 95–103.

Gibson-Harman, K., & Austin, G. (1985). A revised form of the Tennessee Self-Concept Scale for use with deaf and hard-of-hearing persons. *American Annals of the Deaf, 130*(3), 218–225.

Gillies, J. (1968). Variation in drawings of "a person" and "myself" by hearing-impaired and normal children. *British Journal of Educational Psychology, 38*, 86–89.

Gillies, J. (1983). The personal adjustment of severely deaf children: A study using the Lowenthal "World" Technique. *British Journal of Projective Psychology and Personality Study, 28*(2), 23–29.

Harris, D. B. (1963). *Children's drawings as measures of intellectual maturity*. New York: Harcourt, Brace & World.

Henggeler, S. W., Watson, S. M., & Whelan, J. O. (1990). Peer relations of hearing-impaired adolescents. *Journal of Pediatric Psychology, 15*(6), 721–731.

Hiskey, M. S. (1966). *Manual for the Hiskey-Nebraska Test of Learning Aptitude*. Lincoln, NE: Union College Press.

Holcomb, T. K. (1997). Development of deaf bicultural identity. *American Annals of the Deaf, 142*(2), 89–93.

Horn, J. (1989). Models of intelligence. In R. Linn (Ed.), *Intelligence: Measurement, theory, and public policy* (pp. 29–73). Urbana: University of Illinois Press.

Inman, P., & Lian, M. (1991). Conservation and metaphor performance among children with hearing impairments. *Journal of the American Deafness and Rehabilitation Association, 25*(1), 28–41.

Jones, C. (1985). Analysis of the self-concepts of handicapped students. *RASE: Remedial and Special Education, 6*(5), 32–36.

Jones, E., & Badger, T. (1991). Deaf children's knowledge of internal human anatomy. *Journal of Special Education, 25*(2), 252–260.

Kagan, J., Rosman, B. L., Day, D., & Phillips, W. (1964). Information processing in the child. *Psychological Monographs, 78*(1, Whole No. 578).

Kaufman, A. S., & Kaufman N. L. (1983). *Kaufman Assessment Battery for Children*. Circle Pines, MN: American Guidance Service.

Kline, M., & Sapp, G. L. (1989). Carolina Picture Vocabulary Test: Validation with hearing-impaired student. *Perceptual and Motor Skills, 69*, 64–66.

Kluwin, T., Blennerhassett, L., & Sweet, C. (1990). The revision of an instrument to measure the capacity of hearing impaired adolescents to cope. *Volta Review, 92*(6), 283–291.

Knell, S. M., & Klonoff, E. A. (1983). Language sampling in deaf children: A comparison of oral and signed communication modes. *Journal of Communication Disorders, 16*, 435–437.

Koelle, W. H., & Convey, J. J. (1982). The prediction of the achievement of deaf adolescents from self-concept and locus of control measures. *American Annals of the Deaf, 127*, 769–778.

Kretschmer, R. E. (1983). Assessing the hearing impaired child. In S. Ray, M. J. O'Neill, & N. T. Morris (Eds.), *Low incidence children: A guide to psychoeducational assessment*. Sulphur, OK: Ray.

Kusche, C. A., Greenberg, M. T., & Garfield, T. S. (1983). Nonvervbal intelligence and verbal achievement in deaf adolescents: An examination of heredity and environment. *American Annals of the Deaf, 128*(4), 458–466.

Lala, F. J. (1998). Is there room in the DSM for consideration of deaf people? *American Annals of the Deaf, 143*(4), 314–317.

Lane, H. (1992). *The mask of benevolence*. New York: Knopf.

Lane, H., Hoffmeister, R., & Bahan, B. (1996). *A journey into the Deaf-world*. San Diego, CA: Dawn Sign Press.

Layton, T. L., & Holmes, D. W. (1985). *Carolina Picture Vocabulary Test*. Tulsa, OK: Modern Education.

Leiter, R. G. (1952). *Leiter International Performance Scale*. Chicago: Stoelting.

Leiter, R. G. (1969). *Leiter International Performance Scale–Revised*. Los Angeles: Western Psychological Services.

Levine, E. S. (1971). Mental assessment of the deaf child. *Volta Review, 73*(2), 80–105.

Levine, E. S. (1974). Psychological tests and practices with the deaf: A survey of the state of the art. *Volta Review, 76*, 298–319.

Lindhout, D., Frets, P. G., & Niermeijer, M. F. (1992). Approaches to genetic counseling. In R. J. Ruben, T. R. Van De Water, & K. P. Steel (Eds.), *Genetics of hearing impairment* (pp. 223–229). New York: New York Academy of Sciences.

Lucas, C., & Valli, C. (1993). ASL, English, and contact signing. In C. Lucas (Ed.), *Sign language research: Theoretical issues* (pp. 288–307). Washington, DC: Gallaudet University Press.

MacKay-Soroka, S., Trehub, S., & Thorpe, L. (1987). Deaf children's referential messages to mother. *Child Development, 58*(1), 385–394.

Maller, S. (1996). WISC-III verbal item invariance across samples of deaf and hearing children of similar measured ability. *Journal of Psychoeducational Assessment, 14*(2), 152–165.

Maller, S. (1997). Deafness and WISC-III item difficulty: Invariance and fit. *Journal of School Psychology, 35*(3), 299–314.

Mars, H. (1998). *Psychological evaluation of children who are deaf-blind: An overview with recommendations for practice*i (Revised.) [Online fact sheet]. Available: http://www. tr.wou.edu/dbline/eval.htm

Marsharck, M. (1993). *Psychological development of deaf children*. New York: Oxford University Press.

Meadow, K. P. (1983). An instrument for assessment of social-emotional adjustment in hearing impaired preschoolers. *American Annals of the Deaf, 128*, 826–884.

Musgrove, W. J., & Counts, L. (1975). Leiter and Raven performance and teacher ranking: A correlation study with deaf children. *Journal of Rehabilitation of the Deaf, 8*(3), 19–22.

Myklebust, H. R. (1964). *The psychology of deafness* (2nd ed.). New York: Grune & Stratton.

Neville, H., & Mills, D. (1997). Epigenesis of language. *Mental Retardation and Developmental Disabilities Research Reviews, 3*(4), 282–292.

Nihira, K., Foster, R., Shellhaas, M., & Leland, H. (1974). *AAMD Adaptive Behavior Scale*. Washington, DC: American Association of Mental Deficiency.

Nowicki, S., & Strickland, B. R. (1973). A locus of control scale for children. *Journal of Consulting and Clinical Psychology, 40*, 148–154.

Parasnis, I. (1998). Cognitive diversity in deaf people: Implications for communication and education. *Scandinavian Audiology, 27*(Suppl. 49), 109–115.

Paul, P., & Jackson, D. (1993). *Toward a psychology of deafness*. Boston: Allyn & Bacon.

Peperkamp, S., & Mehler, J. (1999). Signed and spoken language: A unique underlying system? *Language and Speech, 42*(2–3), 333–346.

Phelps, L., & Branyan, B. J. (1988). Correlations among the Hiskey, K-ABC Nonverbal Scale, Leiter, and WISC-R Performance Scale with public school deaf children. *Journal of Psychoeducational Assessment, 6*(4), 354–358.

Piers, E., & Harris, D. (1969). *Manual for the Piers–Harris Children's Self-Concept Scale*. Nashville, TN: Counselor Recordings and Tests.

Quay, H. C. (1983). A dimensional approach to behavior disorder: The Revised Behavior Problem Checklist. *School Psychology Review, 12*(3), 244–249.

Quigley, S. P. & Paul, P. V. (1984). *Language and deafness*. San Diego: College Hill Press.

Ratcliffe, K. J., & Ratcliffe, M. W. (1979). The Leiter Scales: A review of the validity of findings. *American Annals of the Deaf, 124*, 38–45.

Raven, J. C. (1960). *Progressive Matrices*. New York: Psychological Corporation.

Raven, J. C. (2000, August). The Raven's Progressive Matrices: Changes and stability over culture and time. *Cognitive Psychology, 4*(1), 1–48.

Ray, S. (1982). Adapting the WISC-R for deaf children. *Diagnostique, 7*, 147–157.

Ray, S., & Ulissi, S. M. (1982). *Adaptation of the Wechsler Preschool and Primary Scales of Intelligence for deaf children*. Natchitoches, LA: Ray.

Ritter, D. R. (1976). Intellectual estimates of hearing impaired children: A comparison of three measures. *Psychology in the Schools, 13*, 397–399.

Rodda, M., Buranyi, G., Cumming, C., & Muendel-Atherstone, B. (1985). Cognitive processing and language in deaf students: A decade of research. In D. S. Martin (Ed.), *Cognition, education, and deafness*. Washington, DC: Gallaudet College Press.

Rotter, J. B. (1966). Generalized expectations for internal versus external control of reinforcement. *Psychological Monographs, 80*(1, Whole No. 609).

Samar, V. (1999). Identifying learning disabilities in the deaf population: The leap from Gibraltar. *NTID Research Bulletin, 4*(1), 1, 3–5.

Samar, V., Parasnis, I., & Berent, G. (1998). Learning disabilities, attention deficit disorders, and deafness. In M. Marsharck & D. Clark (Eds.), *Psychological perspectives on deafness* (Vol. 2, pp. 199–242). Mahwah, NJ: Erlbaum.

Schein, J. (1989). *At home among strangers*. Washington, DC: Gallaudet University Press.

Scherer, P. (1983). Psycho-educational evaluation of hearing-impaired preschool children. *American Annals of the Deaf, 128*(2), 118–124.

Searls, M. (1993). Self-concept among deaf and hearing children of deaf parents. *Journal of the American Deafness and Rehabilitation Association, 27*(1), 25–37.

Sisco, F. H., & Anderson, R. J. (1978). Current findings regarding performance of deaf children on the WISC-R. *American Annals of the Deaf, 123*, 115–121.

Slate, J., & Fawcett, J. (1995). Validity of the WISC-III for deaf and hard-of-hearing persons. *American Annals of the Deaf, 140*: 250–254.

Smith , A. J., & Johnson, R. E. (1977). *Smith–Johnson Nonverbal Performance Scale*. Los Angeles: Western Psychological Services.

Stansfield, M., & Veltri, D. (1987). Assessment from the perspective of the sign language inter-
    preter. In H. Elliot, L. Glass., & J. Evans, *Mental health assessment of deaf clients: A practical
    manual* (pp.). Boston: College Hill Press.

Stutsman, R. (1948). *Merrill-Palmer Scale of Mental Tests*. Los Angeles: Western Psychological
    Services.

Suess, J. F., Cotten, P. D., & Sison, G. F. P., Jr. (1983). The American Association on Mental De-
    ficiency—Adaptive Behavior Scale: Allowing credit for alternative means of communication.
    American Annals of the Deaf, 128, 390–393.

Suess, J. F., Dickson, A. L., Anderson, H. N., & Hildman, L. K. (1981). The AAMD Adaptive
    Behavior Scale norm-referenced for deaf-blind individuals: Application and implication. *Ameri-
    can Annals of the Deaf, 126*, 814–818.

Sullivan, P., & Montoya, L. (1997). Factor analysis of WISC-III with deaf and hard-of-hearing
    children. *Psychological Assessment, 9*, 317–321.

Sullivan, P., & Schulte, L. (1992). Factor analysis of WAIS-R with deaf and hard-of-hearing chil-
    dren. *Psychological Assessment, 4*(4), 537–540.

Sullivan, P. M. (1982). Administration modifications on the WISC-R Performance Scale with dif-
    ferent categories of deaf children. *American Annals of the Deaf, 127*(6), 780–788.

Sullivan, P. M., & Vernon, M. (1979). *Psychological assessment of hearing impaired children, 8*(3),
    271–290.

Tomlinson-Keasey, C., & Kelly, R. R. (1978). The deaf child's symbolic world. *American Annals
    of the Deaf, 123*, 452–459.

Ulissi, S. M., Brice, P. J., & Gibbins, S. (1989). Use of the Kaufman Assessment Battery for Chil-
    dren with the hearing impaired. *American Annals of the Deaf, 134*(4), 283–287.

Uzgiris, I. C., & Hunt, J. M. (1975). *Ordinal Scales of Psychological Development*. Urbana: Uni-
    versity of Illinois Press.

Vernon, M. (1987). Psychological adjustments and psychological assessments of deaf-blind chil-
    dren. In B. Heller & L. Flohr (Eds.), *Psychological interventions with sensorially disabled per-
    sons* (pp. 79–93). Orlando, FL: Harcourt Brace Jovanovich.

Vernon, M., & Andrews, J. (1990). *The psychology of deafness*. White Plains, NY: Longman.

Vostanis, P., Hayes, M., Du Feu, M., & Warren, J. (1996). Detection of behavioural and emo-
    tional problems in deaf children and adolescents: Comparison of two rating scales. *Child: Care,
    Health and Development, 23*(3), 233–246.

Walker-Vann, C. (1998). Profiling Hispanic deaf students: A first step toward solving the greater
    problems. *American Annals of the Deaf, 143*(1), 46–54.

Watson, B. U. (1983). Test–retest stability of the Hiskey–Nebraska Test of Learning Aptitude in a
    sample of hearing-impaired children and adolescents. *Journal of Speech and Hearing Disor-
    ders, 48*(2), 145–149.

Wechsler, D. (1967). *Wechsler Preschool and Primary Scale of Intelligence*. San Antonio, TX: Psy-
    chological Corporation.

Wechsler, D. (1974). *Wechsler Intelligence Scale for Children—Revised*. San Antonio, TX: Psy-
    chological Corporation.

Wechsler, D. (1991). WISC-III: *Wechsler Intelligence Scale for Children—Manual* (3rd ed.) San
    Antonio, TX: Psychological Corporation.

Witters-Churchill, L. J., Kelly, R. R., & Witters, L. A. (1983). Hearing-impaired students' percep-
    tion of liquid horizontality: An examination of the effects of gender, development and train-
    ing. *Volta Review, 85*, 211–225.

Wolf-Schein, E. (1993). Assessing the "untestable" client: ADLO. *Developmental Disabilities Bul-
    letin, 21*(2), 52–70.

Zweibel, A., & Mertens, D. (1985). A comparison of intellectual structure in deaf and hearing
    children. *American Annals of the Deaf, 130*(1), 27–31.

13

ASSESSMENT OF CHILDREN WITH AUTISM

LEE M. MARCUS
SALLY FLAGLER
SUSAN ROBINSON

Tommy is a 5-year-old boy referred to the Student Psychological Services by his kindergarten teacher because of his inattentiveness to group instruction, his lack of focused play, his tendency to get upset when other children intruded on his space, and his reluctance to speak. She thought he might be either emotionally disturbed or, because this was his first year in school, immature in his development. His parents did not express the same concerns, although they have acknowledged that he is "different" from his older siblings. The school psychologist observed Tommy in his class and did cognitive and educational testing, and a speech therapist did a language and communication evaluation. They noted that although many of his scores were within the average range, several fell below average, particularly those involving complex reasoning. The psychologist was struck by Tommy's lack of social interest in his peers and need for routines. The speech therapist noted that despite an adequate vocabulary, Tommy seemed lacking in communicative intent and got "stuck" on certain verbal themes, such as a favorite video.

In this chapter we review critical issues in the assessment of children with autism, including current perspectives on diagnosis and methods for assessing skills and behaviors. Our framework is cognitive-developmental and behavioral and also reflects experiences from clinical and educational settings. Autism has become a more widely known and understood disorder in the past decade. With the expectation and requirement that assessment and services be provided within the public school environment from at least 3 to 21 years of age for the majority of students, diagnostic and prescriptive testing skills now must be part of the training and practice of school psychologists, as well as of clinical, child, and pediatric psychologists. This chapter is aimed at this broad group of practitioners.

DEFINITIONS

With the publication of the fourth edition of the *Diagnostic and Statistical Manual of Mental Disorders* (DSM-IV; American Psychiatric Association, 1994), autism was included as the primary category under pervasive developmental disorders (PDD). Other categories included Asperger syndrome, Rett syndrome, childhood disintegrative disorder, and pervasive developmental disorder not otherwise specified (PDD/NOS). DSM-IV represents the current thinking about the differences, similarities, and scope of these conditions of atypical development and is most often used in clinical and private settings. A new revision (DSM-IV TR; 2000) has attempted to broaden the autism definitions once more by doing such a thing as defining dual diagnoses like autism and schizophrenia. In school settings, state special education guidelines define autism, generally under one single term (autism) and do not differentiate among subcategories of autism. Although there is a reasonable consensus about the broad defining features of PDD, researchers and clinicians differ on whether the term PDD is the proper umbrella term. The term "autism-spectrum disorders" is sometimes used as an alternative to highlight the relevance and saliency of the core condition of autism. In the case illustration presented at the beginning of the chapter, Tommy shows the core features of autism, even though his problems might be considered fairly mild because of his high functioning and verbal skills. In the past, a child like Tommy might not be considered to fall in the autism spectrum, but it is clear from the pattern of learning and behavioral problems that autism is an appropriate diagnosis. Other unresolved issues include whether Asperger syndrome is a separate disorder from high-functioning autism, whether Rett syndrome belongs in this classification even though girls diagnosed with Rett syndrome have a brief period of development in which a few characteristics of autism appear (particularly since the identification of a specific gene related to Rett syndrome), and how frequently childhood disintegrative disorder (essentially late-onset autism with widespread regression) occurs (Schopler, 1998; Volkmar, Klin, & Cohen, 1997).

All too often, in practice, a clinician will make the diagnosis of PDD without specifying whether it is autism, PDD/NOS, or some other category. From the family and service provider perspective, the PDD diagnosis is too indefinite and vague to formulate intervention plans. PDD may not be the best diagnosis because of its all-encompassing nature and the preconceived notions that the label connotes. Parents, particularly those who are assertive and have access to resource material (such as that on the Internet), usually make the translation of an undefined PDD diagnosis into autism but often are at a loss to know what is needed at home, how impaired the child is, and what is required for educational interventions. Because confusion remains about what constitutes the rationale for a PDD diagnosis (e.g., mild symptoms or symptoms in one or two but not all categories), there appears to be a lack of sufficient information on which to base a diagnosis and thereby confusion on merit or generalizability of a diagnosis across settings. At times it seems as though the lack of experience or confidence of the clinician influences this decision, and an inconclusive PDD diagnosis is given as a hedge.

Regardless of the terminology used (PDD or autism spectrum), researchers seem to agree that the incidence of these disorders has increased from the early reported figure of 2 to 4 per 10,000 to 20 per 10,000 and perhaps as high as 50 per 10,000 (Bryson, 1997). The differences between the earlier and current numbers probably reflect several factors: broadening of the definition and the inclusion of very mild cases; improved early identification, due in part to the downward extension of the public school education laws to include very young children; and increased public awareness. The experience of the Treatment and Education of Autism and Related Communication-Handicapped Children (TEACCH) program in North Carolina appears to be mirrored in other states and countries—namely, that the increase in referrals comes primarily from at least three sources: very young children, high-functioning children, and children previously diagnosed with other problems, such as ADHD and bipolar disorder. Tommy is an example of a young child with high-functioning autism, who was referred at a somewhat later age (5 years old) because of the relatively mild degree of impairments. It is premature to speculate about whether the increase in referrals involves a true increase in the population rather than redefinition and early identification. Whatever the reasons, the impact on professionals and families has been significant, necessitating the sharpening of diagnostic and assessment skills, with particular emphasis on assessment of young children and mild, higher functioning students.

ISSUES IN ASSESSMENT OF AUTISM

One issue affecting assessment of autism is the nature of the syndrome itself. The primary defining features of autism include delayed and atypical development in social reciprocity and relatedness, delayed and atypical development, idiosyncratic language and communication skills, and repetitive and restricted behaviors and interests. In addition, a number of problems in cognitive development and functioning that are closely associated with the diagnosis of autism are important for understanding the nature of this condition (Schopler & Mesibov, 1995). There can be considerable variability in the expression of these different characteristics along a continuum of severity and qualitative impairment. For example, one youngster may be extremely aloof with few, if any, communication skills. A second child, like Tommy (described in the vignette at the beginning of the chapter), may have some social interest and ability to communicate but may show obsessive preoccupations and markedly restricted play interests. Despite these different patterns, both children would meet the diagnostic criteria of autism.

In addition to the variability of behaviors associated with the label of autism, problems inherent in the testing of children with autism present a second issue. In the past, the exclusion of such children from the educational mainstream, partly the result of their misclassification as severely emotionally disturbed, prevented school psychologists from developing methods and skills for appropriate evaluations. Contributing to this lack of exposure was the myth that the test information would be invalid because these children could never show their true potential because of their emotional disturbances—the "child in the glass bowl" mystique. In addition, few training opportunities were available in most college preparatory programs. Many times psychologists felt that autistic individuals were untestable. The lack of understanding of the basic nature of the disorder, unclear purpose and preparation, inappropriate expectations, and improper test selection may have played a role in the development of this attitude. Just as professionals, unable to find a clear etiological explanation for autism, assumed in the past that parents were responsible for their child's problems, psychologists and other clinicians may have placed the blame on the child when the problem was more a reflection of the nature of autism and its incompatibility with standard test protocols and test demands. In the end, the child was often described as uncooperative, hyperactive, noncompliant, and willful and thus untestable. More recent training, newer test methods, and a better understanding of the child with autism has helped psychologists view an unsuccessful test session as a criteria for modification instead of failure. The more recent experience in the field of autism suggests that these children can be assessed reliably and meaningfully regardless of the severity of disability (Marcus & Schopler, 1993).

A third factor lies in the interplay between the impairments of autism and the demands of the testing situation. The wide variability among children with autism and the impact of the characteristics of autism on prescribed testing formats and situations markedly influence the psychologist's ability to assess a child. Thus a full understanding of the range of behaviors exhibited in such areas as communication, socialization, attention, and cognitive development will help the psychologist better match the child's presenting characteristics with techniques that can be used to best delineate his or her strengths and deficits.

Severe Communication Deficits

Autistic children have communication and language difficulties that range, expressively, from complete muteness to peculiar jargon and echolalia to fairly complex language functioning (Schopler & Mesibov, 1985). With lower functioning children, comprehension of language is frequently limited to a few very simple commands. Many youngsters require gestures or situation cues in order to understand spoken directions. Occasionally autistic children react negatively to language demands because of their frustration with limited comprehension. Not only are verbal expression and comprehension deficient but other forms of communication (gestural, facial, affective) are usually impaired as well. Examiners expect most children in an assessment situation, whether developmentally delayed or not, to respond to language, initiate and react to conversational speech, express needs clearly, and be aware of the rules of communication. Because the child with autism frequently has few or none of these skills, the likelihood of behavior problems is often increased by language expectations that are too high. Not only are language-related test items likely to produce negative reactions or no response, but also verbal direction of any sort may be met with confusion that is often interpreted as noncompliance. Even when children have apparently well-developed language skills, communication may still be repetitive, insular, and disorganized. Comprehension of more abstract language skills may be significantly limited.

Deficits in Social Judgment and Relating to People

The failure of autistic individuals to develop normal patterns of relating to other people has been well documented (Volkmar, Carter, Grossman, & Klin, 1997). This impairment varies in severity, from total lack of awareness and interest in people and resistance to intrusion to shallow relating skills and inadequate understanding of social rules. What this means for the examiner is that the usual methods of establishing rapport, often perceived as critical for a reliable evaluation, will be generally ineffective. The child may not be familiar with basic social behaviors such as sitting quietly at a table, taking turns, or returning test materials after an item is completed. Most autistic children must learn social rules by direct, specific, repetitive instruction, which may have to be uniquely structured to their understanding of the environment. A testing situation may not allow this type of interaction.

In addition to the frustration of dealing with the communicative and social deficits of autistic children, the examiner may have to struggle with personal feelings of unworthiness or inadequacy. Because the goal of the session may be to acquire a reliable score and set of data, the roadblocks set up by the child because of his or her own impairments can generate emotional reactions on the part of the examiner. In turn, this can color his or her perception of the child and interpretation of the data. The examiner needs to recognize that these behavioral problems (e.g., not staying seated, not responding to questions) are manifestations of the fundamental organically based dysfunctions of autism and not willful acts.

Attention, Organization, and Perceptual Problems

Autistic children tend to be distractible, to have a short attention span (especially for language-related tasks), and to organize themselves poorly in time and space. Perceptual anomalies such as hyper- or hyposensitivity to sounds, preoccupation with visual phenomena, or tactile–kinesthetic abnormalities are common, especially with lower functioning children (Burack, Enns, Stauder, Mottron, & Randolph, 1997; Demeyer, Hingtgen, & Jackson, 1981). Often these children will display oral or self-stimulatory behaviors with the test materials themselves. This creates difficulties for the examiner in a number of ways. The child's attention may be difficult to hold; he or she may become disorganized when faced with a test that has either several sequential steps or multiple stimuli. He or she may repeatedly attempt to lick or smell materials and may attend to sounds outside the room rather than to the examiner's voice. These manifestations of the disorder obviously interfere with smooth test administration, but they need to be recognized diagnostically and handled skillfully during the testing session.

Uneven Pattern of Development

Many autistic children are mentally retarded (Wing & Gould, 1979). However, the child's strengths affect both the test selection and the management of the test situation. It is not uncommon for a child to be able to run freely about the room or climb skillfully up stairs or onto the window sill, yet not understand the command, "sit in your seat." If the examiner judges the child's language comprehension by his or her motor skills, overexpectations and resultant behavioral problems may occur. Similarly, a child may have good toileting skills but be unable to ask to use the toilet, causing the examiner to infer that these skills are deficient. Many of these children have excellent visual memory, visual discrimination, and matching skills but have very poor complex problem-solving and reasoning abilities. The same child who can effortlessly put together a 25-piece jigsaw puzzle may have no concept of temporal events and consequently have great difficulty delaying gratification. Thus the examiner must be prepared to deal with a child who may be functioning at age level in some activities but well below age level in others. In particular, the examiner must understand that the mental retardation is not simply functional (a euphemism for "intact intelligence masked by emotional disturbance") but rather a manifestation of the fundamental developmental disorder associated with autism.

Motivational Deficits

Teachers and parents are often concerned about the autistic child's lack of normal interests and motivation. The examiner must worry about this because, as noted earlier, social reinforcers are unlikely to succeed with these children. The problem is at least twofold: lack of normal interests in such things as praise and affection and a strong, if inconsistent, interest in idiosyncratic objects and events (such as flapping a material, rubbing a surface, staring out a window). This interest may fluctuate because of an unusual sensory response (e.g., preoccupation with a shiny surface), an abnormally strong attachment to a preferred object from home, or a poorly communicated basic biological need such as hunger. The examiner needs to anticipate the unpredictable nature of the range in motivation and the child's response to rewards, as well as to evaluate the relative effectiveness of different types of reinforcers to aid in treatment planning.

Other Atypical Behaviors

Now considered secondary characteristics by the major diagnostic systems, body stereo-typies (e.g., hand flapping, twirling) and their rarer, more severe manifestations (e.g., self-injurious behavior) nevertheless pose obvious obstacles to successful psychological assessment. Some students will perseverate with materials (e.g., tapping a block on a tooth), others with their bodies (e.g., rocking). Interrupting or redirecting the child who is preoccupied with sameness (a ritualistic need to maintain a constant environment) may trigger a variety of responses that can interrupt assessment procedures.

By reviewing the major deficits of autism from the testing perspective, the examiner is taking the first step toward anticipating problems and preparing to conduct the evaluation successfully. As noted earlier, it is important to understand the reality the child has constructed because of limitations of cognition, communication, and perception. Rather than seeing these behaviors as noncompliance, the psychologist needs to keep in mind typical responses a child with autism might exhibit when routines are changed or when under stress. By assuming that the child won't comply, the examiner is forced to rely exclusively on authority and control with a youngster who may be experiencing considerable confusion over expectations. By seeing the behavior as *can't* rather than *won't*, the examiner has many more options to explore. Employing such a shift in perspective helps address the issue of untestability.

Structuring the Testing Environment

The following general guidelines are provided to enable the examiner to use the knowledge of autism to structure the testing environment.

Flexibility in Test Administration

The optimal test situation is one that combines an appropriate instrument (see the next section) with sensitivity to the child's difficulties with communication, attention, and social demands. This requires flexibility in (1) altering sequences of items so that stressful language items are balanced by more enjoyable visual–motor tasks; (2) modifying instructions so that the task is clearly understood; (3) providing frequent breaks when necessary; or (4) simplifying a task to give the child a successful experience. The examiner should show flexibility with the test protocol when necessary, noting these modifications for the record. The observations gathered in interacting with the child and the information obtained from experimenting with test materials and procedures can be as useful as the actual scores. (Issues of standardized administration are discussed later.)

Establishing an Appropriate Structure

Many of the management problems encountered in a test situation can be prevented by structuring the environment and establishing a set of rules and routines not dependent on verbal explanations. The room should be cleared of extraneous materials and should have separate work and play areas (e.g, table and chair on one side, rug or mat with toys on the other). A confused, disorganized student can be led through the routine of completing a task, then allowed to go to the play area for a few minutes. The release from task demands can begin to serve as a reinforcer for work and give the child a predictable, orderly routine without the use of language that may not be understood. A container (finished box) can be placed at one end of the table to demonstrate the idea of task completion. Higher functioning children may be helped by a visual, token, or word system that conveys how many tasks have to be performed before a break. The establishment of such structures and routines recognizes and deals with the child's basic deficits in communication and organization.

Alternative Methods of Communication

As noted previously, verbal language may not be sufficient to convey the rules of the testing situation. The examiner should expect to use dramatic gestures, exaggerated affect, manual prompts (perhaps even mild physical redirection), or other visual concrete aids as means of communicating with many autistic children. Even higher-functioning children or adolescents are not likely to grasp casual conversation and the nuances of social discourse. Verbal language still must be kept uncomplicated, free of idiomatic expressions, and limited to the task at hand. If the examining situation provides sufficient time, experimenting with simple manual signs or a picture system may prove useful diagnostically and may help with behavior management.

OTHER CONSIDERATIONS IN ASSESSMENT

Assessment not only addresses questions of diagnosis but also provides detailed information about skill levels, learning styles, and potential for successful treatment and adaptation. Prior to the categorization of autism as a developmental disorder, the only assessment data considered valid were observation in unstructured settings, parent interviews, or behavior analysis. Despite evidence to the contrary, many psychologists and other diagnosticians considered autistic individuals to be untestable. Now we know that, with more appropriate assumptions about autism and improved assessment methods, comprehensive and useful evaluations can be conducted.

Often assessment is based on data obtained in limited settings, typically a clinic or school site. Although this information is necessary and potentially useful, it is limited and needs to be supplemented by data from other sources, such as the home, classroom, and community. The nature of these data may include interviews, questionnaires, direct observation, and even videotaping. This increased scope of evaluation supports the assumption that the autistic child may function differently in different settings. The autistic child's needs, capabilities, and priorities in one setting, such as the school, may differ from those displayed at another site, such as the child's home. Even within a specific setting, variability in functioning may be noted. The direct testing information gathered in the clinic or school can be applied more meaningfully if considered in this broader context.

A comprehensive assessment must deal with the ramifications of the child's developmental disorder, not only across different settings but also across time. When families seek a professional opinion about their child, they need both diagnostic and prognostic information—that is, what the condition is now and what is likely to happen in the future. With reliable psychological data supplemented by other sources of data, the sensitive clinician can begin to address the question of probable future development. Obviously, such discussion must be tempered by the family's readiness to face these questions, as well as by the certainty of the prognosis, which will vary with the clarity and degree of current impairment. Thus a valid assessment may substantially clarify these issues of chronicity and prognosis.

Once diagnosis and, in some cases, prognostic clarification has been established, there is a need to understand the levels of developmental functioning of the autistic child, including his or her unique pattern of strengths and weaknesses. With younger children the assessment profile should be based primarily on guidelines derived from developmental norms, should use developmentally sequenced materials and activities, and should reflect concepts derived from well-established developmental models and themes (such as means–end, causality, role-taking perspective). At the adolescent age level and beyond, strictly developmental guidelines may have to be gradually replaced by criterion-based assessment of specific, pragmatic skills. The shift from the more developmentally based approaches to those concerned with assessment of behavior and competence in a functional environment reflects the current efforts of special educators in establishing appropriate secondary-level programs for severely handicapped individuals. Regardless of the fundamental assumptions of the assessment approach, the evaluation and analysis of abilities and disabilities within and across specific skill areas should be a basic objective.

Obviously, an assessment that fails to lead to constructive intervention plans is an inadequate assessment. Development of a meaningful Individual Education Plan (IEP), including appropriate educational placement, is mandated by federal law for individuals with autism and other disabilities. Such planning should include the type of assessment described in this chapter. Periodic reevaluations are required and should incorporate the students' needs with appropriate evaluative tools integrated into this assessment strategy. Use of developmental, psychoeducational, and psychological tests allow for the creation of an individualized profile of abilities and deficits that can then be translated into specific teaching programs. Other intervention strategies, such as medication, residential care, and special behavior management techniques, naturally evolve from thoughtful application of these data.

When considered in conjunction with home observations or reports from family members, direct testing information can form the basis of a meaningful set of strategies to help families manage and teach their autistic child. By providing parents with a clear understanding of their child's disability, the clinician takes the first step in giving parents the tools they need to become their child's primary advocate. Unfortunately, many clinicians who carry out the assessment give far less information to parents than to professional colleagues. Withholding assessment information serves no useful purpose and excludes parents from the treatment process, increasing their sense of frustration and helplessness. Parents are not only a major source of relevant data, but they also have been shown to be potentially outstanding teachers and cotherapists with or without professional guidance. The role of the parents cannot be overestimated, either as a source of information or as an important participant in discussion of assessment results (Attwood, 1998; Marcus, Kunce, & Schopler, 1997).

ASSESSMENT OF HIGH-FUNCTIONING
CHILDREN WITH AUTISM

The assessment of children suspected of having autism may emphasize language, socialization, cognitive, and academic abilities, much like the assessment of children with other developmental disabilities. Often, however, it may necessitate the evaluation of other abilities such as flexibility, executive functioning, joint attention, memory, and sensory responses. Such a comprehensive assessment may require the modification of traditional testing procedures, shifts in preconceived ideas about development, and increased reliance on informal and observational information requiring refined clinical judgment across settings. The inclusion of parents and others significant in the environment of the child will be necessary because of the importance of historical data and adaptive behavior in final diagnostic and prescriptive assessment.

A significant factor in a comprehensive approach is to determine what types of tests and procedures might be most successful in gaining information about the child. It may help to organize assessment procedures around age and domain parameters, even though most complex domains are not mutually exclusive; that is, they do not assess only one area. Also, many of the assessment activities and procedures are similar across age ranges. However, a developmental perspective allows the examiner to consider normal developmental issues that are germane to age-specific populations and provides a necessary framework when assessing lower functioning and/or younger children.

In the past decade, there has been growing interest and research on children such as Tommy (described in the chapter-opening vignette) who do not exhibit all the symptoms of classic autism; that is, those who have been loosely grouped into the categories of high-functioning children with autism and/or Asperger syndrome (Rutter & Schopler, 1992; Schopler, Mesibov, & Kunce, 1998). Although there is disagreement about the nomenclature—that is, whether this is one syndrome or two different subclassifications—there is some consensus about tools that might facilitate diagnostic assessment with this population, such as tools that include neuropsychological tasks. Such an assessment can assist in diagnosis and can provide information on a child's preferred learning styles and his or her cognitive strengths and weaknesses. Wide variations in behavior and assessment results have been noted in this population. Behaviors may be more subtle or may not surface in a one-on-one testing situation; therefore, it is advantageous to employ a variety of formal and informal strategies in order to properly assess children suspected of having autism.

Children currently being diagnosed with Asperger syndrome may demonstrate difficulties with social relatedness and social skills, language functioning in social and pragmatic situations, and limited ranges of interest, similar to some degree to those seen in children typically identified as autistic. However, these children with Asperger syndrome have higher cognitive abilities (at least normal IQs) and somewhat more normal basic language skills but more subtle difficulties with language processing. Fine and gross motor deficits also are more common in this group (Wing, 1988). These children seem less aloof than other children with autism, showing some desire to fit in socially and to have friends. Often they are quite puzzled when they are socially unsuccessful.

There also is a small subgroup of this Asperger population who are extremely bright and in whom more functional abilities have been spared. These children may score in the above average or superior range on cognitive and academic testing and show few autistic tendencies. However, they often struggle from year to year, have problems making friends, and may develop secondary symptoms, such as depression or aggression (Klin, Volkmar, Sparrow, Cichetti, & Rourke, 1995). Comprehensive observation within the classroom and in other unstructured situations may pinpoint areas of difficulty that affect their overall performance. This appears to be a population of children who are often misdiagnosed throughout their formal school years, with teachers and parents continually seeking ways to work successfully with them.

There are a variety of assessment instruments pertinent to neuropsychological assessment of higher functioning autistic populations that measure executive functioning. These include (1) tests of flexibility, such as the Wisconsin Card Sorting Test (WCST; Heaton, 1981) and the Trail-Making Tests A and B (Reitan & Wolfson, 1985) and more informal tests such as set shifting and object sorting games (sorting the same objects into different categories); (2) visual–motor tasks, such as figure–ground reversal illusions using such materials as the Escher calendar; (3) tests of planning and organization, such as the Tower of Hanoi/London (Shallice, 1982), the Rey–Osterrieth Complex Figures (Lezak, 1995), maze tasks, and Simon Says (a computer game); (4) tests of inhibition, such as the Stroop Color–Word Test (Trenerry, Crosson, DeBoe, & Leber, 1989), Matching Familiar Figures Test (Kagan, 1964), Visual Search and Attention Test (Trenerry, Crosson, DeBoe, & Leber, 1990), and Continuous Performance Tests (Lezak, 1995) and informal measures, such as odd–even number cancellation tests, and tests that give directions by alternating words with instructional intent—for example, "underline the little words and cross out the big words."

BEHAVIORAL AND SOCIAL ASSESSMENT

Behavioral assessments and social and developmental histories are crucial in the evaluation of autistic children, particularly because accurate diagnosis can only be derived using these types of data. Such information should serve as the foundation upon which other, more standardized data can be integrated to fully understand the autistic child. Much of these data can be derived from scales, checklists, interviews, and observations. However, it is important to have a working knowledge of typical autistic behaviors to correlate with data acquired from these more formal processes. These tools can provide an objective basis for acquiring and reporting such information in a standardized way. They also can be used for intervention evaluations and can allow for cross-setting comparisons of behavior and of evaluations obtained from different personnel.

Behaviorial Assessment Instruments

With the major reliance on clinical judgment, most assessment tools are clinical in nature. There are, however, a few commercially published checklists that directly relate to the behavioral assessment of children with autism. These measures generally include subscales that relate to language, social interaction, functional or adaptive skills, affect, and sensory behaviors. The reliability of the informant and how realistic he or she is about the child are germane to any good behavioral assessment compiled in this manner. It is equally important to be familiar with the instrument and its scoring criteria. What follows is a brief description of the most common measures used to assess behavior.

The Childhood Autism Rating Scale (CARS; Schopler, Reichler, & Renner, 1988) is a 15-item objective measure that can be used in a variety of settings and that yields diagnostic information that can be used as a screening tool or as part of a comprehensive assessment. Scores are obtained on specific subscales such as Relating to People and Verbal Communication, and a total score results in classification into one of three categories: not autistic, mildly to moderately autistic, and severely autistic. Like any single test, the CARS should not be used by itself in making the diagnosis but can be integrated effectively into the total assessment process. The CARS can be applied in several settings and with different sources of information, including direct observation of a developmental or psychological testing situation, parent interview, and observation in home or school setting. Morgan (1988) concluded that the CARS emerged as the strongest of the current scales in terms of demonstrated psychometric properties.

The Ritvo–Freeman Real Life Rating Scale (Freeman, Ritvo, Yokota, & Ritvo, 1986) is a scale for children with infantile autism. The scale can be used by a variety of personnel and looks at five areas of functioning that are rated along a scale of 0 (never demonstrated) to 3 (seen almost consistently). The behavioral traits listed in each of the scales are clearly defined, allowing the examiner to view a variety of behaviors across domains.

The Autism Screening Instrument for Educational Planning (Krug, Arick, & Almond, 1995) has a battery of five procedures used to assess autistic populations. Scores and percentile ranks are listed for each procedure. Norms are somewhat dated.

The Behavioral Rating Instrument for Autistic and Other Atypical Children (BRIAAC; Ruttenberg, Kalish, Wenar, & Wolf, 1977) uses standardized procedures for the observation of low-functioning atypical and autistic children. It contains seven scales that vary from severe to normal behaviors of 3–4-year-olds.

Adaptive Behavior Assessment

A second area that is required for a comprehensive evaluation of children with autism is an assessment of adaptive behavior: How children along the developmental spectrum meet the social and environmental demands in their lives. Most of the adaptive behavior scales focus on two major themes: (1) the degree to which individuals are able to function and maintain themselves independently, and (2) the degree to which they can meet cultural and social demands of society. No single instrument is generally able to assess all areas relevant to adaptive functioning. With childhood and youth autism, it may be important to look at the questions being asked, not at the age guidelines. The clinician may need to know about the history of the child's behaviors that occurred in infancy and early childhood, even though the child may now be of school age. Several examples of adaptive measures are described.

The Adaptive Behavior Inventory for Children (Mercer & Lewis, 1978) is a useful measure. Items deal with family life, school, and interpersonal relationships across a variety of settings, including leisure and domestic settings. There are English and Spanish editions. One criticism of the measure has been that it may discriminate against lower class and ethnic minority populations because it does not take into consideration what is expected within those cultures.

The Vineland Adaptive Behavior Scales (Sparrow, Balla, & Cicchetti, 1984) is a widely used instrument for assessing adaptive behavior. The scale has three versions: a survey form, an expanded form, and a classroom edition that can be used with children from birth through age 19. It has four domains that are combined to provide an adaptive behavior composite standard score. The survey form is an interview instrument and should be used in this capacity. The scale also has a maladaptive section for children aged 5 and older. Although the Vineland is psychometrically sound, experience with autistic children has led the authors to conclude that at times norming procedures are problematic, as fluctuations in the means and standard deviations of the standard scores from age group to age group are skewed. The classroom form can produce higher standard scores and lower age scores than the interview edition when children are low functioning. There also is an estimated-versus-observed rating in the classroom edition that may be misleading, that is, overestimating or underestimating the actual adaptive functioning for autistic children. The expanded version provides more concrete questions that relate to each area of functioning. This may help control the "looseness" of the abridged form. However, it is more time-consuming. The interview edition does allow a competent examiner to expand and gain considerable information on the child being assessed.

The Scales of Independent Behavior—Revised (Braininks, Woodcock, Weatherman, & Hill, 1996) is a relatively new instrument. This scale is highly structured in that it contains 14 main subscales organized into four adaptive behavior clusters, as well as an early-development subscale and a problem-behavior subscale. In addition, there is a short form that can be used for overall screening, which takes 15 to 20 minutes. It can be administered in two different ways, via a checklist or an interview. The norms are more current than those of most other scales and therefore may give lower standard scores than instruments developed earlier. Range between items tends to be very large. Ceilings may misrepresent autistic populations because a child could ceiling out but have splinter skills at higher levels. The scale also groups communication and social skills together under one cluster, which may not be specific enough for autistic populations.

There are a number of other adaptive scales on the market. Most have been used sparingly with autistic populations, so there is little data to determine whether they might be viable instruments. However, regardless of the instrument, the important consideration in assessing adaptive behavior in autistic populations may not be formal scores but what parents and teachers communicate about the child. This information should be expanded to address issues and gain knowledge about rituals, idiosyncratic patterns, and other atypical behavioral markers that might not be represented in formal scores. Such tools also serve as another means to gain early social and developmental history about the child, a crucial element in the diagnosis of autism.

DSM-IV has stated that children with Asperger syndrome may not exhibit clinically significant delays in adaptive behavior (other than social interactions), although the technical version currently published has expanded this concept. Our clinical experience has shown that this is not necessarily true. Although these children may have "average" scores on standardized instruments, the quality of specific adaptive skills, particularly in unstructured and unlearned settings, may be atypical and/or rote. Many times early developmental information will document a pattern of behavior that is atypical, even though the child possesses enough intelligence to learn appropriate social routines. Often, from very early in life, the free-flowing reciprocal interactions necessary for good social engagement are not evident. For example, on the Vineland Adaptive Behavior Scales, it is likely that Tommy's overall score would fall in the deficient range, although his communication standard score might be close to average because of adequate reading skills. Socialization is likely to be his weakest area.

DEVELOPMENTAL AND COGNITIVE ASSESSMENT

Informal Play Assessment

With very young children with disabilities, the use of cognitive measures may raise concerns about validity and reliability. Some may rely too heavily on sensory-motor competence, language abilities, and socialization, thereby underestimating cognitive potential in children having impaired functioning in these areas. They also may lack a variety of tasks that tap perceptual discrimination and memory competence, both precursors for later conceptual development. The sequential developmental nature of the instruments also can misrepresent the uneven profile of autistic children. For example, these children may ceiling out at a low level because of socialization and language difficulties, but they may have perceptual, motor, and memory skills well above the obtained ceiling. With higher functioning children, the converse may be true. Despite the fact that these children may obtain a very high cognitive score on an instrument, this score may not be predictive of classroom and adaptive functioning or of their success in school. Thus more informal procedures that emphasize play-based techniques can be useful to gain a full understanding of the range of functioning within this age group.

An important technique that can be used to gain a comprehensive picture of the young autistic child is a play assessment. Although there is not one set of behaviors that encompasses the many forms of play, there is consensus on common characteristics that seem to occur at different ages. These behaviors can provide meaningful information about the child's developmental levels. Because play changes as children mature, it is equally important to understand normal developmental patterns. Play also has social significance, because it is through play that young children learn how to interact, learn the rules and norms of their culture, and develop a variety of affective and emotional responses to the environment and other people. Systematic play assessment can thus help document ranges in affect, arousal, and engagement, concrete and abstract functioning, and complexity of object and person interactions. Play assessment can therefore provide an excellent opportunity to identify engagement and attachment skills, expand skills that are demonstrated to maximal levels without compromising the integrity of the test format, and document the variance in emergence of skills often seen in children with autism. Because it is enticing, naturalistic, and fun, it often becomes an appropriate avenue for a variety of young children.

A typical play-based assessment process is generally done with a multidisciplinary team of professionals (psychologist, special educator, occupational therapist, physical therapist, speech pathologist) and organized through one facilitator who works directly with the child. The other members of the team note behaviors and suggest alternative strategies or techniques that might be used to elicit responses not spontaneously observed, either through direct quiet verbal remarks or through notes. The members of the team gather data on levels of interaction and communication, categories of play, social skills, cognition, sensorimotor responses and preferences, attentional issues, concept formation and organizational skills, memory, problem solving and motivation, and gross and fine motor manipulation skills. Play also can be used in a one-on-one testing situation to assess affect, executive functioning, and set shifting with higher functioning children.

A formal play assessment usually involves periods of unstructured playtime, normally with the parent and child or a peer, and a more structured set of informal and formal routines with a facilitator. The facilitator observes what the child does spontaneously, integrates into the child's play routines, and then attempts to escalate the child's exhibited play behaviors into higher functional levels. Sequences are often done on the floor, in short segments, and following the child's initiative. During such periods, the examiner can determine if and how the child initiates play, how level of play is exhibited, and what type of interactive patterns, both verbal and nonverbal, are shown. It is preferable that a naturalistic observation (in the home–day care–preschool setting) be done whenever possible.

The parent is an integral part of this assessment, helping the child become comfortable in the testing environment, providing emotional support, and following directions that can enable the child to show maximal performance. Skills can be modeled for the parent during this time, skills that can then be generalized to the home environment. The parent also will be asked to leave at the end of the unstructured session so that the examiner can observe the child's separation and coping behaviors, as well as to signal the transition from an unstructured to a more structured situation. An observational checklist, framed with developmental age ranges, is most often used with such assessments, as it provides a simple guide on what and how to observe a child in play. A sample of such a checklist is included in Appendix 13.1 (Flagler, 1997).

Standardized Developmental Assessment Measures

In addition to the unstructured play-based approach to the assessment of functioning in young children, some criterion-referenced and standardized instruments can provide developmental and readiness information about functioning. These include the Psychoeducational Profile—Revised (PEP-R; Schopler, Reichler, Bashford, Lansing, & Marcus, 1990), the Infant–Preschool Play Assessment Scale (I-PAS; Flagler, 1997), the Carolina Curriculum for Infants and Toddlers/Preschoolers with Special Needs (Johnson-Martin, Attermeier, & Hecker, 1991), the Pre-Linguistic Autism Diagnostic Observation Schedule (PLA-DOS; Dilavore, Lord, & Rutter, 1995), the Mullen Scales of Early Learning (Mullen, 1995), and the Brigance Inventory of Early Development—Revised (Brigance, 1991), among many other scales currently on the market.

The PEP-R (and its predecessor, the PEP) has been used with autistic children for over 25 years. It is designed for use with children functioning at or below the preschool range and within the chronological age range of 6 months to 7 years. The test is divided into two sections: one that assesses developmental functions and one that identifies unusual or atypical behaviors. The developmental functions include imitation, perception, fine and gross motor skills, eye–hand integration, and cognitive verbal and performance skills. Behavioral areas assessed include relating and affect, play and interest in materials, sensory responses, and language abnormalities. In addition to age scores on each developmental function, an overall developmental age score is derived. Behavioral ratings are made on 43 items and scored as either absent, mild, or severe and then marked on a circular graph, providing a visual display of the amount and degree of behavioral abnormality. Once the PEP-R assessment is completed and the scores charted on the profiles, information is obtained that helps with specifying problems and characteristics associated with autism, overall level of developmental functioning, patterns of strengths and weaknesses, strategies that might be used to enhance learning potential and behavioral functioning, and emerging areas that should be targeted for educational programming.

For children in the middle childhood years (ages 8–12), cognitive assessment may involve procedures similar to those for younger populations, particularly if the child is significantly delayed. At this age, many autistic children have been in school long enough to be able to function in a formal testing situation, so standard intelligence tests can be used successfully. Children at this age level also may have developed a broader range of cognitive abilities; they may not need or want to do simplistic tasks that younger children prefer. However, they may have extensive knowledge about areas of specific interest that might not be illustrated in a formal assessment procedure. Their pattern of development typically appears to plateau at this stage, with strengths shown at the concrete comparison level and deficits shown when needing to manipulate material in new or more abstract ways. For these reasons, formal instruments can be used with minor or moderate adaptations, and a clearer picture of cognitive development may be derived. It will continue to be important to measure social and affective functioning in both the home and school settings.

For adolescents with autism (ages 13–18), cognitive assessment is probably only indicated when a formal diagnosis of autism is needed or when marked changes in the child's behavior or output has been observed. It also may be used with higher functioning children. After the age of 14, many school systems no longer require reevaluation, and with the changes in the Individuals with Disabilities Education Act (IDEA), future reevaluations may not encompass traditional assessments at all. However, if an initial assessment is needed, common batteries may range from completely nonverbal instruments (Test of Nonverbal Intelligence; C-TONI-3: Brown, Sherbenou, & Johnson, 1982; Leiter International Performance Scale—Revised; LIPS-R; Roid & Miller, 1997) to those that are more widely used (Wechsler Adult Intelligence Scale—3; Wechsler, 1997; Stanford–Binet-IV; Thorndike, Hagen, & Sattler, 1986). Level of functioning is an important consideration in test selection. With higher functioning adolescents with autism, verbal areas may appear as a relative strength, and thus tests that focus on these areas would be appropriate. In addition, tests that emphasize more complex neuropsychological functioning, for example, Differential Ability Scales (DAS; Elliott, 1990), NEPSY (Korkman, Kirk, & Kemp, 1998) may provide additional information on the overall processing of such students.

With very delayed children at this age level, functional assessment scales and vocationally related information may be relevant. The LIPS-R and C-TONI also can provide good information for this population because the format of every item is the same, no verbal instructions are needed or verbal responses required, and the tests rely on visual discrimination and reasoning, a relative strength for many autistic children. It is important to remember that these scales cater to autistic children's strengths and thus may inflate their overall cognitive scores. As these instruments have selective coverage and do not measure many other domains, they may not encompass the concept of general intelligence or social comprehension. Consequently, ancillary information should be derived from other, more comprehensive cognitive instruments, as well as from general test performance—for example, processing of more abstract questions, appropriate eye gaze, following verbal instructions.

For high-functioning, as well as more delayed, populations, it will be important to look beyond the cognitive and academic assessments that are traditionally completed on these children with autism. With this age group, tools that measure socialization, peer interaction, judgment, executive functioning, and adaptability to changes in the environment may have much more significance and be more relevant than any formal cognitive measures. Observation of peer and social interactions help tremendously with this population.

Cognitive Measures

Cognitive assessment should focus on overall development across domains, as well as on the qualitative nature of thought and processing as children mature. The underlying assumption is that normal development tends to be fairly ordinal and that earlier stages precede later stages in a prescribed order. Thus emphasis will be on what a child has learned and how it is generalized in new situations. There are a variety of formal assessment instruments that commonly are used to assess cognitive processing.

In the Bayley Scales of Infant Development—Second Edition (Bayley, 1993), an assessment measure for children from birth through 42 months of age, scoring procedures may cause a very low ceiling to be exhibited by autistic populations unless testing-of-limits procedures are used. The inclusion of language-based items throughout each item set usually results in the student reaching a ceiling before other areas of strength are demonstrated.

Because of this, the examiner may want to test the limits with the autistic child and administer items until there is a clear ceiling across all areas. Unless an examiner is using a play-based or modified procedure, such limit testing might not be done consistently. The BSID-2 has added a Facet Scales profile that developmentally charts the items on the test into four areas (cognitive, language, social, and motor), providing a visual picture of the scattering of abilities that might be demonstrated by the autistic child. However, there are not an equal number of items at each developmental level or across facets on the test.

The Merrill–Palmer Scale of Mental Tests (Stutsman, 1948), a primarily nonverbal instrument for children 18 to 71 months of age, provides a mental age and potential ratio IQ and is thus often suited to a variety of children with autism. It taps into relative strengths demonstrated by many autistic children (concrete visual discrimination, matching, and assembly tasks) and is colorful and brief in presentation. It tends to highlight the intact abilities of these children whose deficits in abstract and symbolic thinking are so pervasive. Because language and abstract problem-solving requirements are minimal, the results can be deceptively high. For children who become preoccupied with materials, the timing criteria may be detrimental. For others, the content of the test may not provide an opportunity to measure greater cognitive growth or flexibility. Because the repeated tasks do not change over age ranges—that is, they do not become more complex but rather have shorter time limits—it is not clear whether these items tap into higher level thinking skills at older age levels. The Merrill–Palmer Scales are presently being updated, and items are being added to both the floor and ceiling.

The DAS (Elliott, 1990), for children and youth in the 2 years, 6 months–17 years, 11 months age ranges, can be used with individuals with autism who have somewhat higher levels of functioning. It has a variety of batteries, such as lower preschool, upper preschool, and school-age ranges, as well as diagnostic subtests. It also has a lower basal and higher ceiling than other instruments in these age ranges. An extended GCA (general conceptual ability) score can be derived, depending on the subtests that are administered. Comprehension subtests are structured, which makes them adaptable to autistic populations. They provide visual information along with verbal instructions, offering the child a variety of ways to understand the task demands. Many of the subtests focus on receptive functioning as opposed to expressive output. Although the test was not formatted in this way, test modifications (e.g., enlarging pages, cutting out stimuli and responses) can provide added information that may measure discrete traits such as quantitative concepts. It is important to make sure that the correct concept is being measured when modifying the format and that such changes are reflected in the report. The school-age battery expands the nonverbal reasoning preschool cluster to include more reasoning tasks. It also adds a spatial ability cluster. There is a special nonverbal composite that can be used instead of the GCA at all levels. The manual also gives special test considerations for varied populations.

The Kaufman Assessment Battery for Children (K-ABC; Kaufman & Kaufman, 1983) is a measure designed for children in the 2 years, 6 months to 12 years, 6 months age ranges. It has been useful in the assessment of autistic children in that it reduces emphasis on language and provides an opportunity to teach subtest requirements before the actual administration of the test itself. It has quasi-flexible instructions; that is, it can allow the examiner several ways to teach an item, which may let an autistic child's preferred style be included. Although there is a preschool component to the test, it suffers, like most normed tests for this population, from having too few examples for each age range and inflated scores for younger children. Spatial memory and photo series are particularly sensitive to difficulties autistic children display because the students tend to focus on the visual elements of the subtests and disregard or misunderstand the actual task demands. Poor sequencing skills may affect their performances here. On the Triangles subtest, early examples measure visual matching tasks. When the subtest shifts to more abstract reasoning and spatial shifts become more obscure, autistic children begin to show deficits. Verbal working memory is hard to discern using this instrument. The norms are dated, although there are indications that this instrument is being renormed currently. The revisions to this instrument are due out in 2001.

The Stanford–Binet-IV (SB-IV; Thorndike et. al, 1986) may be a viable instrument for the assessment of cognition in people aged 2 years to adult, as opposed to the Stanford–Binet L-M. The new test seems most useful for autistic children who have some language and whose cognitive abilities fall above 50. This test extracts short-term memory and quantitative reasoning from the verbal reasoning subtests, allowing the examiner to measure each area of reasoning independently. The vocabulary subtest allows for measurement of both labeling and definition skills. Because the labeling portion of the test does not extend beyond preschool, and because many autistic children have extremely high labeling abilities, an alternative instrument may be required to accurately measure this particular skill. A simple picture vocabulary test may be a useful measure in this regard.

The quantitative subtests of the SB-IV appear to miss or subsume critical areas of development, causing large gaps or sudden shifts in overall skills. This presents some difficulty for autistic children because it requires them to shift sets, change response styles within the test, and attend to more verbal information. Number series (1, 5 1, 4 1, 3 ___ ___) may tap into a relative strength for autistic children because it emphasizes visual patterns. The clinician can observe how the child approaches this task and what cognitive strategies are employed, as abstract reasoning tasks often are very difficult for many autistic children. The format of this subtest provides children with a visual pattern that seems to help their mental organization.

Relatively speaking, memory is typically a strength for autistic children. The SB–IV allows the examiner to see this strength exhibited in the child. The test measures visual memory, language memory, digit memory, and visual–sequential memory. For children who are significantly impaired cognitively, some split may occur when more than a single attribute is assessed. Then organization becomes a factor. Autistic children tend to see the patterns when they are visually presented but not when they need to shift and reorganize the information. Problem-solving strategies are rudimentary, generally focused on a single attribute. It is not unusual for children to do well on sentence memory tasks, but only when sentences are declarative and concrete. When they become complex, with subordinate phrases attached, or when they begin to use esoteric words, they will rapidly miss major elements in the sentences. With other subtests in this group, sequencing and set shifting provide the most difficulty for autistic populations.

The Wechsler scales (Wechsler Preschool and Primary Scale of Intelligence—Revised; WPPSI-R; Wechsler, 1989; Wechsler Intelligence Scale for Children—Third Edition; WISC-III; Wechsler, 1991; WAIS-III; Wechsler, 1997), for people from 3 years of age through adulthood, can be used with little modification with higher functioning autistic persons (i.e., IQs above 85). It is highly likely that there will be scattering within and between the subscales, but clear patterns have not yet been established. The tests are familiar to examiners, are easily scored, and are commonly understood by professionals in the assessment field. The tests enable an examiner to document children's relative strengths in verbal and visuospatial processing. Because the tests are verbally mediated, even within the performance scales, they may be ineffective for students having difficulties with language processing. Time parameters on the performance subscales may penalize autistic children whose inflexible manner or rigid approach to problem solving does not adjust to increases in speed.

The test does not contain enough flexibility; there are few teaching items, and presentation cannot be modified to assure understanding.

There are other instruments which might have some usefulness with autistic children: The cognitive portion of the Woodcock–Johnson Battery (WJ-R COG; Woodcock & Johnson, 1989) and the Kaufman Adolescent & Adult Intelligence Test (KAIT; Kaufman & Kaufman, 1993a), although they lack validity studies with this population. Recently developed instruments that appear to have some merit for consideration include the Universal Nonverbal Intelligence Test (Bracken & McCallum, 1998), which can be administered without language. It has a variety of memory, problem-solving, and symbolic and nonsymbolic processing subtests; has an abbreviated, extended, and standard battery for children 5–17 years of age; and it contains a guide to gestures that can be used in administration. The LIPS-R, for students aged 2–20, is completely nonverbal, but has not been normed on autistic persons. It has received mixed reviews for use with this group from psychologists using the instrument, partially because of the shift in test parameters within subtests. However, it appears to have merit with other nonverbal children. It is easily administered. Although the comprehensive battery has 20 subtests, it has three quick screens for both ADHD and gifted children in the areas of Visual and Reasoning, Memory and Attention, and IQ). Attention and memory domains have been added to the previous LIPS.

Psychologists trained in evaluating autistic children may, with training, add a neuropsychological component to their assessment protocols. Recent studies and reports (Dawson, 1996; Rourke, 1995; Szatmari, Tuff, Finlayson, & Bartolucci, 1990) have suggested that there may be spared and impaired functioning that can be measured through tests such as the Stroop Color and Word Test (Golden, 1978), Incomplete Sentence Form (Goldstein, 1987), the NEPSY (Korkman, Kirk, & Kemp, 1998), and the WISC-PI (Kaplan, Fein, Framer, Delis, & Morris, 1999) and other information and neuropsychological subtests. Such testing may help support or negate the notion that autism may be a selective disorder of complex information-processing abilities and a disorder of multiple primary deficits that has been forwarded by researchers in recent years (Minshew & Goldstein, 1998).

A wider range of biomedical evaluations is also being done to assess metabolic abnormalities, gastrointestinal problems, and possible reactions to vaccines and poisonings, for example, immunizations and mercury. In children with an early history of lethargy, seizures, and vomiting, there may be a reason to do such extensive testing. However, most current data has established that only a very small group (fewer than 5%) of children with autism have some comorbid disorders (Dykens & Volkmar, 1997). It is also interesting that a skewed population, that is, middle-class, more highly educated parents, seem to be reporting the majority of the incidence of these occurrences. It may be that they are more knowledgeable. Our experience has shown that much anecdotal information is shared via the Internet with only sketchy case histories and little verifiable documentation.

ACHIEVEMENT TESTING

Testing of educational functioning with autistic populations usually can help document uneven skill development, a pattern often exhibited in this group. With younger children, a checklist of readiness skills may provide as much information as most tests, and once again, the developmental profile and the play assessment can document areas of strength and weakness. The PEP-R (discussed earlier) also can help document readiness skills and has been normed on autistic populations.

With school-age populations, achievement tests may provide only one picture of the functional capability and adaptability of autistic children. They can provide data on relative strengths and weaknesses compared with peer groups and can occasionally document splinter skills. It is more common for restricted interests and atypical skill strengths to show up in more preferred activities, like reading a favorite book or completing computer games. What may be exhibited on tests is a finite strength as opposed to an achievement capability, such as a capacity to define many words but a lack of skill in using them. Thus a formal achievement test alone may not provide necessary information on the overall educational functioning of the child. High scores may only indicate learned, rote skills, with little generalization or flexibility evident when similar materials are presented in alternative ways.

A common characteristic found in most autistic students is variability among achievement scores, with many children exhibiting "peaks" and "valleys" in functional abilities. Some autistic children show signs of being hyperverbal and hyperlexic. For others, mathematical calculation skills may be spared, whereas math concepts are more difficult to attain. Reading comprehension may be impaired, whereas decoding skills may be excellent. Problems may develop when language becomes more abstract, when flexibility is required to manipulate information, and when complex organization is required. Memory may be a relative strength so problems and instruments like the Children's Memory Scale (Cohen, 1997) may help disguise areas of strength or difficulty.

For children functioning at early elementary levels, a variety of instruments can be used. These include the Test of Early Reading Ability (TERA-2; Reid, Hresko, & Hammill, 1989), Test of Early Mathematics (TEMA-2; Ginsburg & Baroddy, 1990), Test of Early Written Language (TEWL-2; Hresko, Herron & Peak, 1996), Test of Written Language (TOWL; Hammill & Larsen, 1996), and the Kaufman Survey of Early Academic Skills (Kaufman & Kaufman, 1993b), although all have limits when assessing young children. Many rely on visual components, a relative strength for many autistic children. The Achievement subscales on the K-ABC and the DAS also tap into early educational abilities. Material can be added or modified in these tests that could provide additional information. There are problems with these instruments at younger levels, as most contain a very small percentage of skills at each age level and may therefore not provide an accurate picture of items that autistic children might be able to accomplish in another milieu. For example, a child might receive a scaled score of 5 without passing one item on a particular subtest. The content of the items often is not functionally related to the child's environment and experiences. They also tend to be verbally mediated.

In order to supplement these achievement tests with a more appropriate educational assessment, a curriculum-based evaluation might provide the most useful data for the autistic population. In this way, the child's needs and preferred learning styles can be integrated to the best advantage. The teacher is able to assess, on a continuing basis, whether instructional patterns are understood, are beneficial, and can serve to increase learning. A need for modifications can be readily observed in such a situation and can be implemented before the child incorporates and generalizes an erroneous concept or learned behavior. It is easier to analyze where problems occur in a task because there is flexibility and opportunity for expanded curriculum examples and extended trials. Standardized tests provide only a few selected items in any one area at each level, making such modifications more difficult.

The Brigance Diagnostic Inventory of Early Development—Revised (Brigance, 1991) is a screening instrument that seems useful, and, for lower functioning and elementary students, it is functionally oriented and can provide fairly extensive information on school and home functioning. The Brigance is relatively common in schools, has different levels for various age ranges, and is simple to administer. It provides good guidelines for IEP goals, as long as these items are not used verbatim.

With lower functioning autistic youth at the secondary level, educational assessment should integrate vocationally related skills, as well as socialization and independent living skills and work habits. The Adolescent and Adult Psychoeducational Profile (AAPEP; Mesibov, Schopler, Schaffer, & Landrus, 1988) is specifically designed for this purpose. In addition, supplemental instruments might include scales that have sections on life and work skills and other essential skills. These scales may be relevant for lower functioning students. A vocational rehabilitation counselor could provide more data on transitioning to the workplace and from secondary school.

For higher functioning children, academic achievement is less problematic, as many will function in ways that are similar to nondisabled populations. Most standard instruments can be used, for example, the Woodcock–Johnson Psychoeducational Battery—Revised (Woodcock & Johnson, 1989a), or some tests that have strong diagnostic components, such as Key Math—Revised (Connolly, 1988), Woodcock Diagnostic Reading Battery (Woodcock, 1997). Response requirements, however, are often more concrete than classroom content and organizational requirements. Although responses may meet criteria, several differences in their patterns may be noted. For example, higher functioning children may be more concrete, less able to shift into abstract and open-ended material, less organized, and more mechanical in their responses to learned material and may show less planning and execution of novel tasks. This is a pattern that Tommy, in the case illustration at the beginning of the chapter, is likely to show. Tests such as the Tell Me a Story Apperception Test can provide added information on language organization (Constantino, Malgady, & Rogier, 1988).

CONCLUSIONS

With a thorough knowledge of the characteristics and underlying problems of autism, testing instruments, strategies, and behavior management techniques, psychologists should be able to provide a careful, practical, and comprehensive assessment of the child with autism. Appropriate test selection, coupled with sensitivity to the unique social, communicative, and cognitive and perceptual needs of the autistic child, allows the psychologist to obtain a reliable and valid assessment of skills and to help in treatment and educational planning and allows the child and family to have as productive and meaningful a life as possible.

APPENDIX 13.1. PLAY OBSERVATION CHECKLIST

The following information (adapted from Flagler, 1996) can be used to help examiners when observing children during play. It also can be used when talking with parents about their children's behaviors at home. It also helps to organize an observational situation.

1. *Response to new situations.* Look at the child's reaction to separation from the parent, reluctance to enter new situations, and response to changes in the environment.

2. *General play behaviors.* How much time does the child spend in various categories of play (social, functional, constructive, rough-and-tumble, symbolic)? Which activities are most/least engaging? Does the child demonstrate atypical play? Who controls the play sequences?

3. *Social play*. Does the child primarily look at others when playing? Is there reciprocal language interchange and joint attention? Can the child solve problems? Does the child orient to affective stimuli and recognize them? Can the child relate social stimuli to rewards? Does the child inhibit and wait for his or her turn? When inhibited, what are his or her reactions? Can he or she take a series of turns using verbal or nonverbal prompts effectively?

4. *Sensory-motor responses and preferences*. Can the child regulate sensory input and organize it effectively? Is the child responsive to all stimuli? How does he or she react to tactile interactions or arousal techniques? Does the child have a restricted range of interest in toys, carry an object around, or only show interest in minute parts of toys? Does the child have a perception of gaze direction? Are stereotypical behaviors seen?

5. *Attention*. How does the child react to ancillary auditory and visual stimuli? Can the child attend to a variety of visual and auditory stimuli at one time? How does the child respond to language? Does the child demonstrate rapid shifts in attention?

6. *Concept-formation skills*. Can the child classify and categorize? Can he or she discriminate by color, size, shape, or quantity? Can he or she note similarities and differences? How many attributes can the child use to sort without getting confused? Can he or she combine items that are conceptually the same but different in structure? Can the child sequence auditory and visual models? How many items or events can he or she sequence accurately? Can he or she follow two- or three-step directions? Can he or she sequence picture cards (up to a set of five)? Can he or she count effectively?

7. *Memory skills (long and short term, visual and auditory)*. How many items can a child recall from an initial presentation of numerals or pictures? Is there a preference (visual, auditory, or other)? Can the child recall video characters or cartoons seen in the past?

8. *Problem solving*. How does the child perform a task? Does the child have object permanence? Does the child show foresight when doing things like mazes? Can the child predict where an object will be seen next when it is moved behind a screen? Can the child determine how to get an object that is out of reach? Can the child understand means–ends and cause–effect behaviors with toys? Can the child be taught a new skill and internalize it into his or her play repertoire? Can the child generalize?

9. *Motivation*. Does the child make one or two attempts and give up? How persistent is the child? Is the child perseverative? When he or she becomes frustrated, what behaviors are exhibited?

10. *Fine motor skills*. Can the child manipulate small items? What techniques are used? Can he or she place items correctly? Can he or she open and close containers? Does the child have cross-modal associations? Can the child execute motor planning activities? Does the child demonstrate long-term memory for motor movements? Does he or she show a hand dominance? Does the child exhibit writing skills?

11. *Gross motor abilities*. What is the child's general physical appearance? Is muscle tone normal? What range of movements can the child perform? What positions are used for play? Can he or she walk, run, climb, or manipulate stairs? Does the child have perception of body movements?

12. *Communication*. What is the child's primary mode of communication? Can the child imitate peer or adult language? What type of social communicative skills are seen? Can the child answer abstract and concrete questions? What level of pragmatic skills are seen? What level of complex information processing is seen?

13. *Atypical academic skills areas*. Does the child have advanced reading or math abilities? Is the child particularly talented in art? Does the child exhibit an unusual range of knowledge in any particular area?

14. *Planning and organization.* How does the child plan a series of events? When doing mazes, how does the child determine directions and correct for errors? When given a multi-step task, how does the child complete it? Where does the child place items on paper when drawing?

REFERENCES

Achenbach, T. (1997). *Child Behavior Checklists*. Itasca, IL: Riverside.

American Psychiatric Association. (1994). *Diagnostic and statistical manual of mental disorders* (4th ed.). Washington, DC: Author.

Attwood, A. (1998). *Asperger's syndrome: A guide for parents and professionals*. Philadelphia: Kingsley.

Bayley, N. (1993). *Bayley Scales of Infant Development* (2nd ed.). San Antonio, TX: Psychological Corporation.

Bracken, B., & McCallum, R. S. (1998). *Universal Nonverbal Intelligence Test (UNIT)*. Itasca, IL: Riverside.

Braininks, R., Woodcock, R., Weatherman, R., & Hill, B. (1996). *Scales of Independent Behavior—Revised*. Itasca, IL: Riverside.

Brigance, A. (1991). *Diagnostic Inventory of Early Development—Revised*. North Billerica, MA: Curriculum Associates.

Brown, L., Sherbenou, R., & Johnson, S. (1997). *Test of Nonverbal Intelligence (CTONI-3)*. Itasca, IL: Riverside.

Bryson, S. E. (1997). Epidemology of autism: Overview and issues outstanding. In D. J. Cohen & F. R. Volkmar (Eds.), *Handbook of autism and pervasive developmental disorders* (2nd ed.; pp. 41–46). New York: Wiley.

Burack, J. A., Enns, J. T., Stauder, J. E. A., Mottron, L., & Randolph, B. (1997). Attention and autism: Behavioral and electrophysiological evidence. In D. J. Cohen & F. R. Volkmar (Eds.), *Handbook of autism and pervasive developmental disorders* (2nd ed., pp. 226–247). New York: Wiley.

Cohen, M. (1997). *Children's Memory Scale*. San Antonio, TX: Psychological Corporation.

Connolly, A. (1988). *Key Math—Revised*. Circle Pines, MN: American Guidance Service.

Constantino, G., Malgady, R., & Rogier, J. (1988). *Tell Me a Story Apperception Test Manual*. Los Angeles: Western Psychological Services.

Dawson, G. (1996). Brief report: Neuropsychology of autism. A report on the state of the science. *Journal of Autism and Developmental Disorders, 26,* 179–184.

Dawson, G., Klinger, L., Panagiotides, H., Lewy, A., & Castelloe, P. (1995). Subgroups of autistic children based on social behavior display distinct patterns of brain activity. *Journal of Abnormal Child Psychology, 23,* 569–583.

Demeyer, M. K., Hingtgen, J. N., & Jackson, R. K. (1981). Infantile autism reviewed. *Schizophrenia Bulletin, 7,* 388–445.

Dilavore, P., Lord, C., & Rutter, M. (1995). Pre-Linguistic Autism Diagnostic Observation Schedule (PLA-DOS). *Journal of Autism and Developmental Disorders, 25,* 355–379.

Dykens, E. M., & Volkmar, F. R. (1997). Medical conditions associated with autism. In D. J. Cohen & F. R. Volkmar (Eds.), *Handbook of autism and pervasive developmental disorders* (2nd ed., pp. 388–410). New York: Wiley.

Eaves, R. (1993). *Pervasive Developmental Disorder Rating Scale*. Opelika, AL: Small World.

Eaves, R. (1996). *Pervasive Developmental Disorder Observation Schedule*. Opelika, AL: Small World.

Elliott, C. (1990). *Differential Ability Scales*. San Antonio, TX: Psychological Corporation.

Flagler, S. (1996). *Multidimensional assessment of young children through play*. Lewisville, NC: Kaplan.

Flagler, S. (1997). *Infant–Preschool Play Assessment Scale (I-PAS)*. Atlanta, GA: Kaplan.

Freeman, B., Ritvo, E., Yokota, A., & Ritvo, A. (1986). A scale for rating symptoms of patients with the diagnosis of autism in real life settings. *Journal of the American Academy of Child Psychiatry, 25,* 130–136.

Ginsburg, H., & Baroddy, A. (1990). *Test of Early Mathematics* (TEMA-2). Itasca, IL: Riverside.

Golden, C. (1978). *Stroop Color and Word Test*. Itasca, IL: Riverside.

Goldstein, S. (1987). *Incomplete Sentence Form*. Salt Lake City, UT: Neurology, Learning and Behavior Center.

Hammill, D., & Larsen., D. (1996). *Test of Written Language* (TOWL-3). Itasca, IL: Riverside.

Heaton, R. (1981). *The Wisconsin Card Sorting Test Manual*. Odessa, FL: Psychological Assessment Resources.

Hresko, W., Herron, S., & Peak, P. (1996). *Test of Early Written Language* (TEWL-2). Itasca, IL: Riverside.

Johnson-Martin, N., Attermeier, S., & Hecker, B. (1991). *Carolina Curriculum for Infants and Toddlers/Preschoolers with Special Needs*. Itasca, IL: Riverside.

Kagan, J. (1964). *Matching Familiar Figures Test*. Unpublished manuscript, Harvard University.

Kaplan, E., Fein, D., Frame, J., Delis, D., & Morris, R. (1999). *WISC-PI*. San Antonio, TX: Psychological Corporation.

Karp, S., & Konstadt, N. (1971). *Children's Embedded Figures Test*. Palo Alto, CA: Consulting Psychologist Press.

Kaufman, A., & Kaufman, N. (1983). *Kaufman Assessment Battery for Children*. Circle Pines, MN: American Guidance Service.

Kaufman, A., & Kaufman, N. (1993a). *Kaufman Adolescent & Adult Intelligence Test*. Circle Pines, MN: American Guidance Service.

Kaufman, A., & Kaufman, N. (1993b). *Kaufman Survey of Early Academic Skills*. Circle Pines, MN: American Guidance Service.

Klin, A., Volkmar, J., Sparrow, S., Cichetti, D., & Rourke, B. (1995). Validity and neuropsychological characteristics of Asperger syndrome: Convergence with nonverbal learning disabilities. *Journal of Child Psychology and Psychiatry, 36*, 1127–1140.

Kolb, B., & Whishaw, I. (1995). *Fundamentals of human neuropsychology* (4th ed.). New York: Freeman.

Korkman, M., Kirk, U., & Kemp, S. (1998). *NEPSY*. San Antonio, TX: Psychological Corporation.

Krug, D., Arick, J., & Almond, P. (1995). *Autism Screening Instrument for Educational Planning*. Austin, TX: Pro-Ed.

Leiter, R. (1984). *Leiter International Performance Scale*. Chicago, IL: Stoelting.

Lezak, M. (1995). *Neuropsychological assessment* (3rd ed.). New York: Oxford University Press.

Marcus, L. M., Kunce, L. J., & Schopler, E. (1997). Working with families. In D. J. Cohen & F. R. Volkmar (Eds.), *Handbook of autism and pervasive developmental disorders* (2nd ed.; pp. 631–649). New York: Wiley.

Marcus, L. M., & Schopler, E. (1993). Pervasive developmental disorders. In T. O. Ollendick & M. Hersen (Eds.), *Handbook of child and adolescent assessment* (pp. 346–363). Needham Heights, MA: Allyn & Bacon.

Mercer, J., & Lewis, J. (1978). Adaptive Behavior Inventory for Children. In *The system of multicultural pluralistic*. New York: Psychological Corporation.

Merrell, K. (1994). *Assessment of behavioral, social, and emotional problems: Direct and objective methods for use with children and adolescents*. New York: Longman.

Mesibov, G. B., Schopler, E., Schaffer, B., & Landrus, R. (1988). *Individualized assessment and treatment for autistic and developmentally disabled children: Vol. 4. Adolescent and Adult Psychoeducational Profile (AAPEP)*. Austin, TX: Pro-Ed.

Meyers, J., & Meyers, K. (1995). *Rey Complex Figure Test and Recognition Trial*. San Antonio, TX: Psychological Corporation

Miller, L. (1982). *Miller Assessment for Preschoolers*. San Antonio, TX: Psychological Corporation.

Minshew, N. J., & Goldstein, G. (1998). Autism as a disorder of complex information processing. *Mental Retardation and Developmental Disabilities Research Review, 4*, 129–136.

Morgan, S. (1988). Diagnostic assessment of autism: A review of objective scales. *Journal of Psychoeducational Assessment, 6*, 139–151.

Mullen, E. (1995). *Mullen Scales of Early Learning*. Circle Pines, MN: American Guidance Service.

Mundy, P. (1995). Joint attention and social-emotional approach behavior in children with autism. *Development and Psychopathology, 7*, 63–82.

Ozonoff, S., Rogers, S., & Pennington, B. (1991). Asperger's syndrome: Evidence of an empirical distinction from high-functioning autism. *Journal of Child Psychology and Psychiatry, 32*, 1107–1122.

Reid, D., Hresko, W., & Hammill, D. (1989). *Test of Early Reading Ability (TERA-2)*. Itasca, IL: Riverside.

Reitan, R., & Wolfson, D. (1985). *The Halstead–Reitan Neuropsychological Test Battery: Theory and clinical interpretation*. Tucson, AZ: Neuropsychological Press.

Roid, G., & Miller, L. (1997). *Leiter International Performance Scale—Revised*. Wood Dale, IL: Stoelting.

Rourke, B. P. (Ed.). (1995). *Syndrome of nonverbal learning disabilities: Neurodevelopmental Manifestations*. New York: Guilford Press.

Ruttenburg, B. A., Kalish, B. I., Wenar, C., & Wolf, E. G. (1977). *Behavior rating instrument for autistic and other atypical children* (Rev. ed.). Philadelphia: Developmental Center for Children.

Rutter, M., & Schopler, E. (1992). Classification of pervasive developmental disorders: Some concepts and practical considerations. *Journal of Autism and Developmental Disorders, 22,* 459–482.

Schopler, E. (1998). Premature popularization of Asperger syndrome. In E. Schopler, G. B. Mesibov, & L. J. Kunce (Eds.), *Asperger syndrome or high-functioning autism?* (pp. 385–399). New York: Plenum Press.

Schopler, E. & Mesibov, G. B. (Eds.). (1995). *Learning and cognition in autism*. New York: Plenum Press.

Schopler, E., Mesibov, G. B., & Kunce, L. J. (Eds.). (1998). *Asperger syndrome or high-functioning autism?* New York: Plenum Press.

Schopler, E., Reichler, R. J., Bashford, A., Lansing, M. D., & Marcus, L. M. (1990). *Individualized assessment and treatment for autistic and developmentally disabled children: Vol. 1 Psychoeducational Profile–revised (PEP-R)*. Austin, TX: Pro Ed.

Schopler, E., Reichler, R. J., & Renner, B. R. (1988). *The Childhood Autism Rating Scale* (CARS): For diagnostic screen and classification of autism. New York: Irvington.

Shallice, T. (1982). Specific impairments of planning. *Philosophical Transactions of the Royal Society of London, B298,* 199–209.

Sparrow, S., Balla, D., & Cicchetti, D. (1984). *Vineland Adaptive Behavior Scales*. Circle Pines, MN: American Guidance Service.

Stone, W., & Hogan, K. (1993). A structured parent interview for identifying young children with autism. *Journal of Autism and Developmental Disorders, 23,* 639–652.

Stutsman, R. (1948). *Merrill–Palmer Scale of Mental Tests*. Los Angeles: Western Psychological Services.

Szatmari, P., Tuff., L., Finlayson, A., & Bartolucci, G. (1990). Asperger's syndrome and autism: Neurocognitive aspects. *Journal of the American Academy of Child and Adolescent Psychiatry, 29,* 130–136.

Thorndike, R., Hagen, E., & Sattler, J. (1986). *Stanford–Binet Intelligence Scale-IV*. Itasca, IL: Riverside.

Trenerry, M., Crosson, B., DeBoe, J., & Leber, W. (1989). *The Stroop Neuropsychological Screening Test*. Odessa, FL: Psychological Assessment Resources.

Trenerry, M., Crosson, B., DeBoe, J., & Leber, W. (1990). *Visual Search and Attention Test*. Odessa, FL: Psychological Assessment Resources.

Volkmar, F. R. (1987). Diagnostic issues in the pervasive developmental disorders. *Journal of Child Psychology and Psychiatry, 28,* 365–369.

Volkmar, F. R., Carter, A., Grossman, J., & Klin, A. (1997). Social development in autism. In D. J. Cohen & F. R. Volkmar (Eds.), *Handbook of autism and pervasive developmental disorders* (2nd ed., pp. 173–194). New York: Wiley.

Volkmar, F. R., Klin, A., & Cohen, D. J. (1997). Diagnosis and classification of autism and related conditions: Consensus and issues. In D. J. Cohen & F. R. Volkmar (Eds.), *Handbook of autism and pervasive developmental disorders* (2nd ed., pp. 5–40). New York: Wiley.

Wechsler, D. (1989). *Wechsler Preschool and Primary Scale of Intelligence—Revised*. San Antonio, TX: Psychological Corporation.

Wechsler, D. (1991). *Wechsler Intelligence Scale for Children—Third Edition (WISC-III)*. San Antonio, TX: Psychological Corporation.

Wechsler, D. (1992). *Wechsler Individual Achievement Test*. San Antonio, TX: Psychological Corporation.

Wechsler, D. (1997). *Wechsler Adult Intelligence Scale—III (WAIS-III)*. San Antonio, TX: Psychological Corporation.

Wetherby, A., & Prizant, B. (1993). *Communication and Symbolic Behavior Scales*. Itasca, IL: Riverside.

Wing, L. (1988). The continuum of autistic characteristics. In E. Schapler & G. B. Mesibov (Eds.), *Diagnosis and assessment in autism* (pp. 91–110). New York: Plenum Press.

Wing, L., & Gould, J. (1979). Severe impairments in social interactions and associated abnormalities in children: Epidemiology and classification. *Journal of Autism and Developmental Disorders, 9,* 11–29.

Woodcock, R. (1997). *Woodcock Diagnostic Reading Battery*. Itasca, IL: Riverside.

Woodcock, R., & Johnson, M. (1989a). *Woodcock–Johnson Psycho-Educational Battery—Revised*. Allen, TX: DLM Teaching Resources.

Woodcock, R., & Johnson, M. (1989b). *Woodcock–Johnson Tests of Cognitive Ability*. Itasca, IL: Riverside.

14

ASSESSMENT OF CHILDREN
WITH CHRONIC ILLNESS

JANET R. SCHULTZ
CHERYL CHASE-CARMICHAEL

Greg is a verbal and sociable 9-year-old boy with cystic fibrosis. He was referred for psychological consultation by his pulmonary physician because of several concerns. First, he was resisting taking responsibility for preparing and taking his routine medication and aerosol treatments. He was cooperative if his parents initiated and prepared the materials. Second, he was also eating substantially less than the 120% RDA he needed. He had not gained weight in some time, and his physicians were hoping to avoid a surgically placed tube for nutritional supplementation. Finally, teachers reported that Greg was becoming verbally disruptive during class and having academic problems for the first time in his school career.

When interviewed, both Greg and his parents affirmed these concerns as problem areas. Failure to eat, however, evoked the strongest reaction. Greg's parents felt he made little effort to eat despite their efforts to make his favorite foods and present them in unusually attractive ways. Greg felt they were always pushing him to eat when he didn't feel hungry. The parents, with less energy, reported that Greg was not taking the initiative for the measuring and mixing of the medicine for his nebulizer, nor organizing and counting out his pills for the day or week. They had been told that lots of kids Greg's age do this and felt it was age appropriate. Their concern about school was that Greg had always done pretty well and that his self-esteem might suffer if his grades declined. Greg just said that he never had liked math and "didn't get it". Otherwise, the family was warm and interactive and reported doing many things together. As the only child, Greg received a great deal of adult attention and affection. The family used humor well and generally communicated fairly directly.

A phone conversation with his teacher clarified that although Greg's grades had gone down slightly over the past 2 years, the primary concern was with math and science, which had always been his weakest areas. Greg also was having trouble with carrying out long-range projects that were being introduced for the first time in his 4th-grade class.

Greg was tested and found to have a specific learning disability in math related to both concepts and mechanics. Organization and sequencing were also clear problems for him. Results of the Child Behavior Checklist suggested that although some oppositional behaviors were present, overall behavior was well within the normal range. Based on these findings, Greg's "resistance" was reformulated as part of his organization, sequencing, and math problems. His parents could approach preparing pills and aerosols as a teaching task in which their supervision would be necessary and appropriate. Supportive services in math were arranged at his school, and his regular teacher agreed to help structure the steps for long-term project planning.

Greg's eating was becoming a major power struggle. Behavior analysis indicated that Greg received a great deal of attention for not eating and that meal times were tense and unpleasant. A treatment plan that included using humor at meals and not talking about anyone's intake was set. Behavioral work with the family improved his intake by 50% and returned the pleasure to mealtimes.

Like many children referred with chronic illnesses, Greg presented with several concerns. Although his learning disability most likely did not result from his cystic fibrosis, it was affecting his self-care, as well as his school performance. The frustration of not understanding major subjects at school and the perceived pressure to try harder was contributing to increased oppositionality at home. This exacerbated an already growing conflict and power struggle with his parents. Eating would not have become a major issue had it not been for his medical condition. Children with chronic illnesses often present complex diagnostic questions that reflect the interactions among the biological, psychological, and social aspects of a child's life. In order to identify problems and useful, focused interventions, comprehensive psychological assessment is often indicated.

CHRONIC CONDITIONS IN CHILDHOOD

The purpose of this chapter is to provide a knowledge base about chronic illnesses in children and about psychological approaches and measures relevant to assessing children with such conditions. To this end, the chapter briefly identifies representative chronic conditions and reviews cognitive and psychosocial functions and priorities for assessment. This is followed by an examination of selected measures of developmental, cognitive, behavioral, and social functioning.

With the advent of immunizations, antibiotics, and other modern medical advances, the practice of pediatrics has shifted away from treatment of acute illness toward treatment and management of chronic illnesses. Not only are many of the acute infections of the past preventable, but also many children who would have died at early ages are living into adulthood. The classic example of this group of children are those with cystic fibrosis. In the not too distant past, life expectancy for a child with cystic fibrosis was around 5 years of age, whereas now it is near 30, with great hope for genetic cure in the foreseeable future. Similarly, diseases such as leukemia, which were acute and inevitably fatal, now can be classified as chronic and often curable. Medically fragile babies, such as "micro-premies," who would have died from complications of their prematurity are now growing up. However, lifesaving procedures can contribute to the development of chronic conditions, as in the case of bronchiopulmonary dysplasia following prolonged ventilator dependence. Estimates of prevalence of chronic illness change with definitions, but most data-based estimates have indicated that 10–20% of children suffer from some kind of chronic illnesses (Cadman, Boyle, Szatmari, & Offord, 1987). Many of these children, however, do not experience major daily challenges from their diseases, and it appears that only 10–15% of ill children would be classified as having severe disorders (Gortmaker &

Sappenfield, 1984). This means that more than 1 million children in the United States are affected by severe chronic illnesses, and several million more have milder chronic conditions.

The most common childhood chronic diseases involve pulmonary functioning. Respiratory conditions account for approximately one-fourth of all restrictions on childhood activities (Newacheck, Budetti, & Halfon, 1986). Asthma is the most common respiratory disease of childhood, affecting almost 3 million children (Taylor & Newacheck, 1992). Allergies alone may affect more than 10% of the general population of children (Perrin & MacLean, 1988). Other common disorders include genetic diseases such as cystic fibrosis, hemophilia, and sickle cell disease; congenital conditions such as cardiac disease and some renal dysfunction; and acquired conditions such as arthritis, tumors, leukemia, and epilepsy. Although some common childhood conditions, such as juvenile rheumatoid arthritis, are distributed fairly evenly across ethnic groups, others, such as sickle cell anemia and cystic fibrosis, are associated with specific ethnic groups. The findings from the Ontario Child Health Study (Cadman et al., 1987) indicated that overall boys have a slightly higher rate of chronic illness than girls. Socioeconomic status appears to differentiate groups more significantly than sex, however. In the Ontario study, children in families whose income was classified as below the poverty line had a 24% prevalence of chronic health problems, whereas an 18% prevalence rate was found for children whose families were not as financially limited. Analyzing data from the U.S. 1984 National Health Interview Survey, Newacheck (1989) reported that adolescents living in poverty were 46% more likely than teens from families above the poverty line to be affected by chronic medical conditions that were significant enough to limit typical life activities. Although the scope of this chapter does not allow a description of the medical aspects of chronic illnesses, specific information can be found in most textbooks on pediatrics. Additionally, educational materials can be obtained from the foundations associated with specific diseases, such as the Cystic Fibrosis Foundation, the National Hemophilia Foundation, and the American Cancer Society.

As the previous review indicates, the prevalence of chronic childhood illnesses is significant, and the interactions of specific conditions with biological, social, and psychological factors often contribute to complex developmental and behavioral problems. Knowledge regarding chronic illness is important for psychologists working with children and youth in health settings for several reasons. First, psychologists assessing children with complex medical problems need to be aware of the literature regarding the development of these children. Knowledge of the medical and social factors that may place the children at risk for cognitive, emotional, social, and behavioral problems should inform the assessment. Second, in planning interventions, it is especially useful to have a detailed understanding of the daily treatment requirements, physical limitations, and prognosis with which the child and family live. Third, being informed about a child's medical condition is important for establishing the psychologist's credibility, not only with the child and family but also with the child's physician, who is often the referring agent and a valuable collaborator.

ASSESSMENT DOMAINS

Cognitive Functioning

The earliest studies regarding cognitive effects of chronic illness involved administering IQ tests to small groups of children with chronic conditions and comparing their scores with national norms based on healthy children. There was little attempt to compare the study children with healthy children who were matched for other relevant variables, such as age, birth order, sex, socioeconomic status, ethnicity, or school attendance. As the field matured, more of those factors were taken into consideration, and studies broadened to investigate the effects of various treatments within groups of children with specific diseases. Studying cognitive effects is not a straightforward task, however, because the stress or emotional issues involved in being sick may interact with intellectual development or its measurement in some way. Landtman, Valanne, and Aukee (1968) took advantage of a naturally occurring opportunity to study the intellectual performance of children who had been incorrectly diagnosed as having a cardiac defect. The news was given to the parents and children that the children in fact had no such problem. Retesting soon after this information showed improvement in intelligence scores.

In general, the greater the involvement of the central nervous system in the disease process and/or treatment, the greater likelihood of deleterious cognitive effects. Breslau and Marshall (1985) conducted a 5-year longitudinal study of children with different medical conditions. Those with disorders involving the brain showed more frequent and more severe adjustment and cognitive problems than those children with other conditions. Most of the nonneurological conditions are not associated with major cognitive deficits. Children with cystic fibrosis (Cytryn, Moore, Van, & Robinson, 1973), arthritis (Cleveland, Reitman, & Brewer, 1965), hemophilia (Olch, 1971), or solid tumors (Stehbens, Ford, Kisker, Clark, & Strayer, 1981) have all been identified as functioning in at least the average range of intelligence. In contrast, groups of children with epilepsy (Stores, 1978) or myelomeningocele (Friedrich, Lovejoy, Shaffer, Shurtleff, & Beilke, 1991) have been described as scoring below the average range of intelligence.

Age of onset can also be important. Studies of children with renal failure in infancy that resulted in transplant found that 40% scored more than 1 standard deviation below the mean IQ for healthy children (Najarian et al., 1990). In children with diabetes the picture is complicated by varying effects depending on age of onset and the nature of glycemic control established. Onset before age 5 and poor control (resulting in frequent and/or severe hypoglycemic attacks) are associated with some cognitive impairment (Eeg-Olofsson, 1977; Rovet, Ehrlich, & Hoppe, 1987).

In the case of leukemia, there has been considerable controversy regarding the effects of various illness and treatment variables on cognitive outcome. Children with leukemia have been studied more often and in greater detail than most other chronic illness groups. Most studies of children who have undergone central nervous system prophylaxis involving antineoplastic drugs and craniospinal irradiation have reported cognitive deficits. These procedures, which helped make leukemia a survivable illness, result in a mean deficit of 10 Wechsler IQ points, according to a meta-analysis by Cousens, Waters, Said, and Stevens (1988). That analysis also indicates that the younger the child is at onset, the greater the impact of the treatment is. Mulhern and colleagues (1987) tested survivors of a single central nervous system relapse 6 years later. They found the mean IQ of their group to be below 90, with 20% in the retarded range. Number of radiation treatments, presence of brain pathology, and younger ages were associated with poorer outcomes. Attention/concentration and memory appear to be the most affected areas, regardless of age (see, e.g., Deasy-Spinetta, Spinetta, & Oxman, 1989).

Although a particular illness or treatment may change the base rates of cognitive impairment, there is considerable variation in the cognitive functioning of children within a specific disease group. For many conditions, studies of possible subtle effects on cognition have not been carried out. As in Greg's case (cited at the beginning of the chapter), only an individual assessment can address a specific child's particular cognitive style, level, strengths, and weaknesses.

When evaluating a chronically ill child's academic functioning, there are important issues other than intelligence. Repeated findings have shown that children with chronic medical problems do not do as well in school as their healthy peers (see, e.g., Richman & Harper 1978; Rutter, Tizard, & Whitmore, 1968). First, the child's school attendance must be taken into account. Differing patterns of absences may have differential effects. For example, although a child with leukemia may not have attended school for an extended time, he or she may have been tutored or attended school in the hospital. In contrast, a child with asthma may have missed many days of school but never in blocks of more than a few days, so special services may not have been initiated. Second, teachers and parents often have different expectations for children whom they know have medical problems (Richman, 1976). In the example at the beginning of the chapter, such expectations appeared to have affected Greg's chances of referral for an evaluation for a learning disability. Third, the ever-possible interaction of many factors, such as cognitive delays, medication effects, absences, and emotional distress, needs to be considered. Especially at the time of acute exacerbations or diagnosis, school performance may not have the priority for the child and parents that it holds at other, less emotionally upsetting times.

Two other related facets of the cognitive domain are often relevant when working with children with chronic medical conditions. The first is the child's understanding of concepts related to illness and health. A number of factors are important to this understanding, including the child's general intellectual functioning, level of education, sociocultural background, family religious beliefs, visibility of the condition, and, perhaps most significant, level of cognitive development. Children's conceptualization of their experiences follows a general trend: The younger the child, the more global and magical the thinking. As children mature, they move toward more specific and realistic understanding. Many studies have documented that concepts of illness tend to follow that same developmental course (see, e.g., Berry, Hayford, Ross, Pachman, & Lavigne, 1993; Bibace & Walsh, 1980; Perrin & Gerrity, 1981; Simeonsson, Buckley, & Monson, 1979). Younger children are more likely to overextend the concept of contagion and rely more on external cues (e.g., parents' actions) than internal cues for information about their own state of health. They are also more likely to interpret illness and its treatment as punishment. Brewster (1982) found that younger children (under 7) also are more likely to inaccurately infer the intentions of medical personnel, seeing their actions as deliberately malicious or punitive or, at best, incomprehensible. Between 7 and 10 years of age, children seem to understand that health care providers are trying to help sick children get well but feel that they have little or no appreciation of what the experience is like for the patients. It was only after 10 years old that children consistently reported believing that health care professionals are not only trying to help them but also have empathy for their feelings. Children's understanding of illness-related concepts colors their understanding of their medical condition, its treatment, communication about it, and relationships with caregivers. Their understanding changes both qualitatively and quantitatively over time. This, in turn, often changes the meaning of the condition to the child.

The second, related aspect of the cognitive domain is the knowledge a child has of his or her own condition. Pediatric patients need to know about their own conditions to give them a sense of mastery, to engage them in their own care, and to improve the likelihood of adherence to treatment recommendations. Many patients do not, however, have a clear understanding because of lack of teaching, instruction that is not in tune with the child's development and/or knowledge base, misunderstanding of what has been presented, and conflicting information from various sources such as television, books, parents, medical personnel, friends, and other patients. Although formal paper-and-pencil tests of some disease-specific knowledge (e.g., of AIDS, diabetes, hemophilia) do exist, more often the child's knowledge is assessed informally through conversation and, more behaviorally, by observation of self-care skills.

Psychosocial Functioning

The findings of literature regarding the prevalence of emotional problems in children with chronic illness relative to healthy children generally vary with the age of the studies cited. Older, more anecdotal studies (mostly previous to 1975) report widespread emotional difficulties, especially depression and anxiety in sick children and their mothers. On the other hand, later controlled studies using objective measures tended to find much less emotional disorder. This may reflect not only a difference in design and sampling but also changes in prognosis and medical care over the years.

Epidemiological studies have suggested that up to 30% of children with chronic physical conditions have secondary psychosocial maladjustment (Cadman et al., 1987). In general, studies of adjustment of children with a range of chronic illnesses have found that the majority of those children function well, although not necessarily as well as their healthy peers (see, e.g., Cadman et al., 1987; Wallander, Varni, Babani, Banis, & Willcox, 1988). Major psychiatric disturbance is not common in chronically ill children. On the other hand, chronic illness appears to be a risk factor for milder adjustment problems. Children with chronic medical problems are more likely than healthy peers to have been diagnosed with at least one psychiatric disorder. The probability of such a diagnosis increases when a physical disability is part of the condition (Cadman et al., 1987).

Lavigne and Faier-Routman (1992) carried out a meta-analysis of the empirical literature regarding children with chronic medical conditions. They found that, on average, these children are more likely to score in a problematic direction on adjustment measures as compared with either instrument norms or in-study healthy controls. Most of the studies suggested that internalizing types of symptoms such as anxiety and depression were the most common, whereas externalizing problems such as oppositional defiant or conduct disorders were fewer among sick children. Studies that included clinical interviews and assessments, such as those done by Thompson and his colleagues, found the same trends (Thompson, Hodges, & Hamlett, 1990; Thompson, Gil, Burbach, Keith, & Kinney, 1993). However, their later studies suggested that there was considerable variability, with specific children being categorized as having diagnosable psychological disorders although overall group numbers remained fairly constant (Thompson et al., 1994; Thompson, Gustafson, George, & Spock, 1994). Chronic illness is a significant risk factor for emotional disorders but by itself does not inevitably result in psychological problems.

Having a chronic medical condition alters a person's life experiences and, regardless of the presence of an emotional disorder, can also alter the feelings an individual child or adolescent has about him- or herself. A large collection of sometimes contradictory research findings examines whether children with chronic medical conditions show self-ratings (esteem, competence, or concept) differences from healthy children. Although there is still disagreement in the literature in this regard, the trend suggests that children with appearance differences, particularly involving the face and head (see, e.g., Broder & Strauss, 1989; Pillemer & Cook, 1989), or obvious functional limitations, including motor or orthopedic problems (see, e.g., Orr, Weller, Satterwhite, & Pless, 1984), are more consistently seen as having concerns about themselves, their bodies, and their attractiveness to others. The way a child feels about him- or herself is related to the way he or she is handled by the family system. Families of children with chronic illness provide a major social context for the condition. Illnesses, however, provide challenges for other family members that physically healthy families do not confront. Walker, Van Slyke, and Newbrough (1992) found there to be no more general family conflict in families with a chronically ill child than in those without. Instead, there are problems associated with the specific chronic illness. Some of the problems are physical or logistical, and others are financial. Many parents report, however, that the biggest challenges are the emotional ones, those having to do with the documented stress and the competing demands related to chronic illness (Schilling, Kirkham, Snow, & Schinke, 1986).

Parents and siblings not only are affected by the illness but also influence the individual experience of chronic illness for the affected children. If chronic illness serves as a risk factor for children, their families can function in ways that make the families either risk or protective factors for the children. Rae-Grant, Thomas, Offord, and Boyle (1989), analyzing data from the Ontario Child Health Study, found that serious family problems (marital discord, abuse) and parental problems (physical or mental illness or criminality) were major risk factors for adolescents developing emotional and behavioral disorders. If chronic illness is another risk factor, the two together render the child particularly vulnerable. Rutter (1979) found that children with one risk factor were no more likely to have emotional disorders than those with no risk factors. However, two risk factors for the same child quadrupled the risk. More risk factors increased the risk several times further.

The interaction of physiological and psychological variables can markedly affect medical outcomes, as well as emotional functioning. Strunk, Mrazek, Wolfson-Fuhrmann, and LaBrecque (1985) studied the clinical characteristics associated with death from asthma in a small group of children and teenagers with severe disease. Fourteen variables differentiated children who died from asthma from those who lived. Ten of the 14 variables were psychosocial, four physiological. Depressive symptoms, patient–parent relationship problems, family dysfunction, and parent–staff conflict differentiated the two groups.

On the other hand, families can also provide protective factors for their offspring. A supportive relationship with at least one parent, family closeness, and appropriate limit setting have all been documented as buffers for children with other risk factors (Garmazy, 1983a, 1983b; Rutter, 1985). However, it may be more difficult for families of a chronically ill child to provide such protection. Coping with the practical and emotional demands of a chronic illness is a major task for all family members. Although a discussion of coping is beyond the scope of this chapter, it is often an issue to be considered during the assessment process. Briefly, coping can be thought of as the process of engaging in cognitive and/or behavioral strategies to manage stressful situations. Coping strategies can be thought of as adaptive or maladaptive, although different coping styles can be useful in one situation or phase and not useful in another. Although coping strategies have been classified in a variety of ways, common categories include finding meaning in the experience; using instrumental coping, such as seeking information about the disease and its treatment; deliberate avoidance of thoughts or feelings related to the condition; and seeking social support. Although each member of a family copes individually, there also appears to be family system-wide coping (McCubbin & Patterson, 1982; McCubbin et al., 1983).

Chronically ill children also have relationships outside the home, of course. Peer and social relationships have long been of concern to professionals who work with children with chronic illnesses. Pless and Roghmann (1971) found a higher proportion of social problems in children with physical conditions than in healthy children. Cadman and colleagues (1987) reported that the presence of a physical disability was an important risk factor for developing social problems. Children with chronic medical conditions without a disability were indistinguishable from healthy children in terms of isolation, peer problems, or social activities. Orr and colleagues (1984) found similar results of impairment versus illness in chronically ill adolescents. The disability may serve to publicly set these children apart, as well as to limit normal activity in some way.

Studies of children with visible and invisible disorders suggest that visible differences are more socially relevant (Broder & Strauss, 1989). This seems particularly true if the children are not rated as attractive as their peers. Children with facial differences (e.g., craniofacial anomalies or postsurgery alterations in structure) have repeatedly been shown to have more social difficulty than attractive peers (Tobiasen, 1989; Tobiasen & Hiebert, 1989; Krueckeburg, & Kapp-Simon, 1993a, 1993b).

Noll's research group uses multiple data sources and matched classroom controls to study peer relations in chronically ill children. The group has found that those with cancer had the reputation of being more socially isolated but were not different in measured friendship evaluations or popularity. Similarly, the children reported no differences in loneliness (Noll, Bukowski, Rogosch, LeRoy, & Kulkarni, 1990; Noll, LeRoy, Bukowski, Rogosch, & Kulkarni, 1991). In 1993, Noll, Bukowski, Davies, Koontz, and Kulkarni reported on their 2-year follow-up of 19 previous subjects with cancer, finding similar results, without signs of late-developing social problems.

ASSESSMENT PRIORITIES

Children with chronic illnesses are subject to all the same developmental fluctuations and forces as any other child. The illness may increase the risk of certain kinds of events, changes, and reactions. Also in many instances children had either premorbid problems or less-than-optimal functioning that appeared minimally related to the disease process. This means that the assessment domains relevant to children with chronic illnesses overlap substantially with those pertaining to healthy children. All the detailed areas of cognitive, emotional, adaptive, behavioral, social, and family functions are relevant. In this section we attempt to highlight some of the technical and conceptual differences involved in the assessment of these familiar areas with children with chronic medical conditions. Because family assessment is discussed in depth elsewhere in this book, we do not address it here.

Although commonalities in context, and at times behaviors, are associated with particular chronic illnesses, the assessment of a chronically ill child must still be focused on the individual child and family. This creates a demand for assessment strategies that are both sensitive to the particular concerns relevant to the illness and also flexible enough to detect the individual characteristics of the specific child and family. The central assessment question is the relationship of the disease process to psychological development and adjustment. Within that broad question are many possibilities, and it must be clear prior to the assessment procedures what the referral question is so as to avoid unnecessary procedures or the embarrassment of coming to the end of the evaluation only to find that the intended question remains unanswered. Even when the intended purpose may be clear, it is also important to ascertain whether the reference group is healthy children, children with chronic illness, or other children with the same particular health problem. Is the purpose of assessment to determine how this child and/or family compares with healthy peers? Or is it to evaluate the child's functioning relative to other children with the same condition or perhaps other healthy children in the same family? As in the example of Greg at the beginning of the chapter, two or more reference groups may be relevant for the same referral.

The major purposes of assessment of children with chronic illnesses fall into the following categories: (1) early detection of problems in psychological functioning to prevent secondary problems ("screening"), (2) diagnosing existing cognitive or psychosocial problems, (3) obtaining data to inform the design of treatment or rehabilitation programming, (4) evaluating of treatment outcomes, (5) monitoring over time certain aspects of functioning believed to be directly relevant to the disease process (including the establishment of the child's baseline function), and (6) assessing the child's capacity to participate in or assume control over his or her own health care. These purposes are not mutually exclusive, and many of the same procedures and tools can be helpful for several questions.

The early detection of problems can be approached similarly to the diagnosis of existing problems, although the extent of assessment and implications for intervention are often different. Depending on the referral question, these assessments can apply to almost any area of the child's functioning: cognitive, behavioral, emotional, or social. Family function may be included as well. In any case, multiple sources of information can be helpful in establishing the range of the behaviors noted. Chronically ill children, like all children, should not be assessed in a vacuum, with information coming from the patient alone. Health care providers who know the family well, teachers, the child's regular baby-sitter, parents, and extended family all may add important data and perspective.

Data to inform intervention planning and to permit treatment evaluation often stems from the evaluation that determined the need for treatment. Additional fine-grained behavioral assessment may be helpful in setting measurable treatment goals. Special care must be taken whenever repeating measures, especially for measuring intervention outcome, that the assessment tools used are both adequately reliable and not subject to practice effects. Another element especially important to this kind of assessment is the identification of strengths in the child and the family that can be mobilized to facilitate the desired changes. Monitoring psychological factors to document progress over time has a well-established precedent in the sequential measurement of various medical variables to determine relapse or progress. Many times when a child is ill with a condition for which the treatment can cause as much or more damage to cognition as the disease itself, a baseline assessment is requested. Examples of these treatments include cranial radiation and/or certain types of chemotherapy administration for childhood cancer. When the illness or related events can directly affect cognition, as in the case of sickle cell anemia, HIV infection, or head injuries in boys with hemophilia, repeated monitoring can afford reliable measures of disease progression and/or disease-related damage. Although referrals of this nature are most often made to track cognitive functioning, psychosocial variables can be approached in the same fashion. Commonly, however, emotional and behavioral status appear to be monitored via interviews, impressions, and informal assessment, despite the availability of reliable, valid, and quantitative measures.

The assessment of a child's capacity to participate in or take over his or her own health care requires information regarding several interdependent areas of function. One of the most basic is the child's developmental level as it relates to the nature of the child's understanding of illness, causality, and the role and meaning of the required treatments. Especially with younger children or when there is a question of developmental delay, assessment of various aspects of cognitive development is important in answering this question. Academic skills may be relevant if the treatment requires the use of mathematics or reading skills (e.g., in diabetes management). Knowledge of the child's level of independent functioning as determined by history and observation of parent–child interaction is useful as well. Under some conditions, a measure of the child's adaptive functioning is helpful. The child's skill with the techniques required can be observed and quantified and a teaching plan formulated if other measures indicate success is possible. The success of the teaching is quantified relative to the measured preteaching skills. Then a plan to address maintaining the practice of the skill can be developed in cooperation with the parents and/or other caregivers.

SPECIAL ISSUES WHEN ASSESSING CHILDREN WITH CHRONIC ILLNESS

There are several special considerations in assessing these children and their families. First, knowing the stage of the illness is important in many situations. For example, the effects of congenital heart disease on cognitive development appear to vary with the stage of the condition. Specifically, children whose heart defects have not yet been surgically corrected have cognitive difficulties that may disappear a few months after correction (Linde, Rasof, & Dunn, 1970). Similarly, children with renal disease who receive transplants have been reported to have improvements in IQ scores following the operation (Crittenden, Holliday, Piel, & Potter, 1985). Children who are in an intense treatment phase of their diseases (e.g., those newly diagnosed with leukemia) may also be more overwhelmed and preoccupied by treatment demands than those in a maintenance phase. Parents may also be more distressed closer to the diagnosis, during intense treatment, and, of course, during the terminal phase of the illness (Van Dongen-Melman & Sanders-Woudstra, 1986). It has also been noted that after a diagnosis of a chronic disease, a transition period occurs as parents move from the mode of parenting used in acute physical illnesses to one appropriate to chronic disorders. While the transition is occurring or if it fails to take place as it should, the highly nurturant, sometimes indulgent stance of the acute mode may reduce self-care and/or contribute to the development of undesirable behaviors in the child, often of an oppositional or whiny nature.

Second, if an evaluation of a child with a chronic medical condition involves standardized tests, the interaction of the physical aspects of the disease with the tasks must be considered. In general, chronic illness does not alter the use of standardized tests unless the child has a perceptual, motor, or orthopedic impairment. In that case, two approaches can be taken. One approach is to administer the test in the prescribed fashion, then note what effects the child's condition had on his or her performance. The advantage to this approach is that it allows comparison of the child's functioning with that of a reference group. This approach is often useful for placement or diagnostic decisions. On the other hand, the actual limits of the child's abilities may not have been reached. The second approach, then, is to adapt the testing procedures and/or materials to minimize the impact of the disability on test performance. This approach allows the delineation of relative areas of strength or weakness that can be particularly important in planning interventions such as educational adaptations. The drawback is that decisions are based on clinical judgment without the use of a normative reference group. The referral question can guide which approach or what combination of the approaches is utilized in evaluating a specific child.

A third important consideration when assessing a child with chronic illness is the medication prescribed. As in any assessment, the question of what medication the child is taking needs to be raised early in the process. Certain medications, including corticosteroids (sometimes used in a variety of conditions, including cancer, juvenile rheumatoid arthritis, asthma, and dermatological conditions and after transplants) can change the child's emotional functioning. Parents often complain that their child is tired or more irritable, tearful, or otherwise emotionally labile than when he or she is not taking the steroids (Harris,

Carel, Rosenberg, Joshi, & Leventhal, 1986). Reversible memory deficits have also been described in children taking steroids (Bender, Lerner, & Poland, 1991). Case reports have associated inhaled steroids, commonly used in asthma care, with hyperactivity, aggressiveness, and oppositional behavior (see, e.g., Connett & Lenney, 1991). Other medications for asthma (e.g., theophylline) have been noted, although inconsistently, to change activity level and attention span of their users, especially early in their use (Rachelefsky et al., 1986; Stein & Lerner, 1993). Rappoport and colleagues (1989) and Schlieper, Alcock, Beaudry, Feldman, and Leikin (1991), however, concluded after randomized, placebo-controlled, double-blind studies that these medications yield no significant changes on comprehensive test batteries. Even common over-the-counter medications such as antihistamines taken by children with allergies may affect verbal memory, mental calculations, reaction time, and/or visual perception (Seppala & Visakorpi, 1983). Children under the age of 6 are reportedly at special risk of confusion, delusions, or hallucinations after taking some common decongestants (Lake, Masson, & Quirk, 1988). Medications with the side effects of lethargy, nausea, or headaches (e.g., Imuran, used after transplant surgery) can also alter the outcome of assessment. The medication effects may not be at their peak, but they can still alter performance if the child has chronic malaise. Often, the medication cannot be suspended for the period of the child's assessment. Other times, suspending medication would mean that the data gained is not relevant to the bulk of the child's life when the medication is in use. Therefore, the primary method of handling this problem is to be aware of the possible influences of the child's medicines and to be open to the possibility that medicine may be only one of the contributing forces involved in a problem.

A fourth special consideration is the child's history of hospital admissions and/or surgeries and, with that history, the correlate of school attendance. Preschool children who have been hospitalized repeatedly are especially likely to score lower on developmental screening and adaptive functioning than healthy peers because of regression during hospitalizations and loss of opportunities for normal learning and mastery. When children have missed a great deal of school, they sometimes have reentry difficulties, both socially and academically. Many children's hospitals have school reentry programs to aid in this transition. If the child has not been in the hospital or restricted to the home by physician order, it is often informative to inquire about the decision-making process involved in the child's missing school. As might be expected, high levels of absenteeism have been associated with academic lags.

MEASURES

Developmental and Cognitive Measure

As noted, there are special considerations when using standardized measures with children with chronic medical conditions. These relate to the interaction of physical limitations with measurement. However, cognitive functioning is often central to the assessment of such children. In general, the more physical impairment that is present, the greater the caution that must be used in interpreting and the more frequent the modifications that need to be made.

Both the first (Bayley, 1969) and second editions (Bayley, 1993) of the Bayley Scales of Infant Development (BSID, BSID-II) have been widely used with children with medical problems. Use of the BSID with high-risk infants has been especially widespread. The BSID-II provides scores for the Mental scale, Motor scale, and Behavior Rating scale. This test has no norms for the chronically ill, but its structure provides opportunity for testing the limits of the child's abilities without losing all the advantages of a normed reference group. When considerable scattering on test items or other clinical warning signs are present, the clinician can use the standard presentations to score for reference to norms, whereas additional items can be administered to test the limits. General guidelines for testing a child with physical disability are provided in the manual.

Shoemaker, Saylor, and Erickson (1993) compared Bayley Mental scores and the Minnesota Child Development Inventory (MCDI; Ireton & Thwing, 1974) a true-or-false survey of developmentally significant behaviors that is completed by parents. They found that the MCDI was a useful screening device for high-risk infants, some of whom had chronic physical conditions. Because of low sensitivity, however, the authors recommended using the MCDI diagnostically only in concert with other measures and observations. When screening only is desired, the MCDI may provide a low-cost alternative. The MCDI has also been revised, and this study has not been repeated with the Child Development Inventory, the revised version.

Since the original Wechsler Intelligence Scale for Children (WISC; Wechsler, 1949), all versions of the Wechsler Intelligence Scales have been used extensively with children with chronic illnesses. The WISC-III (Wechsler, 1991) is essentially the "gold standard" for cognitive assessment at this time. It has been particularly useful because of the three IQ scores, four-factor scores, and many subtest scores that allow detailed consideration of information-processing capacities and patterns. Wechsler tests have been used with children with a wide variety of illnesses (see, e.g., Cousens, Ungerer, Crawford, & Stevens, 1991; Hurtig, Koepke, & Park, 1989).

Other than the considerations normally involved in using Wechsler tests, there are no special restrictions or problems noted for use with chronically ill children. If, however, the child has an orthopedic handicap that affects motor speed, the use of the Performance scale is questionable. If it is used, Kaufman suggested using Mazes, not Coding, for computing the Performance IQ. He felt that the psychomotor speed component of Coding made it inappropriate as a contributor to the Performance IQ of children with orthopedic handicaps. In general, if the handicap impedes performance but does not prevent reasonable performance, then it can be used for children under age 9, because most of the variance at younger ages is accounted for by accuracy, not speed (Kaufman, 1979). After age 9, the ratio of accuracy to speed changes, so that solving every nonverbal problem, but too slowly to earn bonus points, results in a maximum score of 11 on some Performance subtests. With the advent of the WISC-III Processing Speed factor, it is likely that this continues to be an issue.

The Stanford–Binet Intelligence Scale has been used with a variety of medically involved populations over several decades. The current SB-IV (Thorndike, Hagen, & Sattler, 1986), is designed for children 2 years and older and has good reliability and validity data. There are no norms for children with chronic illness. However, the *Examiner's Handbook* (Delaney & Hopkins, 1987) contains an outline of which tests can be modified for children with motor impairments. Because of the timed nature of Pattern Analysis, it may need to be omitted. The Bead Memory, Copying, and Memory for Objects scales are allowed to be modified to the point where responses are entirely verbal, if necessary. Other test administration remains unchanged. It is recommended that all modifications be outlined in the narrative report. Emphasis on qualitative rather than the typical quantitative analysis is recommended.

The Kaufman Assessment Battery for Children (K-ABC; Kaufman & Kaufman, 1983) has been used with groups of children with various chronic illnesses. It has been used often by neuropsychologists, so that many of the tested groups have had some sort of neurological impairment. The K-ABC is designed to assess the intelligence and achievement of children from 2½ to 12½ years of age. Reliability coefficients are quite high, and validity has been established with regard to the underlying constructs of sequential and simultaneous processing and its use as an intelligence measure. Exceptional children were included in the standardization population, and the emphasis on process makes this test particularly informative for children with physical differences. The K-ABC has a Nonverbal scale composed of those Mental Processing subtests that can be administered in pantomime and responded to motorically. This special scale is normally reserved for children with special needs, including speech impairment and severe language disorder. For children with physical handicaps affecting the hands or arms, the manual specifies attempting to administer all subtests. Most often affected are Hand Movements, Triangles, and Reading/Understanding. Small modifications are allowed for some of the processing subtests. Standard scores may be prorated on the Mental Processing scales, based on the handicapped child's performance on the remaining K-ABC subtests as necessary. All prorating is to be indicated both on the test form and in the report.

Academic Measures

Measuring academic skills of children with chronic illness is important primarily as part of the process that qualifies school-age children for special educational support. Academic skills evaluation can also be used as part of long-term monitoring and problem identification (see, e.g., Allen & Zigler, 1986; Friedrich et al., 1991). There are, however, no academic measures designed exclusively for children with medical problems. Nor do any of the commonly used assessment tools (e.g., Kaufman Test of Educational Achievement, [K-TEA], Kaufman & Kaufman, 1985; Peabody Individual Achievement Test—Revised [PIAT], Markwardt, 1998; Wechsler Individual Achievement Test [WIAT], Wechsler, 1992; Wide Range Achievement Test—Revised, Wilkinson, 1993; Woodcock–Johnson Psychoeducational Battery—Revised, Woodcock & Johnson, 1990) have norms for this subpopulation. On the other hand, because the question is usually how the child is performing relative to his or her healthy classmates, the issue of specialized norms is less relevant here. No adaptations are specified for children with physical impairments, although some measures (e.g., WIAT, K-TEA) provide cursory guidelines indicating that modifications may be made but that norms may be violated as a result.

Professionals assessing the scholastic achievement of chronically ill children need to ensure that the test chosen will serve the desired purpose. In all cases, but especially when motor impairments are present, the scores must be based on tasks that the child is physically capable of carrying out. This may necessitate modification of the test or its administration, with all such modifications noted in the report. If placement is the issue, care must be taken that the test administered is acceptable to the child's school. When possible, the report should also address the role of the child's illness and/or impairment in both testing and daily learning. If long-term follow-along is the goal, the academic measure chosen should cover a wide age range (e.g., Woodcock–Johnson, WIAT, or PIAT).

Measures of Concepts of Illness

Many of the significant studies addressing the development of concepts related to health and illness used semistructured interviews or a short series of questions nested within a larger, orally presented survey. However, a few instruments have been specifically designed to assess children's concepts related to illness, although none have attained a preeminent position.

One of the earlier scales is the Children's Illness Anxiety Scale, developed by Brodie (1974) to assess three areas: the child's perceptions of illness as punishment; the child's perception of his parent's reaction to his illness; and the child's perception of illness as a disruptive force, particularly with regard to peers and school. It was used with healthy school-age children. Reliability and validity data was not provided, however.

Bibace and Walsh (1980) developed the Concept of Illness Protocol, containing 12 sets of questions, with each set investigating the child's thinking about a single health-related topic. Used with 4- to 11-year-olds, scoring of this orally administered questionnaire provided information regarding the Piagetian category of explanations used. Pilot data had been used as a basis for this protocol, results of which were quite consistent with predictions based on Piaget's cognitive development theory.

Brewster (1982) also used Piagetian developmental stages as a starting point for her work, and she also modified Selman's social-role-perspective research to apply to the role of medical staff, including their intent in carrying out medical procedures. Like many later studies, many of the questions used were similar to those used by Bibace and Walsh, but with the addition of questions relevant to a specific disease such as AIDS (Walsh & Bibace, 1991) or arthritis (Berry et al., 1993). The latter group developed a scoring system for both accuracy of responses and their conceptual level, for which reliability was carefully addressed.

For nonresearch settings, some clinicians use an informal assessment technique of asking the child a few questions like those that have been used in the interview protocols and informally assigning a cognitive category (e.g., undifferentiated, concrete, abstract) to the responses. Some of these questions have included, "How can children keep from getting sick?", "How do children get sick?" (Simeonsson, Buckley, & Monson, 1979), "What is illness?" and "I'm wondering about how you know when you're sick. One day you know you're well and on another day you know you are sick. OK, what's the difference?" (Campbell, 1975; Millstein, Adler, & Irwin, 1981). Assessment of conceptual understanding may be most informative with children under 10, although many teenagers who might be capable of formal operations do not necessarily utilize that kind of thinking with regard to their own condition (Berry et al., 1993).

Measures of Behavioral and Emotional Functioning

Psychosocial functioning of all natures has long been assessed through interviews with the child and family. Some are referral questions or concerns may best be addressed by standardized or projective tests. Although there are many such instruments available, those presented below are selected because of their previous use with children with chronic medical conditions or because of their particular usefulness with this population.

Parent-Completed Inventories

The Achenbach Child Behavior Checklist (CBCL; Achenbach & Edelbrock, 1983a) is a standardized parent-completed rating scale assessing social competence and behavior problems in children and adolescents. There is a special preschool form for 2- and 3-year-olds. (The CBCL also has a Teacher Report Form; Achenbach & Edelbrock, 1983b.) Both versions provide profiles based on subscales. In the 1991 manual, Achenbach suggested that the CBCL be used to screen for behavioral problems in ill children and their siblings, to monitor behavior over time by repeated administrations, and to provide anticipatory guidance for parents whose children are facing treatments or procedures that may alter behavior. It has also been used for screening purposes, as one source of diagnostic information, and to assess treatment outcomes. It has been used extensively with children with various chronic illnesses, to the extent that the CBCL has been referred to as "the gold standard for assessment of psychosocial functioning of children with chronic physical conditions" (Perrin, Stein, & Drotar, 1991; Wallander &Thompson, 1995, p. 126).

Perrin and her coauthors outlined several limitations in the use of the CBCL with chronically ill children, however. Specifically, the items on the CBCL that assess physical symptoms, including the items of the Somatic Complaints scale, do not hold the same meanings or significance for chronically ill as for physically healthy children. Children with many physical symptoms have elevated scores on this scale, regardless of etiology. Additionally, interpreting social competence scores from this measure is difficult when dealing with this population. For example, the social activity items would not be completed if a child is homebound at the time of assessment. This temporary limitation of social activity should not be viewed as reflective of overall social competence. Although the 1991 manual addressed some of those concerns, caution with the Somatic Complaints scale is still recommended. A recent study by Holmes, Respess, Greer, and Frentz (1998) found no signs of confounding of internalization scores with physiological symptoms. They calculated the CBCL scores of diabetic children three different ways: using traditional whole-scale scoring, deleting the Somatic Complaints scale, and deleting nine items tapping physical symptoms considered a priori to be likely in diabetes. The children had mildly elevated scores on six of eight scales relative to healthy controls, regardless of the method of scoring. Homes and colleagues pointed out, however, that the CBCL was designed to detect psychopathology, not subtle or mild behavioral difficulties.

Another caveat was raised by Mulhern, Fairclough, Smith, and Douglas (1992), who noted in a pediatric oncology population that the higher the depression score of patients' mothers on the Beck Depression Inventory (BDI), the more problematic they rated their child's depression on the CBCL. Because agreement among multiple sources of information, including oncology nurses and the patients themselves, was relatively low, there is concern that the high depression scores on the CBCL may be reflective at least in part of the mothers' own mood states. Long, Holden, and Zolten (1991) reported similar results with mothers of children with a variety of chronic disorders, finding a large part of the variance in maternal ratings of child behavior accounted for by the mothers' depression.

Stawski and colleagues (1995) found that the responses of younger adolescents with medical problems to the Youth Self-Report were poorly correlated with responses of their parents to the CBCL. This was not the case for young adolescents referred for psychiatric reasons. As before, agreement among multiple sources of information was relatively low. The authors emphasized the need to include the viewpoints of the patients themselves in their assessments, particularly when dealing with chronically ill children.

In a study of chronically ill children and adolescents, diagnoses derived from the Diagnostic Interview Schedule for Children (DISC; Costello, Edelbrock, Dulcan, Kalas, & Klavic, 1984), an intensive, structured psychiatric interview, were compared with those suggested by the CBCL (Canning & Kelleher, 1994). The researchers concluded that the CBCL should not be used as a screening instrument for children and adolescents with chronic medical problems because of low sensitivity and predictive values. Similarly, Harris, Canning, and Kelleher (1996) found that the CBCL tends to underidentify medically ill children with comorbid psychiatric problems.

The Personality Inventory for Children—Revised (PIC-R; Lachar, 1982; Wirt et al., 1984) is an objective, multidimensional measure of behavior, affect, ability (including an intellectual screening scale), and family functioning. This form is to be completed by an adult informant, with norms established for mothers' responses. There are no norms developed specifically for chronically ill children, however.

This questionnaire has been widely used clinically and in research. Armstrong, Wirt, Nesbit, and Martinson (1982) found high Somatic Concern scores (SOM) for children with cancer but noted that the symptoms reported on the scale are similar to those from the disease and questioned etiology and specificity. Sanger, Copeland, and Davidson (1991) reported similar findings but also noted elevations in two or more PIC scales for over half their pediatric cancer patients. Pritchard, Ball, Culbert, and Faust (1988) attempted to use the PIC to distinguish among 137 children with somatoform disorders, neurological disorders, chronic medical conditions, and no medical problems. (Somatoform disorders included pseudo-seizures, headaches, leg weakness or pain that interfered with walking, headaches, and tics.) Children with somatoform and neurological disorders scored higher than normals on 7 of 13 scales evaluated, but those with chronic medical disorders showed higher scores than healthy school children only on the SOM scale. The somatoform and disorder group did not differ from the neurological group and scored differently from the chronic medical disorder group on only two subscales. The researchers concluded that neither the PIC nor the Somatic Concern scale in particular is useful to differentiate children with somatoform disorders from those with verifiable medical illness.

R. E. K. Stein and her colleagues shortened the Personal Adjustment and Role Skills Scale (PARS-II), which had been developed by Ellsworth and Ellsworth (CAAP, 1982). There have been two major revisions to the PARS-II for children, one of which is now known as the scale and the other as the PARS-III (Walker, Stein, Perrin, & Jessop, 1990). The major difference is that the 28-item PARS-III scale has an Anxiety–Depression subscale. The other five subscales are Peer Relations, Hostility, Dependency, Productivity, and Withdrawal. It applies to 5- to 18-year-olds. The PARS-III has been used by four groups of investigators from the Research Consortium on Chronic Illness in Childhood. Walker, Stein, Perrin, and Jessop (1990) reported that this group found the PARS-III to be reliable and valid in assessing the psychosocial functioning of children with chronic illness and no major cognitive impairments. Although this scale does not appear to be widely used in purely clinical applications, it has the advantage of having been shown to be useful specifically in the assessment of chronically ill children and teenagers. There are no items that assess physical symptoms as a sign of anxiety or depression, avoiding some of the problems with the CBCL and the PIC-R. The PARS-III is also short and could be used for either screening or diagnostic purposes. Harris and colleagues (1996) found that for chronically ill children and adolescents from ages 9 to 18, the PARS-III measures similar constructs as the CBCL but shares its problems of underidentifying psychiatric problems in that population.

Child-Completed Measures

Various measures focus on the health- and illness-related beliefs of children. One of the beliefs frequently addressed is *locus of control*, which reflects the responsibility one takes for one's own well-being. The Nowicki–Strickland Locus of Control Scale (1973) is one of the most well known of these scales. It has been used for general assessment of beliefs and specifically to detect changes in attribution after intervention (Moffatt & Pless, 1983). Parcel and Meyer (1978) developed the Children's Health Locus of Control (CHLC) scale for use with children 7–12 years of age. The 20-item scale comprises three factors, including an internal-control scale that shows an increase with age. There is moderate agreement between the two scales. Another related measure of control, based on a somewhat different theoretical approach, is Connell's (1985) Multidimensional Measure of Children's Perceptions of Control, which was designed as a structured interview that could be altered to accommodate to the situation in question (school, hospital, home, etc.). Three sources of perceived control (Internal, Powerful Other, and Unknown) are assessed. Carpenter (1992) found that children who made attributions of unknown source of control when having blood drawn were more behaviorally distressed than those who attributed control to either other source.

For children under 13, the Self-Perception Profiles for Children and Adolescents (Harter, 1985, 1988) consist of subscales designed to measure a child's perception of his or her competence in five areas: scholastic competence, social acceptance, athletic competence, physical appearance, and behavioral conduct. There is also a global self-worth scale. The adolescent version adds items related to perceived competence in the domains of close friendship, romantic appeal, and job functioning. Harter and others (see, e.g., Morison & Masten, 1991) have reported reasonable reliability and validity. There are no norms for chronically ill children. This measure has been used clinically and in a large number of studies of chronically ill children partly because of the relevance of the areas addressed, especially the sense of athletic competence, which is not included in many other similar scales.

The Piers–Harris Self-Concept Scale (Piers & Harris, 1969) consists of 80 yes-or-no questions presented in the form of, "Is this like you or not like you?" Results include a Global self-concept percentile score and six-factor derived subscales: Behavior, School Status, Physical Appearance, Anxiety, Popularity, and Happiness and Satisfaction. Reliability has been reported in an acceptable range. It has been used in multiple studies with chronically ill children with no particular precautions emerging (see, e.g., Hurtig & White, 1986; Ryan & Morrow, 1986).

When the issue of *body image and comfort with physical appearance* is of particular concern, three scales can be helpful in assessing this concern. The older two have an established track record, allowing knowledge of psychometric properties, and none of the three is entirely focused on anorexia, unlike many body-related scales. The Body Esteem Scale (Mendelson & White, 1985), designed for school-age children and teenagers, requires responses of degree of agreement with various statements about their bodies. The Body Image subscale of the Self-Image Questionnaire for Young Adolescents (Petersen, Shulenberg, Abramowitz, Offer, & Jarcho, 1984) represents 11 items related to the positive and negative feelings held about one's body. The whole questionnaire evaluates the feelings about a variety of aspects of a young person between 10 and 15 years of age. The newest scale is the Body Image Instrument (BII; Kopel, Eiser, Cool, Grimer, & Carter, 1998), a 28-item self-report measure that uses 5-point Likert-type scales with "disagree" and "agree" as end points. It was designed to assess the body image of adolescents who had cancer. There are five subscales, General Appearance, Body Competence, Others' Reaction to Appearance, Value of Appearance (relative importance of appearance), and Body Parts (feelings about specific parts of the body commonly involved in cancer). Its first use was marked by adequate internal reliability and concurrent validity with two other research instruments relating to medical status.

The Children's Depression Inventory (CDI; Kovacs, 1981) is a 27-item self-report inventory developed to measure depression in school-age children and adolescents. It is a widely used measure of depression in children, and extensive reliability and validity have been reported (Helsel & Matson, 1984; Kovacs, 1992; Romano & Nelson, 1988; Smucker, Craighead, Craighead, & Green, 1986). A number of problems in using this measure with chronically ill children have been identified. Worchel, Rae, Olson, and Crowley (1992) found that showing a videotape modeling disclosure significantly altered the level of depression expressed by chronically ill children on the CDI, although not on all measures. This effect was strongest when the examiner was an unfamiliar person. Their conclusion was that the CDI can be useful but should never be interpreted alone. Our experience has suggested that children who are concerned about "impression management" can respond differentially to this task because of the overt nature of its content. Canning and Kelleher (1994) compared CDI scores of chronically ill children and adolescents with the diagnoses derived from intense, structured diagnostic interviews. They concluded that the CDI is not very sensitive nor predictive and should not be relied on as a screening instrument for depression in the medically ill population.

The Millon Adolescent Personality Inventory (MAPI; Millon, Green, & Meagher, 1982) is a theory-grounded personality measure that requires the teenager to answer 150 true-or-false questions and that takes less than one-half hour to complete. Norms were developed for physically healthy 13- to 18-year-olds and included both clinical and nonclinical populations. Reliability and validity appear adequate. The MAPI scales are divided into two groups, one designed to measure enduring personality styles and the other current psychopathology. The advantage in its use with chronically ill children is that it can give information regarding normal functioning, as well as deviance. Although not a lot has been published regarding the use of the MAPI with chronically ill youth, its scales have the potential of being particularly useful for this population. The MAPI was one of the measures recommended by Schweitzer and Hobbs (1995) for use with adolescents with renal failure or transplants. Subscales of Self-Concept, Personal Esteem, Body Comfort, Sexual Acceptance, Family Rapport, and Academic Confidence are particularly relevant to many of the concerns regarding teens with chronic illness. A drawback, however, is the limited validity scale, containing only three items.

There are three apperception—storytelling—tasks that have been used to assess language ability and psychosocial concerns of chronically ill children and adolescents. All of the concerns noted elsewhere (see, e.g., Lanyon & Goodstein, 1971) regarding the reliability and validity of the results of these tests apply when assessing ill children. The Thematic Apperception Test (TAT) developed by Murray (1943) has been used with adolescents, but its developer suggested that only 17 of the 31 cards would be appropriate for use with nonadults, and only 2 depict children. In contrast, all 10 of the pictures of the Children's Apperception Test (CAT; Bellak, 1954) depict children. It should be noted that some of the Children's Apperception Test Supplementary cards (CAT-S) are physician or injury related, providing stimuli with a particular "pull" for children's perceptions. CAT cards, especially the "Animal" versions, are not well received by older children and adolescents, however, because of their "juvenile" appearance.

In the current research literature regarding chronically ill children, the apperception test most often used is the Roberts Apperception Test for Children (RATC; McArthur & Roberts, 1982). There are 27 possible stimulus cards; fewer are shown to each child. This test has the advantage of having standardized scoring methods and norms for 6- to 15-year-olds. The authors have cited relatively high interrater reliability and acceptable split-half reliabilities for the 13 scales. Worchel and colleagues (1992) reported that the Depression scale of the RATC was less affected by the child's familiarity with the examiner than the CDI when used with children with cancer or diabetes.

Although there are scales that are designed to address narrow, usually research, interests, such as the Orthodontic Locus of Control (Tedesco, Albino, & Cunat, 1985) or tests of specific disease-related knowledge, the majority of clinically driven assessments of children with medical conditions involve the use of the same measures that are used with other children. A major limitation is that these tests have not been normed for the population of children with chronic illnesses, a limitation that can result in some spurious findings such as those involving the Child Behavior Checklist Somatic Concerns scale. An area of growth for the field would be the development of such norms or the design and psychometric validation of tests designed for this population. The lack of norms of this kind also calls into question the rather common research practice of comparing the scores of a sample of ill children with the norms derived from the population of children at large and drawing conclusions based on the differences. The use of control groups leads to a sounder comparison base, especially when selection of the controls is done carefully with attention to important variables other than illness. Noll and his colleagues have addressed this concern in their publications stemming from the "Friendship Study," in which numbers of children with chronic illness are compared with children drawn from their own classmates (see, e.g., Noll et al., 1990, 1991).

Another aspect of the choice of comparison groups, even in clinically driven assessments, is the question to be answered. If the question has to do with how a child is functioning in comparison with healthy children against whom he or she may be compared in everyday life, as with the academic performance concerns about Greg in the chapter-opening vignette, the tests used for all children may be the most informative. On the other hand, if the question is the child's ability to contribute to decision making about treatment options compared with other children of his or her age who have the same illness, the healthy-child norms do not inform the interpretation of assessment data. Because of the life-and-death situations involved in these kinds of assessments, the ethical concerns are intensified. Research that would help inform these assessments would be welcome.

For questions that relate closely to the medical disorder, research addressing the psychological course of a condition and its predictable influence on measures administered at various points would be helpful. Although data are available on the general effects of recency of a life-threatening diagnosis or the death of a family member, there is considerably less detail with regard to the typical assessment scores over time. This course-of-illness variable may have important implications for prediction and for degree of deviation of an affected child or adolescent.

In the current health-care atmosphere, it is particularly important to address what kinds of formal assessments are useful and meaningful and under what conditions. Preauthorization requests for psychological testing for any reason are often greeted with suspicion or resistance, if not flat denial. There is a growing need to be able to document the utility of assessments, especially with children with chronic medical conditions, and for psychologists to be clear as to which characteristics can be assessed through interview, observation, parent report, teacher ratings, or formal testing.

Children with chronic medical conditions are at risk for a variety of cognitive, behavioral, social, and emotional problems, but chronic illnesses in and of itself does not create psychopathology. As in Greg's case, children with chronic illnesses are also susceptible to problems that have little or nothing to do with their illnesses. Having a disease does, however, alter life experiences for the child and his or her family, creating greater demands for coping. Assessment of these children must always occur in context, with an awareness of the mutual influences of the family, school, social, and medical systems and a respect for the complexity of the task undertaken.

REFERENCES

Achenbach, T. M., & Edelbrock, C. (1983a). *Manual for Child Behavior Checklist and Revised Child Behavior Profile*. Burlington: University of Vermont, Department of Psychiatry.

Achenbach, T. M., & Edelbrock, C. (1983b). *Manual for the Teacher Report Form of the Child Behavior Checklist and Revised Child Behavior Profile*. Burlington: University Associates in Psychiatry.

Achenback, T. M. (1991). *Manual for Child Behavior Checklist, 4–18 and 1991 Profile*. Burlington: University of Vermont Department of Psychiatry.

Allen, L., & Zigler, E. (1986). Psychological adjustment of seriously ill children. *Journal of the American Academy of Child and Adolescent Psychiatry, 25,* 708–712.

Armstrong, G. D., Wirt, R. D., Nesbit, M. E., & Martinson, I. M. (1982). Multidimensional assessment of psychological problems in children with cancer. *Research in Nursing and Health, 5,* 205–211.

Bayley, N. (1969). *Bayley Scales of Infant Development*. San Antonio, TX: Psychological Corporation.

Bayley, N. (1993). *Bayley Scales of Infant Development—Second Edition*. San Antonio, TX: Psychological Corporation.

Bellak, L. (1954). *The Thematic Apperception Test and the Children's Apperception Test in Clinical Use*. New York: Grune & Stratton.

Bender, B. G., Lerner, J. A., & Poland, J. E. (1991). Association between corticosteroids and psychologic change in hospitalized asthmatic children. *Annals of Allergy, 66,* 414–419.

Berry, S. L., Hayford, J. R., Ross, C. K., Pachman, L. M. H., & Lavigne, J. V. (1993). Conceptions of illness by children with juvenile rheumatoid arthritis: A cognitive developmental approach. *Journal of Pediatric Psychology, 18,* 83–97.

Bibace, R., & Walsh, M. E. (1980). Development of children's concepts of illness. *Pediatrics, 66,* 912–917.

Breslau, N., & Marshall, I. A. (1985). Psychological disturbance in children with physical disabilities: Continuity and change in a five year follow-up. *Journal of Abnormal Child Psychology, 13,* 199–216.

Brewster, A. (1982). Chronically ill hospitalized children's concepts of their illness. *Pediatrics, 69,* 355–362.

Broder, H., & Strauss, R. P. (1989). Self concept of early primary school age children with visible or invisible defects. *Cleft Palate Journal, 26,* 114–116.

Brodie, B. (1974). Views of healthy children toward illness. *American Journal of Public Health, 64,* 1156–1159.

Cadman, D., Boyle, M., Szatmari, P., & Offord, D. R. (1987). Chronic illness, disability, and mental and social well-being: Findings of the Ontario Child Health Study. *Pediatrics, 79,* 805–813.

Campbell, J. D. (1975). Illness is a point of view: The development of children's concepts of illness. *Child Development, 46,* 92–100.

Canning, E. H., & Kelleher, K. (1994). Performance of screening tools for mental health problems in chronically ill children. *Archives of Pediatric and Adolescent Medicine, 148,* 272–278.

Carpenter, P. (1992). Perceived control as a predictor of distress in children undergoing invasive medical procedures. *Journal of Pediatric Psychology, 17,* 757–773.

Cleveland, S. E., Reitman, E. E., & Brewer, E. J., Jr. (1965). Psychological factors in juvenile rheumatoid arthritis. *Arthritis and Rheumatism, 8,* 1152–1158.

Connell, J. P. (1985). A new multidimensional measure of children's perceptions of control. *Child Development, 56,* 1018–1041.

Connett, G., & Lenney, W. (1991). Inhaled budesonside and behavioural disturbances. *Lancet, 338,* 634–635.

Costello, A. J., Edelbrock, C., Dulcan, M. K., Kalas, R., & Klaric, S. H. (1984). *Development and testing of the NIMH diagnostic interview schedule for children in a clinical population: Final report* (Contract # RFP-DB-81-0027). Rocheville, MD: Center for Epidemiologic Studies, NIMH.

Cousens, P., Ungerer, J. A., Crawford, J. A., & Stevens, M. M. (1991). Cognitive effects of childhood leukemia therapy: A case for four specific deficits. *Journal of Pediatric Psychology, 16,* 475–488.

Cousens, P., Waters, B., Said, J., & Stevens, M. (1988). Cognitive effects of cranial radiation in leukemia: A survey and meta-analysis. *Child Psychology and Psychiatry, 29,* 839–852.

Crittenden, M. R., Holliday, M. A., Piel, C. F., & Potter, D. E. (1985). Intellectual development of children with renal insufficiency and end-stage renal disease. *International Journal of Pediatric Nephrology, 6,* 275–280.

Cytryn, L., Moore, P., Van, P., & Robinson, M. E. (1973). Psychology adjustment of children with cystic fibrosis. In E. J. Anthony & C. Koupernik (Eds.), *The child in his family: The impact of disease and death* (Vol. 2, pp. 181–203). New York: Wiley.

Deasey-Spinetta, P., Spinetta, H., & Oxman, J. B. (1988). The relationship between learning deficits and social adaptation in children with leukemia. *Journal of Psychosocial Oncology, 6,* 109–121.

Delaney, E. A., & Hopkins, T. F. (1987). The Stanford-Binet intelligence scale, fourth edition: *Examiner's handbook.* Chicago: Riverside.

Eeg-Olofsson, O. (1977). Hypoglycemia and neurological disturbance in children with diabetes mellitus. *Acta Paediatrica Scandinavia* (Suppl. 270), 91–96.

Ellsworth, R. B., & Ellsworth, S. (1982). *CAAP Scale: The measurement of child and adolescent adjustment.* Palo Alto, CA: Consulting Psychologists Press.

Friedrich, W. N., Lovejoy, M. C., Shaffer, J., Shurtleff, D. B., & Beilke, R. L. (1991). Cognitive abilities and achievement status of children with myelomeningocele: A contemporary sample. *Journal of Pediatric Psychology, 16,* 423–428.

Garmezy, N. (1983a). Resilience in the face of adversity: Protective factors and resistance to psychiatric disorder. *British Journal of Psychiatry, 147,* 598–617.

Garmezy, N. (1983b). Stressors of childhood. In N. Garmezy & M. Rutter (Eds.), *Stress, coping and development in children* (pp. 364–394). New York: McGraw-Hill.

Gortmaker, S. L., & Sappenfield, W. (1984). Chronic childhood disorders: Prevalence and impact. *Pediatric Clinics of North America, 31*(1), 3–18.

Harris, E. S., Canning, R. D., & Kelleher, K. J. (1996). A comparison of measures of adjustment, symptoms, and impairment among children with chronic medical conditions. *Journal of the American Academy of Child and Adolescent Psychiatry, 35,* 1025–1032.

Harris, J. C., Carel, C. A., Rosenberg, L. A., Joshi, P., & Leventhal, B. G. (1986). Intermittent high dose corticosteroid treatment in childhood cancer: Behavioral and emotional consequences. *Journal of American Academy of Child Psychiatry, 25,* 120–124.

Harter, S. (1985). *The Self-Perception Profile for Children.* (Available from Susan Harter, University of Denver, 2040 S. York St., Denver, CO 80208–0204)

Harter, S. (1988). *The Self-Perception Profile for Adolescents.* (Available from Susan Harter, University of Denver, 2040 S. York St., Denver, CO 80208–0204)

Helsel, V. J., & Matson, J. L. (1984). Assessment of depression in children: The internal structure of the Child Depression Inventory (CDI). *Behavior Therapy and Research, 22,* 289–298.

Holmes, C. S., Respess, D., Greer, T., & Frentz, J. (1998). Behavior problems in children with diabetes: Disentangling possible scoring confounds on the Child Behavior Checklist. *Journal of Pediatric Psychology, 23,* 179–185.

Hurtig, A. L., Koepke, D., & Park, K. B. (1989). Relation between severity of chronic illness and adjustment in children and adolescents with sickle cell disease. *Journal of Pediatric Psychology, 14,* 117–132.

Hurtig, A. L., & White, L. S. (1986). Psychosocial adjustment in children and adolescents with sickle cell disease. *Journal of Pediatric Psychology, 11,* 411–427.

Ireton, H., & Thwing, E. (1974). *Manual for the Minnesota Child Development Inventory.* Minneapolis, MN: Behavior Science Systems.

Kaufman, A. (1979). *Intelligent Testing with the WISC-R.* New York: Wiley.

Kaufman, A. S., & Kaufman, N. L. (1983). *Kaufman Assessment Battery for Children.* Circle Pines, MN: American Guidance Service.

Kaufman, A. S., & Kaufman, N. L. (1985). *Kaufman Test of Educational Achievement.* Circle Pines, MN: American Guidance Service.

Kellerman, J., Zeltzer, L., Elienberg, L., Dash, H., & Rigler, D. (1980). Psychological effects of illness in adolescence: I. Anxiety, self-esteem and perception of control. *Journal of Pediatrics, 97,* 126–131.

Kirkham, M. A., Schilling, R. F., Norelius, K., & Schinke, S. P. (1986). Developing coping styles and social support networks: An intervention outcome study with mothers of handicapped children. *Child Care, Health, and Development, 12*(5), 313–123.

Kopel, S. J., Eiser, C., Cool, P., Grimer, R. J., & Carter, S. R. (1998). Brief report: Assessment of body image in survivors of childhood cancer. *Journal of Pediatric Psychology, 23,* 141–147.

Kovacs, M. (1981). Rating scales to assess depression in school-aged children. *Acta Paedopsychiatrica, 46*, 305–315.

Kovacs, M. (1992). *Children's Depression Inventory*. North Tonawanda, NY: Multi-Health Systems.

Krueckeburg, S. M., & Kapp-Simon, K. A. (1993a). Social skills of preschoolers with and without craniofacial anomalies. *Cleft Palate-Craniofacial Journal 30*(5), 475–481.

Krueckeburg, S. M., & Kapp-Simon, K. A. (1993b). Effect of parental factors on social skills of preschoolers with craniofacial anomalies. *Cleft Palate-Craniofacial Journal, 30*(5), 490–496.

Lachar, D. (1982). *Personality Inventory for Children—(PIC): Revised format manual supplement*. Los Angeles: Western Psychological Services.

Lake, C. R., Masson, E. B., & Quirk, A. S. (1988). Psychiatric side effects attributed to phenylpropanolamine. *Pharmacopsychiatry, 21*, 171–181.

Landtman, B., Valanne, E., & Aukee, M. (1968). Emotional implications of heart disease: A study of 256 children with real and "imaginary" heart disease. *Annals Paediatrial Fennial, 14*, 71–92.

Lanyon, R. I., & Goodstein, L. D. (1971). *Personality assessment*. New York: Wiley.

Lavigne, J. V., & Faier-Routman, J. (1992). Psychological adjustment to pediatric physical disorders: A meta-analytic review. *Journal of Pediatric Psychology, 17*, 133–157.

Linde, L. M., Rasof, B., & Dunn, O. J. (1970). Longitudinal studies of intellectual and behavioral development in children with congenital heart disease. *Acta Paediatrica Scandinavia, 59*, 169–176.

Long, N., Holden, S. T., & Zolten, K. H. (1991, April). *Maternal ratings of chronically ill children's behavior: What is being measured?* Paper presented at the Florida Conference on Child Health Psychology, Gainesville.

Markwardt, F. C., Jr. (1998). *PAT-Rnu manual*. Circle Pines, MN: American Guidance Services.

Matson, J. L., Senatore, V., Kazdin, A. E., & Helsel, W. T. (1983). Verbal behaviors in depressed and nondepressed mentally retarded persons. *Applied Research In Mental Retardation, 4*, 79–83.

McArthur, D. S., & Roberts, C. E. (1982). *Roberts Apperception Test for Children Manual*. Los Angeles: Western Psychological Services.

McCubbin, H. I., McCubbin, M. A., Patterson, J. M., Cauble, A. E., Wilson, L. R., & Warwick, W. (1983). CHIP, Coping Health Inventory for Parents: An assessment of parental coping patterns in the care of the chronically ill child. *Journal of Marriage and the Family, 45*, 359–370.

McCubbin, H. I., & Patterson, J. M. (1982). Family stress and adaptation to crises: A double ABCX model of family behavior. In D. Olson & B. Miller (Eds.), *Family studies review yearbook* (pp. 114–153). Beverly Hills: Sage.

Mendelson, B. K., & White, D. R. (1985). Development of self-body esteem in overweight youngsters. *Developmental Psychology, 21*, 90–96.

Millon, T., Green, C. J., & Meagher, R. B. (1982). *Millon Adolescent Personality Inventory*. Minneapolis: National Computer Systems.

Millstein, S. G., Adler, N. E., & Irwin, C. E. (1981). Conceptions of illness in young adolescents. *Pediatrics, 68*, 834–839.

Moffatt, M. E., & Pless, I. B. (1983). Locus of control in juvenile diabetic campers: Changes during camp and relationship to camp staff assessments. *Journal of Pediatrics, 103*, 146–150.

Morison, P., & Masten, A. S. (1991). Peer reputation in middle childhood as a predictor of adaptation in adolescence: A seven-year follow-up. *Child Development, 62*, 991–1007.

Mulhern, R. K., Fairclough, D. L., Smith, B., & Douglas, S. M. (1992). Maternal depression, assessment methods, and physical symptoms affect estimates of depressive symptomatology among children with cancer. *Journal of Pediatric Psychology, 7*, 313–326.

Mulhern, R. K., Ochs, J., Fairclough, D., Wasserman, A. L., Davis, I. S., & Williams, J. M. (1987). Intellectual and academic achievement status after CNS relapse: A retrospective analysis of 40 children treated for acute lymphoblastic leukemia. *Journal of Clinical Oncology, 5*, 933–940.

Murray, H. A. (1943, 1971). *Thematic Apperception Test*. Cambridge, MA: Harvard University Press.

Najarian, J. S., Frey, D. J., Matas, A. J., Gillingham, K. J., So, S. S., Cook, M., Chavers, B., Mauer, S. M., & Nevins, T. E. (1990). Renal transplantation in infants. *Annals of Surgery, 212*, 353–365.

Newacheck, P. W. (1989). Adolescents with special health needs: Prevalence, severity and access to health services. *Pediatrics, 84*, 872–81.

Newacheck, P. W., Budetti, P. P., & Halfon, N. (1986). Trend in activity-limiting chronic conditions among children. *American Journal of Public Health, 76*, 178–184.

Noll, R. B., Bukowski, W. M., Davies, W. H., Koontz, K., & Kulkarni, R. (1993). Adjustment in the peer system of adolescents with cancer: A two-year study. *Journal of Pediatric Psychology, 18,* 351–364.

Noll, R. B., Bukowski, W. M., Rogosch, F. A., LeRoy, S., & Kulkarni, R. (1990). Social interactions between children with cancer and their peers: Teacher ratings. *Journal of Pediatric Psychology, 15,* 43–56.

Noll, R. B., LeRoy, S., Bukowski, W. M., Rogosch, F. A., & Kulkarni, R. (1991). Peer relationships and adjustment in children with cancer. *Journal of Pediatric Psychology, 16,* 307–326.

Nowicki, S., & Strickland, B. R. (1973). A locus of control scale for children. *Journal of Consulting and Clinical Psychology, 40,* 148–154.

Olch, D. (1971). Effects of hemophilia upon intellectual growth and academic achievement. *Journal of Genetic Psychology, 119,* 63–74.

Orr, D. P., Weller, S. C., Satterwhite, B., & Pless, I. B. (1984). Psychosocial implications of chronic illness in adolescence. *Journal of Pediatrics, 194,* 152–157.

Parcel, G. S., & Meyer, M. P. (1978). Development of an instrument to measure children's health locus of control. *Health Education Monographs, 6,* 149–159.

Perrin, E. C., & Gerrity, P. S. (1981). There's a demon in your belly: Children's understanding of illness. *Pediatrics, 67,* 841–849.

Perrin, E. C., Stein, R. E. K., & Drotar, D. (1991). Cautions in using the Child Behavior Checklist: Observations based on research about children with a chronic illness. *Journal of Pediatric Psychology, 16,* 411–421.

Perrin, J. M., & MacLean, W. E., Jr. (1988). Biomedical and psychosocial dimensions of chronic illness in childhood. In P. Karoly (Ed.), *Handbook of child health assessment: Biopsychosocial perspectives* (pp. 11–29). New York: Wiley.

Petersen, A. C., Shulenberg, J. E., Abramowitz, R. M., Offer, D., & Jarcho, H. D. (1984). A self-image questionnaire for young adolescents (SIQYA): Reliability and validity studies. *Journal of Youth and Adolescence, 13,* 93–111.

Piers, E. V., & Harris, O. (1969). *The Piers–Harris Children's Self Concept Scale.* Los Angeles: Western Psychological Services.

Pillemer, F. G., & Cook, K. V. (1989). The psychosocial adjustment of pediatric craniofacial patients after surgery. *Cleft Palate Journal, 26,* 201–207.

Pless, I. B., & Pinkerton, P. (1975). *Chronic childhood disorders: Promoting patterns of adjustment.* Chicago: Year Book Medical.

Pless, I. B., & Roghmann, K. J. (1971). Chronic illnesses and its consequences: Observations based on three epidemiological surveys. *Journal of Pediatrics, 79,* 351–359.

Pritchard, C. T., Ball, J. D., Culbert, J., & Faust, D. (1988). Using the Personality Inventory for Children to identify children with somatoform disorders: MMPI findings revisited. *Journal of Pediatric Psychology, 13,* 237–245.

Rachelefsky, G. S., Wo, J., Adelson, J., Mickey, M. R., Spector, S., Katz, R., Siegel, S., & Rohr, A. (1986). Behavior abnormalities and poor school performance due to oral theophylline usage. *Pediatrics, 78,* 1133–1138.

Rae-Grant, N., Thomas, B. H., Offord, D. R., & Boyle, M. H. (1989). Risk, protective factors and the prevalence of behavioral and emotional disorders in children and adolescents. *Journal of American Academy of Child and Adolescent Psychiatry, 28,* 262–268.

Rappoport, L. Coffman, H., Guare, R., Fenton, T., DeGravo, C., & Twarog, F. (1989). Effects of theophylline on behavior and learning in children with asthma. *American Journal of Diseases of Children, 143,* 368–372.

Richman, L. (1976). Behavior and achievement of cleft palate children. *Cleft Palate Journal, 13,* 4–10.

Richman, L. C., & Harper, D. (1978). School adjustment of children with observable disabilities. *Journal of Abnormal Child Psychology, 6,* 11–18.

Romano, B. A., & Nelson, R. O. (1988). Discriminant and concurrent validity of measures of children's depression. *Journal of Clinical Child Psychology, 17,* 255–259.

Rovet, J. F., Ehrlich, R. M., & Hoppe, M. (1987). Behavior problems in children with diabetes as a function of sex and age of onset of disease. *Journal of Child Psychology and Psychiatry, 28,* 477–491.

Rutter, M. (1979). Protective factors in children's responses to stress and disadvantage: Social competence in children. In M. W. Kent & J. E. Rolf (Eds.), *Primary prevention of psychopathology* (Vol. 3, pp. 217–239). Hanover, NH: University Press of New England.

Rutter, M. (1985). Resilience in the face of adversity: Protective factors and resistance to psychiatric disorder. *British Journal of Psychiatry, 147,* 598–611.

Rutter, M., Tizard, J. & Whitmore, K. (1968). *Handicapped children: A total population prevalence study of education, physical and behavioral disorders.* London: Longmans Green.

Ryan, C. M., & Morrow, L. A. (1986). Self-esteem in diabetic adolescents: Relationship between age at onset and gender. *Journal of Consulting and Clinical Psychology, 54,* 730–731.

Sanger, M. S., Copeland, D. R., & Davidson, E. R. (1991). Psychosocial adjustment among pediatric cancer patients: A multidimensional assessment. *Journal of Pediatric Psychology, 16,* 463–474.

Sanger, M. S., Perrin, E. C., & Sandler, H. M. (1993). Development in children's causal theories of their seizure disorders. *Journal of Developmental and Behavioral Psychology, 14,* 88–93.

Schilling, R. F., Kirkham, M. A., Snow, W. H., & Schinke, S. P. (1986). Single mothers with handicapped children: Different from their married counterparts? *Family Relations: Journal of Applied Family and Child Studies, 35,* 69–77.

Schlieper, A., Alcock, D., Beaudry, P., Feldman, W., & Leikin, L. (1991). Effect of therapeutic plasma concentration of theophylline on behavior, cognitive processing and affect in children with asthma. *Journal of Pediatrics, 718,* 449–455.

Schweitzer, J. B., & Hobbs, S. A. (1995). Renal and liver disease: End stage and transplantation issues. In M. C. Roberts (Ed.), *Handbook of pediatric psychology* (2nd ed., pp. 425–445). New York: Guilford Press.

Seppala, T., & Visakorpi, R. (1983). Psychophysiological measurement after oral atropine in man. *Acta Pharmacologica Toxicologica, 52,* 68–74.

Shoemaker, O. S., Saylor, C. F., & Erickson, M. T. (1993). Concurrent validity of the Minnesota Child Development Inventory with high risk infants. *Journal of Pediatric Psychology, 18,* 377–388.

Simeonsson, R. J., Buckley, L., & Monson, L. (1979). Conceptions of illness causality in hospitalized children. *Journal of Pediatric Psychology, 4,* 77–84.

Smucker, M. R., Craighead, W. E., Craighead, L. W., & Green, B. (1986). Normative and reliability data for the Children's Depression Inventory. *Journal of Abnormal Child Psychology, 14,* 25–39.

Stawski, M., Auerbach, J. G., Barasch, M., Lerner, Y., Zimin, R., & Miller, M. S. (1995). Behavioral problems of adolescents with chronic physical illness: A comparison of parent-report and self-report measures. *European Child and Adolescent Psychiatry, 4,* 14–20.

Stehbens, H., Ford, M. E., Kisker, C. T., Clark, W. R., & Strayer, F. (1981). WISC-R verbal/performance discrepancies in pediatric cancer patients. *Journal of Pediatric Psychology, 6,* 61–68.

Stein, M. A., & Lerner, C. A. (1993). Behavioral and cognitive effect of theophylline: A dose-response study. *Annals of Allergy, 70,* 135–140.

Stein, R. E. K. (1988). *Personal Adjustment and Role Skills–III (PARS-III).* Bronx, NY: Department of Pediatrics, Albert Einstein College of Medicine.

Stein, R. E. K., & Jessop, G. J. (1984). General issues in the care of children with chronic physical conditions. *Pediatric Clinics of North America, 31,* 189–191.

Steinhausen, H. C. (1982). Locus of control among psychosomatically and chronically ill children and adolescents. *Journal of Abnormal Child Psychology, 10,* 609–615.

Stores, G. (1978). School children with epilepsy at risk for learning and behavioural problems. *Developmental Medicine and Child Neurology, 20,* 502–508.

Strunk, R. C., Mrazek, D. A., Wolfson-Fuhrmann, G. S., & LaBrecque, J. F. (1985). Physiologic and psychological characteristics associated with deaths due to asthma in childhood. *Journal of the American Medical Association, 254,* 1193–1196.

Taylor, W. R., & Newacheck, P. W. (1992). Impact of childhood asthma on health. *Pediatrics, 90,* 657–662.

Tedesco, L. A., Albino, J. E., & Cunat, J. J. (1985). Reliability and validity of the Orthodontic Locus of Control Scale. *American Journal of Orthodontics, 88,* 396–401.

Thompson, R. J., Jr., Gil, K. M., Burbach, D. J., Keith, B. R., & Kinney, T. R. (1993). The role of child and maternal processes in the psychological adjustment of children with sickle cell disease. *Journal of Consulting and Clinical Psychology, 61,* 468–474.

Thompson, R. J., Jr., Gil, K. M., Keith, B. R., Gustafson, K. E., George, L. K., & Kinney, T. R. (1994). Psychological adjustment of children with sickle cell disease: Stability and change over a 10 month period. *Journal of Consulting Psychology, 62,* 856–860.

Thompson, R. J., Jr., Gustafson, K. E., George, L. K., & Spock, A. (1994). Change over a 12-month period in psychological adjustment in children and adolescents with cystic fibrosis. *Journal of Pediatric Psychology, 19*, 189–204.

Thompson, R. J., Jr., Hodges, K., & Hamlett, K. W. (1990). A matched comparison of adjustment in children with cystic fibrosis and psychiatrically referred and nonreferred children. *Journal of Pediatric Psychology, 15*, 745–759.

Thorndike, R. L., Hagen, E. P., & Sattler, J. M. (1986). *The Stanford–Binet Intelligence Scale: Fourth Edition Guide for Administration and Scoring*. Chicago: Riverside.

Tobiasen, J. M. (1989). Scaling facial impairment. *Cleft Palate Journal, 26*(3), 249–254.

Tobiasen, J. M., & Hiebert, J. M. (1989). Reliability of esthetic ratings of cleft impairment. *Cleft Palate Journal, 26*(3), 313–317.

Van Dongen-Melman, E. W. M., & Sanders-Woudstra, A. R. (1986). Psychological aspects of childhood cancer: A review of the literature. *Journal of Child Psychology and Psychiatry, 27*, 145–180.

Walker, D., Stein, R., Perrin, E., & Jessop, D. (1990). Assessing psychological adjustment of children with chronic illnesses: A review of the technical properties of the PARS-III. *Journal of Developmental and Behavioral Pediatrics, 11*, 116–121.

Walker, L. S., Van Slyke, D., & Newbrough, J. R. (1992). Family resources and stress: A comparison of families with children with cystic fibrosis, diabetes, and mental retardation. *Journal of Pediatric Psychology, 17*, 327–344.

Wallander, J. L., & Thompson, R. J., Jr. (1995). Psychosocial adjustment of children with chronic physical conditions. In M. C. Roberts (Ed.), *Handbook of pediatric psychology* (2nd ed., pp. 124–142). New York: Guilford Press.

Wallander, J. L., Varni, J. W., Babani, L., Banis, H. T., & Willcox, K. T. (1988). Children with chronic physical disorders: Maternal reports of their psychological adustment. *Journal of Pediatric Psychology, 13*, 197–212.

Walsh, M. E., & Bibace, R. (1991). Children's conceptions of AIDS: A developmental analysis. *Journal of Pediatric Psychology, 10*, 273–286.

Wechsler, D. (1949). *Manual for the Wechsler Intelligence Scale for Children*. San Antonio, TX: Psychological Corporation.

Wechsler, D. (1991). *WISC-III: Wechsler Intelligence Scale for Children: Manual*. San Antonio, TX: Psychological Corporation.

Wechsler, D. (1991). *Wechsler Intelligence Scale for Children—Revised*. San Antonio, TX: Psychological Corporation.

Wechsler, D. (1992). *Manual for Wechsler Individual Achievement Test*. San Antonio, TX: Psychological Corporation.

Wilkinson, G. S. (1993). *The Wide Range Achievement Test 1993 Edition Administration Manual*. Wilmington, DE: Wide Range.

Wirt, R. D., Lachar, D., Klinedienst, J. K., & Seat, R. D. (1984). *Multidimensional description of child personality: A manual for the Personality Inventory for Children* (Rev. ed.). Los Angeles: Western Psychological Services.

Woodcock, R. W., & Johnson, M. B. (1989, 1990). *Manual for Woodcock–Johnson Psychoeducational Battery—Revised*. Allen, TX: DLM Teaching Resources.

Worchel, F. F., Rae, W. A., Olson, T. K., & Crowley, S. L. (1992). Selective responsiveness of chronically ill children to assessments of depression. *Journal of Personality Assessment, 59*, 605–615.

15

ASSESSMENT OF EXECUTIVE FUNCTIONS IN CHILDREN WITH NEUROLOGICAL IMPAIRMENT

GERARD A. GIOIA
PETER K. ISQUITH
STEVEN C. GUY

Jenny is an 8-year-old girl in the second grade who was struck by a car while riding her bicycle in her neighborhood. Unfortunately, she was not wearing her helmet that afternoon 6 months ago. She was unconscious for 2 days and was unable to learn any new information for a period of 5 to 7 days following her accident (posttraumatic amnesia). She was unable to recall the accident or any events leading up to her injury. In fact, her last memory of that day is having breakfast with her father at a local restaurant. Her recovery in the rehabilitation hospital was slow but steady over a 2-month period, after which time she returned home. Everyone was impressed at her quick physical recovery, and Jenny even began school 2 weeks into the school year. Her teachers and parents quickly observed, however, that she had trouble attending during group instruction in the classroom, had increased frequency of emotional outbursts with peers and adults, and was very unorganized with her school materials and personal belongings.

On interview, her parents reported that she has always been somewhat fidgety and talkative in class but that she has never exhibited the degree of overactivity and impulsivity that she has during the past school year. She has no overt physical signs of the injury, and although she may become more fatigued in the afternoon and evening, she is able to walk and run without much difficulty, and her speech is clear and fluent. Her teacher and parents, however, are very concerned about her functioning, because she was an excellent student prior to the injury, and they do not understand why she is having so much trouble given her apparent remarkable recovery. Jenny has begun to dislike school and often asks to stay home.

Phillip is a 14-year-old ninth-grader referred for evaluation because of poor academic performance and motivation during the fall of his ninth-grade year. His parents report that he is apathetic toward school and that, despite educational and cognitive evaluations that suggest superior intellectual potential, he is failing most of his classes. His parents also report that he was an A student throughout elementary school but that his grades began to fail once he reached middle school and have steadily declined to their current level of failure. Phillip reports, and his parents confirm, that it has nothing to do with his ability to understand the work, but it is more a problem with completing work, starting work at the last minute, or poorly organized work. Phillip actually completes about half of his homework as assigned but often does not turn it in or cannot find it. He complains that he is bored at school and cannot tolerate sitting in class. Relevant history is remarkable for several diagnoses. Phillip was diagnosed at the age of 7 with Tourette syndrome, which originally manifested as a chronic sniffing tic that was attributed to allergies. He later began to demonstrate eye blinking, shoulder shrugging, and throat clearing tics, and he was given the diagnosis of Tourette syndrome. Approximately 1 year later, Phillip was also noted to be somewhat overactive and anxious and was notably impulsive both at home and at school. He was diagnosed with attention-deficit/hyperactivity disorder, combined type. Since that time, his tics have waxed and waned. He demonstrates no negative social impact of the tics. Phillip is a popular student but tends to have only a small select group of friends. He is a good athlete and plays lacrosse and football. His tics are only a problem during periods of high stress, such as during examinations or at the beginning of each school year. His attentional difficulties and overactivity have decreased in the past 2 to 3 years, and he has not been taking stimulant medication.

Regarding academic difficulties, Phillip reports difficulty starting long-term projects and often puts them off until the last minute. Additionally, he frequently starts projects without much thought as to how the steps should be sequenced. As a result, he often has to start over, and it takes him much longer to complete a task than predicted. This causes significant frustration for Phillip and his parents. His handwriting has always been poor, and when he is working or taking notes, his work is even sloppier. In his haste to complete work, he often makes careless errors that go unchecked. When his parents have tried to help him, he quickly becomes angry and insists on doing the work his own way, regardless of the cost. He often attempts to solve problems via trial and error rather than strategically. His parents report that his desk, locker, and book bag are disorganized and full of old papers and "useless junk." He often forgets to write down homework assignments or loses the assignment sheets.

These case studies illustrate the complex assessment picture presented by children with neurological impairment. The purpose of this chapter is to focus on one aspect of assessment, the executive functions, that are at the core of each of these scenarios. This is an expanding area of interest in neuropsychology, psychology, and education, with substantial relevance to many neurological disorders of childhood (Barkley, 1997; Benton, 1991; Denckla & Reiss, 1997; Mateer & Williams, 1991; Pennington, 1997). We have chosen to focus on this critically important aspect of the child's functioning from both an assessment and intervention perspective. Our task is to describe the critical set of executive functions that is relevant not only to neuropsychologists but also to clinical child, pediatric, and school psychologists who work with children with neurological impairments. This neuropsychological mechanism of regulatory control plays a fundamental role in the child's cognitive, behavioral, and social-emotional development and has substantial implications for everyday social and academic functioning. Disorders of specific subdomains of the executive functions are found in a variety of clinical conditions due to the vulnerability of the brain during development. This functional domain is equally applicable to the assessment of all children with neurological impairment, including those with developmental origins (e.g., learning disabilities, attention-deficit/hyperactivity disorder, autism/pervasive developmental disorder, mental retardation) and acquired etiologies (e.g., traumatic, infectious, toxic, metabolic, neoplastic encephalopathies).

Given the potentially wide scope of this chapter, it is important to clarify what is *not* covered here. This chapter does not describe all neurological conditions or all possible aspects of psychological/neuropsychological assessment of children with neurological impairments, as this is far too broad a task. The reader is referred to a number of authoritative works that review the many different types of neurological disorders in childhood (Berg, 1996; Spreen, Risser, & Edgell, 1995). Furthermore, many aspects of general neuropsychological assessment of children have been covered quite effectively in other references (see, e.g., Baron, Fennell, & Voeller, 1995; Bernstein & Waber, 1990; Pennington, 1991; Rourke, Fisk, & Strang, 1986). The intent of this chapter is to provide the reader with an understanding of a specific area of neuropsychological functioning that has broad relevance to the everyday functioning of the child with developmental and acquired neurological impairment. To this end, we examine definitions and the historical, theoretical, and descriptive aspects of executive function and review assessment approaches and instruments. Assessment of executive function can be carried out through a variety of methods, including traditional psychometric performance tests, quasi-experimental measures, observational tools, interview, and structured behavior rating scales. We also consider formal and informal methods of assessing these critical functions.

Returning to the two cases at the beginning of the chapter, Jenny is having difficulties at home with poor control of her impulses and difficulties following through on everyday chores and tasks. She is weepy and forgetful at times, particularly when asked to perform jobs that involve more than one step. With her peers, Jenny is happy and effusive but emotionally unpredictable, and she frequently yells at her friends over seemingly minor disagreements. She is also more aggressive with her younger sister and has been repeatedly punished for hitting and yelling at her. Her parents report that it appears Jenny has fewer friends as of late and is not invited to as many outings as before her accident. She has been referred for further assessment regarding difficulties in behavioral adjustment and school learning. Jenny's history is not at all uncommon among children with mild to moderate traumatic brain injury. Although motor and orthopedic disturbances heal relatively quickly, cognitive disturbances often are masked by the stringent routine of inpatient rehabilitation setting and outpatient rehabilitation schedules. Additionally, as parents are usually relieved by their child's recovery and are more attuned to their physical needs, the cognitive difficulties usually associated with traumatic brain injury are ignored or rationalized as a product of hospitalization.

If a child's history of traumatic brain injury does come to light during a parent interview, then it is essential to elicit a clearer picture of the severity of the injury and change in function since the injury in order to determine its potential impact. In Jenny's case, the dramatic change in function was clear. She demonstrated difficulties in several of the subdomains of executive functioning, including the abilities to inhibit, sustain, and organize. She also demonstrated problems with emotional control and working memory. In a case such as Jenny's, a thorough neuropsychological evaluation is essential to document her profile of strengths and weaknesses to assist with clinical management. In other cases of traumatic brain injury, however, even though the injury may be seemingly mild and the dysfunction more subtle, the impact on daily functioning may be substantial.

As we can see in the second case, Phillip also demonstrates difficulties within many of the subdomains of executive functions, including difficulties in sustaining performance, in inhibiting competing thoughts and actions, in flexibly shifting his problem-solving approach, in organizing complex information and his environment, in initiating tasks, in planning, and in self-monitoring his performance. These difficulties have a profound effect on his academic performance despite his excellent cognitive potential. The assessment challenge is to determine the severity and nature of his difficulties in order to develop appropriate intervention strategies. As we discuss later, executive dysfunction is a common aspect of Tourette syndrome.

HISTORY AND DEFINITION OF THE EXECUTIVE FUNCTIONS

Though the concepts related to goal-directed behavior have been described in some fashion for decades (Bianchi, 1922; Luria, 1966), the term "executive control" is attributed to the cognitive psychologist Ulric Neisser (1967), who described the orchestration of basic cognitive processes during goal-oriented problem solving (Welsh & Pennington, 1988). This early definition is important because it began the differentiation of "basic" cognitive functions from the "executive," or directive, cognitive control functions.

More recent authors have viewed the executive functions as a collection of related yet distinct abilities that provide for intentional, goal-directed, problem-solving action. Fuster (1985) discussed the critical subfunctions of the prefrontal cortex necessary for performing long-term tasks via the "mediation of cross-temporal contingencies." In his conceptualization, executive functions are necessary for the organization of goal-directed behavior over a time dimension. These executive functions are highlighted by delayed tasks, which require the ability to hold information actively in mind as it is operated on in the service of a future goal. Fuster described three key components of this system, including the temporally retrospective function of working memory, the temporally prospective function of anticipatory set, and interference control. In Fuster's (1989) view, cells within the prefrontal regions of the brain become activated for a sustained period of time during these cognitive activities, bridging the temporal delay between events. In their classic treatise on functions associated with the frontal lobes, Stuss and Benson (1986) provided a set of related capacities for intentional problem solving, including anticipation, goal selection, planning, monitoring, and use of feedback. Their hierarchical model highlights important aspects of the executive functions that relate to the highest levels of cognition, including anticipation, judgment, self-awareness, and decision making. Welsh and Pennington (1988) characterized the early development of the executive functions in terms of "the ability to maintain an appropriate problem-solving set for attainment of a future goal" (p. 201). Denckla (1994) defined the critical features of the executive functions for active problem solving as follows: providing for delayed responding, future orientation, strategic action selection, intentionality, anticipatory set, freedom from interference, and the ability to sequence behavioral outputs.

Although different aspects of the executive functions have been discussed by various authors, most would agree that the term is an umbrella construct for a collection of interrelated functions that are responsible for purposeful, goal-directed, problem-solving behavior. A useful metaphor for conceptualizing their general purpose is as a conductor of an orchestra in which the component "instruments" of the orchestra are the "basic" domain-specific cognitive functions (e.g., language, visuospatial functions, memory) and in which the conductor serves as the directing system—making intentional decisions regarding the final output of the music and recruiting the necessary components in reaching the intended goal. Thus the executive functions are defined as the control or self-regulatory functions that organize and direct all cognitive activity, emotional response, and overt behavior. In cognitive and educational psychology, the executive functions are described in terms of metacognition, the domain-general functions that serve an oversight role.

Specific subdomains that make up this collection of regulatory or management functions include the following abilities: initiating behavior, inhibiting competing actions or stimuli, selecting relevant task goals, planning and organizing a means to solve complex problems, shifting problem-solving strategies flexibly when necessary, and monitoring and evaluating behavior. The working memory capacity to hold information actively "on-line" in the service of problem solving is also described within this domain of functioning (Pennington, Bennetto, McAleer, & Roberts, 1996). Finally, the executive functions are not exclusive to cognition; emotional control is also relevant to effective problem-solving activity.

Basic behavioral definitions for each of eight subdomains of the executive functions are provided in Table 15.1. A brief example that illustrates the types of dysfunctional behaviors for each area of executive function is also provided. These eight areas are not exhaustive of the entire spectrum but include the major components described in the literature.

TABLE 15.1. Behavioral Definitions for Executive Function Subdomains

Subdomain	Definition	Expression of dysfunction
Initiate	Beginning a task or activity	Has trouble getting started on homework or chores
Inhibit	Not acting on an impulse or appropriately stopping one's own activity at the proper time	Has trouble "putting the brakes" on behavior; acts without thinking
Shift	Freely moving from one situation, activity, or aspect of a problem to another as the situation demands	Gets stuck on a topic or tends to perseverate
Plan	Anticipating future events, setting goals, and developing appropriate steps ahead of time to carry out an associated task or action	Starts assignments at the last minute; does not think ahead about possible problems
Organize	Establishing or maintaining order in an activity or place; carrying out a task in a systematic manner	Has a scattered, disorganized approach to solving a problem; is easily overwhelmed by large tasks or assignments
Self-monitor	Checking on one's own actions during, or shortly after finishing, the task or activity to assure appropriate attainment of goal	Does not check work for mistakes; is unaware of own behavior and its impact on others
Emotional control	Modulating/controlling one's own emotional response appropriate to the situation or stressor	Is too easily upset, explosive; small events trigger big emotional response
Working memory	Holding information in mind for the purpose of completing a specific and related task	Has trouble remembering things, even for a few minutes; when sent to get something, forgets what he or she is supposed to get

NEUROANATOMIC ORGANIZATION
OF THE EXECUTIVE FUNCTIONS

The developmental course of the executive functions parallels the protracted course of neurological development, particularly with respect to the prefrontal regions of the brain. A commonly held view of the neuroanatomic organization of the executive functions, however, is that they are seated *solely* in the prefrontal region. This position is an oversimplification of the complex organization of the brain. Although damage to the frontal lobes can result in significant dysfunction of various executive subdomains (Anderson, 1998; Asarnow, Satz, Light, Lewis, & Neumann, 1991; Eslinger & Grattan, 1991; Fletcher, Ewing-Cobbs, Miner, Levin, & Eisenberg, 1990), the executive functions do not simply reside in the frontal lobes. Nevertheless, an understanding of this phylogenetically unique neuroanatomic region is important in any discussion of the executive functions. The neuro-anatomical essence of the frontal lobes is their dense connectivity with other cortical and subcortical regions of the brain. The prefrontal system is highly and reciprocally interconnected through bidirectional connections with the limbic (motivational) system, reticular activating (arousal) system, posterior association cortex (perceptual/cognitive processes and knowledge base), and the motor (action) regions of the frontal lobes (see e.g., Johnson, Rosvold, & Mishkin, 1968; Porrino & Goldman-Rakic, 1982). This central neuroanatomic position underlies the regulatory control that the frontal systems exert over the perceptual coding/conceptual processes of the posterior cortex, attentional, and emotional functions subserved by the subcortical systems (Welsh & Pennington, 1988).

It is worth mentioning the intentional use of the term frontal "system" as opposed to frontal "lobe" in this discussion. The concept of frontal system explicitly acknowledges and directly incorporates the frontal lobe's interconnections with the cortical and subcortical regions of the brain. The relevance of this concept is that a disorder *within any component* of the frontal system network can result in executive dysfunction (Mesulam, 1981). Conditions that render the frontal systems vulnerable to dysfunction include: disorders affecting the connectivity of the brain, such as cranial radiation and white matter development (Brouwers, Riccardi, Poplack, & Fedio, 1984); lead poisoning affecting synaptogenesis (Goldstein, 1992); direct trauma to the prefrontal regions in traumatic brain injury (Fletcher et al., 1990); dysfunctional neurotransmitters, such as dopamine in Tourette syndrome and ADHD (Rogeness, Javors, & Pliska, 1992; Singer & Walkup, 1991); disorders of the posterior cortex, including learning disabilities (see the next section); and disorders of the arousal mechanism, such as that seen in brain injury and severe depression. Thus executive dysfunction can arise from damage to the primary frontal regions, as well as to the densely interconnected secondary posterior or subcortical areas. Understanding this network is a crucial point for the functional control aspects of the executive functions that are discussed later. The associated basic cognitive "partners" must be present in order for the executive regulatory functions to have any operational purpose. Thus a close complementary and contributory relationship (Kaplan, 1988) of the anterior cerebral region with the posterior and subcortical structures is necessary.

DEVELOPMENTAL SPECTRUM

The developmental course of the executive functions across childhood has been an intriguing area of research (see e.g., Levin et al., 1991; Passler, Isaac, & Hynd, 1985; Welsh & Pennington, 1988). A key developmental feature of the executive control functions is their protracted ontogenetic course in comparison with other cognitive functions—paralleling the prolonged pattern of neurodevelopment of the prefrontal regions of the brain. Although earlier views of the executive functions argued for their emergence in early adolescence (Golden, 1981), studies in developmental psychology suggest a much earlier trajectory. The development of attentional control, future-oriented intentional problem solving, and self-regulation of emotion and behavior can be observed beginning in infancy and continuing through the preschool and school-age years (Welsh & Pennington, 1988). Examples of this work include studies of the development of goal-directed, planful problem-solving behaviors in 12-month-old infants using an object-permanence and object-retrieval paradigm (Diamond & Goldman-Rakic, 1989). A comparative study with intact infant monkeys and frontally operated adult monkeys found these behaviors to be localized specifically to the frontal lobes (Diamond & Goldman-Rakic, 1985). Eighteen-month-old children exhibit the self-control abilities to maintain an intentional behavior and inhibit behavior incompatible with attaining a goal (Vaughn, Kopp, & Krakow, 1984). These examples demonstrate the utilization of early intentional self-control behaviors by infants and toddlers for the purpose of goal-directed problem solving. The executive self-control at these early ages is variable, fragile, and bound to the external stimulus situation, whereas increasing stability is gained between 18 and 30 months of age. Developmental studies of children through adolescence demonstrate a time-related course of development for specific subdomains of executive function, including inhibitory control (Passler et al., 1985), flexible problem solving (Chelune & Baer, 1986; Levin et al., 1991; Welsh, Pennington, & Grossier, 1991), and planning (Klahr & Robinson, 1981; Levin et al., 1991; Welsh et al., 1991). As is the case with most dimensions of psychological and neuropsychological development, the emergence of executive control functions during development can vary across individuals in terms of when specific subdomains emerge and to what ultimate degree.

Developmentally, the executive control functions must be considered not only in terms of their own unique developmental progression but also in light of the type and nature of the age- relevant functions with which they are intimately associated (e.g., language, memory, visual–spatial processes). For example, preschoolers are working on different cognitive tasks than are school-age children, who in turn are working on different tasks than are adolescents. Thus the early executive control functions would not be expected to take the same form in preschoolers as in older age groups. Certain general similarities may appear in terms of the structure of executive functions (e.g., initiating, sustaining, inhibiting, shifting, planning, organizing/strategizing, monitoring), but several aspects are different and result in different behavioral manifestations. First, the types of representations or information being operated on are very different for the younger child (e.g., simpler language structures, more immediate time frame, more concrete representations). Second, various executive functions, though not absent, may be at earlier stages of development and therefore not fully operational. The interaction of simple task demands and immature executive functions in early development may make it difficult to observe such functions in their less mature form. In the adult, such functions reflect easily initiated, well-planned and organized, flexible, abstract thought processes that can be sustained over a long period of time, considering multiple possibilities, inhibiting the inappropriate and selecting the appropriate actions in pursuit of an established goal, all the while monitoring the adequacy and efficiency of the process.

Executive functions of self-awareness and control develop in parallel with the domain-specific content area or functional areas as described by Stuss and Benson (1986). For example, as basic memory skills (e.g., immediate memory span, encoding or retrieval) develop, the child develops a concurrent "metamemory" knowledge about how to strategically use and control these memory abilities for particular tasks or situations (Brown, 1975). An important corollary is that if the basic ability does not develop, then the associated "meta" knowledge and control skill (i.e., the executive function) would not develop as fully. This point relates directly to the interest in metacognition in learning disabilities (Pressley & Levin, 1987; Siegel & Ryan, 1989; Swanson, Cochran, & Ewers, 1990; Wong, 1991) and the development of self-control strategies within the context of specific processes (e.g., reading disorder, writing process). Part of the assessment and intervention in learning disabilities, therefore, must include the control strategies (e.g., recognizing the critical "problem" situation, planning and evaluating the use of specific learning strategies), in addition to the primary domain-specific content or processing disorder (e.g., decoding words, extracting meaning from sentences).

CLINICAL MANIFESTATION OF EXECUTIVE FUNCTION DISORDERS

With a working understanding of executive functions and their developmental course, we now turn to how deficits in the executive functions, broadly and in specific subdomains, may present as clinical symptoms or disorders or contribute to other disorders such as ADHD and Tourette syndrome. Deficits in executive functions are characteristic features in a variety of clinical disorders. For example, inhibitory control is a primary element of dysfunction in ADHD (Barkley, 1997). Children with learning disabilities can vary in their ability to organize and plan long-term tasks (Denckla, 1989). Problem-solving rigidity has been associated with acquired brain injuries (Ylvisaker, Szerkeres, & Hartwick, 1992) and lead poisoning (Bellinger, Hu, Titlebaum, & Needleman, 1994; Gioia, Guy, & Isquith, 1997). Executive dysfunction has been reported in other disorders, including leukemia (Waber et al., 1994), Tourette syndrome (Denckla et al., 1991), psychiatric disorders (Rothenberger, 1992), and developmental disorders such as pervasive developmental disorder (Klin, Volkmar, Sparrow, Cicchetti, & Rourke, 1995).

At the outset, it is important to acknowledge and emphasize that there is no singular, core disorder of executive function. Clearly defining a singular executive disorder is difficult for several reasons. First, there is considerable variation in how subdomains of executive function are defined in the research domain. Some authors perceive little general agreement among researchers as to the subdomains of executive function, with agreement on only four or five central components (Eslinger, Biddle, & Gratten, 1997). Among nine clinical practitioners, however, Gioia, Isquith, Guy, and Kenworthy (2000) found good agreement for the eight executive function subdomains presented in Table 15.1 with 75% or better agreement as to approximately 100 behavioral descriptors of these domains. Second, Pennington (1997) point out that disorders with different neuroanatomical bases can present with similar broad manifestations of executive function deficits (e.g., treated phenylketonuria, ADHD, autism, and fragile-X syndrome in women). On the other hand, a single clinical syndrome such as ADHD may reflect different executive function deficits, such as inhibiting and sustaining. Unlike a domain-specific function such as language, in which a commonality of deficits is seen in a clinical syndrome, executive function deficits can present differently within a syndrome or similarly across syndromes. Third, although neuropsychologists attempt to measure executive function in a variety of disorders in an effort to define the domains, there is not yet a full complement of sensitive and reliable measures with good specificity (Pennington et al., 1996). Further, although using the same measure of executive function, various researchers define the task requirements differently. For example, the Wisconsin Card Sorting Test (Heaton, Chelune, Talley, Kay, & Curtiss, 1993) is sometimes referred to as a measure of mental flexibility or shifting but is also referred to as a test of concept development, idea generation, abstraction (see, e.g., Berg, 1948), or attention (Mirsky, 1989). Such a measure may indeed involve several components of executive function, rendering a relatively pure interpretation difficult. Thus it is not a simple task to define the clinical manifestation of executive function deficits, as they may be broad, variable, and difficult to measure accurately both within and across clinical syndromes.

In this context, there is some general agreement as to basic components of executive function. Most researchers agree that working memory, mental flexibility or shifting, and inhibition are essential characteristics of executive function. In a factor analytic study, for example, Pennington and colleagues (1997) identified separable working memory, shifting, inhibiting, and planning components. Pennington's findings support the notion that executive function subdomains may contribute differentially to different disorders. The researchers found that individuals with ADHD, autism, early-treated phenylketonuria, and women with fragile-X syndrome exhibited similar within-group profiles but different between-group profiles on executive function measures. Participants with autism were most impaired on shifting set, followed by the women with fragile-X syndrome and, last, by those with ADHD. Inhibitory control problems were greatest for the ADHD group, whereas the autistic group was not different from controls. For planning, the autistic group was most impaired. Such patterns of findings suggest that, with further study, we may be able to more clearly define subdomains of executive function, develop more specific ways to measure executive function clinically, and define how these executive function subdomain deficits manifest in clinical disorders.

As we attempt to measure executive functioning in children, it is important to appreciate that deficits in one or more subdomains of executive function may not be visible until later in adolescence or adulthood. Eslinger and colleagues (1997) point out that, although executive functions are several steps removed from fundamental psychological development, they are highly influenced by such development. The explicit emergence of executive function is variable and susceptible to influence by a number of factors, including domain-specific abilities, environmental demands, and a variety of insults to the developing brain. As we have noted, there is a prolonged developmental course for the executive functions, in part attributable to the continued integration of prefrontal circuitry with all brain systems into late adolescence. Further, the demand for complexity and organization of cognitive processes increases with age. Thus two factors are at work that can obscure behavioral manifestations of deficits in executive function until later in the developmental trajectory: normal biological development and naturally increasing environmental demands on the executive functions as the child ages.

In summary, there is no singular disorder of executive function but rather a variety of presentations that involve one or more aspects of executive function, including a number of common syndromes that reflect different patterns of executive dysfunction. These syndromes may be developmental in origin, such as learning disabilities or ADHD, or acquired, such as traumatic brain injury or cranial radiation as treatment for leukemia. We now discuss some of these syndromes that characteristically involve executive function.

The "Dysexecutive" Child

Deficits in one or more aspects of executive function may be the primary presenting problem in a clinical setting. Many children present in a clinical setting with difficulties in academic, social, or behavioral functioning that do not meet criteria for a standard clinical syndrome (e.g., ADHD, learning disabilities, Tourette syndrome). When assessment can rule out deficits in specific cognitive domains (e.g., language, attention, visuospatial, motor), executive difficulties alone may be suspected. As we show in our review, parents, teachers, and children themselves often report a coherent cluster of behavioral characteristics that suggest an executive basis for functional deficits (Gioia, 1992). For example, similar to the case of Phillip in the chapter-opening vignette, parents who complain that their child is disorganized in all that he or she does, loses papers for school even when completed, misses the point of reading materials, and has trouble writing a coherent answer on paper may be describing a child who fails to organize behavior, thinking, or output. Similarly, a child who is described as lazy, unmotivated, unable to get work done, underactive, confused about how to begin tasks, or a "couch potato" may have initiation deficits.

The timing of manifestation of a child's executive difficulties is also important to assess. As Holmes (1987) describes in her discussion of the natural history of learning disabilities, the demand for executive functions is very limited until the upper elementary grades and, most notably, the middle school years. This is due to changes in environmental demands and expectations: As children make the adjustment from learning specific academic skills (e.g., reading, writing, calculating) to applying these skills for learning content areas (e.g., literary analysis, report writing, algebra), the demand for the executive functions increases dramatically. Further, the organizational support and structure of elementary schools are reduced as children enter middle school, a context in which increasing executive problem-solving independence is expected of the child. Suddenly, children who had previously been good students without any academic problems become poor performers in school. The parents' first complaint about a seventh-grader may be that he was always a good student but that his grades have dropped steadily since fifth grade. This reflects the natural impact of an executive deficit in academics. Socially, these children may also experience increasing difficulties as they enter middle school. The middle school environment is a demanding social milieu that requires intact executive function to grasp the gist of social interactions, inhibit impulsive responses to challenges, and effectively regulate emotions.

Attentional Disorders

As can be presumed from the nature of executive function, there is a close link with attentional functioning (Barkley, 1997; Mirsky, 1989). Indeed, executive function deficits may be most noticeable, and perhaps most measurable, as expressed via the attentional system. An intact executive system is necessary to support the ability to initiate, sustain, inhibit, shift, and direct the child's attention (Denckla, 1989). A child who cannot initiate attention or is slow to do so may never manage to focus on what someone is saying or on what he himself is doing. Disorders of sustaining attention and performance are characteristic of the inattentive type of ADHD. Isquith and Gioia (1999) recently demonstrated that deficits in initiating, sustaining, planning, organization, and working memory are likely functional underpinnings of the inattentive subtype of ADHD, whereas deficits in inhibiting, shifting, self-monitoring, and emotional control are strongly related to the combined subtype of ADHD. Barkley (1990, 1997) also gives thorough consideration to inhibitory control as a central problem in ADHD.

Language Disabilities

The development of language is an important aspect of, and possibly a precursor to, the development of executive controls, as proposed by Vygotsky and Luria (Rieber & Carton, 1987; Tinsley & Waters, 1982). Verbal formulations play a role in inhibitory control and working memory and, subsequently, executive function in general (Denckla & Reiss, 1997). An internalized language system allows the child to delay responses, in turn increasing working memory and allowing for mediation of multistep problem solving (Welsh & Pennington, 1988). The language system presumably also aids in generating appropriate strategies for problem solving. It may help children to remain focused on tasks and to direct their attentional systems according to plans or set goals. When the language system is impaired, there is a greater likelihood that the child will also manifest some degree of executive deficit. Clinically, we are often asked to sort out whether a child has a language deficit or an executive deficit. Language and executive disorders can be difficult to tease apart, as they are inextricably linked.

Hydrocephalus

Children with this type of neurologic condition, with or without myelomeningocele, can present with a variety of symptoms, depending on site, onset, duration, and shunting (Baron, Fennell, & Voeller, 1995). Although Wills (1993) notes that executive functioning is often overlooked in this population, general descriptions of hydrocephalic children's behaviors reflect problems in sustaining attention and inhibiting distraction (Fennell, Eisenstadt, Bodiford, Redeiss, & Mickle, 1987) and increased disinhibition in general. One often cited characteristic of hydrocephalic children is disinhibited, automatic, so-called "cocktail party chatter" (Tew, 1979), although this is not entirely supported in the literature (Byrne, Abbenduto, & Brooks, 1990).

Epilepsy

The cognitive characteristics of epilepsy are highly varied and multifactorially determined. Cognitive dysfunction varies depending on timing (during an epileptic event, postictally, or between events), location of seizure focus, onset of seizures, type and severity of seizures, and medications. Certainly, children with epilepsy are at significantly greater risk for learning difficulties, with 5%–50% exhibiting problems (Aldenkamp, 1987; Thompson, 1987). Although documentation with regard to the rate of executive function problems in children with epilepsy is limited, there is likely a rate commensurate with this estimate of learning problems. Research in this area is difficult, given the multiple variables that influence functioning over time, within an individual and between groups.

Childhood Cancer

Although the direct effects of childhood cancer on executive function are not known, there is considerable research on the cognitive profiles of children who undergo treatments for cancers such as leukemia. As such treatment typically involves various toxic agents that are designed to interrupt cell function (radiation, chemotherapy agents), there is evidence of a variety of "late effects" or cognitive difficulties that emerge later in development, long after chemotherapy and radiation have been terminated (Brouwers et al., 1984; Waber et al., 1994). Of particular interest in children treated with cranial irradiation is a consistent finding of initiation deficits (Einsiedel, Weigl, & Gutjahr, 1979; Ross, 1982; Stehbens et al., 1991; Waber et al., 1994) and perhaps also of organization deficits (Waber et al., 1994).

Brain Injury

Children with traumatic brain injury are perhaps the most widely studied population with executive function difficulty (Ylvisaker, 1998). Problem-solving rigidity (Ylvisaker, Szekeres, & Hartwick, 1992), social interaction deficits (Eslinger et al., 1997; Eslinger & Grattan, 1991), disinhibition, and planning deficits (Levin et al., 1994; Scheibel & Levin, 1997) have all been described in children who sustained traumatic brain injury. In this acquired disability, the greatest impact of executive deficits may not be seen in children at the time of injury but may emerge later with the dramatic increase of environmental, academic, behavioral, emotional, and social demands on the executive system during adolescence. Problems in the social realm of functioning for this group are often the most distinctive features (Ackerly, 1964; Eslinger et al., 1997; Eslinger & Damasio, 1985; Marlowe, 1992). Executive function deficits can result in a demanding, self-centered personality, lack of social tact, impulsive speech and behaviors, disinhibition, apathy and indifference, and a lack of empathy (Eslinger, 1997). Prospective case studies (Ackerly, 1964; Grattan & Eslinger, 1991) show the onset of marked behavioral, social, and emotional problems in children who sustained, and appeared to "recover" from, brain injury as children.

Tourette Syndrome

Tourette syndrome has been the focus of much research in the past few years (Singer & Walkup, 1991). In particular, a number of researchers specifically examined executive functions in Tourette syndrome (Denckla et al., 1991). Theoretically, inefficient functioning of the inhibitory control system can account for the inability to inhibit tics. Some recent work (Schuerholz, Baumgardner, Singer, Reiss, & Denckla, 1996), however, found difficulties largely on word generation fluency in children with Tourette syndrome, suggesting possible initiation deficits in addition to inhibitory deficits. However, children with Tourette syndrome exhibit fewer deficits in executive function than those with the comorbid condition of ADHD (Harris et al., 1995). Thus the picture may not yet be entirely defined as to which subdomain(s) of executive function are at risk for impairment in Tourette syndrome.

ASSESSMENT OF EXECUTIVE FUNCTIONS

In considering whether or not a child has difficulty in the executive domain, suspected executive difficulties need to be viewed within the larger context of a neuropsychological framework (Bernstein & Waber, 1990). Although it may be possible to identify isolated executive deficits or strengths based on tests, observations, behavioral ratings, or interviews, confirmation requires that problems in other domain-specific functions be understood. These domain-specific functions include attention, language, visual/nonverbal processing, sensory inputs, motor outputs, and learning and memory. For example, the child who, on copying a complex figure, produces a disorganized figure with distortions, repetitions of details, or no apparent grasp of the overall structure may be doing so because of executive function difficulties such as organization or inhibition problems or because of visual–perceptual or visuoconstructional deficits. Before executive function deficits can be confirmed, the underlying specific functions (in this case, visual–perceptual functions) must be shown to be intact (Denckla, 1996). The child must be able to process visual information both at the primary vision level and at the cognitive–perception level, must be able to grasp simpler figures that do not require higher level organization, and must be able to produce these simpler figures from a cognitive representation through the graphomotor system. If the latter functions are intact, then the problem can be presumed to be within the executive domain. On assessment in this case, one might rule out perception and reproduction problems for simpler figures with a task such as the Test of Visual–Motor Integration (VMI; Beery, 1967, 1982, 1997) as a control for copying a more complex figure such as the Rey–Osterrieth Complex Figure (Rey, 1964). Denckla (1996) argues for the use of a domain-specific control task (e.g., VMI) as a covariate for the more complex task (e.g., Rey–Osterrieth Complex Figure). When the specific function is controlled for, the remaining difficulty can more surely be attributed to an executive problem, such as organization, planning, or inhibition.

Not only must requisite skills in the underlying domain-specific content area be intact, but the executive problem should also be seen in *more than one* content area. Because executive functions are theoretically domain-general or overarching, a deficit in an executive function should influence performance across two or more specific domains. Disorganization in performance on one task might suggest an executive problem with organization but is not solely sufficient. Instead, the organization problem should be observable in other domains, such as in language (e.g., tangential expression, difficulty formulating a clear goal-oriented message) or in behavior on a day-to-day basis (e.g., difficulty keeping one's room or belongings organized). In the case of the disorganized copy of the complex figure, a disorganized approach to problem solving on other tasks, such as the Block Design subtest of the Wechsler scales (Wechsler, 1991) or in the recall of a Story Memory task (e.g., Wide Range Assessment of Memory and Learning; Sheslow & Adams, 1990) might be seen. The child might also be described as disorganized in work habits or as unable to keep his or her room reasonably organized. Confirmation of a suspected deficit in one or more of the executive functions requires *both* that the more basic domain-specific functions be adequate for the task *and* that the deficit be demonstrated across more than one specific domain. To fully examine whether a problem is broad, as in the case of executive functions, or domain-specific, a neuropsychological framework is important in guiding assessment.

A GENERAL NEUROPSYCHOLOGICAL ASSESSMENT MODEL

A neuropsychological model provides a theoretically based framework for assessment of cognitive and behavioral functions within which executive functions can be integrated and more thoroughly assessed (Bernstein & Waber, 1990). Such a model, to be useful, must be theoretically consistent, allow for integration of the wide variety of cognitive functions, explain patterns of deviation from normal or typical functions, and translate to assessment methods and tools. The model should also, in turn, suggest methods for intervention or accommodation. Given that neuropsychology evolved, in part, from the study of cognitive functions and the underlying neurological substrate, a model of neuropsychology might also be expected to refer to brain function at some level. Indeed, for a period of time in the history of neuropsychology, neuropsychological assessment was primarily a diagnostic tool that attempted to localize suspected structural lesions (Reitan, 1958). With the advent of neuroimaging and other diagnostic techniques, however, this role for neuropsychology has declined substantially. Instead, current neuropsychological assessment typically plays a much greater role in functional diagnosis and treatment or intervention planning (Lezak, 1995). It is difficult, particularly with children, to translate from function to structure (e.g., from neuropsychological test performance profile to brain structures). Although a neuropsychological model can be helpful conceptually for generating hypotheses, it is risky to assume that deficits on one or more tests implicate specific brain structures, particularly in the case of developmentally based disorders. (For a thorough discussion of this issue and a functional model of brain–behavior relationships in children, see Rudel, Holmes, & Pardes, 1988, and Bernstein & Waber, 1990.) For children whose neurological difficulties are of a congenital rather than an acquired nature, neuropsychology can play an essential role in describing the child's pattern of cognitive strengths and weaknesses and the functional impact on academic, social, emotional, and behavioral domains. With a growing focus within neuropsychology on rehabilitation (Meier, Benton, & Diller, 1987), assessment will likely play an increasing role in predicting recovery or improvement, planning interventions, measuring change over time, and documenting effects of interventions.

There are various approaches to neuropsychological assessment with different historical roots. Each model has advocates and opponents, as well as advantages and limitations. Although there are fixed test batteries such as the Halsted–Reitan Neuropsychological Test Battery (Reitan & Wolfson, 1993) and, at the opposite end of the spectrum, pure clinical hypothesis-testing models (Kaplan, 1988), many clinicians rely on similar sets of measures in a flexible form that allow for both psychometric analysis and qualitative, hypothesis-driven observations. Neuropsychological assessment is not a collection of tests but a conceptual framework for understanding specific domains of cognitive, social, and emotional function and their integration. Although a wide array of tests are available, a great deal of information about a child's cognitive functioning comes from careful observation of the process rather than test scores in isolation (Rudel et al., 1988). The child who offers a one-word correct response to a Similarities item on the Wechsler scales (Wechsler, 1991) gets full credit, yet he or she arrived at a correct solution quite differently from the child who explains his or her answer in detail. Both types of responses suggest problem-solving or verbal capacities quite different from those of yet another child who circumlocutes, or talks around the answer, until arriving at a satisfactory solution. In assessing executive function, it is essential to make careful observations about *why* a child did well or poorly rather than simply that they did or did not arrive at a correct solution.

Neuropsychological assessment typically involves examination of several domains of cognitive function. The amount of time required, number of tests, and depth of evaluation in each area depends on the referral question, history, and examiner's observations. A child with clearly intact spontaneous language and clear, well-formulated responses to questions likely would not need a comprehensive examination of language. On the other hand, a circumlocutory child or a child with long verbal response latencies requires further exploration in the language domain. As a context for evaluating executive functions, we offer a brief overview of domains typically examined in a neuropsychological evaluation.

General Cognitive Functioning

In order to place specific functions in context, it is important to include assessment of the child's general cognitive or intellectual ability as it relates to each area. Although it is not necessarily the case that children with higher IQ scores should have better executive functioning than those with lower IQ scores, the greater knowledge base and problem-solving capacity that defines strong performance on intelligence tests likely also leads to a decreased requirement for executive functions. A larger repertoire of problem-solving approaches means the child is less likely to have to generate novel strategies, to monitor for success or failure, and to shift strategies as much as does a child with lower IQ who has a more limited knowledge of problem-solving strategies. For this reason, it is important to have an assessment of the child's overall cognitive ability, typically derived from all or part of a standardized intelligence test battery such as the Wechsler scales (Wechsler, 1991), Differential Ability Scales (Elliot, 1990), or Stanford–Binet (Thorndike, Hagen, & Sattler, 1986).

Both quality of performance and subtest patterns on standardized tests can suggest executive dysfunction. As noted, just as overall cognitive ability may influence the degree to which executive functions are called into play on test performance, deficits in executive functions can also influence performance on intellectual assessment batteries. Tasks requiring active problem solving with novel material or efficiency and speed of performance, such as the Performance subtests of the Wechsler scales (Wechsler, 1991), are more susceptible to the influence of executive difficulties than are rote verbal measures (Gioia, 1993). This is a result of the demand that each subtest places on the executive functions. Although some verbal subtests on the WISC-III require language formulation, most verbal subtests primarily tap rote verbal knowledge. Executive functions are invoked in limited fashion when tasks require existing knowledge or vocabulary. The Performance subtests, on the other hand, involve novel, complex, speeded problem solving, the very same demand situations that tap executive function. Thus reduced scores on some or all of the Performance measures might suggest problems with initiating ideas or strategies for problem solving or with working memory, inhibiting attentional pull to details, or organization. For a full discussion of subtest patterns, see Rudel, Holmes, and Pardes (1988).

Attention

Attention is a well-studied complex phenomenon that is closely linked with and highly influenced by executive function (Barkley, 1997; Isquith & Gioia, 1999). This is perhaps the most difficult specific domain to separate from executive function. At the outset, attention is not a unitary phenomenon (Mirsky, 1989): It involves many basic and higher level components that are referable to several brain systems. A review of the attentional system starts with arousal, a child's tonic level or general state of alertness. In the extreme case, coma or unconsciousness reflects gross underarousal and likely damage to the reticular activating system in the brain stem. At the opposite extreme, overarousal can be seen as chronic hypervigilance associated with anxiety disorders or thyroid disorders (e.g., Graves disease) that artificially activate the sympathetic nervous system. Among more moderate cases, the underaroused child may be less able to attend to simple tasks yet may perform well on tasks that are more challenging and stimulating and require greater mental effort. The classic example of such a condition is evident when a child can repeat more digits backward than forward, the latter task in most cases being less challenging than the former.

Arousal is assessed by observation across the testing setting and by history. Is the child generally lethargic, slow moving, and underactive? Is the arousal level influenced by external, environmental factors, such as something the child finds exciting? For example, one child seen for evaluation was described repeatedly as having a pervasive developmental disorder. He presented with flat affect, poor eye contact, and monotone vocal production. On evaluation, the child presented as described and was slow moving, inattentive, and physically floppy or hypotonic. When given challenging tasks or when the examiner infused the assessment session with energy via rapid pacing and vocal intonation, the child became much more aroused and demonstrated average performance on most tasks, producing good vocal intonation and prosody and maintaining adequate eye contact. Further, although his performance on complex figure copying and story memory tasks was previously grossly impaired, administration of similar tasks while the child was aroused produced average results. In essence, the child was tonically underaroused but could be "jazzed up" by external means. As this case illustrates, the diagnostic implications and subsequent interventions are quite different for a child who is underaroused versus a child with the complex features of pervasive developmental disorder.

With general level of arousal as a backdrop, attention can be examined globally and in detail. Observations during conversation and testing can show fluctuations in ability to sustain attention. Does the child become fatigued across the evaluation or respond with better sustained attention to certain tasks than others? Or does the child attend initially at the outset of a task, then fade quickly? For example, on a lengthy verbal learning test on which the child must listen to and repeat a word list five times, many attentionally disordered children will initially increase the number of words they report but decrease reported words dramatically after a few trials. Qualitatively, these same children often complain of boredom by the third trial. Continuous performance tasks, such as the Gordon Diagnostic System (Gordon, 1983; Gordon, McClure, & Aylward, 1996), the Test of Variables of Attention (TOVA; Greenberg & Kindschi, 1996), or other continuous performance tests, can be helpful in formally examining sustained visual attention.

More demanding tasks might require higher level attentional functions, such as rapidly shifting attention or dividing attention. Any task of complexity may require attention to multiple elements and thus demand flexibility in shifting one's attention between the multiple stimulus components. Can the child shift attention from one set or problem to another? Can he or she divide attention between simultaneously competing stimuli? This might be seen in a complex-figure copying task, in which the child has to attend to the overall structure, as well as the details.

Language and Language-Related Processing

Assessment of basic language functions typically involves examining basic expressive functions, such as rate and fluency of speech, articulation, voice volume, intonation, prosody, syntax, grammar, vocabulary usage, word finding, and fluency of language formulation, as well as the receptive functions involved in registration and comprehension of language. Additionally, pragmatic use of language in social interaction is important. Although many formal tests exist for most of these areas, observation through conversational interaction often serves as a clinical screen for problems. As the Wechsler scales are more a test of verbal knowledge than of language functions per se, the neuropsychological evaluation typically includes a sampling of measures that involve more focused or complex language processing, such as naming and word retrieval tests (e.g., Boston Naming Test; Kaplan,

Goodglass, & Weintraub, 1983), sentence repetition or formulation tasks, and comprehension tasks (e.g., the Verbal Comprehension subtest of the Differential Abilities Scale, Elliot, 1990; the Comprehension of Instructions subtest from the NEPSY, Korkman, Kirk, & Kemp, 1998).

The relationship between language and executive function is complex in a bidirectional fashion. In one direction, deficits in executive function domains may interfere with language production. Problems of initiation can be seen in latencies to respond to questions or in word-retrieval difficulties (Ylvisaker, 1993). Organization problems are typically expressed as disorganized verbal output, with frequent, sometimes random, topic changes. Disinhibition may present as inappropriate verbosity or inappropriate or irrelevant questions. For example, one child who could discuss famous guitarists in a rote, one-sided monologue was unable to maintain an organized topic outside of that area and tended to ask inappropriate questions of the examiner. Problems sustaining attention can be seen in the child who frequently loses track of what he or she was saying. In the opposite direction, language deficits can interfere with executive function. As children develop language skills, they increasingly rely on an internal monologue to self-monitor, to generate strategies for problem solving, to direct attention, and to select desired behaviors. They use language, then, to assist in organizing information, in choosing where and when to pay attention, and in inhibiting inappropriate behaviors. We need only to think of the internal discussion we have with ourselves when a rude driver cuts us off during the morning traffic rush. Although the impulse may be to hit the other driver, our internal language system helps direct our thoughts toward better solutions and allows us to inhibit aggressive action. In children, language and executive disorders often go hand in hand. It is not uncommon to find marked language problems in impulsive, aggressive children.

Visual/Nonverbal Processing

This area involves the ability to process at the primary visual and perceptual level, to decode simple and complex visual stimuli, and to grasp the structure or meaning of the material. On the output end of the process, the child must be able to reproduce visual stimuli either from memory, as in a clock drawing, or from a present stimulus, such as design copying (e.g., VMI; Beery, 1997). More complicated "constructional" tasks such as the WISC-III Block Design subtest (Wechsler, 1991) further ask the child to comprehend and reproduce more complex designs from component parts. Although there are many individual tests for examining minute aspects of visual perception and reproduction, the more process-oriented neuropsychological evaluation relies on starting at more difficult integrative levels and assuming that the basic functions are intact. For example, if a child can adequately reproduce a complex figure drawing, it is reasonable to assume intact ability to copy simpler designs (e.g., VMI). Should problems be apparent on the copy production of the complex figure, there are many tests that break down visual information processing into simple recognition and matching, rotation of figures, comprehension for degraded stimuli, and so on. It is useful to note whether the child can comprehend meaningful visual information, such as pictures of familiar objects versus more abstract, nonverbal/visual materials such as the Rey–Osterrieth Complex Figure (Rey, 1964) or Block Design (Wechsler, 1991) items.

The overlap between visual/nonverbal functioning and executive functions is often seen in children with inhibitory control and organizational difficulties. Classically, the child who copies the complex figure in a highly disorganized manner but, on production from memory, demonstrates a good grasp of the gestalt and organization displays a problem with disinhibition, characterized by an impulsive, poorly planned approach to the figure. If, however, the child shows the same pattern of performance for the figure during recall as during copying, then organization may indeed be a problem. Self-monitoring difficulties may be displayed on this type of task as a failure to recognize errors. During testing, the child who makes a noticeable error on a Block Design and makes no move to correct it can be challenged to find the error or to compare his or her work with the stimulus after formal administration. If the child finds the error on a second, closer look, he or she likely was not monitoring his or her production carefully.

Learning and Memory

Learning, the complex phenomenon of being able to acquire new skills and knowledge, and the requisite memory processes are inextricably linked with executive functions (Schneider & Pressley, 1989). On assessment, it must first be shown that basic memory processes are intact. These are typically defined as the ability to encode, store, and retrieve stimuli of any type (e.g., visual, verbal, olfactory, motor). A stimulus must first be perceived, reflecting intact visual/nonverbal and language functions, then held in immediate memory sufficiently long to be encoded into storage. Later, information is retrieved from storage as needed. Although "memory" difficulties are often reported in children ("He doesn't remember when I ask him to do three things"), instead these are often problems of executive function, attention, language, or even behavior that can adversely affect memory processing or performance. Assuming these areas are adequate to the task, we can then examine the memory functions. A typical approach assesses immediate memory via repetition for limited amounts of rote information (e.g., digits, letters, visual sequences, sentences). Story memory tasks check for encoding by requiring immediate report of the story after hearing it, then check retrieval by requiring another report of the story after a delayed period. Although a significant decrement in recall might suggest storage difficulties, cues or recognition testing most often show the problem to be one of encoding or retrieval. Storage deficits are rare in children unless they have clear neurological damage to the temporal lobes, such as with some seizure disorders, tumors, or infectious encephalopathies (e.g., Herpes encephalitis). Other memory storage difficulties can be seen in children who have undergone cranial irradiation therapy for leukemia, although this may be partially attributable also to steroid treatments (Waber et al., 1995). There is also some indication in the literature of storage deficits in severely traumatized children who perform poorly on memory tasks (Gurwitch, Sullivan & Long, 1998; Stein, Koverola, Hanna, Torchia, & McClarty, 1997). The current literature suggests a decrease in temporal lobe volumes, specifically hippocampal volumes, with protracted trauma (Bremner & Narayan, 1998; Golier & Yehuda, 1998; Joseph, 1998).

As noted, the association between executive function and memory makes the two difficult to separate. Sustaining attention and concentration for the duration of the information is a prerequisite to encoding. Beyond simply attending to the material, the child must initiate encoding strategies for efficient storage. Efficient strategies will likely invoke organization systems and may involve a plan to remember the material. The child must also inhibit distraction by minor aspects of the information while attending to essential features. On the retrieval side of the equation, initiation of retrieval strategies is necessary, with more efficient retrieval typically reflecting more planful and organized search strategies.

To illustrate the association between memory and executive function, a repeated-trial word-list learning task can be administered, such as the California Verbal Learning Test—

Children's Version (CVLT-C; Fridlund & Delis, 1994). Immediate memory is demanded on the first trial, and number of words recalled is often commensurate with digit-span-forward performance. With repeated presentations, the child is asked to compare what he or she has already encoded with the rapidly presented list to fill in the missing information. The child who plans to remember and initiates an active encoding strategy will be more successful than the child who passively listens. In the case of the CVLT-C, there is a clear semantic organization inherent in the task that the child can use to organize and "chunk" the words, facilitating performance on the task. Children with sustained attention problems often show an inverted "U" pattern of recall: They increase the number of words recalled until about the third trial, after which time, they show a decrease in the number of words recalled. Typically, they also often complain about this type of task. The CVLT-C and other verbal learning tasks (e.g., Rey Auditory Verbal Learning Test; Rey, 1964) also require storage and retrieval after a delay and measure perseverations and intrusions, both of which may reflect disinhibition.

Motor and Sensory Functions

The motor output system and sensory input system are of interest to the evaluator. One can learn much about the child's motor system through general observation, beginning in the waiting room: Can the child navigate the hallways? Does he or she drift to one side or another? Can he or she maintain posture while seated at the testing table? During testing, key behaviors to be observed include pencil grasp, fluidity of letter making, ability to grasp and manipulate small objects, and differences in use and control with each hand. Formal tests can document fine motor speed, control, strength, and laterality. Tactile sensory functioning is less directly observable but may be of interest. A variety of formal test procedures in this area are available, including subtests from the sensory-motor domain of the NEPSY (Korkman et al., 1998), as well as from the children's adaptation of the Halstead–Reitan Neuropsychological Battery (Knights & Norwood, 1980).

As with other domain-specific functions, executive function provides a supervisory role in the integration of motor outputs and sensory inputs. Motor impersistence, though infrequent, may reflect a general inability to sustain output in a neurologically impaired child. Motor disinhibition is commonly seen in the impulsive–overactive child. Many times one is asked to differentiate between a problem of primary graphomotor production (i.e., the child can't adequately form the letters) and an impulsive approach to handwriting (i.e., the child can form basic letters but rushes quickly through writing tasks). Motor overflow or disinhibition of motor outputs in the face, mouth, or opposite hand is commonly seen in children for whom writing is difficult (Denckla, 1985). Thus motor planning difficulties may reflect an executive function component. Neuroanatomically, the motor production system and aspects of the executive system (e.g., inhibitory, organizational) reside in close cortical proximity to each other. It is, therefore, not surprising that the presence of dysfunction in one system is frequently accompanied by dysfunction in the other.

Academic Skills

Academic skills are an outcome of the underlying cognitive processes rather than a domain-specific function per se. That is, reading, writing, and calculation are developed skills that rely on a variety of specific brain systems that, in turn, must be functional. At a basic level, the auditory processing system must register sounds, allow for the segmentation of sounds into basic units (i.e., phonemes), associate the phonemes with the visual symbol (i.e., letters and letter combinations), and translate the associations into graphic units (Rudel et al., 1988). The graphemes are produced motorically via an integrated fine motor system. Similarly, calculation requires the ability to perform symbolic translations with numbers, as well as an understanding of number concepts. Increasingly, many more systems are invoked as the child eventually applies basic academic skills to more complex mathematical concepts and more complex, integrated reading and writing tasks to learn and to communicate.

Executive functions are implicated differently at various stages of academic development. Clearly the ability to inhibit plays a large role in the acquisition of early academic skills. For example, inhibitory deficits are seen in the child who is responding to other stimuli in the classroom rather than to the learning task at hand. Another example is the child who impulsively attends to only the first letter of a word rather than fully decoding all the critical phonemic elements, thus erroneously "reading" the word. While the child is acquiring the basic technical skills of reading and writing, he or she must have the ability to sustain overpractice so that the skills become automatic. Once successfully automatized, the skills require little attention and effort from the child. At this point, the focus in school typically shifts to applying these basic skills to learning more advanced reading, writing, and calculating skills. Such advanced application of basic skills requires more of the executive system, particularly for organization and integration of novel information, written output, and thinking in general. Hence, children with executive/organizational difficulties are more likely to present with problems during later elementary grades, when this change in educational demand takes place (Holmes, 1987).

Social/Emotional/Behavioral Functioning

As in most assessments, it is helpful to have information about the child's social skills, emotional status, and day-to-day behaviors. Many assessment methods are available for evaluating children's social, emotional, and behavioral functioning, and a number of these have been described elsewhere in this book. Executive functions play an important and often readily apparent role in the modulation of behavior, emotions, and social interaction. An evaluator can learn much about a child's likely executive functioning through observation of general behavior and through parent and teacher reports.

Many parents report clear characteristics of general disinhibition: The child is "always into things," acts before thinking, races through homework carelessly, intrudes into adult conversations repeatedly, and requires continual supervision in order to stay out of trouble. Organizational problems may be similarly described by parents: The child is messy, has a messy room, locker, and desk, can never find her homework even when it has been completed, and doesn't remember where things are or doesn't follow through on routine chores or activities. Parents who describe their child as "drifty," fading from tasks, having difficulty finishing homework that is within his or her mastery level, or "zoning out" may be describing problems with sustaining attention and effort. Planning deficits may be reported as difficulties in figuring out what things are needed for a project, starting activities without all the requisite materials, or having problems completing projects on time for school. Children who get "stuck" on one topic or become overly focused on a peripheral point or minor detail may have difficulty shifting attention. Such children may be rigid in their use of problem-solving strategies, leaving them at risk for social problems. Finally, initiation difficulties are often seen in children who are described as "couch potatoes" or as generally lethargic: "He sits around all day, but if you invite him to do something, he'll get up and join you." Children with initiation deficits also may have trouble knowing where or how to begin on homework, but once they begin, they perform well.

There can be a close relationship between the child's emotional functioning and his or her executive function. The child who is poorly regulated in the cognitive realm of problem solving may also have a difficult time maintaining an age-appropriate degree of control over his or her emotional responses to stress. The child may tend to overreact out of proportion to the stressor. Of course, anxiety can also disrupt efficient executive problem solving through a variety of mechanisms: by reducing the child's working memory capacity, by decreasing the freedom to think flexibly about alternative problem solutions, or by having an adverse impact on organized systematic problem solving. Depression resulting in decreased arousal contributes to poor initiation and difficulties with sustained performance, as well as to decreased working memory and problem-solving flexibility. Thus the executive functions have a bidirectional relationship with emotional functioning—they contribute to the regulation of emotion and behavior while also being influenced by one's emotional state.

In summary, neuropsychology provides a conceptual framework for assessment that encompasses a wide range of cognitive functions. There are several different models for approaching the assessment, and each model offers valuable tools and techniques. Against this background of testing fundamental domain-specific cognitive functions, we now consider the assessment of executive function in some detail.

SPECIAL ISSUES IN THE ASSESSMENT OF THE EXECUTIVE FUNCTIONS

Although the collection of behaviors and processes known as the executive functions may be defined in a relatively straightforward manner, their precise assessment can be very challenging. A clear understanding of the differences between assessment of the "basic" domain-specific content areas of cognition (e.g., memory, language, visuospatial) and the domain-general or "control" aspects of cognition and behavior is essential. What may appear as a problem with the expression of language may be due less (or not at all) to the basic aspects of linguistic functioning (e.g., vocabulary, syntax, semantics) than to poor metalinguistic functions (e.g., formulating and maintaining an organized, planful approach to the topic of conversation). There is no test or battery that singularly assesses executive function. By necessity, there is always a "domain-specific" content area regulated by the executive control process. Returning to our orchestral metaphor, the conductor (executive function) must have players (cognitive processes) to direct in order to make "cognitive" music. Teasing apart executive functions from domain-specific functions is part of the challenge of the neuropsychological assessment.

Dynamic Essence

Historically, clinical assessment of the executive functions has been challenging, given their dynamic essence (Denckla, 1994). Any assumption that the executive functions are static abilities amenable to traditional testing is simply false and can lead to their misrepresentation. In many respects, fluid, strategic, goal-oriented problem solving is not as amenable to paper-and-pencil methods as are the more domain-specific functions of language, memory, motor, and visual/nonverbal abilities. Furthermore, the structured and interactive nature of the typical assessment situation may relieve the demands on the executive functions and thereby reduce the opportunity to observe critical behaviors associated with the executive functions (Bernstein & Waber, 1990). That is, in many testing situations, the examiner provides the structure, organization, guidance, and plan, as well as the cueing and monitoring necessary for optimal performance by the child, thus serving as that child's external executive control (Kaplan, 1988; Stuss & Benson, 1986). A child with significant executive dysfunction can perform appropriately on well-structured tasks of knowledge on which the examiner is allowed to cue and probe for more information, thus relieving the child of the need to be strategic and goal-directed.

Novelty—Familiarity Dimension

Recognizing the different stimulus conditions that are provided within the comfort of the controlled setting of testing (which may be very necessary to identify the child's knowledge and abilities) versus those existing within the child's "real" day-to-day world is critically important. Frequently, the more novel and/or complex the task, the greater the demand for the executive functions. The more familiar, automatic, and simple the task, the less the child needs to recruit his or her executive functions. What may be a complex, novel task for one child may be a relatively familiar and automatic task for another, requiring that these children recruit vastly different degrees of executive control functions toward solving that particular problem. The ultimate application of assessment data to formulate credible practical recommendations and intervention strategies demands a clear understanding of this issue. Assessing the child's behavior and responses under greater and lesser degrees of examiner-determined control and structure can help clarify the child's executive control competence. This point stresses the importance of an intraindividual approach to assessment as opposed to a simply normative model.

A paradox in the assessment of the executive functions is that some individuals with significant deficits in specific executive function subdomains may, in fact, perform appropriately on many purported "tests of executive function" yet have significant problems making simple real-life decisions (Stuss & Buckle, 1992). It is critical to remember that all tests are multifactorial, requiring for any particular individual greater and/or lesser degrees of domain-specific content knowledge and experience (the novelty–familiarity issue) and thereby demanding varying degrees of organization, planning, inhibitory control, or flexibility. For example, a child may be able to perform appropriately on the Wisconsin Card Sorting Test (Heaton et al. 1993), which requires flexibility in problem solving, yet may fail miserably in strategically modifying his or her approach to completing a set of math problems in the classroom. In the assessment of the executive functions, it is particularly important to remember Teuber's (1964) classic statement, that "absence of evidence is not evidence of absence." One may not be collecting the relevant data to document the full essence of strengths and weaknesses in the array of executive functions.

An additional complicating factor in the assessment of the executive functions in children is that most existing standardized clinical measures are downward extensions of adult measures that have not been constructed with developmental change in mind. Given the extensive literature in developmental psychology documenting changes of strategic behavior and knowledge from infancy through adolescence (Welsh & Pennington, 1988), recognition of these effects in the use of assessment instruments is of critical importance. There is, of course, a related priority for the construction of instruments that are sensitive to developmental effects.

As is more fully addressed in the discussion that follows, assessment requires a variety of approaches to characterize fully the profile of the executive functions for a given child. The examiner must (1) maintain systematic observations of the ways that the child manages task demands within the context of the assessment situation, including his or her social behavior during interviews, in the waiting room, and during testing; (2) recruit reliable reports of critical problem-solving behaviors in the child's "real world"; and (3) provide psychometrically and developmentally appropriate tests for direct observation of executive problem-solving performance.

METHODS OF ASSESSING THE EXECUTIVE FUNCTIONS

We now consider the various methods of assessing each of the different subdomains of executive function. Table 15.2 provides a representative sample of the measures currently available to assess these functions in children and adolescents. When examining the psychometric properties of the performance measures, the examiner must recognize that there is an inherent confound that limits the utility of the test–retest indices. As discussed earlier, measures of executive functioning assess the individual's ability to solve problems or complete tasks with novel and complex demands. Once a person has been exposed to a novel problem-solving task, the practice effect limits interpretation of retest performance as "executive." In other words, the second administration is no longer "novel," and therefore the nature of the task demands is likely somewhat different from an executive problem-solving perspective. Caution is also warranted regarding the validity indices of the measures. As Pennington (1997) points out, the consistency, severity, and profile of executive function deficits vary across the developmental disorders, creating challenges in establishing discriminant validity of the measurement tools. Nonetheless, most tasks have been found to adequately discriminate between clinical and normal samples and have strong clinical utility. Perhaps as important as the derived standard scores, which offer only partial information, these tests also yield rich qualitative observations of a child's problem-solving capabilities.

The ability to initiate is described as beginning a task or activity or the process of generating responses or problem-solving strategies. Performance measures that tap this ability often involve the rapid generation of responses such as words or designs (e.g., Controlled Oral Word Association, Benton & Hamsher,1989; Design Fluency, Jones-Gotman & Milner, 1977; NEPSY, Korkman, Kirk, & Kemp, 1998). For example, verbal fluency tests require the examinee to say as many words as possible that begin with a certain letter or are within a certain category (e.g., animals, foods). The design fluency tasks require a participant to draw as many different designs as possible in a given time period. This function can be also be readily evident through observation during the assessment process, as children with initiation difficulties often require additional cues from the examiner to start a task. Furthermore, caregivers often report that children with initiation difficulties have trouble getting started on homework or chores and require prompts or cues in order to begin. It is important to emphasize that problems with initiation are not the result of noncompliance or disinterest in the task. The child typically has an interest in the task or activity and wants to succeed but cannot get started.

A child's inability to sustain performance and attention is a common reason for referral for evaluation and treatment. Not surprisingly, there are a variety of methods to assess

TABLE 15.2. Representative Tests and Subdomains of Executive Function

Executive subdomains	Measure	Publisher/reference	Age range (years)	Description	Psychometric properties	Comments
Initiate (shift, self-monitor)	Verbal Fluency (e.g., FAS; Category Fluency)	Unpublished; Gaddes & Crockett (1975)	6–13	Rapidly generate words based on letter/category cue.	Interscorer reliability excellent. Test–retest reliability = .70–.88. Validity considered moderate to good.	This measure has been useful in studying ADHD and Tourette syndrome
Initiate (shift, self-monitor)	Five-Point Test	PAR (Ruff, 1988)	6–adult	Rapidly generate different designs.	Test–retest = .36–.76.	
Sustain; inhibit	Test of Variables of Attention (TOVA)	Universal Attentional Disorders (Greenberg & Kindschi, 1996)	4–adult	11.5–21.6-minute continuous performance measure.	Studies suggest good at discriminating children with ADHD from normal participants. Adequate test–retest reliability.	Multiple performance scores allow assessment of several subdomains of executive function—min. practice effects.
Sustain; inhibit	Gordon Diagnostic System	Gordon (1983)	4–adult	3 subtests—Vigilance, Delay, Distractibility.	Test–retest reliability (2–45 days): Delay .60–.77; Vigilance .72–.84; Distractibility .67–.85. Numerous validity studies of ADHD vs. controls.	Good normative sample and research base. Shorter vigilance task makes utility with adolescents questionable.
Sustain; working memory	Children's Paced Auditory Serial Addition Test (CHIPASAT)	Johnson et al., (1988); Dyche & Johnson (1991)	8–15	Serial addition task.	Split-half reliability good. Significant practice effects. Moderately correlated to other attention tests.	Intact math calculation skills required.
Inhibit (strategic search)	Matching Familiar Figures Test	Welsh, Pennington, & Grossier (1991)	7–12	Matching target figures from group of nearly identical stimuli.	Internal consistency: response time = .89; error = .62.	Limited sample of normal children.

EF component	Test	Source	Age	Task	Reliability	Comments
Inhibit; shift	Stroop Test	Stoelting Co. (Golden, 1978)	8–adult	Requires inhibiting and shifting from automatic perceptual set to novel set.	Test-retest = .75–.90. Significant practice effects.	Quick and easy to administer measure (5 minutes).
Shift (inhibit/sustain); hypothesis testing	Wisconsin Card Sorting Test	Psychological Assessment Resources (Heaton et al., 1993)	6½–adult	Matching cards to stimulus features that change. Constant feedback provided by examiner.	Inter-intrascorer reliability excellent. Practice effects skew test-retest results.	Good measure of problem-solving flexibility and of a child's ability to benefit from feedback from environment.
Shift/sustain	Trail Making Test	Reitan Neuropsych. Laboratory (Reitan & Wolfson, 1985)	9–15, 15–adult	Maintain an alternating number/letter sequence.	Interrater reliability = .90–.94. Significant practice effects.	Questionable discriminatory power with children. Confound with automatic knowledge of letter and number sequences.
Shift	Contingency Naming Test	Taylor (1989)	6–16 yrs	Naming of colored shapes according to rules and mental set shifting.	Norms based on control participants in research projects: factor analysis loads on EF factor. Test distinguishes between normal and children with early brain insults. Predicts achievement and attention.	Various clinical populations studied, including ALL, meningitis, traumatic brain injury, low birth wt.
Concept formation; hypothesis testing	Category Test	Reitan Neuropsych. Laboratory (Reitan & Wolfson, 1985)	5–8, 9–14, 15–adult	Deduction of principles utilizing feedback.	Split-half reliability good. Test-retest reliability variable.	Long-standing history of use with neurological disorders. Tends to be related as much to global dysfunction as to EF.

(continued)

341

TABLE 15.2. *continued*

Executive subdomains	Measure	Publisher/reference	Age range (years)	Description	Psychometric properties	Comments
Organize; plan	Rey–Osterrieth Complex Figure (ROCF)	Psychological Assessment Resources; Bernstein & Waber (1996)	5–14	Drawing/copy and recall of complex visual figure.	Newest scoring criteria interrater reliability = .87–.95. Test–retest not calculated. Good discrimination between clinical and normal samples.	This task has a detailed but excellent scoring system that allows for qualitative and quantitative interpretation. Excellent measure of how children approach and solve complex novel problems.
Organize (inhibit; sustain)	California Verbal Learning Test—Children's Version (CVLT-C)	Psychological Corporation (Fridland & Delis, 1994)	5–16	Recall and storage of repeatedly presented verbal list with organizational demands.	Moderate to high internal consistency. Practice effects result in questionable test–retest reliability.	Good measure of strategic information processing. Provides indices that examine organizational components of verbal learning.
Plan (inhibit; working memory)	Tower of Hanoi	Welsh et al. (1991)	3–12	Disc transfer task requiring systematic planning of sequence of steps to reach goal state.	Interrater reliability good. Practice effects evident.	Limited normal sample. Has been used in a number of clinical studies, including PKU, LD, ADHD.
Plan (inhibit; working memory)	Tower of London	Krikorian, Bartrok, & Gay (1994)	6–adult	Same as above except number of discrete number of moves required.	Moderately correlated with other measures of executive functions.	Larger normative sample.
Inhibit; shift; emotional control; initiate; working memory; plan/organize; organization of materials; monitor	Behavior Rating Inventory of Executive Function (BRIEF)	PAR; Gioia, Isquith, Guy, & Kenworthy, (2000)	5–18	Parent and teacher report–behavioral checklist.	Demonstrate appropriate reliability (internal consistency, test–retest), consistent factor structure; convergent/divergent validity with other behavior rating scales; differing profiles of dysfunction with variety of populations	Focus on behavioral manifestation of executive function; good companion to performance-based tests; multiple domains assessed

Construct	Test	Source	Age	Subtests/description	Psychometric properties	Comments
Planning	Das–Naglieri Cognitive Assessment System (CAS)	Riverside Publishing (Naglieri & DAS, 1997)	5–17	3 subtests that assess planning—Matching Numbers, Planned Codes, Planned Connections	Average reliability for the Standard Battery Planning Scale is .88. Construct, concurrent, predictive, and discriminant validity are reported.	This task has a detailed Planning scale as part of the overall cognitive battery, which includes attention, successive, and simultaneous processing. Well-standardized measure.
Initiate; sustain; inhibit; shift; hypothesis testing; plan; organize	Delis–Kaplan Executive Function Scale (D-KEFS)	Psychological Corporation (Delis, Kaplan, & Kramar, 2001)	8–15, 16–adult	Renorming of 10 existing tests within single battery across a wide age span.	Large, national normative study.	Consists of a variety of subtests similar to those described above, many with additional process-oriented variables, including: a Trail Making Test; Verbal Learning Test; Design Fluency; Stroop Test; Tower Test; Sorting Test; Verbal Fluency; Twenty Questions; Word Context; Proverb Test.
Plan; inhibit; sustain; initiate; shift	NEPSY attention/ executive domain	Psychological Corporation (Delis, Kaplan, & Kramar, 2001)	3–12	6 subtests within general battery.	Nationally stratified normative base. Moderate to high reliability.	Based on Luria's model. Child-friendly tasks. First attempt to assess at preschool ages.

this function. Continuous performance measures are popular methods that require the child to maintain attention on a nonstimulating or minimally reinforcing task (TOVA, Greenberg & Kindschi, 1996; Gordon Diagnostic System, Gordon, McClure, & Aylward, 1996; Gordon, 1983) for an extended period of time. Other tests of sustaining require intense concentration under difficult task demands. For example, the Children's Paced Auditory Serial Addition Test (CHIPASAT; Dyche & Johnson, 1991; Johnson, Roethig-Johnston, & Middleton, 1988) requires the examinee to mentally add two consecutive digits, which are steadily presented over a period of time. Still another method to assess a child's ability to sustain is through caregiver reports, as numerous opportunities exist in daily activities to observe these behaviors. A common complaint about children who cannot sustain is that they cannot "stick to" an activity for an age-appropriate amount of time (e.g., has trouble completing tasks, switches from one activity to another). In the context of the evaluation, frequent requests by the child for breaks may be a sign of difficulties sustaining attention and effort.

The ability to inhibit is a critical trait for success in school and home. Measures to assess this subdomain examine the ability to not act on (inhibit or resist) an impulse and/ or to appropriately stop one's own activity at the proper time. Several continuous performance measures described previously provide distracting stimuli in an effort to measure the child's ability to ignore the conflicting or distracting information. Additionally, some tests examine the ability to wait or withhold a response until all information is processed. For example, a subtest on the Gordon Diagnostic System (Gordon, 1983; Gordon, McClure, & Aylward, 1996) requires the child to wait at least 7 seconds between responses in order to score points. If the child does not wait the allotted time, then he or she does not receive the point, and the interval is repeated. An impulsive child who is eager to gain points typically cannot inhibit responses and typically will not attain as many points as a child who is able to estimate the necessary delay period and learn the most effective way to gain points. On the Matching Familiar Figures Test (Welsh, Pennington, & Grossier, 1991), the examinee is asked to match a target figure with its exact mate from among a set of nearly identical figures. The child's performance is based not only on accuracy but also on the time taken in responding. The longer the time to respond, the better the ability to process all relevant information and to inhibit an incorrect response. Other measures examine the ability to suppress a natural, prepotent response (e.g., Stroop Test; Stroop, 1935). The ability to inhibit is also readily observed in daily activities, with common examples of disinhibition including acting without thinking, being easily distracted, and being unable to sit still. Parents and teachers typically possess a wealth of information about a child's ability to inhibit his or her responses, and rating scales are effective means of gathering information about this subdomain.

The ability to shift one's problem-solving strategy during complex tasks is a key aspect of executive function. Thinking flexibly and being able to switch or alternate attention is an essential component of novel problem solving. The most common performance measure used to assess this ability is the Wisconsin Card Sorting Test (Heaton et al., 1993), on which children match cards and receive feedback regarding their accuracy after every response. Once the correct matching strategy is determined and maintained for 10 consecutive responses, the matching principle changes unbeknownst to the child. The child must flexibly develop a new strategy to perform adequately. In their day-to-day lives, children who are rigid or inflexible may exhibit problems transitioning from one situation, activity, or aspect of a problem to another as the situation demands. Caregivers often describe these children as "getting stuck" on a topic or as being highly perseverative.

The ability to plan involves anticipating future events, setting goals, and developing appropriate steps ahead of time to carry out an associated task or action. Planning involves imagining or developing a goal or end state and then strategically determining the most effective method or steps to attain that goal. This often involves the sequencing and stringing together of steps in order to most efficiently move toward an end state. The ability to plan had previously been considered a skill of later development, but research has illustrated its active use even in preschool children. A variety of "tower" tasks have been developed that can measure this subdomain (e.g., Tower of Hanoi, Welsh et al., 1991; NEPSY Tower, Korkman et al., 1998). These tasks require the child to reach a goal (replicating a tower model) via a self-generated sequence of planned steps. The ability to plan or strategically solve problems can also be observed in a variety of other measures. For example, the WISC-III Object Assembly subtest provides the opportunity to directly observe a child's strategy when problem solving. Does the child stop to determine the gestalt or whole and then use that knowledge to guide performance? Does the child begin by randomly shuffling the puzzle pieces and then arranging them via trial and error? Does he or she use an efficient strategic approach (e.g., lining up the internal details on the pieces, placing recognizable pieces where they should eventually be placed and organizing around them), or does he or she use the external or less salient information (e.g., shape of the pieces)? The ability to plan can also be assessed from caregiver observations. For example, parents and teachers may complain about the child's lack of planning ability, tendency to start assignments at the last minute, or failure to think ahead about possible problems.

The ability to organize complex amounts of information is a subdomain that becomes increasingly important as demands for independent functioning increase. Organization involves establishing and maintaining order within an activity or carrying out a task in a systematic manner. The way in which information is strategically organized can play a critical role in how it is learned, remembered, and retrieved (Schneider & Pressley, 1989). Numerous information processing tasks are available that involve presenting the participant with a complex or seemingly overwhelming amount of information and then observing how the child responds to the problem. Although there are no direct tests of organization, tasks such as the Rey–Osterrieth Complex Figure can be scored for organization (Bernstein & Waber, 1996; Stern et al., 1994), and the CVLT-C provides an index of semantic versus serial clustering (Fridlund & Delis, 1994) . The child's approach provides critical information about how he or she is able to organize in the face of complexity. Common reports from caregivers that suggest disorganization in a child include a scattered approach to solving problems, being easily overwhelmed by large tasks or assignments, or having difficulties organizing personal belongings.

The ability to self-monitor is typically not assessed via a discrete performance measure but rather by direct examiner observation and caregiver reports. The ability to self-monitor includes checking on one's own actions during or shortly after finishing a task to assure appropriate attainment of a goal. Children who do not self-monitor often rush through assignments without checking their work for mistakes. Additionally, such children may be unaware of how their actions affect others in a social context.

Emotional control is the manifestation of the executive functions within the emotional realm. It is closely associated with the ability to inhibit and modulate responses. Emotional control is not a characteristic that can be directly assessed, but it is readily observed at home, school, and during assessment. The Behavior Rating Inventory of Executive Function (BRIEF; Gioia, Isquith, Guy, & Kenworthy, 2000) and other behavioral checklists are the most effective methods to measure this function. The inability to modulate one's own emotional response may manifest as the child's overblown emotional reactions to seemingly trivial events or as a general affective reactivity. Such children are often described as emotionally explosive.

Working memory is the process of holding information in mind for the purpose of completing a specific and related task. Working memory is essential in order to follow complex instructions, complete mental arithmetic, or perform tasks with more than one step. A variety of assessment tasks directly or indirectly tap this subdomain. Digit-repetition tasks, specifically in the reverse order, are a common method to assess working memory. In the reverse format, a child must hold the information in mind while actively performing an operation on that information (i.e., manipulating the digits in a different order). Tasks requiring the ability to mentally compute arithmetic problems, such as the CHIPASAT (Dyche & Johnson, 1991) or the Wechsler Scales Arithmetic subtest (Wechsler, 1991), also tap working memory. Several research tasks have been developed to assess working memory; however, they are not yet available in standardized, norm-referenced forms (e.g., Sentence Span, Counting Span; Siegel & Ryan, 1989). Problems of working memory may also be observed by parents and caregivers. A common observation made by parents is that their child often has trouble remembering things for even a few minutes or, when sent to get something, forgets what he or she was supposed to get.

Structured Behavior Rating Scales

A rich tradition exists of utilizing structured behavior rating systems in the assessment of psychological and neuropsychological functions (Achenbach, 1991; Conners, 1989; Reynolds & Kamphaus, 1994). The use of rating scales, completed by parents and teachers, that measure overt behavior is an often-used and well-proven method for the assessment of various domains of social, emotional, and behavioral functioning in children. The need exists for other methodologies in addition to performance tests to assess the executive functions. Observations of the child at home or in school by adult caregivers provide an essential source of information in the assessment of executive functions. Given the difficulties and complexities involved in performance assessment of executive function, an ecologically valid system of assessing the everyday self-regulatory behaviors of children serves as an important adjunct to the clinical evaluation and treatment of executive dysfunction. One such measure, the Behavior Rating Inventory of Executive Function (BRIEF), was designed to assess the behavioral manifestations of executive functions in children aged 5 to 18 years (Gioia, Isquith, Guy, & Kenworthy, 2000; Isquith, Gioia, & Guy, 1998).

The BRIEF assesses eight interrelated subdomains of executive function: Inhibit, Shift (Flexibility), Emotional Control, Initiate, Working Memory, Plan/Organize, Organization of Materials, and Monitor. More general domains of executive function (e.g., self-regulation, anticipation) for which specific behaviors could not be generated were not included. Other possible domains (e.g., goal setting, strategic problem solving) were incorporated within the eight existing domains (e.g., planning, shift). Items were generated primarily from behavioral descriptions of executive difficulties during clinical interviews with parents and teachers, ensuring good face and content validity. Item-category membership was validated by the sorting decisions of nine clinical neuropsychologists, as well as by statistical analyses (item-total correlation analyses, principal factor analyses, and interrater agreement). The correlations between parent and teacher informants are moderate, with an overall mean of .32 for the normative sample, which is similar to the literature on consistency among parent–teacher informants (Achenbach, McConaughy, & Howell, 1987). The subscales and their representative items are provided in Table 15.3.

The construct validity of the BRIEF was examined using common factor analysis while exploring undimensional versus multidimensional solutions. Parent ratings of 852 clini-

TABLE 15.3. BRIEF Subdomains and Sample Items

Subdomain	Sample items
Inhibit	Interrupts others. Acts too wild or "out of control." Has trouble putting the brakes on his/her actions.
Shift	Does same thing over and over for no apparent reason. Resists change of routine, foods, places. Gets stuck on one topic or activity.
Emotional control	Overreacts to small problems. Has explosive, angry outbursts. Angry or tearful outbursts are intense but end suddenly.
Initiate	Is not a self-starter. Has trouble getting started on homework or chores. Lies around the house a lot (couch potato).
Working memory	Has trouble with chores or tasks that have more than one step. When sent to get something, forgets what he/she is supposed to get. Has trouble remembering things, even for a few minutes.
Organization of materials	Leaves playroom a mess. Cannot find things in room or school desk. Leaves a trail of belongings wherever he/she goes.
Plan/organize	Does not bring home homework, assignment sheets, materials, etc. Becomes overwhelmed by large assignments. Does not plan ahead for school assignments.
Monitor	Does not check work for mistakes. Is unaware of how his/her behavior affects or bothers others. Leaves work incomplete.

cally referred and 1,419 normative students and teacher ratings of 475 clinically referred and 720 normative students were examined. The eight scales were submitted to a principal factor analysis with oblique rotation. Examination of one-, two-, three-, and four-factor solutions yielded a similar factor structure for the parent and teacher clinical and normative groups. The two-factor solution was the most theoretically and statistically sound (accounting for between 74–83% of the variance across the four analyses). Across parent and teacher groups, Factor 1, a metacognitive problem-solving factor, is defined by the subdomains Initiate, Working Memory, Plan/Organize, Organization of Materials, and Monitor. Factor 2, a behavior-regulation factor, is defined by Inhibit, Shift, and Emotional Control. Correlations between the two factors ranged from .56–.71. The overall stability of the two-factor solutions across clinical and normative samples for the parent and teacher scales provides strong support for the underlying factor structure of the BRIEF. The present findings also provide support for a limited multidimensional model of executive function.

To establish a measure of convergent and discriminant validity, the BRIEF was examined in relationship to a general measure of behavior in children (Child Behavior Checklist [CBCL]/Teacher Report Form [TRF]; Achenbach, 1991). Correlations ranged between .3 and .6, indicating an appropriate low to moderate relationship. Principal factor analysis with oblique rotation of the Parent and Teacher Forms of the BRIEF and Achenbach (1991) forms resulted in a four-factor structure with most of the BRIEF scales separating from the TRF and CBCL scales (Gioia, Isquith, & Guy, 1998). The BRIEF structure was again defined by a "metacognitive problem-solving" factor (BRIEF Initiate, Working Memory, Plan/Organize, Organization of Materials, Monitor scales [with Attention scale of TRF], a "behavior regulation" factor (BRIEF Inhibit, Shift, and Emotional Control), a CBCL/TRF externalizing factor, and a CBCL/TRF "internalizing" factor. The Inhibit Scale had a co-loading on the CBCL/TRF externalizing factor. In a second study, the BRIEF was successful in differentiating between a diagnostically mixed clinical group and a matched initial normative group (aged 5–13 years) on all executive function domains (Isquith, Pratt,

Guy, & Gioia, 1999). That is, there were significant differences with large effect sizes between clinical and normative groups on all domains of the BRIEF. Pratt, Campbell-LaVoie, Isquith, Gioia, and Guy (2000) recently demonstrated that children with inattentive versus combined subtypes of ADHD exhibit distinct clinical scale patterns on the BRIEF as opposed to children with reading disorders and controls. Children with reading disorders exhibited primarily working memory and task planning/organization difficulties.

Observational Procedures

In addition to formal tasks that assess the executive functions, the examiner can also apply a systematic set of observational procedures for any task or test that the child is administered (Ylvisaker & Gioia, 1998; see also Table 15.4). The goal of these procedures is to identify the child's control processes in performing a given task. These procedures can accompany virtually any task when there is interest in documenting the inherent executive functions and thus can be used in real-world or informal contexts, as well as in the testing setting.

Before the beginning of the task, the examiner assesses the child's self-awareness of his or her own ability as it relates to that task. This gives an indication of whether the child is accurately appreciating the type of task that lies ahead. The child is then asked what his or her goal is for the task and the strategies he or she plans to use to achieve the goal. Once the task is underway, observe the child's ability to initiate necessary problem-solving activities, especially when a problem arises. This gives a good understanding of his or her

TABLE 15.4. Observational Procedures for Assessing Executive Functions during Task Performance

Before beginning a task

1. *Self-awareness of ability*: Ask the child whether the task will be easy or difficult and to explain the choice of answer. If relevant, ask for a prediction of performance.
2. *Goal setting, strategic behavior*: Ask the child what his or her goal is and to explain plans for achieving that goal.

During the task

1. *Initiation*: If appropriate, create opportunities for initiation (e.g., provide insufficient materials, requiring the child to initiate a request).
2. *Inhibition*: If appropriate, create some distractions that would require active inhibition from the child.
3. *Sustain*: Observe the length of time that the child persists on the tasks, those that are well within their abilities and those that are more difficult.
4. *Self-monitoring*: Ask the child how he or she is doing.
5. *Strategic behavior/ problem solving*: If appropriate, create obstacles that would require active, flexible problem solving from the child.

After completion of the task

1. *Self-evaluation*: Ask the child how he or she did and how the results compare with the prediction.
2. *Strategic behavior and problem solving*: Ask what the child did to succeed; list relevant strategic procedures; ask the child whether he or she used them or whether they might be useful.

skill in initiating strategic behavior to solve the problem. In order to assess the child's ability to inhibit inappropriate stimulation during the task, observe his or her skill at not attending to nontask activity. It may also be necessary to create distraction (e.g., auditory, visual) and observe the child's response. Documenting the length of time the child remains on the task can give information regarding his or her capacity to sustain. During the task, note whether the child is aware of mistakes that are made. Also, questioning the child about his or her performance provides information regarding self-monitoring skill. As stated, when obstacles occur during the task, observe the child's ability to be flexible and try a different strategy. When the task is completed, asking the child to evaluate his or her performance as it relates to his or her goal and prediction assesses self-evaluation skills. Asking for a summary of what worked and didn't work can be useful to understand how well the child appreciates the full scope of his or her problem-solving efforts.

A creative play observation strategy has been employed in a number of research projects with preschool and school-age children to assess goal-oriented play schemas that have much relevance to "real world" executive functions (Ewing-Cobbs et al., 1999; Landry, Denson, & Swank, 1997; Landry, Smith, Miller-Loncar, & Swank, 1998). Ewing-Cobbs and colleagues (1999) demonstrated that the complexity and duration of age-appropriate play activities was significantly disrupted by traumatic brain injury in infants and preschoolers. Similarly, Landry and colleagues have demonstrated deficits in the child's ability to independently formulate play goals and to sustain goal-directed activity in both social and nonsocial situations for children who have Down syndrome, complications associated with prematurity, and hydrocephalus associated with spina bifida. Thus such ecologically valid executive behaviors as sustained attention, task initiation, task maintenance, and goal regulation can be assessed in children's everyday exploratory play behavior, even in infants and preschoolers. Assessment methods such as these, though early in their development, deserve much more attention as ecologically valid procedures to tap the child's profile of executive function.

IMPLICATIONS FOR PRACTICE

An understanding of the executive functions is necessary in conceptualizing the full complexity of developmental and acquired neurologic disorders in children. Mental ability is not simply the knowledge of "domain-specific" content that the child demonstrates on a test. It also involves the general supervisory performance across domains; that is, how the child executes such knowledge and skill in a sustained, appropriately inhibited, systematic, organized, and planful manner with flexibility and monitoring of the adequacy of the performance, all toward the attainment of the end goal. Certain testing conditions facilitate the assessment of the executive functions, whereas others limit the opportunity. The examiner must know the difference and, in fact, intentionally manipulate these conditions to tease apart the executive control behaviors from the "domain-specific" aspects of performance. The psychologist should consider the use of several different assessment methodologies toward this end. In addition to standardized tests, the observational procedures and behavior rating scales can be used in assessing the "real world" aspects of the executive functions. The more general psychological assessment can contribute to the identification of possible executive dysfunction in children with neurological impairment. Given the specialty training typically required to perform a comprehensive neuropsychological evaluation, referral for more in-depth testing of the executive functions (and their concurrent "domain specific" partners) would be warranted should further definition be necessary.

An appropriate assessment of the profile of executive functions in a given child has significant implications for treatment. With knowledge of the child's strengths and weaknesses in the executive subdomains, including an understanding of the contributory role of environmental factors, the clinician is in a very favorable position to develop and implement treatment plans that target essential elements. For example, a child with significant organizational deficits, such as Phillip in the chapter-opening vignette, would benefit from a targeted approach that facilitates his learning through the use of metacognitive strategies and problem-solving routines (Ylvisaker, 1998). This would include teaching specific organizational techniques directly to Phillip, modeling the use of these strategies by important people in his world (e.g., parents, teacher, peers), and providing the necessary environmental opportunities for the development of these executive routines in frequent and varied real-world, everyday situations and contexts. Assessment of executive functions thus extends the psychologist's understanding and provision of interventions for children with neurocognitive and learning difficulties.

REFERENCES

Achenbach, T. (1991). *Manual for the Child Behavior Checklist/4–18 and 1991 profile*. Burlington: University of Vermont, Department of Psychiatry.

Achenbach, T., McConaughy, S., & Howell, C. (1987). Child/adolescent behavioral and emotional problems: Implications of cross-informant correlations for situational specificity. *Psychological Bulletin, 101*, 213–232.

Ackerly, S. S. (1964). A case of perinatal bilateral frontal lobe defect observed for thirty years. In J. M. Warren & K. Akert (Eds.), *The frontal granular cortex and behavior* (pp. 192–218). New York: McGraw-Hill.

Aldenkamp, A. P. (1987). Learning disabilities in epilepsy. In A. P. Aldenkamp, W. C. J. Alpherts, H. Meinardi, & G. Stores (Eds.), *Education and epilepsy: Proceedings of an international workshop on education and epilepsy* (pp. 21–38). Amsterdam: Swets and Zeitlinger.

Anderson, V. (1998). Assessing executive functions in children: Biological, psychological and developmental considerations. *Neuropsychological Rehabilitation, 8*, 319–349.

Asarnow, R. F., Satz, P., Light, R. V., Lewis, R., & Neumann, E. (1991). Behavior problems and adaptive functioning in children with mild and severe closed head injury. *Journal of Pediatric Psychology, 16*, 543–555.

Barkley, R. A. (1997). *ADHD and the nature of self-control*. New York: Guilford Press.

Barkley, R. A. (1990). *Attention-deficit hyperactivity disorder: A handbook for diagnosis and treatment*. New York: Guilford Press.

Baron, I. S., Fennell, E. B., & Voeller, K. K. S. (1995). *Pediatric neuropsychology in the medical setting*. New York: Oxford University Press.

Beery, K. E. (1967). *Developmental Test of Visual–Motor Integration: Administration and scoring manual*. Chicago: Follett.

Beery, K. E. (1982). *Revised administration, scoring and teaching manual for the Developmental Test of Visual–Motor Integration*. Cleveland, OH: Modern Curriculum Press.

Beery, K. E. (1997). The *Visual–Motor Integration Test—Fourth Edition: Administration, scoring and teaching manual*. Austin, TX: Pro-Ed.

Bellinger, D., Hu, H., Titlebaum, L., & Needleman, H. L. (1994). Attentional correlates of dentin and bone lead levels in adolescents. *Archives of Environmental Health, 49*, 98–105.

Benton, A. (1991). Prefrontal injury and behavior in children. *Developmental Neuropsychology, 7*, 275–282.

Benton, A., & Hamsher, K. (1989). *Multilingual aphasia examination*. Iowa City: AJA Associates.

Berg, B. O. (Ed.). (1996). *Principles of child neurology*. New York: McGraw-Hill.

Berg, E. A. (1948). A simple objective technique for measuring flexibility in thinking. *Journal of General Psychology, 39*, 15–22.

Bernstein, J. H., & Waber, D. P. (1990). Developmental neuropsychological assessment: The systemic approach. In A. A. Boulton, G. B. Baker, & M. Hiscock (Eds.), *Neuromethods: Vol. 17. Neuropsychology* (pp. 311–371). Clifton, NJ: Humana.

Bernstein, J. H., & Waber, D. P. (1996). *Developmental scoring system for the Rey–Osterrieth Complex Figure.* Odessa, FL: Psychological Assessment Resources.

Bianchi, L. (1922). *The mechanism of brain and the function of the frontal lobes.* Edinburgh, Scotland: Livingstone.

Bremner, J. D., & Narayan, M. (1998). The effects of stress on memory and the hippocampus throughout the life cycle: Implications for childhood development and aging. *Developmental Psychopathology, 10,* 871–875.

Brouwers, P., Riccardi, R., Poplack, D., & Fedio, P. (1984). Attentional deficits in long-term survivors of childhood acute lymphoblastic leukemia (ALL). *Journal of Clinical Neuropsychology, 6,* 325–336.

Brown, A. L. (1975). The development of memory: Knowing, knowing about knowing and knowing how to know. In H.W. Reese (Ed.), *Advances in child development and behavior* (Vol. 10, pp. 103–152). New York: Academic Press.

Byrne, K., Abbenduto, I., & Brooks, R. (1990). The language of children with spina bifida and hydrocephalus: Meeting task demands and mastering syntax. *Journal of Speech and Hearing Disorders, 55,* 118–123.

Chelune, G. J., & Baer, R. L. (1986). Developmental norms for the Wisconsin Card Sorting Test. *Journal of Clinical and Experimental Neuropsychology, 8,* 210–228.

Conners, C. K. (1989). *Manual for Conners' Rating Scales.* North Towanda, NY: Multi-Health Systems.

Delis, D. C., Kaplan, E. F., & Kramer, J. H. (2001). *Delis-Kaplan Executive Functional Scales (D-KEFS).* San Antonio, TX: Psychological Corporation.

Denckla, M. B. (1985). Revised neurological examination for subtle signs. *Psychopharmacology Bulletin, 21,* 773–790.

Denckla, M. B. (1989). Executive function: The overlap zone between attention deficit hyperactivity disorder and learning disabilities. *International Pediatrics, 4,* 155–160.

Denckla, M. B. (1994). Measurement of executive function. In G. R. Lyon (Ed.), *Frames of reference for the assessment of learning disabilities: New views on measurement issues* (pp. 117–142). Baltimore: Brookes.

Denckla, M. B. (1996). A theory and model of executive function: A neuropsychological perspective. In F. R. Lyon & N. A. Krasnegor (Eds.), *Attention, memory, and executive function* (pp. 263–278). Baltimore: Brookes.

Denckla, M. B., Harris, E. L., Aylward, E. H., Singer, H. S., Reiss, A. L., Reader, M. J., Bryan, R. N., & Chase, G. A. (1991). Executive functions and volume of the basal ganglia in children with Tourette's syndrome and attention deficit hyperactivity disorder. *Annals of Neurology, 30,* 476.

Denckla, M. B., & Reiss, A. L. (1997). Prefrontal-subcortical circuits in developmental disorders. In N. A. Krasnegor, G. R. Lyon, & P. S. Goldman-Rakic (Eds.), *Development of the prefrontal cortex: Evolution, neurobiology and behavior* (pp. 283–293). Baltimore: Brookes.

Diamond, A., & Goldman-Rakic, P. S. (1985). Evidence for involvement of prefrontal cortex in cognitive changes during the first year of life: Comparison of human infants and rhesus monkeys on a detour task with transparent barrier. *Neurosciences Abstracts, 11,* 832.

Diamond, A., & Goldman-Rakic, P. S. (1989). Comparison of human infants and rhesus monkeys on Piaget's AB task: Evidence for dependence on dorsolateral prefrontal cortex. *Experimental Brain Research, 74,* 24–40.

Dyche, G. E., & Johnson, D. A. (1991). Development and evaluation of the CHIPASAT, an attention test for children: II. Test–retest reliability and practice effects for a normal sample. *Perceptual and Motor Skills, 72,* 563–572.

Einsiedel, E., Weigl, I., & Gutjahr, P. (1979). The psychosocial status of children surviving a long time with acute lymphoblastic leukemia. *Therapiewoche, 29,* 8669–8673.

Elliot, C. (1990). *Differential ability scale: Administration and scoring manual.* San Antonio, TX: Psychological Corporation.

Eslinger, P. J., Biddle, K. R., & Grattan, L. M. (1997). Cognitive and social development in children with prefrontal cortex lesions. In N. A. Krasnegor, G. R. Lyon, & P. S. Goldman-Rakic (Eds.), *Development of the prefrontal cortex: Evolution, neurobiology and behavior* (pp. 295–335). Baltimore: Brookes.

Eslinger, P. J., & Damasio, A. R. (1985). Severe disturbance of higher cognition after bilateral frontal lobe ablation. *Neurology, 35,* 1731–1741.

Eslinger, P. J., & Grattan L. M. (1991). Perspectives on the developmental consequences of early frontal lobe damage: Introduction. *Developmental Neuropsychology, 7,* 257–260.

Ewing-Cobbs, L., Landry, S. H., Prasad, M., Steubing, K., Leal, F., & Canales, D. (1999). Exploratory play: Assessment of executive functions in young children with brain injury and physical abuse. *Journal of the International Neuropsychological Society, 5,* 127.

Fennell, E. B., Eisenstadt, T., Bodiford, C., Redeiss, S., & Mickle, J. (1987). The assessment of neuropsychological dysfunction in children shunted for hydrocephalus. *Journal of Clinical and Experimental Neuropsychology, 9,* 25–26.

Fletcher, J. M., Ewing-Cobbs, L., Miner, M. E., Levin, H. S., & Eisenberg, H. (1990). Behavioral changes after closed head injury in children. *Journal of Consulting and Clinical Psychology, 58,* 93–98.

Fridlund, A., & Delis, D. (1994). *California Verbal Learning Test–Children's version.* San Antonio, TX: Psychological Corporation.

Fuster, J. M. (1985). The prefrontal cortex, mediator of cross-temporal contingencies. *Human Neurobiology, 4,* 169–179.

Fuster, J. M. (1989). *The prefrontal cortex: Anatomy, physiology, and neurophysiology of the frontal lobe.* New York: Raven Press.

Gaddes, W. H., & Crockett, D. J. (1975). The Spreen-Benton Aphasia Tests: Normative data as a measure of normal language development. *Brain and Language, 2,* 257–280.

Gioia, G. A. (1992). Executive/organizational learning disorder: Description of a unique neuropsychological subtype. *Journal of Clinical and Experimental Neuropsychology, 14,* 119.

Gioia, G. A. (1993). The tower of Hanoi task and developmental executive dysfunction. *Journal of Clinical and Experimental Neuropsychology, 15,* 88.

Gioia, G. A., Guy, S.C., & Isquith, P. K. (1997). Neuropsychological outcome of childhood lead poisoning: Effects of chronicity on executive regulatory function. *Journal of the International Neuropsychological Society, 3,* 56.

Gioia, G. A., Isquith, P. K., & Guy, S. C. (1998). The regulatory role of executive control processes in children's behavioral, social, and emotional functioning. *Journal of Neuropsychiatry and Clinical Neurosciences, 9,* 663.

Gioia, G. A., Isquith, P. K., Guy, S. C., & Kenworthy, L. (2000). *Behavior Rating Inventory of Executive Function.* Odessa, FL: Psychological Assessment Resources.

Golden, C. (1978). *Stroop Test.* Wood Dale, IL: Stoelting.

Golden, C. J. (1981). The Luria–Nebraska Children's Battery: Theory and formulation. In G. W. Hynd & J. E. Obrzut (Eds.), *Neuropsychological assessment and the school-age child* (pp. 277–302). New York: Grune & Stratton.

Goldstein, G. W. (1992). Developmental neurobiology of lead toxicity. In H. L. Needleman (Ed.), *Human lead exposure* (pp. 125–135). Ann Arbor, MI: CRC Press.

Golier, J., & Yehuda, R. (1998). Neuroendocrine activity and memory-related impairments in posttraumatic stress disorder. *Developmental Psychopathology, 10,* 857–869.

Gordon, M. (1983). *The Gordon Diagnostic System.* DeWitt, NY: Gordon Systems.

Gordon, M., McClure, F. D., & Aylward, G. P (1996). *Gordon Diagnostic System Interpretive Guide—Third Edition.* Dewitt, NY: GSI.

Grattan, L. M., & Eslinger, P. J. (1991). Frontal lobe damage in children and adults: A comparative review. *Developmental Neuropsychology, 7,* 283–326.

Greenberg, L. M., & Kindschi, C. L. (1996). *TOVA clinical guide.* Los Alamitos, CA: Universal Attention Disorders.

Gurwitch, R. H., Sullivan, M. A., & Long, P. J. (1998). The impact of trauma and disaster on young children. *Child and Adolescent Psychiatric Clinics of North America, 7,* 19–32.

Harris, E. L., Schuerholz, L. J., Singer, H. S., Reader, M. J., Brown, J. E., Cox, C., Mohr, J., Chase, G. A., & Denckla, M. B. (1995). Executive function in children with Tourette syndrome and/or attention deficit hyperactivity disorder. *Journal of the International Neuropsychological Society, 1,* 511–516.

Heaton, R. K., Chelune, G. J., Talley, J. L., Kay, G. G., & Curtiss, G. (1993). *Wisconsin Card Sorting Test Manual: Revised and expanded.* Odessa, FL: Psychological Assessment Resources.

Holmes, J. M. (1987). Natural histories in learning disabilities: Neuropsychological difference/

environmental demand. In S. J. Ceci (Ed.), *Handbook of cognitive, social and neuropsychological aspects of learning disabilities* (Vol. 2, pp. 303–319). Hillsdale, NJ: Erlbaum.

Isquith, P. K., & Gioia, G. A. (1999). The nature of executive function in ADHD. *Clinical Neuropsychologist, 13,* 222.

Isquith, P. K., Gioia, G. A., & Guy, S. C. (1998) Assessment of executive functions in children: Development of the Behavior Rating Inventory of Executive Functions (BRIEF). *Journal of the International Neuropsychological Society, 4,* 29.

Isquith, P. K., Pratt, B., Guy, S. C., & Gioia, G. A. (1999). Initial clinical validity of the Behavior Rating Inventory of Executive Function. *Journal of the International Neuropsychological Society, 5,* 117.

Johnson, D. A., Roethig-Johnston, K., & Middleton, J. (1988). Development of an attentional test for head injured children: I. Information processing capacity in a normal sample. *Journal of Child Psychology and Psychiatry, 29,* 199–208.

Johnson, T. N., Rosvold, H. E., & Mishkin, M. (1968). Projections from behaviorally defined sectors of the prefrontal cortex to the basal ganglia, septum, and diencephalon of the monkey. *Experimental Neurology, 21,* 20.

Jones-Gotman, M., & Milner, B. (1977). Design fluency: The invention of nonsense drawings after focal cortical lesions. *Neuropsychologia, 24,* 659–670.

Joseph, R. (1998). Traumatic amnesia, repression, and hippocampus injury due to emotional stress, corticosteroids and enkephalins. *Child Psychiatry and Human Development, 29,* 169–185.

Kaplan, E. (1988). A process approach to neuropsychological assessment. In T. Boll & B. K. Bryant (Eds.), *Clinical neuropsychology and brain function: Research, measurement and practice* (pp. 125–167). Washington, DC: American Psychological Association.

Kaplan, E., Goodglass, H., & Weintraub, S. (1983). *Boston Naming Test* (2nd ed.). Philadelphia: Lea & Febiger.

Klahr, D., & Robinson, M. (1981). Formal assessment of problem-solving and planning processes in preschool children. *Cognitive Psychology, 13,* 113–148.

Klin, A., Volkmar, F. R., Sparrow, S. S., Cicchetti, D. V., & Rourke, B. P. (1995). Validity and neuropsychological characterization of Asperger syndrome: Convergence with Nonverbal Learning Disabilities syndrome. *Journal of Child Psychology and Psychiatry, 36,* 1127–1140.

Knights, R. M., & Norwood, J. A. (1980). *Revised smoothed normative data on the neuropsychological test battery for children* [Mimeograph]. Ottawa, Ontario, Canada: Carleton University, Department of Psychology.

Krikorian, R., Bartok, J., & Gay, N. (1994). Tower of London procedure: Standard method and developmental data. *Journal of Clinical and Experimental Neuropsychology, 16,* 840–850.

Korkman, M., Kirk, U., & Kemp, S. (1998). *NEPSY: A developmental neuropsychological assessment.* San Antonio, TX: Psychological Corporation.

Landry, S. H., Denson, S. E., & Swank, P. R. (1997). Effects of medical risk and socioeconomic status on the rate of change in cognitive and social development for low birth weight children. *Journal of Clinical and Experimental Neuropsychology, 19,* 261–174.

Landry, S. H., Smith, K. E., Miller-Loncar, C. L., & Swank, P. R. (1998). The relation of change in maternal interactive styles to the developing social competence of full-term and preterm children. *Child Development, 69,* 105–123.

Levin, H. S., Culhane, K. A., Hartmann, J., Evankovich, K., Mattson, A. J., Harward, H., Ringholz, G., Ewing-Cobbs, L., & Fletcher, J. M. (1991). Developmental changes in performance on tests of purported frontal lobe functioning. *Developmental Neuropsychology, 7,* 377–395.

Levin, H. S., Mendelsohn, D., Lily, M. A., Fletcher, J. M., Culhane, K. A., Chapman, S. B., Howard, H., Kusneirk, L., Bruce, D., & Eisenberg, H. M. (1994). Tower of London performance in relation to magnetic resonance imaging following closed head injury in children. *Neuropsychology, 8,* 171–179.

Lezak, M. (1995). *Neuropsychological Assessment* (3rd ed.). New York: Oxford University Press.

Luria, A. R. (1966). *Higher cortical functions in man.* New York: Basic Books.

Marlowe, W. (1992). The impact of right prefrontal lesion on the developing brain. *Brain and Cognition, 20,* 205–213.

Mateer, C. A., & Williams, D. (1991). Effects of frontal lobe injury in childhood. *Developmental Neuropsychology, 7,* 359–376.

Meier, M. J., Benton, A. L., & Diller, L. (Eds.). (1987). *Neuropsychological rehabilitation.* New York: Guilford Press.

Mesulam, M.–M. (1981). A cortical network for directed attention and unilateral neglect. *Annals of Neurology, 10,* 309–325.

Mirsky, A. F. (1989). The neuropsychology of attention: Elements of a complex behavior. In E. Perecman (Ed.), *Integrating theory and practice in clinical neuropsychology* (pp. 75–91). Hillsdale, NJ: Erlbaum.

Neisser, U. (1967). *Cognitive psychology.* New York: Appleton-Century-Crofts.

Passler, M. A., Isaac, W., & Hynd, G. W. (1985). Neuropsychological development of behavior attributed to frontal lobe functioning in children. *Developmental Neuropsychology, 1,* 349–370.

Pennington, B. F. (1991). *Diagnosing learning disorders: A neuropsychological framework.* New York: Guilford Press.

Pennington, B. F. (1997). Dimensions of executive functions in normal and abnormal development. In N. A. Krasnegor, G. R. Lyon, & P. S. Goldman-Rakic (Eds.), *Development of the prefrontal cortex: Evolution, neurobiology and behavior* (pp. 265–281). Baltimore: Brookes.

Pennington, B. F., Bennetto, L., McAleer, O. K., & Roberts, R. J. (1996). Executive functions and working memory: Theoretical and measurement issues. In G. R. Lyon & N. A. Krasnegor (Eds.), *Attention, memory and executive function* (pp. 327–348). Baltimore: Brookes.

Porrino, L., & Goldman-Rakic, P. S. (1982). Brainstem innervation of prefrontal and anterior cingulate cortex in the rhesus monkey revealed by retrograde transport of HRP. *Journal of Comparative Neurology, 205,* 63–76.

Pratt, B., Campbell-LaVoie, F., Isquith, P. K., Gioia, G. A., & Guy, S. C. (2000). The comparative development of executive function in elementary school children with reading disorder and attention-deficit/hyperactivity disorder. *Journal of the International Neuropsychological Society, 6,* 127.

Pressley, M., & Levin, J. R. (1987). Elaborative learning strategies for the inefficient learner. In S. J. Ceci (Ed.), *Handbook of cognitive, social, and neuropsychological aspects of learning disabilities* (Vol. 2, pp. 175–212). Hillsdale, NJ: Erlbaum.

Reitan, R. M. (1958). Validity of the Trail Making Test as an indicator of organic brain damage. *Perceptual and Motor Skills, 8,* 271–276.

Reitan, R. M., & Wolfson, D. (1985). *The Halstead-Reitan Neuropsychological Test Battery: Theory and clinical interpretation.* Tucson, AZ: Neuropsychology Press.

Reitan, R. M., & Wolfson, D. (1993). *The Halstead–Reitan Neuropsychological Test Battery: Theory and clinical interpretation.* Tuscon, AZ: Neuropsychology Press.

Rey, A. (1964). *L'examen clinique en psychologie.* Paris: Press Universitaires de France.

Reynolds, C. R., & Kamphaus, R. W. (1994). *Behavior Assessment System for Children.* Circle Pines, MN: American Guidance Service.

Rieber, R. W., & Carton, A. S. (Eds.). (1987). *The collected works of L. S. Vygotsky* (Vol. 1). New York: Plenum Press.

Rogeness, G. A., Javors, M. A., & Pliska, S. R. (1992). Neurochemistry and child and adolescent psychiatry. *Journal of the American Academy of Child and Adolescent Psychiatry, 31,* 765–781.

Ross, J. W. (1982). The role of the social worker with long-term survivors of childhood cancer and their families. *Social Work Health Care, 7,* 1–13.

Rothenberger, A. (1992). The role of the frontal lobes in child psychiatric disorders. In A. Rothenberger (Ed.), *Brain and behavior in child psychiatry* (pp. 34–58). New York: Springer-Verlag.

Rourke, B. P., Fisk, J. L., & Strang, J. D. (1986). *Neuropsychological assessment of children: A treatment-oriented approach.* New York: Guilford Press.

Rudel, R. G., Holmes, J. M., & Pardes, J. R. (1988). *Assessment of developmental learning disorders.* New York: Basic Books.

Ruff, R. (1988). *Ruff Figural Fluency Test.* San Diego, CA: Neuropsychological Resources.

Scheibel, R. S., & Levin, H. S. (1997). Frontal lobe dysfunction following closed head injury in children: Findings from neuropsychology and brain injury. In N. A. Krasnegor, G. R. Lyon, & P. S. Goldman-Rakic (Eds.), *Development of the prefrontal cortex: Evolution, neurobiology and behavior* (pp. 241–263). Baltimore: Brookes.

Schneider, W., & Pressley, M. (1989). *Memory development between 2 and 20.* New York: Springer-Verlag.

Schuerholz, L., Baumgardner, T., Singer, H. S., Reiss, A., & Denckla, M. B. (1996). Neuropsychological status of children with Tourette's syndrome with and without attention deficit hyperactivity disorder. *Neurology, 46*(4), 958–965.

Sheslow, D., & Adams, W. (1990). *Wide Range Assessment of Memory and Learning: Administration manual.* Wilmington, DL: Wide Range.

Siegel, L. S., & Ryan, E. B. (1989). The development of working memory in normally achieving and subtypes of learning disabled children. *Child Development, 60,* 973–980.

Singer, H. S., & Walkup, J. T. (1991). Tourette syndrome and other tic disorders. *Medicine, 70*(1), 15–32.

Spreen, O., Risser, A. H., & Edgell, D. (1995). *Developmental neuropsychology.* New York: Oxford University Press.

Stehbens, J. A., Kaleita, T. A., Knoll, R. B., McLean, W., O'Brien, R., & Hammond, D. (1991). CNS prophylaxis of childhood leukemia: What are the long-term neurological, neuropsychological, and behavioral effects? *Neuropsychology Review, 2,* 147–177.

Stein, M. B., Koverola, C., Hanna, C., Torchia, M. G., & McClarty, B. (1997). Hippocampal volume in women victimized by childhood sexual abuse. *Psychological Medicine, 27,* 951–959.

Stern, R., Singer, E., Duke, L., Singer, N., Morey, C., Daughtrey, E., & Kaplan, E. (1994). The Boston qualitative scoring system for the Rey–Osterrieth Complex Figure: Description of interrater reliability. *Clinical Neuropsychologist, 8*(3), 309–322.

Stroop, J. R. (1935). Studies of interference in serial verbal reactions. *Journal of Experimental Psychology, 18,* 643–662.

Stuss, D. T., & Benson, D.F. (1986). *The frontal lobes.* New York: Raven.

Stuss, D. T., & Buckle, L. (1992). Traumatic brain injury: Neuropsychological deficits and evaluation at different stages of recovery and in different pathological subtypes. *Journal of Head Trauma Rehabilitation, 7,* 40–49.

Swanson, H. L., Cochran, K. F., & Ewers, C. A. (1990). Can learning disabilities be determined from working memory performance? *Journal of Learning Disabilities, 23,* 59–67.

Taylor, H. G. (1989). Learning disabilities. In E. J. Mash and R. A. Barkley (Eds.), *Treatment of childhood disorders* (pp. 347–380). New York: Guilford Press.

Teuber, H.-L. (1964). The riddle of frontal lobe function in man. In J. M. Warren & K. Akert (Eds.), *The frontal granular cortex and behavior* (pp. 410–444). New York: McGraw-Hill.

Tew, B. (1979). The "cocktail party syndrome" in children with hydrocephalus and spina bifida. *British Journal of Disorders of Communication, 14,* 89–101.

Thompson, P. J. (1987). Educational attainment in children and young people with epilepsy. In J. Oxley & G. Stores (Eds.), *Epilepsy and education* (pp. 15–24). London: Medical Tribune Group.

Thorndike, R. L., Hagen, E. P., & Sattler, J. M. (1986). *Stanford–Binet Intelligence Scale—Fourth Edition.* Chicago, IL: Riverside.

Tinsley, V. S., & Waters, H. S. (1982). The development of verbal control over motor behavior: A replication and extension of Luria's findings. *Child Development, 53,* 746–753.

Vaughn, B. E., Kopp, C. B., & Krakow, J. B. (1984). The emergence and consolidation of self-control from eighteen to thirty months of age: Normative trends and individual differences. *Child Development, 55,* 990–1004.

Waber, D. P., Isquith, P. K., Kahn, C., Romero, I., Sallan, S., & Tarbell, N. (1994). Metacognitive factors in the visuo-spatial skills of long-term survivors of acute lymphoblastic leukemia: An experimental approach to the Rey–Osterrieth Complex Figure. *Developmental Neuropsychology, 10,* 349–368.

Waber, D. P., Tarbell, N. J., Fairclough, D., Atmore, K., Castro, R., Isquith, P., Lussier, F., Romero, I., Carpenter, P. J., Schiller, M., & Sallan, S. E. (1995). Cognitive sequelae of treatment in childhood acute lymphoblastic leukemia: Cranial radiation requires an accomplice! *Journal of Clinical Oncology, 12,* 2490–2496.

Wechsler, D. (1991). *Wechsler Intelligence Scale for Children—Third Edition.* San Antonio, TX: Psychological Corporation.

Welsh, M. C., & Pennington, B. F. (1988). Assessing frontal lobe functioning in children: Views from developmental psychology. *Developmental Neuropsychology, 4,* 199–230.

Welsh, M. C., Pennington, B. F., & Grossier, D. B. (1991). A normative-developmental study of executive function: A window on prefrontal function in children. *Developmental Neuropsychology, 7,* 131–149.

Wills, K. E. (1993). Neuropsychological functioning in children with spina bifida and/or hydrocephalus. *Journal of Child Clinical Psychology, 22,* 247–265.

Wong, B. (1991). The relevance of metacognition to learning disabilities. In B. Wong (Ed.), *Learning about learning disabilities* (pp. 231–258). New York: Academic Press.

Ylvisaker, M. (1993). Communication outcome in children and adolescents with traumatic brain injury. *Neuropsychological Rehabilitation, 3,* 367.

Ylvisaker, M. (Ed.). (1998). *Traumatic brain injury rehabilitation: Children and adolescents* (2nd ed.) Boston: Butterworth-Heinemann.

Ylvisaker, M., & Gioia, G. A. (1998). Cognitive assessment. In M. Ylvisaker (Ed.), *Traumatic brain injury rehabilitation: Children and adolescents* (2nd ed., pp. 159–179) Boston: Butterworth-Heinemann.

Ylvisaker, M., Szekeres, S., & Hartwick, P. (1992). Cognitive rehabilitation following traumatic brain injury in children. In M. G. Tramontana & S. R. Hooper (Eds.), *Advances in child neuropsychology* (pp. 168–218). New York: Springer-Verlag.

PART IV

Ethical and Legal Issues

16

ETHICAL AND LEGAL ISSUES IN ASSESSMENT OF CHILDREN WITH SPECIAL NEEDS

WILLIAM A. RAE
CONSTANCE J. FOURNIER
MICHAEL C. ROBERTS

Edward is a 6-year-old who has a mild hearing loss and seizures that are partially controlled by medication. School personnel have assessed him. Both his cognitive ability and adaptive functioning are reported in the mentally retarded range. He has been eligible for special education under health impaired, and has been in a cross-categorical multiage classroom that goes up through age 7. He has an Individualized Educational Plan meeting scheduled in 2 weeks. His parents want to submit a second opinion about his adaptive and cognitive functioning from their family psychologist. Furthermore, they would like their son to be fully included in the regular education setting.

Assessment of children with physical, mental, and emotional disabilities requires extraordinary attention to ethical issues, not only because of the special vulnerabilities of these children but also because of the complicated and chronic nature of their conditions. Assessment of children and adolescents with special needs involves more than psychological testing. These assessments necessitate a qualitative and developmental approach in which the psychologist adapts the test administration and interpretation in order to meet the unique needs of the child. In addition, assessment of children with special needs often takes place within an institutional setting in which the psychologist has conflicting roles. These roles include being an advocate for the child, an employee of an institution, and a supportive helping professional for the child and family. It should be noted that existing ethical guidelines are written primarily for adult clientele; the application to children is not always straightforward. Regardless of these complexities, the psychologist assessing children with special needs must always consider the rights, welfare, and best interests of the child and family.

    This chapter is based upon the most recent edition of the *Ethical Principles of Psychologists and Code of Conduct* by the American Psychological Association (APA; 1992).

Additional guidance was obtained from the *Standards for Educational and Psychological Testing* (APA, American Educational Research Association [AERA], & National Council on Measurement in Education [NCME], 1998) regarding the administration or interpretation of psychological tests. Regardless of the good advice provided in these references, federal and state laws prescribe many of the practice guidelines. At the same time, historically there have been no explicit guidelines established by professional organizations to deal with the competencies specific to low-incidence assessment (Strichart & Lazarus, 1986). The psychologist must make a thoughtful decision about how to apply the highest of ethical standards within the context of real-world constraints. Even with the best of intentions of the psychologist, ethical dilemmas will occur, requiring a thoughtful decision process.

The purpose of this chapter is to discuss some of the relevant ethical and legal issues pertaining to psychological and developmental assessment of children with special needs. We discuss the ethical considerations that arise before, during, and after the assessment and legal issues that pertain to assessment of children with special needs. Emerging issues in assessment and its impact on practice are also described. Finally, we provide practical suggestions on how a busy psychologist can make good ethical decisions.

ETHICAL ISSUES

Before the Assessment

Before initiating contact with a child or adolescent for assessment, the psychologist should attempt to fully inform the child and family as to the nature and purpose of the assessment. Any risks or benefits of the evaluation procedure should be explained. Most young children lack the cognitive ability and experience to understand the potential risks and benefits of an assessment process. Providing informed consent for any child and family can be problematic, but greater challenges exist with a child with a disability that require special considerations by the psychologist. For example, the child with mental retardation or a learning disability may have significant difficulties understanding the conceptual underpinnings of the risks and benefits. In the same way, the child with emotional disturbance may not be able to fully understand because of interfering distress. The psychologist must have an awareness of the child's level of understanding and be prepared to modify the explanation of the assessment techniques accordingly.

Generally, for appropriate informed consent, four essential conditions must be met. First, the participants must be competent to make a decision about the assessment. Second, participation in the assessment must be voluntary. Third, participants must be knowledgeable about the nature and purpose of the assessment. Finally, the consent must be appropriately documented. Children and others who are legally incapable of giving informed consent must have a legally authorized person provide the consent. Although in most instances children are incapable of giving legal consent, the psychologist should attempt to inform the child about the proposed assessment in a manner commensurate with his or her psychological capacity. Seeking such assent does not mean that the child must agree, but if the child does not assent, the psychologist must consider what might be in the child's best interests and then decide how to proceed accordingly. Regardless, the decision to perform the assessment is only made after appropriate consent has been obtained from the child's parent or guardian (Canter, Bennett, Jones, & Nagy, 1994).

Although there is no legal requirement that the child must assent to the assessment, a child who agrees to voluntarily participate may be more cooperative, which could lead to more valid results. In fact, it is not uncommon for an older adolescent and/or a child with a behavior disorder to refuse to be evaluated. Under these circumstances the psychologist should attempt to develop a cooperative relationship with the child or adolescent in which coercion is kept to a minimum. There are times when state-mandated procedures do not require consent—usually by court order or during an emergency. There are other times when parents choose not to give consent. In these cases the public agency, such as the school, may use the hearing procedures as described in the federal regulations pertaining to parents' rights. When there is a difference between government mandates and parental wishes, mediation may be needed. The psychologist must be careful not to consciously or unconsciously exploit the power differential in his or her relationship with the child and family to unfairly compel participation in the assessment. For example, a psychologist speaking for an authoritative institution (i.e., the school) might intimidate the child and family into agreeing to the assessment. In this instance, voluntary informed consent was not truly obtained.

The psychologist is faced with a perplexing dilemma in attempting to obtain informed consent or assent while not knowing the child's capacity to understand the risks and benefits. In fact, often the purpose of the assessment of children with special needs is to determine their cognitive, social, and emotional capabilities. Unfortunately, the assessment of competence is poorly articulated legally (Melton & Ehrenreich, 1992). In practice, competence often is not determined. For example, in a survey of pediatric psychologists it was reported that the child's competence to understand confidentiality issues was often not assessed (Rae & Worchel, 1991). At the same time, it is important that the psychologist have some notion of the child's cognitive abilities prior to obtaining assent to the evaluation. The psychologist must help the child to understand the assessment process by providing terminology and examples compatible with the child's developmental abilities and life experience. The Piagetian stages of cognitive development may provide a helpful construct for understanding the child's capacity to understand the nature and purpose of the assessment (Koocher & Keith-Spiegel, 1990). For children with normal intelligence, consent appears to be fully informed by about age 15 (Gustafson & McNamara, 1987).

The psychologist should explain the nature and purpose of the assessment in a manner that is understandable, clear, and unambiguous. Answering questions and being responsive to the concerns of the child or family is helpful for avoiding misunderstandings later in the assessment process. Although documentation of the informed consent is necessary, it is not sufficient to provide only a written form as a substitute to having a formal discussion of the nature and purpose of the assessment with all involved (Peterson, 1996). Unfortunately, an inherent ethical dilemma occurs when using projective tests with children. Because projective tests often present ambiguous stimuli with accompanying diminished face validity, the child is kept unaware as to the purpose and objective of the test, which appears to be a direct violation of providing informed consent (Schweighofer & Coles, 1994). Explaining the assessment process to the child and family sometimes requires creatively giving examples of the types of activities that take place during the assessment so that they can fully understand the assessment process. Many psychologists find it helpful to have a brochure describing the basic aspects of the assessment process that can be given to the child and family.

As part of the informed consent process, the psychologist should discuss the limits of confidentiality before the assessment begins. The child and family should understand under what circumstances personal information can be revealed to outside parties. In addition to explaining the legally mandated requirement to break confidentiality in cases, for example, of child abuse or neglect or the ethical requirement to break confidentiality in cases, for example, of danger to self or others, it is important that the limits of confidentiality be discussed. For example, parents often believe that any personal information shared during an assessment is privileged and that the child and family are protected from having their disclosures revealed during legal procedures without their consent. The psychologist should explain to the child and family that privileged communication is a legal concept that differs from state to state, and the psychologist should explain how it might affect that child and family in their particular state (Gustafson & McNamara, 1987; Koocher & Keith-Spiegel, 1998). The discussion of confidentiality should be undertaken with the child and family members at the initial contact. The parents and the child should sign a statement acknowledging the mutual understanding of confidentiality.

Assessment of children with special needs often requires helping the child and family understand the potential for conflict in the psychologist's role during the assessment. Assessments of children with special needs usually are performed under the auspices of a third party, such as a school, governmental agency, or other institutional entity in order that educational placement be expedited, curriculum be designed, or the child receive entitled resources (e.g., Social Security payments). When assessment is performed without a third party involved, the psychologist should explain to the family that no written or oral information can be communicated to schools, physicians, mental health agencies, insurance providers, and/or others without the written approval of the parents. In contrast, if a third partly is involved, the psychologist must clarify the nature of the relationship between the psychologist, the child, the family, and the third party requesting the evaluation. The psychologist must provide a reasonable description of his or her role with the child and family and the probable uses of the interview and testing data. The way in which confidential or sensitive information will be disclosed must be completely explained. For example, it is important for the school psychologist or educational diagnostician to explain how, when, and to whom information will be communicated, such as during an education team meeting.

There are times when the parents may feel that the psychologist is not supportive of their child's special needs. For example, parents who are advocates for their child with special needs might feel that because the psychologist is "working for the school," he or she does not necessarily represent the best interests of their child. It is important that the psychologist clarify the nature of his or her responsibilities before the assessment takes place. All parties should work together to ensure a cooperative assessment process. Another example involves the use of diagnostic labels. Many parents believe that diagnostic labels might not adequately capture the complexity of the strengths and weaknesses of their child with special needs, but school psychologists are often compelled to provide a label in order to access mandated special education services. Regardless of the ethical dilemma, the psychologist should always try to minimize the invasion of the child's privacy and to contribute to the welfare of the child and family.

During the Assessment

Although it is possible to be competent without being ethical, it is impossible to be ethical without being competent (Weiner, 1989). The psychologist must be competent in the ability to assess children with special needs based on his or her education, training, or experience. Even when an assessment may require a modification of standard testing procedures, the psychologist should take reasonable steps to ensure competent work and that no harm befalls the child or family. Psychologists must be familiar with all aspects of psychological tests administered, including a working knowledge of reliability, validity, normative standardization, and appropriate administration techniques. When assessing children with special needs, the psychologist identifies which assessment techniques or norms may not be applicable to that population and modifies the interpretation of the findings according to the uniqueness of the child. In addition, the competent psychologist will be sensitive to other human differences in addition to the child's identified disability, including age, race, gender, national origin, religion, sexual orientation, or socioeconomic status.

Unlike in other areas of psychological practice, changes have rapidly occurred in assessment techniques and assessment technology that require the psychologist to stay professionally current (Weiner, 1989). There can be a great temptation to practice outside of limits of training or experience when assessing children with special needs. In fact, more than 15% of pediatric psychologists have admitted that they have sometimes administered a psychological test with which they had limited experience (Rae & Worchel, 1991). The temptation to practice outside the limits of training partially stems from the fact that the assessment of children with special needs often requires that the psychologist adapt assessment techniques to the special population because standardized protocols do not exist for many of these low-incidence populations. As a result, the psychologist's interpretation and judgment is crucial to a competent assessment. Under these circumstances, the psychologist could easily overestimate his or her ability to appropriately assess the child with special needs. In institutional settings such as schools, the psychologist may be the expert regarding the educational implications of a particular type of disability (e.g., low vision) but not be expert or competent in psychological assessment of those children.

The psychologist must meet a reasonable standard of competence. Some psychologists have been known to use "vanity" credentials to purportedly extend their areas of competence. For example, a psychologist may attend a 3-hour workshop in assessment of children with hearing impairments and then profess to have the skill to appropriately perform complex evaluations of children in this population. In this case the psychologist might not be able to provide an appropriate standard of care and/or may not have adequate awareness of what should be an appropriate standard of care because of limited experience. In addition, subtle pressures exist for psychologists to perform evaluations beyond their areas of competence because of institutional requirements (i.e., a school district being required to conduct the evaluation) or because of monetary incentives (i.e., a patient paying out of pocket to see a private-practice psychologist). Koocher (1993) provides a number of examples of competence issues, including providing trainees with inadequate supervision, using undertrained testing assistants, and inappropriate use of computerized testing printouts. Psychologists should always be careful in their adaptations of assessment administration or interpretation to special populations, and they should always obtain consultation and/or supervision if they are practicing in an area with which they have had limited experience.

Psychologists are ethically required to take into account both test factors and characteristics of the assessed child that might affect the psychologist's judgments and/or reduce the accuracy of the interpretations. Psychologists must be familiar with the psychometric properties of their assessment instruments, including reliability, validity, and standard error of measurement (Koocher, 1993). Although assessing children with complex disabilities requires a qualitative-developmental approach, it is important that the psychologist not go beyond the data of the psychometrics of the tests used. The psychologist must be thoroughly familiar with which tests might be appropriate and which tests have become obsolete for the assessment purpose.

Reliability issues can be problematic with special populations. Tests are standardized in their administration, scoring, and interpretation, but the psychologist assessing children with special needs must often adapt the standardized procedures to fit the individualized needs of the child. In addition, many children with special needs have inconsistent response patterns from one testing session to another that could reduce reliability. For example, the behavior of the child with autism who may be cooperative one day but agitated and uncooperative on another day would create reliability problems. In the same way, the validity of the test administered to a child with special needs might be questionable. The psychologist must take great care to be sure that the normative sample is appropriate; children with special needs are often not included in the standardization samples of common psychological tests. By their nature, children with special needs are unique and may not be able to be meaningfully compared with a general population included in the normative standardization sample. In addition, the construct validity of an instrument requires that the population be specific, because the basis of construct validity is the match between the posited construct and the presumed representative data obtained from the assessment instrument. One could argue that without convincing evidence of population generalizability, it is impossible to interpret the meaning of the psychological construct with any specific special population (Laosa, 1991).

During a thorough assessment of the child with special needs, the situational context of the child's behavior must also be taken into account. Because of the importance of obtaining information on such things as adaptive functioning from significant others in the child's environment (e.g., teachers, peers, parents), the psychologist must recognize that each informant may have a particular bias about the child. For example, the regular education teacher who feels that the child with special needs is an extra burden in his or her classroom might tend to rate the child more negatively. Psychologists must also be aware of their own bias during the assessment process and take care in monitoring their objectivity during the scoring and in the interpretation of the assessment results (Peterson, 1996). Psychologists must continue to scrutinize the empirical evidence that might justify the use of a particular test with children with special needs and must also recognize any test bias that might have a differential impact on the child being tested.

Interpretation of the assessment data involves integrating all relevant information, including history, behavioral observations, and test results, into a complete picture of the child's functioning. Frequently psychologists will rely on testing alone to provide the bulk of information about the child needed to develop a diagnostic formulation. Using psychological test data as the sole basis for applying a diagnostic label should be done with great caution, and the psychologist should be sensitive to potential alternatives, because the label can have serious consequences for the client (Koocher & Keith-Spiegel, 1998). With the proliferation of diagnostic nosology (e.g., the *Diagnostic and Statistical Manual of Mental Disorders*, Fourth Edition; American Psychiatric Association, 1994) and mandated special education categories (e.g., the Individuals with Disabilities Education Act), labeling the child becomes an important part of the assessment. At the same time, the psychologist must realize that tests are only designed to show that child's performance at a given point in time. Interpreting the test involves understanding why the person performed that way and is tempered by the behavioral observations and by the history obtained about the child and family. Labeling is a shortcut for helping to communicate among professionals, but it should not be used as a substitute for a thorough understanding of the child's performance during the assessment. The child's welfare should always be the primary goal when considering a diagnostic label.

After the Assessment

Confidentiality is one of the most common ethical dilemmas for psychologists (Peterson, 1996). Although confidentiality dilemmas most often occur within the context of a therapeutic relationship, the confidentiality required for an assessment of a child with special needs can be equally problematic. Although assessment is usually time limited and circumscribed in scope, misunderstandings can occur as to the use of the assessment information. The issue of confidentiality is usually more of a problem for parents than for children, who are accustomed to adults being knowledgeable about many of the private details of their lives. At the same time, older teenagers have greater sensitivity to confidentiality issues (Gustafson & McNamara, 1987). Psychologists have an obligation to respect the confidentiality rights and privacy of the child and family. In written reports and oral communications, only that information germane to the purpose of the assessment should be revealed.

Confidentiality is also complicated during the assessment process because the nature of the evaluation requires that the psychologist understand the situational context of the child's environment. In this regard, the psychologist must obtain information either formally or informally from family and/or the child's peer group. When obtaining information from parents, it is very important to clarify how the information will be used and to clarify any potential role conflicts. Parents may not provide a candid history if they feel that the information they provide will not be helpful to their child. Often psychologists working in a school setting can get information about peer interactions from the observations of the teacher, but more direct assessments are often helpful. The use of peer-referenced assessment strategies can be helpful but can pose additional ethical dilemmas in such areas as obtaining parental permission and child assent, and the potential harmful ramifications of negative peer nominations must be considered (Gresham & Little, 1993).

Psychologists should always provide the child and family with an explanation of the assessment results using language that is reasonably understandable. This explanation does not have to be provided by the psychologist personally, but the psychologist is responsible for seeing that feedback is given unless the setting prohibits it. In fact, the 1974 Family Educational Rights and Privacy Act (FERPA) and subsequent federal guidelines clearly specify that parents should be given access to all the assessment information about their child. At the same time, psychologists can have conflicting roles in that they are agents for the school system, which creates a problem of dual loyalty (Bersoff, 1995). This potential for a dual relationship could create a situation in which the psychologist might skew feedback in order to support an institutional need. For example, the psychologist might consciously or unconsciously temper the assessment results in a way that might be supportive of placement in a particular type of special education class that is available in the school district rather than meeting the child's needs with another type of placement.

Although the patient and family have the legal right to the assessment results, ethical guidelines indicate that releasing raw test results to unqualified persons is not ethical (APA, 1992). Matarazzo (1990) has described a continuum of the psychological assessment information, but when defining test scores, he describes scores as either raw (e.g., the items answered correctly on a test) or standardized (e.g., percentile scores, IQ scores). Tranel (1994) has argued that because unqualified persons more easily misinterpret them, standardized scores should not be routinely released. In addition, IQ scores (standardized or percentile) should be included in psychological reports only after careful consideration of the consequences. Without proper understanding of such psychometric concepts as standard error of measurement, standard deviation, reliability, and validity, parents or other unqualified persons could misinterpret the assessment data, which could result in negative consequences for the child. The psychologist must be very careful when providing oral or written feedback of the assessment test results to ensure that the results will not be misinterpreted or misused. Record keeping can provide additional dilemmas for the psychologist. He or she is responsible for maintaining appropriate confidentiality in the creation, storage, transfer, and disposal of records, including written, recorded, or computerized records. Any documentation (e.g., reports or letters) should include only information that is germane to the purposes of that documentation. In the same way, it is important to purge any obsolete test data from files, because their release might be misleading and potentially detrimental to the child. The psychologist is responsible for fulfilling the record-keeping requirements of governmental agencies, insurance companies, and other organizations or entities to which the psychologist may have some obligation. The psychologist is at risk for disciplinary or legal action if records are carelessly treated (Tranel, 1994). Finally, because of the trend toward freer client access to records, reports should be written and files should be maintained with the assumption that the child or family will eventually see the record (Koocher & Keith-Spiegel, 1998).

LEGAL ISSUES

Understanding legal issues as applied to assessment is an ongoing endeavor. There are several legal avenues that influence assessment of children. Four major sources of lawmaking and interpretation are germane to assessment of children: (1) the Constitution of the United States of America, (2) federal statutes, (3) federal administrative regulations, and (4) case law (Fiedler & Prasse, 1996; Jacob-Timm & Hartshorne, 1998). It should be recognized that the Constitution is the primary source of law that influences statutes, regulations, and case law. Pertinent federal statutes include the Individuals with Disabilities Education Act (IDEA), the Rehabilitation Act of 1973 (Public Law 93–122), sometimes called Section 504, and the Family Educational Rights and Privacy Act (FERPA). Federal administrative regulations can come from several sources, with the Office of Special Education and Rehabilitation Services (OSERS) as a key source related to special education assessment. In addition to the federal influences, there are state adaptations and adoptions of the federal mandates that must be considered by the practitioner in each state (Woody, LaVoie, & Epps, 1992). For the psychologist who assesses children and adolescents, special education mandates and considerations must be kept in mind. Even if the assessment is in a private practice setting, there may be professional interface with schools, and therefore key statutes and case law that are related to assessment must always be considered.

Federal Statutes

Individuals with Disabilities Education Act

From its early history, and with additional laws and acts, assessment has been a concern of the Individuals with Disabilities Education Act (IDEA). The original act, called the Education for All Handicapped Children Act, also referred to as Public Law 94-142, addressed assessment in several ways. The act included Protection in Evaluation Procedures (PEP), which contained several mandates for assessment. (See Table 16.1 for specifics.) Assessment within the educational setting must address multiple needs. Assessment is done not only to qualify a child for special services and to help in determining the most appropriate placement but also to address the student's underlying strengths and needs (National Council on Disability, 1996). In addition, assessment must also provide a benchmark by which progress is measured. These various requirements of the assessment process and outcome have been refined and expanded by later versions of the IDEA statute.

TABLE 16.1. Assessment Mandates from Public Law 94-142: Protection in Evaluation Procedures (PEP)

1. Tests selected and administered to be racially and culturally nondiscriminatory.
2. Students should be assessed in their native language or primary mode of communication.
3. Tests must be validated for the purposes for which they are utilized.
4. Trained personnel must administer tests utilizing the procedures standardized for each test.
5. Assessment must include information about specific educational needs, not just a general intelligence quotient.
6. Placement and program decisions must be based on performances on more than one measure.
7. A multidisciplinary team must assess the student, and the team must include at least one member who has specialized knowledge in the area of the suspected disability.
8. The student must be assessed in all areas related to the suspected disability, including health, vision, hearing, social and emotional status, general intelligence, academic performance, communication skills, and motor skills.

In 1986, additional standards for assessment were developed in Public Law 99-457. In this updating of the basic special education law, the mandate is made explicit for multidisciplinary evaluation, as well as for procedures for measuring progress. In addition, it provides for delivery of services to the preschool-age population, with the same evaluation mandates required by PEP. In 1990, the name of the law was changed to reflect the person-first philosophy (e.g., "individuals with disabilities" rather than "handicapped children") and two categories were added: traumatic brain injury and autism. This law also required that transition plans be developed for students who are 16 years of age or older. The transition considerations include the student's further education, including higher education, vocational placement, and living arrangements. The transition plan has an impact on assessment, as there must be consideration of current skill levels, as well as skills requiring development as the transition occurs. This suggests that assessment must include multifaceted aspects of the student, such as adaptive living skills, mobility skills, vocational skills (and/or potential), social skills, and ability to utilize academic skills in daily activities.

In 1997, IDEA was renewed, with a new assessment procedure mandated for students with behavioral concerns. This is called "functional assessment" and is intended to investigate the environmental and social context of behaviors as an integral piece of the assessment of the individual. The functional assessment includes, but is not limited to, observation and recording of multiple skills in multiple settings. For example, the student's ability to solve a social dilemma might be assessed in the classroom, in the lunchroom, at home, and in after-school activities. Examining patterns of strengths and needs, as well as the influence of the setting, contributes to the overall assessment and can help direct intervention and placement. Although it is currently required only for students with behavioral disorders, functional assessment will likely become an essential part of all assessment for special education services in the future.

The six guiding principles in IDEA are as follows: (1) zero reject, (2) nondiscriminatory evaluation, (3) appropriate education, (4) least restrictive environment, (5) parent participation, and (6) procedural due process. Zero reject is the principle that supports all children having access to education, regardless of the degree of a disabling condition. Nondiscriminatory evaluation refers to assessment that is nonbiased in regard to gender, age, ethnic origin, geographic locale, socioeconomic status, and/or handicapping condition. (Other aspects of the nondiscriminatory assessment principle are discussed later.)

Appropriate education refers to providing the education that meets the educational needs of the student rather than trying to fit the student into a prescribed program. Least restrictive environment (LRE) is the delivery of services in the educational setting that best meets the educational needs of the student. For the most part, the LRE is within the local educational agency; however, at times the LRE is in another setting better suited to the child's educational needs. For example, all schools must be accessible to persons with wheelchairs, so a student with this type of mobility need should be able to be served in his or her home school. On the other hand, for some children with low-incidence conditions that require extensive specialized training (e.g., braille training), the LRE may be in an area center program or a state school. Parent participation is legally mandated at several points in the assessment process, especially in giving informed consent and during the report and subsequent decision that is made as a result of the assessment outcome. Procedural due process is again mandated by federal statute. One particular aspect of procedural due process is that the parents are entitled to a second, independent assessment of their child if necessary.

All six principles of IDEA have an impact on assessment, but especially in nondiscriminatory evaluation, which involves four essential elements. First, the evaluation must include multiple sources of information. The multiple-source requirement under IDEA prescribes that assessment must include evaluation and/or reports from several professionals. Typically these include the regular education teacher, the special education teacher, the parents, and the psychological examiner. With students who have low-incidence conditions, others involved in the assessment may include physicians, mobility experts, experts in the specific impairment condition (e.g., low-vision experts), speech therapists, occupational therapists, physical therapists, dietitians, and other specialists as needed. In addition, the student must be assessed in multiple settings, not just in one classroom. Second, the evaluation process must be timely. Timely evaluation refers to the legal mandate that assessment must occur within a prescribed period of time from the initiation of the referral. Third, the testing tools must be reliable and valid for the population for which they are used. If not, adaptive and accommodation issues should be addressed. Fourth, the child must meet the criteria needed for certification. That is, the assessment procedures must take into account the legal aspects that must be met in order for a child to qualify for special services. For example, for a child to qualify for services under the low-vision or blind category, the assessment report must contain documentation of the child's visual impairment.

Section 504

The Rehabilitation Act of 1973 (Public Law 93-122) produced what is commonly called Section 504. This law is broadly based and provides equal access to programs and services, as well as forbidding discrimination against persons with disabilities solely on the basis of that disability. Although the law was not necessarily developed for school-age children, there is increasing use of Section 504 in school settings. In particular, many school systems are choosing to serve children under Section 504 mandates if they do not qualify for services under IDEA. This suggests that the children served by Section 504 must already be assessed as having a disability. Section 504 does not offer the legal protections and due process available in IDEA. As such, it is generally felt that providing services under IDEA is a first choice and that Section 504 can be utilized as a second choice, or in some cases an additional choice. College students frequently wish to utilize Section 504 because IDEA is not in effect for them. If the student has had a previous assessment for IDEA, then obtaining services under Section 504 becomes easier. Many institutions are developing criteria to establish what can be considered a disability under Section 504. This may affect assessment procedures in the future, especially for transition evaluations. It may also create a new cadre of students who require assessment in order to qualify for services.

Family Educational Rights and Privacy Act

In 1974, the Family Educational Rights and Privacy Act (FERPA), also commonly called the Buckley amendment, was enacted. This law provides for parents, and in some cases the students themselves, to inspect and as necessary challenge school records. Furthermore, identifiable information cannot be released without parent consent. Several aspects of this act that have been addressed in case law are important to consider in the assessment process. (See the next section.) Although the act is most applicable to educational agencies, there may be aspects that affect the private practitioner as well. For example, if the private practitioner's report is used as a part of the educational assessment, that report is subject to FERPA, even though it was generated outside of the school setting. This law may create ethical dilemmas in several spheres for the practitioner, especially in regards to securing test materials, confidentiality, and maintenance of records. In particular, institutional requirements, educational laws, and ethical standards must be carefully considered in the confidentiality of assessment records.

Case Law

Several lessons to be learned from case law are already addressed when ethical practices are followed. Assessment that follows ethical guidelines must meet several parameters. Butcher and Pope (1993) address the ethical considerations that capture these essential elements: nondiscrimination, comprehensive assessment, valid assessment, appropriate and timely assessment, appropriate use of tools, independent assessment, and right to information. In examining case law as it relates to assessment of children, both the historical perspective and the influence of federal statutes must be kept in mind. In Table 16.2, we briefly describe several pertinent cases that have influenced assessment.

For the psychologist assessing children, case law and ethical guidelines create possible dilemmas and require deliberate and thoughtful consideration. One example of such an occurrence is in the area of FERPA and ethical guidelines. For the psychologist engaged in private practice, raw test data and test protocols would be held as confidential material. If the psychologist is in a school setting, the parents have the right to examine this information; the same information could be made available to an independent examiner. This holds true even if the psychologist keeps the materials in a file separate from the student's cumulative folder (*John K. and Mary K. v. Board of Education for School District #65, Cook County*, 1987; *Parents Against Abuse in Schools (PAAS) v. Williamsport Area School District*, 1991).

In some cases, case law may dictate the type of assessment or the conditions in which assessment procedures can be utilized (*Guadalupe Organization, Inc. v. Tempe Elementary School District No. 3*, 1972; *California Association of School Psychologists v. Superintendent of Public Instruction*, 1994). Arguably one of the most interesting aspects of case law and assessment is the limitation of assessment procedures within ethnic populations (*Larry P. v. Riles*, 1972). The recovery aspects related to misclassification and inappropriate placement are also addressed in case law (*Hoffman v. Board of Education of the City of New York*, 1979; *Brantley v. Independent School District*, 1996).

TABLE 16.2. Chronological Listing of Key Court Cases Related to Assessment in Special Education

Case	Implication
Plessy v. Ferguson, 1896	"Separate but equal" education established.
Brown v. Board of Education, 1954	"Separate but equal" education struck down; established precedence for education of special populations.
Hobson v. Hansen, 1967	Placement is inappropriate if determined by assessment that is biased or based on norms that do not reflect the student.
Diana v. State Board of Education, 1970	Bias in assessment can occur if testing not done in child's native language, resulting in illegal discrimination.
Pennsylvania Association for Retarded Citizens (PARC) v. Pennsylvania, 1971	Children with special needs are accorded due process and equal protections, and therefore are no longer excluded from public education.
Mills v. Board of Education of District of Columbia, 1972	No child can be excluded from public education; must have alternative educational services provided with constitutionally adequate hearing, periodical review of status, progress, and adequacy of the alternative placement.
Larry P. v. Riles, 1972	Students cannot be placed on the basis of a single criteria, especially an IQ test. Standardized but invalid testing violates IDEA, Title VI of Civil Rights Act of 1964, Section 504, and equal protection clause. In 1984, IQ tests in California were banned for identifying African Americans for any services except gifted and talented programs.
Guadalupe Organization, Inc. v. Tempe Elementary School District, 1972	Requires assessment of children in their primary language or use of nonverbal measures; includes assessment of adaptive behavior and interview of child's parents in their home setting.
Woolman v. Walter, 1977	Standardized testing services can be provided by public school personnel in non–public school setting; however, teaching and remedial services are provided only in public school or neutral setting.
Hoffman v. Board of Education of the City of New York, 1979	In cases of assessment malpractice in which misclassification and/or misplacement of students has occurred, courts typically award compensatory education.
Parents in Action in Special Education v. Hannon, 1980	Found that biased items by themselves do not necessarily cause inappropriate placement because other determinates are utilized in placements.
Riley v. Ambach, 1980	Standard, statewide formulas for determining learning disabilities should be used for guidance only.
Aguilar v. Felton, 1985	Title I programs carried out by public school personnel on non–public school premises violated the Establishment Clause of the First Amendment (overturned in 1997).
Fay v. South Colonie Central School District, 1986	In the absence of notification to the contrary, school personnel can assume the noncustodial parent has access to the child's school records.

(continued)

TABLE 16.2. *continued*

Case	Implication
John K. and Mary K. v. Board of Education for School District #65, Cook County, 1987	Test protocols cannot be considered private notes and therefore are subject to disclosure to parents; raw data must be provided to second professional when parents are seeking an independent evaluation.
Cordrey v. Euckert, 1990	Decisions regarding provision of extended-year services can be based on the "expert opinion" of the professional conducting individual assessment when empirical data is not available.
Parents Against Abuse in Schools (PAAS) v. Williamsport Area School District, 1991	Information, once reported about a student, is not private and is part of the student's educational record, regardless of whether it is separately stored.
California Association of School Psychologists v. Superintendent of Public Education, 1994	Unsuccessful attempt to overturn California's statewide ban on IQ testing with African American children.
Crawford v. Honig, 1994	Allows African American children to be given IQ tests with parental consent.
Brantley v. Independent School District, 1996	Compensatory education awarded for damages due to misclassification and placement.
Agostini v. Felton, 1997	School can provide Title I interventions by public school personnel on non–public school premises.

Note. Data from Fiedler & Prasse (1996); Fischer & Sorenson (1996); Jacob-Timm & Hartshorne (1998); Lantzy (1992); National Council on Disability (1996); Woody, LaVoie, & Epps (1992).

Although the case law is typically applicable in regard to statutes related to IDEA, there are implications for the private practitioner as well. This is especially true if the private practitioner's assessment report is utilized in the educational setting. Certainly understanding case law as it relates to assessment is the responsibility of the psychologist, whatever the practice setting.

SPECIAL TOPICS IN ASSESSMENT

Computer-Assisted Assessment

The psychologist is responsible for insuring that any test or assessment procedure is accurate and that interpretations are valid. The use of computers to assist the psychologist in assessment has been very beneficial. Not only are computational errors minimized, but also testing can be tailored to special populations. Unfortunately, computerized assessment can also have some serious drawbacks. The psychologist may be less vigilant about the test's psychometric properties, may be less familiar with how interpretations are derived, may neglect to integrate qualitative data in the interpretation, and may rely more on the computer-generated report (Cottone & Tarvydas, 1998). Unfortunately, the neatly typed computer-generated report promotes a serious impression of infallibility that can lead to misuse (Jacob & Brantley, 1989). The use of computer assistance in scoring and interpretation still requires clinical judgment on the part of the psychologist. In this way, decisions can be made with full sensitivity to the nuances of administering and interpreting tests in a way that is unique to each person being assessed (Bersoff & Hofer, 1991). In most cases, the computer-generated report should be regarded as a tentative (or suggested) interpretation that is considered by the psychologist in relation to history, interview, and other clinical data (Matarazzo, 1986). With special populations requiring modifications of administration, scoring, or interpretation, the importance of professional judgment cannot be underestimated.

Limited Access to Assessment

With the advent of managed care and limited institutional resources for assessment in the schools, psychological assessment and treatment have been limited. This limitation of access to services has ethical implications, because it is clearly unethical to withhold services from a client who needs them. In particular, managed care companies often provide financial incentives for providers who hold down costs by limiting access to care (Roberts & Hurley, 1997). In the same way, school districts are increasingly under pressure to contain costs, while at the same time being mandated to provide services under Public Law 94–142 (Koocher & Keith-Spiegel, 1998). Some managed care companies have even tried to limit access by restricting the kinds of assessments they will provide. For example, several managed care organizations will not pay for evaluation of specific diagnostic categories such as attention-deficit/hyperactivity disorder (Roberts & Hurley, 1997). The psychologist must be vigilant to economic pressures that might influence appropriate assessment and ultimately contribute negatively to the welfare of the child and family.

Assistive Technology

As technology and medical interventions grow, so do considerations of how they might affect assessment. Assistive technology is a relatively new arena that has an impact on assessment. Examples of assistive technology might include electronic language boards, computer-assisted expressive skills, computer-assisted presentation of academic skills, mobility assistance, such as wheelchairs and other apparatus, and other medical technology, such as respirators and organ pumps. There are several ethical issues to consider. First, the psychologist must consider how the assistive technology might affect the assessment of the child's true score. When assistive technology is utilized, either by the examiner or the child, the question of what is being tested must be asked. Second, the psychologist must be knowledgeable regarding the skills needed to utilize the assistive technology, as well as the limitations this technology might impose. For example, if the child utilizes an electronic language board that has limited responses, using a psychological measure that requires complex responses may not adequately assess the child's receptive or expressive language. Therefore, a poor result might be due to an artifact of the technology rather than to the limitations of the child. In the same way, the child on assisted breathing will need specifically timed breaks, so utilizing a timed test may or may not be appropriate. The psychologist must exercise his or her clinical judgment with assistive technologies in much in the same way that other modifications and adaptations to the assessment are judged.

Invasions of Privacy and Dignity of Children with Special Needs

The psychologist needs to consider the privacy and dignity of children, with particular sensitivity to children with special needs. One issue affecting the privacy and dignity of children with special needs is the amount of information the assessor needs. Although some information is clearly needed to proceed with assessment, some situations are less clear than others. In order to conduct appropriate assessment, the psychologist must know about medical conditions that clearly affect the choice of assessment tools and procedures. For example, if the child has low vision or hearing problems, foreknowledge would assist the psychologist in the assessment process. There are other situations in which the issue of the student's right to privacy versus obtaining the best possible performance is less well delineated. For example, knowing if the child needs specific breaks in order to care for a colostomy device might be important in the timing of the assessment procedures. It could also be argued that this information is not essential to the overall assessment process because all children may require bathroom breaks, and thus this type of information may not need to be divulged to the psychologist. Deciding what information is needed is not an easy task. This is especially true in low-incidence situations in which specific conditions may or may not impinge on the assessment procedures. As the psychologist, it is important to discuss fully with the parents and child the parameters of the assessment procedures and to enlist their assistance in deciding which information is most vital to obtain the best possible performance from the child.

Another issue is the inherent differential in the relationship between the psychologist and the child. Although obtaining informed assent should be a standard practice, with some children this may not be possible. Whether the child may want to participate in the process may not be fully known. There may be circumstances in which the child is tested regardless of his or her opinion. Sensitivity to the dignity of the child must be a major concern of the psychologist. For example, using a measure on which the child clearly fails every item is not only demeaning to the child, but it is also not valid. Children, as do adults, want to be seen as doing well. In the assessment process, there must be opportunity for the child to show strengths and skills rather than just weaknesses and failures. The psychologist has a responsibility to respect the child's abilities and allow for the child's preferences within the assessment process.

GUIDELINES FOR MAKING ETHICAL DECISIONS

Many models for ethical decision making are available (Cottone & Tardyvas, 1998; Jacob-Timm & Hartshorne, 1998; Rae & Fournier, 1999); however, the psychologist assessing children with special needs may face unusual and challenging situations. In some ethical decisions, the choice may be relatively simplified as the psychologist applies an ethical guideline to a practice. This decision is less difficult if the statutes and case law for the situation are in agreement with the ethical guidelines. For example, the psychologist must obtain informed consent from parents or legal guardians before assessing a child. This action is supported by ethical guidelines and by statutes and legal rulings regarding assessment of children.

Ethical dilemmas, defined as two or more competing ethical guidelines and/or legal aspects, are more difficult. For example, even though informed consent is obtained in both private and school settings, the reporting of assessment results differs in each setting. In a private practice, the information may be shared only with the parents and the child. In a school setting, the information must be shared not only with the parents and the child but also with the educational team responsible for provision of services. In the same way, institutional and legal mandates might require assessment of a child, but there may be situations in which this decision might conflict with the parents' wishes and/or the best interests of the child and family.

General considerations in ethical decision making when working with children and families include the setting in which the psychologist practices, the intended audience for the assessment findings, and the statutes and court cases germane to the decision. A four-step model for ethical decision making described by Rae and Fournier (1999) may be helpful for the psychologist in regard to assessment. The first step requires that the psychologist gather information. This includes deciding which rules and guidelines, both ethical and legal, apply to the situation. The second step involves generating possible decisions and examining them for implications and untoward outcomes. At this step, the psychologist must also take into consideration the context in which the decision is made (e.g., school setting vs. private practice, information for educational placement vs. examining therapeutic progress). Often it is helpful to evaluate decisions in terms of possible positive and negative outcomes for the child. For example, releasing a report from a private practice to the school system means that it will become part of the child's educational file. The implications of this release of information must be discussed with the parent and child, and any negative impact of the loss of confidentiality must be weighed against the child receiving appropriate educational services. The third step is to implement the best possible choice under the circumstances. Here the psychologist must consider appropriate time lines and the "how" of implementation. For example, the need to send reports to schools in order to meet an educational placement deadline may require the psychologist to contact the parents immediately to discuss release of information and get their signatures, rather than waiting until the next scheduled meeting. The fourth step is to evaluate the decision and look for avenues for avoiding such ethical dilemmas in the future. This step can help the psychologist modify practices that may inadvertently contribute to ethical dilemmas. For example, having the discussion regarding release of information procedures and general implications as part of the initial contact with the parents and child may expedite the process at a later date.

One important responsibility of the psychologist is to develop a network of colleagues. Consultation with colleagues should be ongoing throughout the ethical decision-making process. In addition, psychologists may contact their state psychology boards, as well as their national boards, to assist in the decision-making process. Ethical guidelines are blueprints for the psychologist and are meant to be followed as closely as possible. There must be recognition that situations may occur that do not fit the plan. Conscientious decision making, as well as continuous updating of his or her ethical and legal knowledge base, is essential for the psychologist.

SUMMARY

Assessment of children and adolescents with special needs is a complex but important endeavor. Responsibilities to the child, family, and various institutions or agencies serving the child require the psychologist to be current in ethics and legal considerations, as well as competent in the assessment process. Utilizing practices with careful, considered assessment tools is not a guarantee that all ethical and legal considerations are met. The burden of proof is on the examiner to document and insure that best practices are followed. Not only is this important to the psychologist, but the most important factor is that the needs of the child are met with the highest standards of ethical and competent assessment practices.

REFERENCES

American Psychiatric Association. (1994). *Diagnostic and statistical manual of mental disorder* (4th ed., Rev.). Washington, DC: Author.

American Psychological Association. (1992). Ethical principles of psychologists and code of conduct. *American Psychologist, 47*, 1597–1611.

American Psychological Association, American Educational Research Association, & National Council on Measurement in Education. (1998). *Standards for educational and psychological testing*. Washington, DC: Author.

Agostini v. Felton, No. 96–522 (U.S. filed June 23, 1997).

Aguilar v. Felton, 473 U.S. 402, 105 S. Ct. 3232, 87 L. Ed. 2d 290 (1985), *rev'd sub nom.* Agostini v. Felton, No. 96–522 (U.S. filed June 23, 1997).

Bersoff, D. N. (1995). School psychology as "institutional psychiatry." In D. N. Bersoff (Ed.), *Ethical conflicts in psychology* (pp. 284–285). Washington, DC: American Psychological Association.

Bersoff, D. N., & Hofer, P. J. (1991). Legal issues in computerized psychological testing. In D. N. Bersoff (Ed.), *Ethical conflicts in psychology* (pp. 291–294). Washington, DC: American Psychological Association.

Brantley v. Independent School District, No. 625, 24 IDELR 696 (D. Minn. 1996).

Brown v. Board of Educ., 347 U.S. 483 (1954).

Butcher, J. N., & Pope, K. S. (1993). Seven issues in conducting forensic assessments: Ethical responsibilities in light of new standards and new tests. *Ethics and Behavior, 3*, 267–288.

California Association of School Psychologists v. Superintendent of Public Instruction, 21 IDELR 130 (N.D. Cal. 1994).

Canter, M. B., Bennett, B. E., Jones, S. E., & Nagy, T. F. (1994). *Ethics for psychologists: A commentary on the APA Ethics Code*. Washington, DC: American Psychological Association.

Cordrey v. Euckert, 917 F.2d 1460 (6th Cir. 1990).

Cottone, R. R., & Tarvydas, V. M. (1998). *Ethical and professional issues in counseling*. Upper Saddle River, NJ: Prentice-Hall.

Crawford v. Honig, 37 F.3d 484 (9th Cir. 1994).

Diana v. State Board of Education, Civ. Act. No. C-70–37 (N.D. Cal. 1970), *further order* (1973).

Family Educational Rights and Privacy Act of 1974, 20 U.S.C. § 1232.

Fay v. South Colonie Central School District, 802 F.2d 21 (2nd Cir. 1986).

Fiedler, C. R., & Prasse, D. P. (1996). Legal and ethical issues in the educational assessment and programming for youth with emotional or behavioral disorders. In M. J. Breen & C. R. Fiedler (Eds.), *Behavioral approach to assessment of youth with emotional/behavioral disorders* (pp. 23–79). Austin, TX: Pro-Ed.

Fischer, L., & Sorenson, G. P. (1996). *School law for counselors, psychologists, and social workers*. White Plains, NY: Longman.

Gresham, F. M., & Little, S. G. (1993) Peer-referenced assessment strategies. In T. H. Ollendick & M. Hersen (Eds.), *Handbook of child and adolescent assessment* (pp. 165–179). Boston: Allyn & Bacon.

Guadalupe Organization, Inc. v. Tempe Elementary School District No. 3, Civ. No. 71–435 (D. Ariz. 1972).

Gustafson, K. E., & McNamara, J. R. (1987). Confidentiality with minor clients: Issues and guidelines for therapists. *Professional Psychology: Research and Practice, 18*, 503–508.

Hobson v. Hansen, 269 F. Supp. 401, 515 (D. D.C. 1967), *aff'd. sub nom*, Smuck v. Hobson, 408 F.2d 175 (D.C. Cir. 1969).

Hoffman v. Board of Education of the City of New York, 49 N.Y.2d 121, 424 N.Y.S.2d 376 (1979).

Individuals with Disabilities Act of 1997, U. S. C. § 1400.

Jacob, S., & Brantley, J. C. (1989). Ethics and computer-assisted assessment: Three case studies. *Psychology in the Schools, 26*, 163–167.

Jacob-Timm, S., & Hartshorne, T. S. (1998). *Ethics and law for school psychologists* (3rd ed.). New York: Wiley.

John K. and Mary K. v. Board of Education for School District #65, Cook County, 504 N.E.2d 797 (Ill. App. 1 Dist. 1987).

Koocher, G. P. (1993). Ethical issues in the psychological assessment of children. In T. H. Ollendick & M. Hersen (Eds.), *Handbook of child and adolescent assessment* (pp. 51–61). Boston: Allyn & Bacon.

Koocher, G. P., & Keith-Spiegel, P. C. (1990). *Children, ethics, and the law: Professional issues and cases*. Lincoln: University of Nebraska Press.

Koocher, G. P., & Keith-Spiegel, P. (1998). *Ethics in psychology: Professional standards and cases* (2nd ed.). New York: Oxford University Press.

Lantzy, M. L. (1992). *Individuals with Disabilities Education Act: An annotated guide to its literature and resources, 1980–1991*. Littleton, CO: Rothman.

Laosa, L. M. (1991). The cultural context of construct validity and the ethics of generalizability. *Early Childhood Research Quarterly, 6*, 313–312.

Larry P. v. Riles, 343 F. Supp. 1306 (D.C. N.D. Cal. 1972), *aff'd.*, 502 F.2d 963 (9th Cir. 1974), further proceedings, 495 F. Supp. 926 (D.C. N.D. Cal. 1979), *aff'd.*, 502 F.2d 693 (9th Cir. 1984).

Matarazzo, J. D. (1986). Computerized clinical psychological test interpretations: Unvalidated plus all mean and no sigma. *American Psychologist, 41*, 14–24.

Matarazzo, J. D. (1990). Psychological assessment versus psychological testing: Validation from Binet to the school, clinic, and courtroom. *American Psychologist, 45*, 999–1017.

Melton, G. B., & Ehrenreich, N. S. (1992). Ethical and legal issues in mental health services for children. In C. E. Walker & M. C. Roberts (Eds.), *Handbook of clinical child psychology* (pp. 1035–1055). New York: Wiley.

Mills v. Board of Education of District of Columbia, 348 F. Supp. 866 (1972), *contempt proceedings*, 551 Educ. of the Handicapped L. Rep. 643 (D. D.C. 1980).

National Council on Disability. (1996). *Improving the implementation of the Individuals with Disabilities Education Act: Making schools work for all of America's children*. Washington, DC: Author.

Parents in Action in Special Education (P.A.S.E.) v. Hannon, 506 F. Supp. 831 (N.D. Ill. 1980).

Parents Against Abuse in Schools (PAAS) v. Williamsport Area School District, 594 A.2d 796 (Pa. Commw. Ct. 1991).

Pennsylvania Association for Retarded Citizens (PARC) v. Pennsylvania, 334 F. Supp. 1257 (E.D. Pa. 1971), 343 F. Supp. 279 (E.D. Pa. 1972).

Peterson, C. (1996). Common problem areas and their causes resulting in disciplinary actions. In L. J. Bass, S. T. DeMers, R. P. James, C. Peterson, J. L. Pettifor, R. P. Reaves, T. Retfalvi, N. P. Simon, C. Sinclair, & R. M. Tipton (Eds.), *Professional conduct and discipline in psychology* (pp. 71–89). Washington, DC: American Psychological Association.

Plessy v. Ferguson, 163 U.S. 537 (1896).

Rae, W. A., & Fournier, C. J. (1999). Ethical and legal issues in the treatment of children and families. In S. W. Russ & T. H. Ollendick (Eds.), *Handbook of psychotherapies with children and families* (pp. 67–83). New York: Kluwer Academic/Plenum Press.

Rae, W. A., & Worchel, F. F. (1991). Ethical beliefs and behaviors of pediatric psychologists: A survey. *Journal of Pediatric Psychology, 16*, 727–745.

Riley v. Ambach, 551 Educ. of the Handicapped L. Rep. 688 (E.D. N.Y. 1980), *rev'd*, 668 F.2d 635 (2nd Cir. 1981), *further proceedings*, 508 F. Supp. 1222 (E.D. N.Y. 1982).

Roberts, M. C., & Hurley, L. K. (1997). *Managing managed care*. New York: Plenum Press.

Schweighofer, A., & Coles, E. M. (1994). Note on the definition and ethics of projective tests. *Perceptual and Motor Skills, 79*, 51–54.

Strichart, S. S., & Lazarus, P. J. (1986). Low-incidence assessment: Influences and issues. In P. J. Lazarus & S. S. Strichart (Eds.), *Psychoeducational evaluation of children and adolescents with low-incidence handicaps* (pp. 1–15). Orlando, FL: Grune & Stratton.

Tranel, D. (1994). The release of psychological data to nonexperts: Ethical and legal considerations. *Professional Psychology: Research and Practice, 25*, 33–38.

Weiner, I. B. (1989). On competence and ethicality in psychodiagnostic assessment. *Journal of Personality Assessment, 53*, 827–831.

Woody, R. H., LaVoie, J. C., & Epps, S. (1992). *School psychology: A developmental and social systems approach*. Boston: Allyn & Bacon.

Woolman v. Walter, 433 U.S. 229, 97 S. Ct. 2593 (1977).

INDEX

AAMD Adaptive Behavior Scale, 260
ABILITIES Index, 25
Abstract reasoning, 283
Abuse, 156–164, 171–172
Academic
  achievement, 228, 229
  functioning, 296, 318
  performance, 317, 320
  problems, 156
  skills, 229, 230, 335
Accommodation, 86, 92
Accountability, 2, 37, 40, 41, 42, 43, 48, 74
Achenbach Child Behavior Checklist (CBL),
    71, 75, 164, 167, 260, 261, 292, 305,
    306, 307, 310, 347
Achievement, 61, 285
Acquired Immune Deficiency Syndrome
    (AIDS), 183
Adapt testing procedures, 301
Adaptation, 74, 86, 87, 88, 216
Adaptive
  behavior, 20, 158, 205, 206, 207, 216, 220,
    230, 244
    delays, 229
  devices, 230
  functioning, 184, 302
  skills, 194
Adaptive Behavior Inventory for Children, 277
Adolescence, 54, 57, 61, 69, 71, 72, 104, 105,
    112, 169, 211, 213, 323, 338, 366
Adolescent and Adult Psycho-educational
    Profile (AAPEP), 286
Adolescent Coping Orientation for Problem
    Experience, 259
Adolescent Sexual Concerns Questionnaire,
    164
Age equivalent, 54, 55, 74, 75, 101
Age-appropriate, 349
Aggression, 156, 163

AIDS, 297, 305
Albinism, 228
Animal abuse, 171
Animism, 95
Anxiety(ies), 10, 169, 212, 219
Arena assessment , 20
Arousal, 331, 332, 337
Arthritis, 211
Artificialism, 95
Asperger syndrome, 268, 275, 278
Assessment of Developmental Levels by
    Observation, 259
Assessment of the Preterm Infant's Behavior,
    198
Assessment, Evaluation, and Programming
    System for Infants and Children, 198
Assistive technology, 372
Asthma, 73, 294, 296, 298
Attachment, 193, 195
Attention, 57, 189, 210, 214, 215, 216, 271,
    326, 329, 331, 332, 334, 339, 344
Attention (deficit) disorders, 253, 326
Attention-deficit/hyperactivity disorder
    (ADHD), 164, 318, 322, 324, 325,
    326, 372
Attribution of change, 43, 45
Atypical development, 20, 66, 269, 272
Auditory impairments, 60, 61
Augmentative communication, 206
Autism, 22, 55, 60, 65, 71, 72, 98, 103, 104,
    105, 111, 132, 135, 267–290, 318,
    325, 364, 367
Autism Screening Instrument for Educational
    Planning, 277
Autism-spectrum disorders, 268
Autonomous, 106

Basic concepts, 56, 57
Basic Reading Rate Scale: Braille Edition, 241

Basic School Skills Inventory, 237
Batelle Developmental Inventory, 190, 198, 234, 235
Bayley Infant Neurodevelopmental Screen, 198
Bayley Scales of Infant Development, 19, 57, 188, 189, 190, 235, 243, 254, 281, 302
Bayley Scales of Infant Development—Second Edition, 194, 198, 205
Behavior
  disorders, 107, 155
  rating, 346, 349
  setting, 122, 123
Behavior Assessment System for Children (BASC), 71, 75
Behavior Problem Checklist (BPC), 71
Behavior Rating Inventory of Executive Function (BRIEF), 345, 346, 347, 348
Behavior(al), 9, 10, 53, 69, 73, 83, 84, 85, 87, 93, 209, 334, 338, 364
  assessment, 89, 276
  characteristics, 53
  concerns, 168
  disorders, 129
  functions(ing), 228, 305, 329, 336, 346
  measures, 260
  observations, 233, 364
  regulation, 193
  style, 10
Behavioral Rating Instrument for Autistic and Other Atypical Children, 277
Behavioral Screening Questionnaire (BSCQ), 71
Behavioral Style Questionnaire (BSQ), 66, 75
Bender–Gestalt Test (BGT), 61
Bioecological model, 3
Biomedical assessment, 23
Biophysical model, 3
Birth weights, 178
Bladder and bowel control, 210
Blind Learning Aptitude Test, 239, 244
Blind/blindness, 9, 225–246
Body Esteem Scale, 308
Body Image Instrument (BII), 308
Boehm's Test of Basic Concepts—Revised (BTBC-R), 57
Boston Naming Test, 332
Braille, 57, 230, 233, 260
Braille Unit Recognition Battery: Diagnostic Test of Grade 2 Literacy Braille, 241
Brain injury, 132, 157–158, 319, 324, 328, 367
Brazelton Neonatal Behavioral Assessment Scale (BNBAS), 194, 198
Brigance Diagnostic Comprehensive Inventory of Basic Skills, 241
Brigance Diagnostic Inventory of Early Development, 280, 285

Cain–Levine Social Competence Scale, 66
California Verbal Learning Test, 334

Cancer, 309, 327
Caregiver(s), 155, 159, 162–164, 169–170, 196, 192
Carolina Curriculum for Infants and Toddlers with Special Needs—Second Edition, 236, 243
Carolina Curriculum for Infants and Toddlers/ Preschoolers with Special Needs, 280
Carolina Picture Vocabulary Test, 257
Carolina Record of Individual Behavior, 27, 100, 101, 108, 109
Case law, 366, 369
Case studies, 47, 171
Cattell Infant Intelligence Scale, 254
Causal reasoning, 113
Causality, 94, 96, 113, 274
Centering, 88
Cerebral palsy, 2, 21, 22, 46, 48, 93, 205, 206, 207, 208, 209, 213, 225, 252
Challenging behavior, 133
Child
  abuse, 171, 361
  neglect, 361
Child Behavior Checklist (CBCL), 71, 75, 242, 260, 261, 292, 305, 306, 307, 310, 347
Child Sexual Behavior Inventory (CSBI), 164, 168–169
Child(ren), 71, 366
Childhood, 105
Childhood Autism Rating Scale, 276
Childhood Trust Events Survey, 164, 165
Children with disabilities, 156
Children's Adaptive Behavior Scale (CABS), 66
Children's Apperception Test (CAT), 309
Children's Depression Inventory, 308
Children's Health Locus of Control Scale, 69, 308
Children's Illness Anxiety Scale, 305
Children's Locus of Control Scale, 75, 259
Children's Memory Scale, 285
Children's Paced Auditory Serial Addition, 344
Children's Perception of Social Interactions, 69
Choice-pointing responses, 216
Chronic
  conditions, 293, 360
  illness, 213, 292–315
Chronolog(s), 122, 123, 124
Classification, 18, 35, 55, 66, 88, 89, 96, 98
Classroom behavior, 71
Classroom Environment Scale (CES), 126
Cleft lip and palate, 182
Clinical
  assessment, 3, 5, 6, 8, 12, 17, 23, 25, 27, 35, 36, 41, 48, 53, 54,76, 171–172
  epidemiology, 54, 76
  interviews, 94, 144
  judgment, 3, 18, 23, 372

Clinician(s), 40, 158, 195, 197, 218
Code for Instructional Structure and Academic
      Response—Mainstream Version (MS-
      CISSAR), 136
Code for Instructional Structure and Student
      Academic Response (CISSAR), 136
Cognition, 22, 54, 56, 57, 63, 93, 94, 127,
      129, 190, 193, 228, 229
Cognitive, 84, 91, 92, 184, 205, 214, 216, 218
   assessment, 254, 280, 281
   competence, 250
   -developmental theory, 91
   functions(ing), 187, 214, 300, 302, 329,
      331, 359
   structures, 90
   style, 230
Cognitive Abilities Scale, 235
Coloured Progressive Matrices, 60, 75, 256
Columbia Mental Maturity Scale (CMMS),
      55, 65, 75, 217
Communication, 22, 53, 54, 56, 63, 65, 72,
      93, 102, 128, 129, 158, 191, 192, 193,
      206, 218
   board, 207
   disorders, 22, 155
   skills, 65
Communication and Symbolic Behavior
      Scales, 193
Communicative functioning, 205, 214, 216
Community, 73, 162, 220
Comorbid disorders, 284
Compensatory devices, 73
Comprehensive Receptive and Expressive
      Vocabulary Test (CREVT), 63
Computer-assisted assessment, 371, 372
COMTASK, 103
Concept Assessment Kit, 95
Concept of Illness Protocol, 305
Concepts of illness, 296, 304
Concrete operations, 88, 91, 95, 96, 98, 104, 111
Conduct disorder, 105
Confidentiality, 12, 172, 362, 365
Congenital, 182, 213, 214
   cataracts, 226
   glaucoma, 227
   heart disease, 301
   limb anomalies, 206
Connective tissue disease, 211, 212
Conservation, 89, 92, 93, 94, 95, 96, 98, 112,
      257
Construction of reality, 86, 87
Continuous Performance Tests, 276
Continuous quantity, 83
Continuum
   of care-taking casualty, 20, 21
   of central nervous system, 20, 21, 22
Controlled Oral Word Association, 339
Cooperative play, 111

Coordination of secondary schemes, 189
Cortical blindness, 228
Counting span, 346
Cranio-facial anomalies, 178, 182
Criterion-referenced, 45, 57, 121, 193, 280
   tests, 233, 243
Critical events, 231
Critical Events Checklist, 231
Cued speech, 249, 257
Cultural diversity, 11
Cultural identity, 251
Culture-fair, 60
Curriculum-based
   measurements, 19
   tests, 233
Cystic fibrosis, 292, 293

Daily living skills, 231
Day care environment, 159, 185
Deaf, 9, 93, 248–262
Deaf culture, 262
Deaf–blind, 252, 260
Deafness, 103, 104
Decalage, 92, 94
Decentration, 90, 98, 110
Declarative/imperative communication
      behaviors, 95
Deferred imitation pretense, 94
Dental age, 54
Denver Developmental Screening Test-Ii, 198
Depression, 158, 169
Design Fluency, 339
Detroit Test of Learning, 239
Development(al), 66, 73, 83, 84, 86, 87, 91
   age, 280
   assessment, 56, 176, 177
   concerns, 168
   delay(s), 60, 142, 176, 196, 300
   disability(ies), 18, 21, 22, 186, 251, 275
   history, 71, 253, 261
   milestones, 229, 230
   monitoring, 185
   screening, 302
   stage, 91
   tasks, 213
   tests, 274
Developmentally appropriate, 339
Devereux Behavior Rating Scales—School
      Form (DCBS-SF), 71
Devereux Scales of Mental Disorders (DSMD),
      71, 72
Deviation IQ, 74
Diabetes, 226, 297, 309
Diagnosis, 3, 17, 35, 164, 177, 184, 207, 211,
      234, 274, 275, 276, 281, 330
Diagnostic Achievement Battery, 239
*Diagnostic and Statistical Manual of Mental
      Disorders* (DSM-IV), 18, 267, 268, 278

Diagnostic Classification of Mental Health and Developmental Disorders of Infancy and Early Childhood, 25
Diagnostic information, 273
Diagnostic Interview Schedule for Children, 306
Diagnostic Reading Scales, 239, 244
Difference scores, 55
Differential Ability Scales (DAS), 60, 75, 281, 282, 285, 331
Diplegia, 208
Disability(ies), 4, 5, 25, 145, 147, 208, 269, 299, 301, 360, 363, 368
Dissociation, 22, 169
Down syndrome, 19, 54, 69, 128, 129, 178, 181, 182, 196, 349
Drawings, 94, 104, 105, 219
DSM-PC—Child and Adolescent Version, 18
Duchenne Muscular Dystrophy (DMD), 214
Dyslexia, 60

Early childhood, 54, 57, 65, 66, 69, 72, 125, 126, 192
Early Childhood Environment Rating Scale (ECERS), 126
Echolalia, 90, 270
Echolalic tendencies, 229
Ecobehavioral, 84, 85, 121, 122, 195
  assessment, 89, 120–140
  science, 3, 120, 121
  strategies, 6, 53
Ecobehavioral System for Complex Analyses of Preschool Environments (ESCAPE), 137
Ecobehavioral System for the Contextual Recording of Interactional Bilingual Environments (ESCRIBE), 137
Ecological, 124, 213
  psychology, 121
  systems, 145
  validity, 44, 45, 46
Eco-map, 146, 148, 149
Educational planning, 234
Environmental force units (EFU), 134
Egocentric errors, 88
Egocentrism, 99, 104, 111, 112
Emotion(al), 73, 205, 209
  disorders, 71, 129
  disturbance, 61, 93, 111, 158, 360
  functioning, 195, 228, 305, 336, 337
Emotional-social, 216
Encephalopathy, 184
Enuresis, 158
Environment, 228, 229, 231, 233, 234
Environment(al), 4, 5, 73, 86, 87, 120, 135, 155, 157, 161, 187, 193, 248, 367
  demands, 325, 326, 328
  factors, 350
Epidemiological studies, 155, 297

Epilepsy, 2, 21, 295, 327
Ethical
  decision making, 373, 374
  dilemmas, 373
  guideline(s), 369, 373, 373
Ethical Principles of Psychologists and Code of Conduct, 359
Etiology, 22, 211, 214
Evaluating of treatment outcomes, 300
Executive functions(ing), 275, 276, 279, 317, 319
Exosystem, 4
Expressive communication, 63, 109
Expressive language, 155, 206, 228
Expressive One-Word Picture Vocabulary Test (EOWPVT), 65, 75
Eye movement, 61
Eye–hand coordination, 158

Factual statements, 36, 43
Fagan Test of Infant Intelligence (FTII), 189, 190, 198
Failed realism, 104
False equilibrium, 91
Family (ies), 2, 17, 28, 40, 42, 43, 141, 144, 156, 160–162, 181, 182, 183, 184, 186, 187, 212, 218, 220, 221, 261, 297, 298, 299, 300, 305, 310, 360, 361, 362, 365, 372, 374
  -centered, 186, 187, 218
  context assessment, 141–150
  culture, 143, 144, 146, 147, 148
  focused, 186
  functioning, 141, 144, 147, 307
  interactions, 143
  interviews, 145
  life cycle model, 142
  needs, 231
  resources, 231
  systems, 147
Family Educational Rights and Privacy Act, 369
Family Environment Scale, 147, 148
Family Need Survey, 231
Family Resource Scale, 231
Fetal alcohol effects (FAE), 180
Fetal alcohol syndrome (FAS), 180
Field of vision, 232
Fine Motor Scale of the Peabody Developmental Scales, 194
Fine motor skills, 194, 280, 287
Flexibility in test administration, 272
Formal operations, 88, 91, 93, 94, 95, 98, 99, 104, 111
Fortuitous realism, 104
Fragile-X syndrome, 325
Free-play, 131
Full scale IQ, 55

Functional
  analysis of behavior, 120, 121
  assessment, 367
  limitations, 72, 73, 297
  skills, 233

Gait, 209
General Cognitive Index (GCI), 60
Genogram, 145, 146, 148, 149
Gesell Developmental Scales, 19, 198
Gestational age, 178, 179
Gesture(s), 10, 101, 192, 193, 258, 261, 273
Goal Attainment Scaling, 37, 38, 40, 47, 48, 230
Goodenough–Harris Drawing Test, 255
Gordon Diagnostic System, 332, 340
Grade equivalent, 74, 75
Griffiths Developmental Scales, 19
Gross Motor Scale of the Peabody Developmental Scales, 194
Gross motor skills, 280

Halo effect, 215
Halsted–Reitan Neuropsychological Test Battery, 330, 335
Hand Test, 260
Hard of hearing, 248–262
Head injuries, 300
Headbanging, 163
Head-pointing device, 207
Health, 53, 73, 162, 169, 179
  conceptions, 92
  promotion, 72
Health-related, 73
  conditions, 53
Hearing
  idioms, 251
  impairment, 8, 22, 60, 94, 105, 108, 125, 126, 129, 146, 156
  loss, 249
Hemophilia, 294, 297, 300
Hiskey Nebraska Test of Learning Aptitude, 254, 256
HIV/AIDS, 178, 184, 185, 300
Home Observation for Measurement of the Environment for Infants and Toddlers (HOME), 125, 126, 198, 254
Horizontal stressors, 142
Hospitalization, 165, 176, 183
House-Tree-Person Test, 255
Human figure drawing, 103, 258
Hydrocephalus, 210, 327
Hyperactivity, 130, 158, 180
Hyperarousal, 164
Hypercholesterolemia, 147
Hyperreactivity, 164
Hypertension, 164
Hypertonia, 194

Hypothyroidism, 54
Hypotonia, 194
Hypotonic, 332

Illinois Test of Psycholinguistic Abilities (ITPA), 56
Imaginary Audience Scale, 101, 112
Incomplete Sentence Form, 284
Independent living skills, 286
Individual differences, 66, 107
Individualized Education Plan, 35, 37, 44, 186, 359
Individualized Family Service Plan (IFSP), 35, 186, 187
Individualized Habilitation Plan, 35
Individualized Program Plan, 35
Individuals with Disabilities Education Act (IDEA), 1, 2, 187, 190, 226, 281, 364, 366, 367, 371
Infancy, 57, 84, 88, 103, 104, 125, 126, 176, 188, 194, 197, 323, 338
Infant, 66, 74, 94, 103, 104, 177, 178, 180, 181, 182, 183, 184, 186, 188, 191, 192, 194, 195, 196, 197, 220, 231, 234
Infant–Preschool Play Assessment Scale, 280
Infant Psychological Development Scale, 94, 95, 198, 254
Inferential statements, 36, 43
Informal Assessment of Developmental Skills for Visually Handicapped Students, 236, 241
Informed consent, 12, 360, 361, 373
Instructional Environment Scale (TIES), 127
Instructional
  needs, 230
  planning, 243
Intellectual functioning, 211, 212
Intellectual realism, 104
Intelligence, 53, 55, 56, 61, 63, 65, 83, 85, 86, 113, 157, 188, 206, 210, 216
Interaction, 188, 191, 195, 197, 218, 228, 229
Interdisciplinary, 40, 161, 164, 172, 182
Inter-individual differences, 7, 28, 85
Internalizing, 71, 72
International Classification of Diseases (ICD-10), 18, 23, 24
International Classification of Functioning and Disability (ICIDH2–B2), 4, 23, 24
International Classification of Impairments, Disabilities, and Handicaps (ICIDH), 23
Intervention, 17, 35, 36, 37, 38, 40, 41, 42, 43, 45, 47, 54, 74, 83, 84, 85, 92, 103, 113, 154, 157, 168, 176, 177, 184, 185, 187, 205
  cycle, 42, 44
  efforts, 46

Interview Questions for Alternative
Caregivers, 164, 170
Interview(ing), 3, 372, 195, 196, 219
Intra-individual differences, 7, 28, 85
Intra-ventricular Hemorrhage (IVH), 179
Invariance of stage development, 86, 87
IQ, 65, 93, 158, 189, 190, 331, 365

Joint attention, 193, 275
Juvenile rheumatoid arthritis (JRA), 211, 212,
214, 294

Kaufman Adolescent & Adult Intelligence Test
(KAIT), 284
Kaufman Assessment Battery for Children
(KABC), 61, 75, 216, 217, 256, 282,
285, 303, 304
Kaufman Survey of Early Academic Skills,
285
Kaufman Test of Educational Achievement,
304
Kent Infant Development Scale, 198
Key Math—Revised, 286

Language, 57, 60, 112, 190, 191, 337
age, 54
competence, 257
comprehension, 193, 271
delays, 157
development, 104, 107, 187, 228
disabilities, 327
disorder, 22
expression, 193
functions, 332
impairments, 60, 209
tasks, 55
Latency-age, 71
Learning, 209, 329, 334
disability(ies), 21, 22, 60, 61, 63, 93, 136,
211, 253, 293, 296, 322, 324, 326,
360
disorders, 55
styles, 273
Least restrictive environment, 368
Legal issues, 357–375
Leiter International Performance Scale, 75,
254, 256, 281
Leiter International Performance Scale—
Revised (LIPS-R), 60
Leukemia, 295, 296, 301, 327, 334
Linguistic competence, 250
Locus of control, 69, 307
Lowenthal "World" Technique, 260

MacArthur Communicative Development
Inventories, 192
Magnetic resonance imaging (MRI), 157
Manning theory, 137

Manual
prompts, 273
signs, 273
Matching Familiar Figures Test, 259, 344
Mathematics, 229, 230
Matson Evaluation of Social Skills with
Youngsters, 242
McCarthy Scales of Children's Abilities
(MSCA), 56, 57, 60
Meadow–Kendall Social Emotional
Assessment Inventory, 259
Mean length of utterance (MLU), 192
Means–end, 274
Medication, 292, 296, 301, 302, 318, 359
Memory, 189, 196, 217, 275, 283, 287, 319,
320, 321, 323, 325, 329, 331, 334,
337, 338, 346
Meningocele, 209
Mental
age, 54, 65, 84, 96, 107
combinations, 189, 106
development, 103
health, 71, 258
imagery, 87
operations, 98
retardation, 17, 21, 22, 55, 56, 60, 61, 63,
66, 69, 71, 91, 93, 94, 96, 98, 101,
102, 103, 105, 107, 111, 123, 129–
132, 135, 142, 155, 179–180, 182,
209, 225, 271, 318, 360
Merrill–Palmer Scales of Mental Development
(MPSMD), 57, 254, 282
Microencephaly, 180
Middle Childhood Temperament
Questionnaire, 69, 75
Miller Assessment for Preschoolers (MAP), 57
Millon Adolescent Personality Inventory, 309
Minnesota Child Development Inventory,
303
Minnesota Multiphasic Personality Inventory,
244
Mirror task, 105
Mobility, 17, 72, 130, 231
Modification(s), 74–75, 216
Modifying instruction, 272
Moral
dilemma, 106, 107
judgment, 88, 93, 100, 105, 106, 107, 113
reasoning, 106, 107, 108
Morphemes, 192
Mother–child relationship, 144, 181
Motivation, 214, 219, 279, 287, 317
Motivational deficits, 271
Motor, 184, 188, 218
development, 225, 228
impairment, 8, 61, 76, 93, 94, 143, 205–
208, 212–216
skills, 57, 193–194, 271, 338

Movement disorder, 208
Mullen Scales of Early Learning, 190, 280
Multidimensional, 28
Multidimensional Measure of Children's
    Perception of Control, 308
Multidisciplinary
    evaluation, 367
    team, 206, 220
Multiple disabilities, 155, 216, 253
Multiple-choice formats, 216
Muscular Dystrophy, 210
Musculo-skeletal system, 205
Mutism, 156
Myelomeningocele, 209, 295, 327

National Health Interview Survey—Disability
    Supplement (NHIS-D), 72, 73
National Health Interview Survey (NHIS), 72,
    73, 294
National Household Education Survey, 73
National Longitudinal Transition Study, 73
Neglect, 154, 156–158, 160–164, 171–172
NEPSY, 281, 284, 335, 339, 345
Neural tube defect, 206, 209
Neurological
    disorders, 319
    dysfunction, 156–157
    impairment, 61, 157, 210, 317–355
Neuromuscular diseases, 206
Neuropsychological, 2, 157
    assessment, 330
    functions, 346
    impairments, 184
Noncategorical approach, 22, 73
Nondiscriminatory assessment, 367
Nonverbal, 1, 6, 10, 19, 60, 61, 65, 101, 128,
    220, 248, 253, 261
Norm-referenced, 45, 76, 121, 185, 229, 230
Norm-referenced measure, 244
Novelty–familiarity dimension, 338
Nowicki–Strickland Locus of Control Scale,
    75, 307
Nowicki–Strickland Locus of Control Scale
    for Children (NSLCS), 69, 259

Object
    concept, 88, 94
    means, 94
    permanence, 93, 94, 189, 196, 323
    play, 111
Observation, 3, 161, 187, 195–196, 207, 248
Operational, 110, 113
Operative representation, 87, 89
Optic Nerve Atrophy, 227
Oral communication, 129, 257
Ordinal Scales of Psychological Development,
    236
Ordinality, 84, 86

Oregon Project for Visually Impaired and
    Blind Preschool Children, 236, 243
Orthodontic Locus of Control, 310

Paired-story, 106
Pantomime, 258
Pantomiming responses, 216
Parallel play, 111
Parent forms, 243
Parent interview, 229–231
Parent locus of control, 147–148
Parent(s), 10, 25, 36, 37, 38, 40, 66, 71,
    156, 158, 160–164, 167, 169, 172,
    177, 183, 196, 197, 206, 212–213,
    218, 225, 231, 253, 261, 267, 274,
    275, 279, 292, 293, 298, 300, 301,
    317, 318, 319, 336, 346, 347, 350,
    361, 362, 364, 365, 368, 369, 373
Parent–child interaction, 196–197, 231, 300
Parenting stress, 148
Parenting Stress Index (PSI), 142, 147, 164,
    169–170
Peabody Individual Achievement Test—
    Revised, 304
Peabody Picture Vocabulary Test, 257
Peabody Picture Vocabulary Test—Third
    edition (PPVT-III), 65, 75, 217
Peer play, 100, 109, 110
Peer(s), 69, 91, 93, 101, 103, 104, 105, 107,
    109, 131–132, 159, 211, 213–214,
    232, 267, 350, 364
Pendulum task, 95, 98, 100
Percentile(s), 53, 54, 74
Perception, 214, 280
Perceptual-motor, 206–207
Perceptual-performance, 217
Perinatal causes, 208
Person perception, 100, 105, 108, 109
Personal Adjustment and Role Skills (PARS-
    II), 307
Personal Adjustment and Role Skills for
    Children—II (PARS-II), 307
Personal Adjustment and Role Skills—III
    (PARS-III), 307
Personal functioning, 10, 54, 65, 69, 250
Personality, 65, 112, 219, 228, 229
Personality Inventory for Children—Revised, 307
Person–environment interaction, 4
Person-perception, 101, 105
Pervasive developmental disorder, 318, 324
Phenylketonuria, 69, 325
Piaget, 83, 84, 86, 188
Piagetian developmental stages, 305, 361
Pictorial Test of Intelligence (PTI), 60, 217
Piers–Harris Children's Self Concept Scale, 75,
    259
Piers–Harris Self-Concept Scale (PHSCS), 69,
    219, 308

Play
    assessment, 191, 197, 216, 278, 279
    development, 127
Play Observation Checklist, 286
Population(s), 46, 53, 54, 72, 73, 74, 76, 132,
        154, 158, 181, 220
Positioning devices, 20
Postnatal causes, 208
Post-traumatic stress disorder (PTSD), 157,
        164, 169
Pragmatics, 192, 193
Prefrontal system, 322
Prenatal
    causes, 208
    substance exposure, 178, 179
    substance use, 180
Preoperational, 87, 88, 91, 94, 95, 101, 105,
        114
Preschool, 69, 88, 126, 205, 220, 302, 323, 349
    assessment, 220
    children, 57, 65, 69, 158, 214, 231
    environment, 153
Preschool and Primary Self-Concept Scale
        (PPCS), 66
Preschool Language Scale, 3, 193
Preschool Observation System for Social
        Interaction—Research Edition, 129
Pretend play, 110
Primary circular reactions, 189
Problem Behavior Analysis (PROBA), 127
Problem solving, 83, 110, 229, 230, 271, 283,
        287, 319, 320, 321, 323, 337, 339,
        344, 348, 349
Projective techniques, 65, 361
Propositional logic, 90, 94
Psychiatric epidemiology, 72
Psychoeducational Profile—Revised (PEP-R),
        280, 284
Psychoeducational tests, 2, 274
Psychometric, 6, 23, 41, 84, 85, 90, 91, 93,
        133, 190, 211
Psychosocial functioning, 72, 84, 297, 306
Public Law 99–457, 367
Purdue Home Inventory, 126

Quadriplegia, 208
Qualitative, 84, 86, 91, 93
    assessment, 89
    -developmental, 6, 9, 83–113, 254, 257,
        363
    strategies, 53
Quantitative, 74, 75, 84, 85, 216
    assessment, 53–80, 89
    strategies, 54
Quebec Classification, 5
Questionnaire on Resources and Stress, 147
Questions about Animal-Related Experiences,
        164, 171

Range of mental retardation, 359
Raven's Progressive Matrices (RPM), 36, 61,
        75, 256
Reading, 55, 69, 158, 211, 218, 229, 230
    age, 54
    comprehension, 158
    disorder, 324
Reality construction, 88, 93
Reasoning, 91, 92, 158, 267, 271
Reasoning skills, 229, 230
Receptive and Expressive Emergent Language
        Scale—2 (REEL-2), 63, 65, 193
Receptive
    communication, 63, 110
    language, 206, 228, 248
    vocabulary, 55, 56, 65
Referential communication, 95, 102, 103,
        109, 257, 258
Referral, 177, 195, 217, 220
Relevance of change, 44, 45
Reliability, 60, 66, 69, 144, 186, 220
Renal disease, 301
Repetitive behaviors, 269
Representational
    competence, 88, 94, 104
    systems, 192
Reproductive casualty, 20, 21
Respiratory disease, 294
Respiratory distress syndrome (RDS), 178
Retinitis pigmentosa, 228
Retinoblastoma, 228
Retinopathy of prematurity, 227
Rett syndrome, 1, 94, 268
Reversibility, 90, 96, 98
Revised Behavior Problem Checklist, 75,
        260
Revised Brigance Diagnostic Inventory of
        Early Development, 236, 243
Rey Auditory Verbal Learning Test, 335
Rey–Osterrieth Complex Figure, 276, 329,
        333, 335, 345
Rhythmic habit patterns, 25, 27
Ritvo–Freeman Real Life Rating Scale, 277
Roberts Apperception Test for Children
        (RATC), 309
Rocking, 163
Role taking, 104, 101, 108, 113, 274
Rossetti Infant-Toddler Language Scale,
        193

Scales of Independent Behavior, 194, 278
School, 71, 73, 124–125, 158, 160–163, 205,
        212, 232, 310
    entry, 213
    functioning, 71
    readiness, 57
Scoliosis, 211
Screening, 3, 162, 206, 300, 306, 307

Secondary
  circular reactions, 189
  complications, 226
  conditions, 2, 17, 73, 209, 275
Section 504, 368
Seizures, 209, 218
Self-Esteem Inventory, 219
Self-Image Questionnaire for Young
    Adolescents, 308
Self-injurious behavior, 133, 225, 272
Self-monitor(ing), 345, 349
Self–other differentiation, 103, 104, 105,
    111
Self-Perception Profiles for Children and
    Adolescents, 308
Self-report, 71, 167
Self-stimulation, 132–133
Sensorimotor, 87, 91, 92, 95, 100, 101, 104,
    108, 109, 188, 193, 254, 278, 287,
    279
  period, 88, 94, 96, 100, 109
Sensory
  abilities, 57
  functions, 335
  impairment, 76
  reactivity, 57
  responses, 275
Sentence span, 346
Seriation, 88, 89, 92, 98
Severe communication deficits, 270
Sexual
  abuse, 155, 163, 169
  functioning, 210
Sibling(s), 28, 145, 164, 267, 298, 306
Sickle cell anemia, 294, 300
Sign
  communication, 129, 192
  language, 87, 248, 251, 257, 260
Significance of change, 44, 45, 46
Single-participant design, 47
Skeletal age, 54
Slosson Intelligence Test—Revised, 60
Smith–Johnson Nonverbal Performance Scale,
    254
Social
  behavior delays, 229
  behaviors, 230
  characteristics, 53, 69, 84, 93
  comparison, 46
  competence, 10, 66
  desirability, 219
  development, 22
  functioning, 54, 65, 69, 195, 218, 250, 336
  intelligence, 112
  interaction, 71, 193, 215
  judgment, 270
  maturity, 55, 66
  play, 129

  services, 72
  skills, 228, 229
  validation, 45, 46
Social Skills Rating System, 238, 243
Somatic symptoms, 164
Spacing, 130–131
Spasticity, 194, 208
Spatial relationships, 230
Special
  education, 61, 127, 249, 370
  needs, 73, 359, 373
Specific language impairment, 60
Specimen record, 123
Speech-language disabilities, 63, 155
Spina bifida, 93, 209–210, 214, 349
Spinal cord injury, 213
Stage concept, 84, 86
Standardized
  assessment, 3, 172, 179, 185, 195, 197,
    207, 280, 301
  scores, 54
  tests, 233
Standardized/standardization, 86, 112, 122,
    187, 190–192, 216, 219, 220
Standards for assessment, 367
Standards for Educational and Psychological
    Testing (APA), 360
Stanford–Binet Intelligence Scale, 60, 61, 303,
    331
Stanford–Binet IQ, 188, 190
Stanford–Binet-IV, 56, 216, 281, 283
State(s), 25, 27, 108, 109, 181, 187, 197
Stereotyped responses, 234
Story memory task, 329
Strange Situation paradigm, 196
Strengths and weaknesses, 7, 215, 319, 338,
    362
Stroop Color-Word Test, 276, 284, 344
Surveillance, 72, 73, 74
Surveys, 72, 73
Symbolic
  play, 100, 104, 110, 112
  representation, 84, 86
Syncretism, 95
Syntax, 192

Tactile exploration and manipulation, 234
Tantrums, 158
Teacher forms, 243
Teacher(s), 36, 37, 69, 71, 158, 161, 167,
    170, 206, 218, 232, 261, 267, 292,
    317, 336, 346, 347, 350, 365, 368
Tell Me a Story Apperception Test, 286
Temperament and Atypical Behavior Scale
    (TABS), 66
Tennessee Self-Concept Scale, 219, 259
Tertiary circular reactions, 189
Test modification, 215–216, 362

Test of Adolescent Language, 240
Test of Early Mathematics, 285
Test of Early Reading Ability, 285
Test of Early Written Language, 285
Test of Language Development (TELD), 238
Test of Language Development—2nd Edition, 240
Test of Language Development—Primary, 3rd Edition (TOLD-P3), 63, 75
Test of Nonverbal Intelligence (TONI), 60, 281
Test of Variables of Attention (TOVA), 332, 344
Test of Visual-Motor Integration (VMI), 329, 333
Test of Written Language, 285
The Carolina Record of Individual Behavior, 109
Thematic Apperception Test (TAT), 309
Theory of mind (TOM), 110–111
Total communication, 249, 250, 252, 261
Tourette syndrome, 318, 322, 324, 326
Tower of Hanoi, 276, 345
Trail Making Tests A and B, 276
Transactional model, 4, 196
Transdisciplinary Play-Based Assessment, 191, 197
Trauma Symptom Checklist for Children (TSCC), 164, 169
Traumatic injury, 226
Trisomy-21, 83
Two-word utterance, 192

Unit of analysis, 134
Universal Nonverbal Intelligence Test, 284

Validity, 60, 65, 87, 88, 164, 186
Verbal, 60, 65, 128, 188, 193, 205, 210, 216, 218–219
Verbal IQ, 55
Verbalism, 228
Vertical stressors, 142

Vineland Adaptive Behavior Scales—Expanded, 242
Vineland Adaptive Behavior Scale (VABS), 66, 75, 194, 244, 260, 277, 278
Vineland Social Maturity Scale (VSMS), 66
Visual
  abilities, 271, 338
  acuity, 232
  cues, 230
  impairment, 8, 10, 22, 93, 98, 102, 225–246
  memory, 271
  processing, 333
  -spatial, 323, 337
Visual Search and Attention Test, 276
Vocalization, 128, 192

Wechsler Adult Intelligence Scale (WAIS)/Revised, 55, 61, 63, 75, 240, 257, 281, 283
Wechsler Individual Achievement Test (WIAT), 304
Wechsler Intelligence Scale for Children (WISC)/3rd Edition, 7, 53, 55, 56, 60, 61, 75, 83, 212, 252, 255, 257, 283, 284, 303, 333, 345
Wechsler intelligence scales, 60, 216, 244, 329, 330, 331, 332, 346
Wechsler Preschool and Primary Scale of Intelligence (WPPSI), 56–57, 60, 217, 237, 243, 255, 257, 283
Williams syndrome, 22, 98, 104, 111
Wisconsin Card Sorting Test, 276, 324, 338, 344
Woodcock Diagnostic Reading Battery, 286
Woodcock–Johnson Psycho-educational Battery (WJB), 284, 286

Young children, 128, 184, 191
Youth Risk Behavior Survey, 73

Zone of proximal development, 84